W9-BRW-986

Emergency Numbers

CHILDREN'S DOCTOR: _____

CHILDREN'S DENTIST: _____

POISON CONTROL CENTER: _____

AMBULANCE: _____

FIRE: _____

POLICE: _____

Emergencies

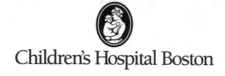

Children's Hospital Boston

MEDICAL EDITORS

Alan D. Woolf, M.D., M.P.H.

Margaret A. Kenna, M.D. ■ Howard C. Shane, Ph.D.

PROJECT EDITOR

Kathleen Cahill Allison

SENIOR EDITOR

Sandra Sardella White

PLANNING CONSULTANT
James C. Lewis

ASSOCIATE EDITOR
Heidi Vanderheiden

EDITORIAL ASSISTANT
Kelleen McGee

WRITERS
Kathleen Cahill Allison
Susan Gilbert
Suzanne LeVert
Sandra Sardella White

A Merloyd Lawrence Book
PERSEUS PUBLISHING
Cambridge, Massachusetts

The
Children's
Hospital
Guide to
Your Child's Health
and
Development

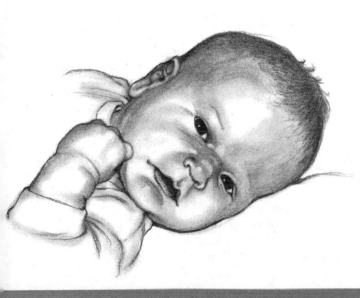

with a Foreword by

T. Berry Brazelton, M.D.

Children's Hospital Boston
300 Longwood Avenue
Boston, MA 02115
www.childrenshospital.org
E-mail addresses:
    For parents and families of patients: famres@a1.tch.harvard.edu
    For physicians: connect@a1.tch.harvard.edu

(617) 355-6000	Main switchboard
(800) 355-7944	Call Center (information and referrals)
(617) 355-6279	Center for Families (parent and family information)
(617) 730-0443	TTY machine at reception desk
(617) 355-7198	Interpreter services
(617) 355-5209	International services

Production Editor: Patricia Jalbert-Levine
Copy Editor: Patricia E. Boyd
Designer: Cia Boynton
Composition: Boynton Hue Studio

A CIP record for this book is available from the Library of Congress.

ISBN 0-7382-0241-X

Perseus Publishing is a member of the Perseus Books Group.
Find us on the World Wide Web at http://www.perseuspublishing.com

Perseus Publishing books are available at special discounts for bulk purchases
in the U.S. by corporations, institutions, and other organizations. For more
information, please contact the Special Markets Department at HarperCollins
Publishers, 10 East 53rd Street, New York, NY 10022, or call 1-212-207-7528.

Printed in the United States of America.

First printing, December 2000

1 2 3 4 5 6 7 8 9 10–03 02 01 00

Dedicated to the health and welfare of the children of the world.
They are truly our tomorrow.

Illustrations

Kay Life
Jaye Schlesinger

Medical Consultants

David Acker, M.D., Obstetrics, Brigham and Women's Hospital

David Ansel, M.D., Children's Medical Associates

Mary Ellen Avery, M.D., Newborn Medicine

Johnye Ballenger, M.D., Pediatrics

Charles F. Barlow M.D., Neurology

William R. Beardslee, M.D., Psychiatry

Marjorie Beeghly, Ph.D., Child Development

Charles B. Berde, M.D., Ph.D., Anesthesia

Henry Bernstein, D.O., Pediatrics

T. Berry Brazelton, M.D., Pediatrics

William Camann, M.D., Anesthesia, Brigham and Women's Hospital

Jean Ciborowski, Ph.D., General Pediatrics

Sharon Collier, R.D., Nutrition

Evelyn Corsini, L.I.C.S.W., Social Work

Allen C. Crocker, M.D., General Pediatrics

Roseann Cutroni, M.S., R.D., Gastroenterology/Nutrition

David R. Demaso, M.D., Psychiatry

David A. Diamond, M.D., Urology

Christopher P. Duggan, M.D., Gastroenterology/ Nutrition

Eric C. Eichenwald, M.D., Newborn Medicine

Richard A. Ferber, M.D., Neurology, Psychiatry

Lynne R. Ferrari, M.D., Anesthesia

Gary Fleisher, M.D., Emergency Medicine

Stephen E. Gellis, M.D., Dermatology

Tal Geva, M.D., Cardiology

Suzanne Graca, M.S., C.C.L.S., Child Life

John W. Graef, M.D., General Pediatrics

Holcombe E. Grier, M.D., Hematology/Oncology

Gerald B. Healy, M.D., Otolaryngology and Communication Disorders

John T. Herrin, M.B.B.S., F.R.A.C.P., Nephrology

Laurie Higgins, R.D., Nutrition

James R. Kasser, M.D., Orthopedic Surgery

Elaine Kaye, M.D., Dermatology

Constance H. Keefer, M.D., General Pediatrics

Gerald P. Koocher, Ph.D., Psychology

Bruce R. Korf, M.D., Ph.D., Genetics

Marc R. Laufer, M.D., Gynecology

Karen Levine, Ph.D., Psychology

Harvey Levy, M.D., Genetic/Metabolism

Frederick H. Lovejoy, Jr., M.D., Medicine

David S. Ludwig, M.D., Ph.D., Endocrinology

Dennis P. Lund, M.D., Surgery

Barbara Jean Magnani, M.D., Laboratory Medicine

Joseph A. Majzoub, M.D., Endocrinology

Frederick Mandell, M.D., Medicine

Bruce Masek, Ph.D., Psychiatry

D. Louisa Mayer, Ph.D., Ophthalmology

Kenneth McIntosh, M.D., Infectious Disease

Lyle J. Micheli, M.D., Sports Medicine

Marilyn Warren Neault, Ph.D., Otolaryngology and Communication Disorders

Howard Needleman, D.M.D, Dentistry

Shari Nethersole, M.D., General Pediatrics

Ellis J. Neufeld, M.D., Ph.D., Hematology/ Oncology

Eli H. Newberger, M.D., General Pediatrics

Edward J. O'Rourke, M.D., Infectious Diseases

Judith S. Palfrey, M.D., General Pediatrics

Irene Paresky, M.B.A., Physicians' Organization

Philip A. Pizzo, M.D., Medicine

Leonard A. Rappaport, M.D., General Pediatrics

Wanessa P. Risko, M.D., D.Sc., General Pediatrics

Richard M. Robb, M.D., Ophthalmology

Sari Rotter, M.D., General Pediatrics

Amy Ryan, M.D., General Pediatrics

Lynda C. Schneider, M.D., Immunology

Michael W. Shannon, M.D., M.P.H., Emergency Medicine

Judy Shaw, R.N., M.P.H., General Pediatrics

Catherine A. Sheils, M.D., Pulmonary Medicine

Stephen Shusterman, D.M.D., Dentistry

Lewis Silverman, M.D., Hematology/Oncology, Dana Farber Cancer Institute

Ann Stadtler, M.S.N., C.P.N.P., Touchpoints Project

Jane E. Stewart, M.D., Infant Follow-Up Program

Robert P. Sundel, M.D., Rheumatology/Arthritis

Edward Z. Tronick, Ph.D., General Pediatrics

Susan B. Twombly, M.S., Child Care Center

David K. Urion, M.D., Neurology

W. Allan Walker, M.D., Gastroenterology/ Nutrition

Katherine Weinberg, Ph.D., Child Development

Joanne Wolfe, M.D., Hematology/Oncology, Dana Farber Cancer Institute

Joseph Wolfsdorf, M.D., Endocrinology

Contents

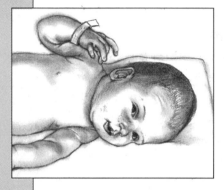

PART TWO

Your Child Age-by-Age

3 YOUR BABY'S FIRST MONTH   54

4 YOUR BABY'S FIRST YEAR   94

6 YOUR PRESCHOOL CHILD   215

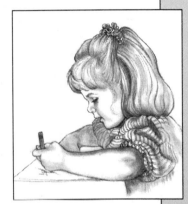

7 YOUR SCHOOL-AGE CHILD   248

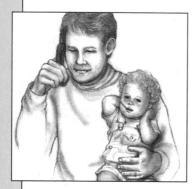

PART THREE
Getting Help

8 YOUR CHILD'S DOCTOR AND HEALTH PLAN

9 LEAVING YOUR CHILD IN THE CARE OF OTHERS

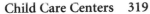

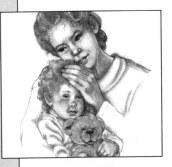

PART FOUR
Childhood
Illness and Injury

10 WHAT TO EXPECT WHEN YOUR CHILD IS SICK

11 PREPARING FOR AND HANDLING EMERGENCIES 367

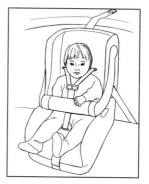

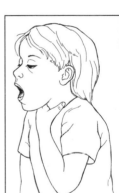

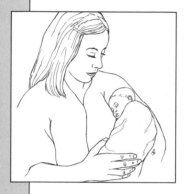

PART FIVE
Guide to Common Childhood Illness, Injury, and Conditions

APPENDIX

Foreword

by T. Berry Brazelton, M.D.

Parenting has grown far more complex in recent decades. It is harder to raise kids now, because there are many new stresses in parents' lives. Women feel split in half between work and home life and find it difficult to resolve the split. Men have also been forced to split themselves in two. They are more involved with their children and home but are still expected to be successful breadwinners. TV and other media, including the Internet, are also stresses for parents. They compete with parents for the hearts and minds of their children. To offset the values often passed along by today's culture—qualities such as greed, power, and aggression—parents are challenged to look to the values, ethics, and traditions from their own ethnic backgrounds.

Parents need sound, authoritative help to handle these stresses and challenges and to find their own solutions. With this in mind, the *Children's Hospital Guide to Your Child's Health and Development* is a welcoming, reinforcing, respectful approach to parenting that can help parents and children make their journey together. It guides parents from pregnancy and childbirth onward through their child's first smile, first step, and first day of school. Created in collaboration with parents nationwide and Children's Hospital doctors and child development experts, the guide offers authoritative information and practical advice on all aspects of parenting, as well as up-to-date medical expertise on all the most common childhood conditions and illnesses. The panel of more than 80 doctors and pediatric specialists at Children's Hospital who participated in the creation of this book are among the most thoughtful and talented people in the United States, and when these professionals put their minds to children, parents receive the best guidance available.

Parenting is complicated and always challenging. When parents ask me for advice concerning a problem they are having with their child, I tell them, "Look at your child. See what your child is trying to tell you." We can learn as much from our children as they can from us.

For instance, an infant who is on the verge of walking can be a difficult child indeed. Parents can usually sense his frustration. He's regressing. He's up and down all night, screaming every 3 or 4 hours. Look at him trying to walk. He's driving forward. He wants to get there. He is showing us what he wants. This is the kind of moment that I call a "touchpoint."

It is at these moments, just before a spurt in development—when he seems to be regressing—that you can understand your child. Understand his language. See what he is doing. What is he telling you? Notice how his face lights up when he plays with his toys. Isn't it going to be exciting when he walks!

In this book, at each age, we describe some of the most important of these moments for children. At about 8 months, for example, your baby suddenly develops stranger awareness. Parents are disturbed when their child screams at the approach of her grandmother or her baby-sitter. If parents can understand that their child's fear signals a cognitive burst—a major stride in the child's learning—it's an important achievement. The baby now recognizes the baby-sitter as a stranger and can also make fine distinctions between her mother and grandmother. If the parents can make contact at this point, they'll be rewarded when they see the baby's eyes light up.

These are passionate moments. I like to say to parents, "Value passion wherever you find it." Instead of getting angry at a child when he displays anger or passion, turn to him and think, "Oh, isn't it great you care so much!"

Children who care. Parents who care. Doctors who care. In a spirit of cooperation, caring, and collaboration, the parents and doctors who helped create this book defined its mission in terms of families who share a common need for the most comprehensive, accessible, and up-to-date medical and parenting information available. Parents told us they need to know quickly and confidently what to do when a child's fever soars or appetite sags. First-time parents, in particular, need information on coping with minor ailments, serious illness, childhood tantrums, and difficult transitions. This guide makes all such information readily available.

Parents have less support from family and community than they used to. They may have no extended family nearby to turn to for help and may have no neighbor or friend who can assist with daily child-rearing challenges. This book helps all parents fill the gap by offering practical, caring advice on health and child-rearing concerns. Parents will still want to build their own network of family, physicians, nurses, teachers, and other parents. All these people with their combined experience, compassion, skills, and love will, together with the expertise, information, and resources in this book, help parents everywhere raise healthy, happy children.

How to Use This Book

Organization

The front half of the *Children's Hospital Guide to Your Child's Health and Development* (Parts 1 through 4) is a guide to your growing child's development and needs. The second half (Part 5) is an alphabetically organized guide to common childhood illnesses, injuries, and chronic conditions. Chapter 11, Preparing for and Handling Emergencies, is trimmed with a red border for easy access. There is also a section of parent resources and a glossary of medical terms.

▌ Part 1, Setting the Stage, describes what you can do to have a healthy pregnancy. It explains what to expect when you meet your new baby for the first time.

▌ Part 2, Your Child Age-by-Age, is a practical, easy-to-read guide to parenting a baby and young child. This section describes a child's physical, emotional, and intellectual development and provides useful step-by-step information for caring for your child and providing a stimulating and nurturing environment.

▌ Part 3, Getting Help, describes how to choose a doctor and health plan for your child and provides a step-by step plan for choosing high-quality child care.

▌ Part 4, Childhood Illness and Injury, provides general guidelines on what to do when your child is sick. This section describes safety and emergency precautions that every family with children should take.

▌ Part 5, Guide to Common Childhood Illness, Injury, and Conditions, is an alphabetical arrangement of the most common childhood health concerns. It includes easy-to-understand descriptions of the condition and a "Signs and Symptoms" list. The guide also explains how diagnosis is determined and the treatment and steps that parents can take to care for an ill child.

A "When to Call the Doctor" box appears under every topic and is designed to provide guidelines that help you determine whether or how soon your child requires medical attention. In these boxes you will find symptoms grouped in varying degrees of urgency. If, for example, your child is experiencing symptoms listed under "Call the Doctor Immediately," your child may require immediate evaluation and treatment and you should call your child's doctor right away. Less urgent symptoms that still require a call to the doctor are listed under "Call the Doctor Today." Sometimes, these boxes include a directive to "Call for Emergency Help." The symptoms listed here are life-threatening; if your child is experiencing them, you should call 911, or, if you don't have 911 in your area, call for an ambulance and provide first aid as needed. The box may also refer you to the appropriate page in Chapter 11, Preparing for and Handling Emergencies, that provides step-by-step first aid guidance.

Remember that the directives listed in the "When to Call the Doctor" boxes are simply guidelines. If you suspect anything unusual or uncommon in your child's condition or you are worried, by all means contact your doctor right away or seek emergency help.

Finding Information Fast

If you are looking for a specific topic in the book, there are three ways to find what you are looking for: the table of contents, the index, and the alphabetical listing in Part 5, Guide to Common Childhood Illness, Injury, and Conditions.

To find a topic in the book, it's a good idea to ask yourself whether the topic relates to everyday concerns about caring for your child (e.g., feeding, child development, discipline) or a medical concern. Child care topics such as discipline and nutrition, which change as a child ages, will appear in each chapter for each age group. Medical topics (e.g., ear infection, fever, joint pain, learning disorders) appear in alphabetical order in Part 5, Guide to Common Childhood Illness, Injury, and Conditions. Throughout the book, some medical topics appear in **bold italics.** Such a treatment indicates that the reader can turn to Part 5 for more information on that subject. Emergencies such as drowning, allergic shock, and choking are covered in Chapter 11, Preparing for and Handling Emergencies (the red-bordered pages of the book).

Finding Information Not in This Book

For more information beyond that provided in this book, turn to the Parent Resources in the back of the book. Here you will find the names, addresses, phone numbers, and Web sites of organizations that supply information, contacts, and support groups for families of children with a wide variety of conditions and problems.

PART ONE
SETTING THE STAGE

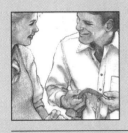

CHAPTER 1
BEFORE BABY ARRIVES

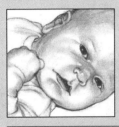

CHAPTER 2
MEETING YOUR NEW BABY

1 Before Baby Arrives

A HEALTHY PREGNANCY

DECISIONS TO MAKE BEFORE BABY ARRIVES

GETTING READY FOR BABY (LAYETTE)

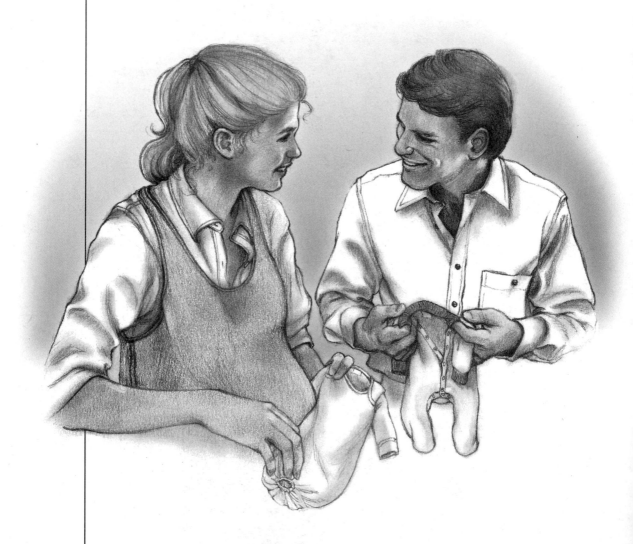

D o you spend time imagining what your baby's tiny face will look like? Do you wonder what it will feel like to hold your own infant in your arms? Do you worry about whether you will know how to care for a newborn baby? Right now, before your baby is born, is the perfect time to prepare yourself and your home for the big changes ahead. A baby's health and safety depend on you, his parent, and that responsibility begins before birth and during pregnancy, when there is a lot to do to ensure a happy, healthy start.

A Healthy Pregnancy

The day a baby is born, he's already been growing, developing, and even learning for about 9 months. During those months, there are many things you can do to keep your growing fetus safe, well nourished, and protected from environmental hazards.

Parents-to-be are bombarded with information about things that may or may not affect a healthy pregnancy. But don't worry, having a healthy pregnancy is mainly a matter of living a healthy lifestyle: getting regular prenatal checkups, eating right, and avoiding substances that might cause harm to the developing fetus. Always ask your doctor, pharmacist, or nurse-midwife about any drugs or medications you are taking if you think you may be pregnant or are planning to become pregnant.

Five Ways to a Healthy Pregnancy

1. Set up a regular schedule of visits with a doctor or nurse trained in obstetrics or prenatal care.
2. Stop using tobacco, alcohol, or other drugs or medications (even aspirin) unless your doctor preapproves the use of a medication, knowing you are pregnant.
3. Begin taking 0.4 milligrams (mg) of folic acid (contained in most multivitamin tablets) to help prevent neural tube defects even before you become pregnant.
4. Eat a balanced diet rich in vegetables, whole grains, and low-fat dairy products.
5. Protect yourself from infection (see p. 11).

Your Prenatal Care

Women who get regular prenatal care are more likely to have a healthy baby. Even a healthy woman with an uncomplicated pregnancy needs to visit a trained medical professional regularly during pregnancy. Most women receive their prenatal care and give birth under the care of a medical doctor who is certified as an obstetrician/ gynecologist (ob/gyn), a family practice physician, or a certified nurse-midwife. Doctors and nurse-midwives often work together, and many health plans provide a team of professionals including a doctor, nurse-midwife, physician's assistant, nutritionist, and childbirth educator who will guide you and monitor your progress throughout your pregnancy and childbirth. If you have health problems or risk factors, your best choice will include an obstetrician who has experience in high-risk pregnancies.

Kinds of Health Professionals

The following describes the kinds of health professionals you may encounter and their training.

Obstetrician/gynecologist (ob/gyn): This is a medical doctor who specializes in women's reproductive health. Obstetrics training applies to caring for pregnant women and delivering their babies. Doctors in this specialty have completed 4 years of residency in their specialty in addition to 4 years of medical school. They also must pass a rigorous written and oral exam in their specialty that qualifies them as board certified. Some obstetricians have further fellowship training in maternal and fetal health, which prepares them to treat high-risk pregnancies.

Certified nurse-midwife: This is a registered nurse with additional training and certification in the treatment of healthy pregnant women. A nurse-midwife has trained in a maternity hospital and is qualified to care for women with uncomplicated pregnancies and deliveries. Nurse-midwives are often the primary health professionals overseeing uncomplicated childbirth in hospitals. They may also work in birthing centers designed to help women have "natural childbirth," which limits the use of drugs and technology as much as possible. Some nurse-midwives work closely in practices with obstetricians. Others work more independently but are affiliated with an obstetrician who is available in case of complications or an emergency.

Doula, labor assistant, or lay midwife: Not medically trained, these care providers are available to perform a variety of support services, including supporting a laboring mother through the childbirth experience. Doulas, labor assistants, and lay midwives do not deliver the baby, but they can be valuable during childbirth and afterward in providing support and informed advice. They often stay with the mother throughout labor to provide active labor coaching, encouragement, labor massage, acupressure, and help with labor positions. They may also provide help at home after the baby is born.

How Often Will You Visit?

If you have always been relatively healthy, you will now be seeing your doctor or nurse more frequently than you ever have before. Check your schedule and that of your birth partner. If you are working, you will need to set up a series of appointments that fit your work schedules. If you have young children, you will be able to bring them to some of the visits, but you may find that for other visits, you need to arrange for child care. Each health plan or doctor is different, but a typical schedule of visits will be something like this:

- First 28 weeks: every 4 to 6 weeks
- Week 28 to 36: every 2 to 3 weeks
- Week 36 to delivery: weekly

During your prenatal visits, your doctor or nurse will monitor your health and that of the developing fetus. The purpose of these visits is to discover any emerging health problems as early as possible so that your doctor can intervene early if difficulties arise. You should also use these visits to ask questions about what to expect and what complications you need to look out for. If a problem or complication emerges, or if you begin your pregnancy with an existing health problem, you probably will see your doctor more frequently than will women without such problems.

If you have a health problem or you have had complications in a previous pregnancy or if your lifestyle jeopardizes your fetus's health, you may hear the term "high risk" to describe your pregnancy. This term refers to pregnancies with a complicating factor that poses a risk to the health of the fetus or the mother.

WHEN TO CALL THE DOCTOR
Problems During Pregnancy

Women experience various discomforts and other symptoms during pregnancy, ranging from nausea to fatigue and from constipation to heartburn. Most of these symptoms are normal. Talk with your doctor or nurse about safe ways to relieve these more common discomforts. Some symptoms, however, are more troubling and may indicate a problem with the pregnancy. Call your doctor or nurse immediately if you notice any of the following:

- Headaches, swelling of the hands and face, dizziness, blurred vision, sudden or uneven weight gain, and abdominal pain, which are all potential symptoms of high blood pressure
- Prolonged pain in the abdominal or pelvic area, which may indicate problems such as premature labor or miscarriage
- Vaginal bleeding in the first trimester, which may be a sign of miscarriage. Later in pregnancy, it can indicate various complications.
- Vaginal discharge that is watery, bloody, or mucous, which may indicate premature labor
- Regular contractions or uterine tightening, which may indicate premature labor

Medications: Things to Consider

If you have a health problem, even a minor one for which you take medication, discuss with your doctor whether you may continue to use that medication during pregnancy. Never discontinue your medicine without checking with your doctor. Your doctor may recommend trying a nondrug treatment (such as cutting down on acid foods and alcohol to prevent heartburn) before resorting to medication. Many medications have not been tested on pregnant women, and no one knows whether they may affect the fetus's health. Others have been shown to cause serious birth defects. So try to avoid the use of medications unless specifically recommended by a doctor who knows you are pregnant.

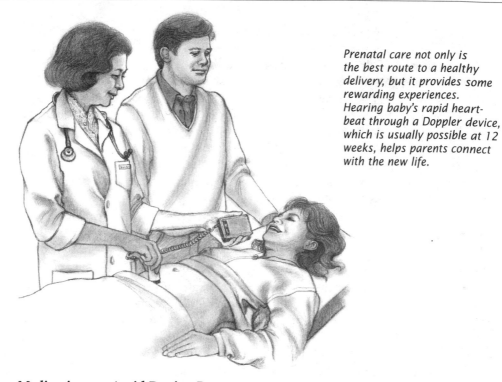

Prenatal care not only is the best route to a healthy delivery, but it provides some rewarding experiences. Hearing baby's rapid heart-beat through a Doppler device, which is usually possible at 12 weeks, helps parents connect with the new life.

Medications to Avoid During Pregnancy

Because some drugs take days, weeks, or even months to clear from your body, try to stop taking medications even before you become pregnant. The following are among the medications to avoid during pregnancy.

- Androgens (used to treat endometriosis)
- Anticoagulants (used to prevent blood-clotting)
- Anticonvulsants (used to treat seizure disorders)
- Antidepressants (fluoxetine, paroxetine, and other selective serotonin reuptake inhibitors)
- Antithyroid drugs (used to treat an overactive thyroid gland)
- Aspirin or ibuprofen (used to treat pain and fever)
- Barbiturates (used to treat anxiety, pain, and sleeplessness)
- Benzodiazepines (used to treat anxiety and sleeplessness)
- Chemotherapy agents such as methotrexate (used for cancer treatment)
- Diethylstilbestrol (DES, used to treat problems with menstruation, menopause, and breast cancer)
- Estradiol (used in oral contraceptives)
- Isotretinoin (used to treat acne)
- Lithium (used to treat manic depression and bipolar disorder)

▌ Nonsedating antihistamines (terfenadine, astemizole used for allergies)

▌ Streptomycin (antibiotic used to treat tuberculosis)

▌ Tetracycline (antibiotic used to treat various infections)

Medications That Can Be Taken Safely During Pregnancy

It is safest to avoid taking any medication during pregnancy. But if you have a medical condition that requires treatment, these medications have been found to be relatively safe during pregnancy. Always consult your doctor before taking any medication.

▌ Acetaminophen (for pain and fever)

▌ Antibiotics
(for bacterial infection)
- Ampicillin
- Erythromycin
- Penicillin

▌ Antiemetics
(for nausea)
- Chlorpromazine
- Meclizine
- Promethazine
- Trimethobenzamide

▌ Antihistamines
(for allergy and cold symptoms)
- Chlorpheniramine
- Diphenhydramine

▌ Antihypertensives
(for high blood pressure)
- Hydralazine
- Labetalol
- Methyldopa

▌ Bronchodilators
(for asthma)
- Albuterol
- Metaproterenol
- Salmeterol
- Terbutaline

▌ Cold medications
- Guaifenesin

▌ Phenylephrine nasal spray

▌ Prednisone

Alcohol, Drugs, and Environmental Hazards

Giving up habits such as smoking, drinking, or drug use is not easy. But if you're looking for a reason to quit, pregnancy is one of the best. It's a good idea to quit even before becoming pregnant, to avoid any possibility that the fetus will be exposed to a harmful substance. Still, quitting at any time is better than not quitting at all. The effects on the fetus are dose-related—in other words, drinking several drinks at one time is more likely to have an effect than having one drink. But because no one knows what level—if any—is safe, the best choice is to abstain.

Alcohol

Alcohol reaches the fetal bloodstream rapidly in a concentration equal to that in the mother's bloodstream. Women who drink heavily during pregnancy are more likely to miscarry than women who don't. One consequence of heavy drinking, fetal alcohol syndrome, is the most common cause of mental retardation in babies. Children born with fetal alcohol syndrome often have long-term problems with physical and intellectual development. Even moderate drinking—one or two drinks a week—may cause problems for some babies, such as learning or attention disorders and speech delays.

Caffeine

Caffeine is a stimulant drug that crosses into the fetal bloodstream. You can safely have one or two cups of coffee or other beverages containing caffeine each day without worry, but try to stop there. No evidence links caffeine with birth defects, but there is some still-debated evidence that heavy caffeine consumption (more than three cups a day) may contribute to infertility and miscarriage. Many beverages, including soda pop, coffee, and tea, contain caffeine. Also containing caffeine are various over-the-counter drugs and natural remedies, including diet aids and products that promote alertness and energy. Check the label.

Tobacco

One of the best things you can do for yourself and your future child is to quit smoking or using any nicotine-containing substance, including chewing tobacco and even the nicotine chewing gums and patches designed to help you quit smoking. The nicotine in tobacco readily crosses the placenta and reaches the developing fetus. Nicotine is an addictive substance that causes fetal blood vessels to constrict so that less nourishment and oxygen reach the fetus. Women who smoke are more likely to have complications such as miscarriage, vaginal bleeding, ectopic pregnancy (when the fertilized egg lodges in the fallopian tube), stillbirth, premature birth, and low-birth-weight babies. Low-birth-weight babies have more health problems than normal-weight babies. Children whose mothers smoked during pregnancy are more likely to develop lung problems, including asthma. They are also more likely to develop learning disabilities.

QUESTIONS PARENTS ASK
Quitting Smoking

Q: I'm a smoker. I'm trying to get pregnant. Is it okay to wait until I am pregnant before I quit? Knowing I am definitely pregnant will give me the motivation I need to quit.

A: Quit before you become pregnant if you can. You may find that it takes longer than you expect to quit, and as a result, the fetus will be exposed to the toxic effects of tobacco. Give yourself plenty of time to quit before getting pregnant. You may need the aid of a nicotine-containing substitute (patch, gum, or nasal spray) and a counseling group. Seek your doctor's advice. Remember, even secondhand smoke can be harmful to you and your fetus.

Illegal Drugs

Depending on which drugs you use, the consequences of even a single exposure can have serious effects on mother and fetus. One of the most common consequences of drug use is premature birth and low birth weight. Babies born smaller than average tend to have more health problems than other babies. Using addictive drugs like cocaine or heroin during pregnancy can cause your fetus to become addicted to the drug and experience painful withdrawal symptoms at birth. Get help from your doctor to detoxify yourself from these harmful substances.

Environmental Hazards

Chemicals in the environment or the workplace can also cause harm to the fetus (see accompanying charts). Some agents may prevent normal development or cause birth defects. If you're concerned that you might be exposed to a harmful substance on the job, talk to your employer about switching to another job temporarily. If you have a question about the potential danger of a substance, ask your doctor.

■ PREGNANCY WORKPLACE HAZARDS

Occupation	Toxin
Health care workers	Anesthetic gases, infectious agents, mercury, ethylene oxide, radiation, cancer chemotherapy, formaldehyde
Pharmacists	Anesthetic gases, radionuclides, cancer chemotherapy
Residential construction	Solvents, methylene chloride, lead
Agriculture	Pesticides
Smelting, alloy manufacture, battery making	Lead, arsenic, cadmium
Veterinary	Anesthetic gases, infectious agents, pesticides, radiation
Laboratory workers	Solvents, radionuclides
Painters	Heavy metals, solvents, methylene chloride
Semiconductor industry	Glycol ethers, xylene, toluene, trichloroethylene, arsine gas, heavy metals, thallium, phenols
Dry cleaning	Trichloroethylene, trichloroethane, solvents

THINGS TO AVOID DURING PREGNANCY

Hazard	Effects on Baby
Legal substances that may cause harm	
Alcohol	May cause fetal alcohol syndrome (mental retardation). Increases risk of miscarriage. May lead to learning disorders or delays.
Tobacco	Nicotine causes fetal addiction and constriction of fetal blood vessels, so that less nourishment and oxygen reach the fetus. Increases risk of complications, such as vaginal bleeding, ectopic pregnancy, stillbirth, premature birth, and low-birth-weight babies.
Medications	Some prescription and nonprescription medications can cause complications, including miscarriage and birth defects (see p. 6).
Environmental hazards	
Lead	May cause birth defects. Avoid scraping paint and varnish in homes and buildings built before the early 1970s. Have your tap water checked for heavy metals, especially if you drink well water. Other exposures to avoid include the products or by-products of industries such as brass foundries, plumbing, shipbuilding, printing, stained-glass window-making, and pottery glazing. If you are concerned, have a blood test for lead levels.
Pesticides, herbicides	Depending on the substance, these chemicals may contribute to complications of pregnancy and birth defects. Avoid exposure to pesticides, insecticides, herbicides, and fertilizers.
X rays	Medical X rays, in large doses, can cause slowed growth and mental retardation. Avoid X rays, especially in early pregnancy.
Industrial chemicals	Several industrial chemicals, including formaldehyde, PCBs, carbon monoxide, and various industrial solvents, may harm the health of your fetus. Ask your employer about any exposure to industrial chemicals at your workplace.
Illegal drugs	
Cocaine, crack	May cause premature birth, fetal death, low birth weight, fetal or newborn addiction, growth retardation, smaller head size, irritability.
Marijuana	Carbon monoxide in smoke may prevent fetus from getting enough oxygen.
Heroin	May cause premature birth, fetal or newborn addiction, low birth weight.
PCP (angel dust)	May cause low birth weight, poor movement control.
LSD	May cause birth defects.
Amphetamines, Ecstasy (MDMA)	May cause miscarriage, birth defects, newborn addiction.
Inhalants: glue, solvents	May cause birth defects, mental retardation.

Avoiding Infection

You can't hide inside a plastic bubble during pregnancy to protect yourself and your fetus from infection, but you can take some steps to reduce your risk of exposure. Protecting yourself from infection during pregnancy is important for several reasons. Not only is coming down with a cold or the flu unpleasant and draining during pregnancy, but certain infections are dangerous (see p. 12). Protect yourself from all infections, if only to avoid the risk of taking medications to treat your symptoms.

You can take the following measures to avoid infection:

▌Wash your hands frequently, particularly if you have been around people with colds or the flu. Don't shake hands with or kiss someone who is ill.

▌If you have sick children, cuddle them as much as you always do, but avoid kissing them on the face and eating and drinking from the same plates, cups, and utensils.

▌Have sex only with a mutually monogamous partner (someone not having sex with anyone else), free of sexually transmitted disease.

▌To avoid contracting toxoplasmosis (see p. 12), avoid contact with cats and litter boxes. Don't garden in soil where cats roam.

▌Don't eat raw meat, unpasteurized milk, raw eggs, or unwashed vegetables.

▌Keep your immune system healthy by eating a balanced diet, exercising moderately, getting enough sleep, and keeping your stress level low.

▌If you do get sick, don't take medication without your doctor's advice.

▌If you work in a health care facility, you may want to be reassigned away from contact with patients who have cytomegalovirus (CMV) (see p. 12) or other infections potentially harmful to your fetus. Talk to your supervisor and your doctor.

Infections Known to Harm the Fetus

Some diseases are preventable by vaccination or through immunity acquired by having had the disease previously. Talk with your doctor about whether you have been vaccinated or previously had the following diseases and if not, what steps you should take to avoid them. Vaccination during pregnancy is not recommended.

▌Chicken pox (varicella vaccine as needed)

▌Influenza vaccine (as needed)

▌Hepatitis B vaccine (as needed)

▌Measles, mumps, and rubella (get vaccinated before you become pregnant if you have not had the disease)

▌Pneumococcal vaccine (as needed)

▌Tetanus-diphtheria booster (needed every 10 years)

Traveling can expose you to infectious diseases not found in the United States. Check with your doctor about vaccinations if you plan to leave the country during your pregnancy.

Many infections cannot be prevented by vaccination. The following are some infections that are potentially dangerous to a developing fetus and cannot be prevented by vaccines.

Cytomegalovirus   This virus is a common infection that may or may not cause symptoms in adults and cannot be prevented by vaccination. In a baby, cytomegalovirus can cause serious health conditions, including birth defects, mental retardation, jaundice, hearing loss, and microcephaly (very small head, often accompanied by mental retardation). Your best defense is to take steps to avoid infections during pregnancy (see p. 11). If you have symptoms including fever, tiredness, swollen lymph glands, or sore throat during your pregnancy, tell your doctor. Often no symptoms appear. But even if a woman becomes infected when she is pregnant, more than 85 percent of fetuses are not affected by the virus.

Toxoplasmosis   Caused by a parasite that lives in some animals, including house cats, toxoplasmosis causes only mild symptoms in adults. But if a fetus becomes infected, it may be born prematurely or too small. It may also have a fever, jaundice, nervous system problems, or eye problems. The mother and the fetus can be treated with antibiotics. Women can get toxoplasmosis by eating or handling raw or undercooked meat, especially lamb, or by coming into contact with cat feces. Pregnant women should eat only well-cooked meat and should wash hands thoroughly after handling raw meat. Litter boxes should be changed every 24 hours, but not by the pregnant woman. If you are pregnant, do not allow your cat on your bed or hold your cat close to your face, especially if your cat spends time outside. Wash your hands after handling your cat, and wear gloves when gardening in areas where cats prowl. Wash your hands after gardening.

Sexually Transmitted Diseases   A sexually transmitted disease (STD) is an infection passed from one person to another during sex. If you or your partner have a sexually transmitted disease, it may affect your pregnancy, the health of your baby, or even your fertility (your ability to get pregnant). STDs often have no symptoms, so ask your doctor about getting tested before you become pregnant.

Some sexually transmitted diseases, such as herpes, HIV (human immunodeficiency virus, which causes AIDS), and hepatitis B, may be passed on to a baby during pregnancy or birth, causing serious health problems. The STDs most dangerous to your fetus's health are HIV, herpes, syphilis, gonorrhea, human papilloma virus (genital warts in the mother), and chlamydia, a common bacterial infection. Be sure to tell your doctor if you think there is a possibility you or your partner has an STD.

Eating for Two: Good Nutrition During Pregnancy

Don't panic. If you are eating a normal diet now, you probably don't need to make any big changes. All your baby really needs is enough calories and a healthy variety of foods. It's a good idea to boost your intake of low-fat dairy products to increase your calcium intake and to eat more vegetables and fruits to boost your intake of vitamins. Now is the time to cut down on french fries and bone up on broccoli and yogurt. Gradually, you will need to eat more calories to feed your growing fetus. Pregnancy is not the time to go on a weight-loss diet. Dietary aids or diet supplements can be dangerous during pregnancy and should be avoided.

A few nutrients, including folic acid, calcium, iron, and protein, are particularly important for pregnant women. You can get most of these nutrients by eating a balanced diet—except folic acid, which you can get in a multivitamin. Women with special diets, such as vegetarians who eat no dairy products, will need to take special steps to make sure they are getting the nutrients they and their developing fetuses need. Other than folic acid, vitamin supplements are not necessary for women who eat a well-balanced diet. Consult your doctor before taking any vitamin supplements, because excess amounts of certain vitamins, including vitamins A and D, can cause birth defects.

Folic Acid

You need to start taking folic acid even before you become pregnant, to help prevent neural tube defects from developing in the fetus. An example of a neural tube defect is **spina bifida** (see Part 5), which is caused by the failure of the neural tube to close during pregnancy. Folic acid is most important in the first few weeks of pregnancy— a time when many women are not yet aware that they are pregnant. Most daily multivitamin pills contain the recommended amount (0.4 mg).

Iron

Your body must now produce more blood to deliver nutrients to the fetus. To do this, you need iron. The National Academy of Sciences recommends that pregnant women get 30 mg of iron in their daily diets. Foods high in iron include red meats, dried beans, enriched cereals, and dried prunes. Any prenatal supplement will also supply iron. Some women have a tendency to become anemic during pregnancy. In this case, your doctor may recommend that you take an iron supplement. If you are not anemic, iron supplements are not essential; you can get the iron you need from food.

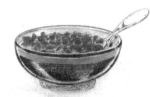

Calcium and Phosphorus

The developing bones of the fetus require extra calcium and phosphorus during pregnancy. Your extra need for these nutrients will continue if you breast-feed. Some evidence shows that calcium may help prevent high blood pressure and preeclampsia during pregnancy. You will need about 1,200 mg each of calcium and phosphorus per day. To get these minerals, eat plenty of low-fat dairy products every day. One extra quart of low-fat milk daily will meet this need. Other foods rich in calcium include sardines and green, leafy vegetables. Nondairy foods rich in phosphorus include meat, poultry, fish, legumes, and whole-grain cereals (see chart on the next page). Most people don't have trouble meeting the daily requirement for phosphorus, since this mineral is easily absorbed by the body. But if you have a hard time getting enough calcium-rich foods in your diet, consult your doctor about taking a calcium supplement.

Protein

The calories you eat come mainly in three forms: fats (butter and oils, 9 calories per gram), carbohydrates (grains and sugars, 4 calories per gram), and proteins (meats, fish, dairy, beans, 4 calories per gram). Although women's bodies need more protein during pregnancy than they normally do, most American women eat plenty of protein. If you are a vegetarian, you may need to take steps to make sure you are getting sufficient proteins in the right proportions.

▬ RECOMMENDED DAILY ALLOWANCES (RDA) FOR PREGNANT WOMEN

Nutrient	RDA[1]	Food Source
Protein	60 g	Meat, fish, poultry, eggs, milk/milk products, soy products (such as tofu), other legumes
Calcium	1,200 mg	Milk/milk products; sardines and salmon with bones; collard, kale, mustard, and turnip greens
Phosphorus	1,200 mg	Meat, milk/milk products, poultry, fish, whole-grain cereals, legumes
Magnesium	320 mg	Legumes, whole-grain cereals, milk/milk products, meat, green vegetables
Iron	30 mg	Red meat, liver, broccoli, dried beans and peas, enriched cereals, prune juice
Zinc	15 mg	Meat, liver, oysters and other seafood, milk/milk products, whole-grain cereals
Iodine	175 mcg	Seafood, iodized salt
Selenium	65 mcg	Fish, meat, breads, whole-grain cereal
Vitamin A	800 mcg	Green, leafy vegetables; dark yellow vegetables (e.g., sweet potatoes and carrots); whole milk/milk products; liver
Vitamin D	10 mcg	Fortified milk, fish liver oils, absorption of sunshine through the skin
Vitamin E	10 mg	Vegetable oils; whole-grain cereals; wheat germ; green, leafy vegetables
Vitamin C	70 mg	Citrus fruits (e.g., grapefruit, orange, lemon), strawberries, broccoli, tomatoes
Vitamin K	65 mcg	Green, leafy vegetables; liver; egg yolks
Thiamin (B_1)	1.5 mg	Whole-grain or enriched breads and cereals, fish, pork, poultry, lean meat, liver, milk/milk products, peas
Riboflavin (B_2)	1.6 mg	Milk; whole-grain or enriched breads and cereals; fish; liver; green, leafy vegetables
Niacin	17 mg	Whole-grain or enriched cereals, meat, liver, poultry, fish
Vitamin B_6 (pyridoxine)	2.2 mg	Beef, beef liver, pork, fish, whole-grain cereals, bananas, beans, nuts
Folic acid	0.4 mg	Spinach, cabbage, beets, Brussels sprouts, beans, lentils, chick peas, green peas, berries, oranges, liver
Vitamin B_{12}	2.2 mcg	Milk/milk products, eggs, liver, meat, fish, poultry

Source for RDAs: Food and Nutrition Board, National Academy of Sciences, 1998.
1. *Abbreviations:* g (gram), mg (milligram, one-thousandth of a gram), mcg (microgram, one-millionth of a gram).
Note: Routine multivitamins are not necessary, except for women who cannot meet the guidelines shown on the chart. Iron and folic acid are the only items that usually cannot be met by diet alone.

Weighing In for a Healthy Baby

Gaining weight during pregnancy is normal and healthy. But being obese (or excessively thin) can cause health problems.

Women need to gain weight during pregnancy. Most women gain few, if any, pounds during their first trimester of pregnancy, and that's normal. But if you haven't started to gain weight at a rate of about a pound a week during your second trimester, tell your doctor or nurse-midwife. Research suggests that the second trimester is the most important time for gaining weight. Weight gained at this time improves your chances of giving birth to a larger, healthier baby.

Overall, if you are normal weight for your height, you will need to gain about 25 to 35 pounds during your pregnancy. If you are underweight, 28 to 40 pounds is recommended. If you are overweight, you don't need to gain as much—15 to 25 pounds is a healthy amount. To gain weight, you need to eat more calories. But for most women, particularly once your appetite increases in later pregnancy, eating more is no problem. The problem is not overdoing it! The average woman needs to eat about 300 more calories a day to gain the right amount of weight for her baby to develop properly. You may have a hard time eating these extra calories during your first trimester, when you may feel nauseous or experience morning sickness, but this usually balances out in later pregnancy, when your appetite increases.

Since your baby will weigh only 6 to 10 pounds at birth, most of the weight you gain is not baby. It's extra fluid, fat, and other tissues. Most women will need to work at losing a few pounds of fat during the months after childbirth.

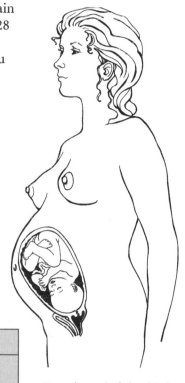

Near the end of the third trimester of pregnancy, the baby makes up only a fraction of the weight a woman gains. Increases in vital fluids, such as blood and stores of nutrients, are needed to supply the placenta.

▬ DISTRIBUTION OF WEIGHT GAIN DURING PREGNANCY

Pounds Gained	Where Weight Is Gained
7	Mother's fat, protein, and other nutrients
4	Blood
2	Amniotic fluid
4	Other fluids (including extra water)
2	Increased breast size
2	Increased size of uterus
1.5	Placenta
7.5	Baby
30.0	**Total weight gain during pregnancy**

Source: American College of Obstetricians and Gynecologists, *Planning for Pregnancy and Beyond*, 2nd ed. © American College of Obstetricians and Gynecologists, 1995.

Exercise

If you're not in great shape, don't worry. You don't have to be an athlete to have a baby. But exercise during pregnancy can help you alleviate stress and feel strong and healthy, and it will help control your weight during the months to come. The best time to start an exercise program is before you become pregnant. But even if you did not exercise before pregnancy, starting a program of daily walking or other moderate exercise is a great way to improve your health and well-being during this time.

Just about any exercise is good. It depends on what you like to do. Walking, stair climbing, aerobics, running, rowing, weight lifting are all OK. However, once you become pregnant, be sure to keep the intensity of your workouts moderate and avoid activities that involve jerky, bouncing movements, such as high-impact aerobics, or the possibility of serious falls, such as horseback riding or downhill skiing. Talk with your doctor about your exercise regimen.

Some women should not exercise during pregnancy, because they have medical conditions that could complicate their pregnancies. Some of the high-risk conditions that may prevent you from exercising include high blood pressure, premature rupture of membranes, premature labor during previous pregnancy, incompetent (weak) cervix, persistent bleeding in your second or third trimester, and slow fetal growth. Ask your doctor about these conditions. Women with other health conditions, such as thyroid, lung, or heart disease, should consult their doctors before exercising during pregnancy.

Decisions to Make Before Baby Arrives

As your baby's due date nears, you will have many things to do to get ready for his or her arrival. It's worthwhile to think now about the decisions you'll need to make about childbirth, breast-feeding or bottle-feeding, returning to work, and your child's regular medical care. Now is also the time to make sure you have the equipment on hand that you'll need when your new daughter or son comes home.

Choosing Your Birth Partner

Every pregnant woman, married or single, needs someone to rely on during pregnancy, labor, and childbirth. As your due date nears, you will be thinking about what to do when your contractions begin and who will help you get to the hospital or birthing center. (Don't even think about driving yourself!) Pregnancy and childbirth are no time to go it alone. The father of the baby is the usual choice for a birth partner, but in some cases, the father may not be available. If this is the case, choose someone close to you who you know will be there when you need help and support. Choose a sister, mother, or friend—whoever you feel is willing to give you the time and attention you need—who will be there at the crucial time during labor and childbirth. You and your birth partner can decide exactly what role he or she will play during pregnancy and childbirth. The most valuable role a birth partner plays is to provide love and support to the pregnant and laboring mother and to be there at the crucial moments. Other common responsibilities include the following:

▌ Attending childbirth classes during pregnancy

▌ Being available and supportive during pregnancy

▌ Joining you in living a healthy lifestyle during pregnancy

▌ Making plans with you for the time when labor begins

▌ Helping prepare the baby's room or sleeping area

▌ Shopping for baby clothes and equipment

▌ Taking you to the hospital or birthing center

▌ Providing support and encouragement during labor and childbirth

▌ Notifying friends and relatives after childbirth

▌ Taking you and your baby home

Creating a Birth Plan

Some expectant parents choose to create a birth plan—a list of preferences regarding the choices to be made during labor and delivery. These choices include such things as what role your birth partner will play, whether you want anesthesia, and if so, what kind, and whether you want a boy baby to be circumcised. Childbirth classes are often the best way to get the information you need to create a birth plan. They cover various topics, including diet and exercise, but their main focus is labor and childbirth. They will discuss how to know whether you are in labor, breathing exercises to relieve the pain of contractions, laboring positions, anesthesia choices, and fetal monitors (electronic devices used to listen to the baby's heart rate during labor and delivery). Some childbirth classes will help you create your birth plan that includes deciding on the setting where you will give birth, whom you want with you, and what medications you will or will not take.

Discuss your choices in advance with people whose opinions you trust, including your health care practitioner, to make sure your choices are compatible with the procedures of the hospital or birthing center where you will

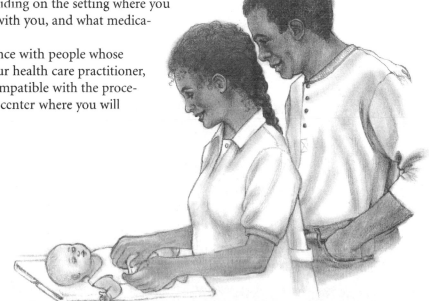

A childbirth class prepares mothers- and fathers-to-be for labor and allows both to practice techniques, such as swaddling and diapering on a doll—techniques that will soon become second nature.

be giving birth. But remember that choices you make while you are comfortably at home may not be the same as choices you will make when you are in the middle of labor and delivery. Consider your choices carefully ahead of time, but remain flexible and open-minded to the other options. Consider the following questions when creating your birth plan:

▌ Whom do you want to be present during your labor? (Birth partner? Obstetrician? Midwife? Other friends or family members?)

▌ Will your birth partner play an active role (coaching? massaging?) during labor, or more of a background role?

▌ What do you want with you during labor? (Music tapes? Camera or video recorder?)

▌ Do you want to be able to walk and labor in different positions during childbirth, or do you expect to be more comfortable in bed?

▌ Do you think you will want pain medication during labor?

▌ Do you think you will want anesthesia during labor? If you prefer to avoid pain medication or anesthesia, what natural pain relief method do you plan to use? (Breathing exercises? Massage? Hypnosis? Other?)

▌ Have you learned and practiced these techniques?

▌ If you decide to use pain medication or anesthesia, do you understand the available options and their uses and risks?

▌ Would you choose to have an episiotomy (an incision under the vagina that increases the size of the opening to prevent tearing of tissues) only if necessary? Let your doctor or nurse-midwife know in advance.

▌ If a cesarean delivery is needed, do you want your birth partner present?

▌ After birth, do you want to postpone noncritical procedures (e.g., washing the baby, warming the baby) until after you have held your baby?

▌ Immediately after birth, do you want to try breast-feeding?

▌ After birth, do you want to keep the baby in your room, or would you prefer to place the baby in the nursery some of the time so you can rest?

▌ After recovery, do you prefer to go home as soon as possible or stay two nights in the hospital?

Returning to Work?

Whether you return to work after you have your baby will depend on your financial situation, your personal preference, the flexibility of your employer, and your child care options. More than half of mothers of young children are employed outside the home, and the numbers are increasing. Fathers, too, must determine how to balance

WHAT TO TAKE TO THE HOSPITAL

Be prepared with a suitcase containing the following items.

For labor:

- Hard candies (to moisten your mouth)
- Lip balm (to moisten your lips)
- Socks (to keep your feet warm)
- Reading materials about childbirth or other subjects
- Camera or video recorder

For the rest of your stay:

- One or two nightgowns (choose a button-down-the-front style or a nightgown designed for breast-feeding if you plan to breast-feed)
- Robe and slippers

- Hair brush, shampoo, and other hair grooming items
- Toothbrush and toothpaste
- A few dollars and change
- Telephone numbers of people you may want to contact
- Pad and pen
- Glasses and contact lenses
- Sanitary napkins
- Nursing bra
- Clothes to wear home (you will still need clothes with a maternity waistline)
- One set of baby clothes: T-shirt, one-piece suit, booties or socks, hat, and warm outer bunting if the weather is cold

their work commitments and their new family responsibilities. If your plan is to return to work, take steps now to pave the way and make the transition smooth. Also, give yourself permission to change your mind or readjust your plans once the baby is born. Be prepared for the possibility that once you have your baby, you may not want to return to work as quickly as you expect to now.

Planning Ahead

If you are anticipating returning to work, plan now by taking some of the following steps:

- *Talk to your boss.* Once you feel comfortable telling your employer about your pregnancy, talk with your supervisor about your options.
- *Know your rights.* If you think you may want extra time off, the federal Family and Medical Leave Act allows fathers and mothers to take up to 12 weeks off (usually without pay) to care for a new baby, an adopted baby, or a foster child. If your employer provides health benefits, it must continue to do so during this time. And remember, an employer cannot legally fire you, lay you off, or demote you because you are pregnant.
- *Consider unpaid leave.* Many employers are now granting extended unpaid leave of 6 months to a year. Inquire about this option if you want it and can afford it.

■ *Consider your options.* Is your employer flexible about your hours when you return to work? Are there any options for working part time after the baby is born, such as job sharing? Does your employer provide access to any on-site or nearby day care facilities? What about working at home?

■ *Factor in breast-feeding.* Women who choose to breast-feed are more likely to decide they need more time at home with their infants. If you breast-feed and work, you will need to obtain a good breast pump (see p. 68) to express milk during your work hours.

■ *Begin exploring child care options.* Find out what state-licensed day care centers are in your area, and visit them or inquire about baby-sitters who will come to your home (see Chapter 9 for more information on finding quality child care).

■ *Talk with your spouse in advance.* Discuss sharing child care responsibilities, including making arrangements for an in-home caregiver or finding a child care center, drop off and pick up at day care, dressing and preparing the child for day care, and covering for each other if you must work late or travel on business. Recognize that these activities will become a big part of your life if you are a working parent.

Breast or Bottle?

One of the most important decisions you can make is how you will feed your baby. This is a decision you should make in advance so you can learn what you need to know about how to feed your child before your baby arrives hungry and ready to be fed. Most major health organizations, including the American Academy of Pediatrics, recommend breast-feeding. Breast-feeding has many benefits for baby and some for parents as well. (See pp. 48 and 62–69 for more on breast-feeding.)

Some women choose not to breast-feed, and in rare cases (e.g., if the mother must take certain medications or if the mother is HIV positive), a woman cannot breast-feed. Infant formulas are not identical to breast milk, but they are approximately as nutritious (for a comparison, see p. 68). Parents who bottle-feed can create similar feelings of closeness to their baby as those who breast-feed.

Choosing Your Child's Doctor

Many parents choose their baby's doctor before the baby is born. You can choose either a pediatrician (a specialist in caring for children) or a family physician. If you choose your baby's doctor ahead of time, the doctor can examine the baby in the hospital within the first 24 hours after birth, even before you take your baby home. If you have not yet chosen a doctor for your child, the staff physician or the nurse practitioner at the hospital where you give birth will do the first exam (see p. 39) before you go home. Consult your health plan about who will do the baby's first exam. See Chapter 8 for a complete discussion of choosing your health plan and choosing your child's doctor.

Getting Ready for Baby (Layette)

Although it's tempting to buy loads of baby clothes and equipment before your baby is born, first make sure you have the basic items that are crucial to a new infant's safety, health, and comfort. And remember, you may receive gifts and hand-me-downs after the baby arrives.

"Layette" is a word you may never have used before but will encounter now as you shop to prepare for your baby. It means a complete set of clothes and equipment for a newborn baby. Here are just the essentials, the things you need to have on hand when you bring your baby home.

What Should My Baby Wear?

Buy only a bare minimum in "newborn" sizes; many babies are already too big for this size at birth, and they grow fast. Most babies wear a size a few months larger than their age. So buy most clothes in the 6- to 9-month range. They will be loose at first but will soon fit well.

Your List of "Must Have" Clothes

Here are basic items of clothing you will need:

- 4 to 8 undershirts (side-opening snap shirts are easiest; pullover "onesies" that snap at the crotch stay tucked in better)
- 4 pairs of socks or booties (newborns should not wear shoes)
- 4 sleepers, either blanket sleepers or gowns (flame retardant)
- 4 zip- or snap-front playsuits with feet (fewer for babies born in warm climates, more for cold-weather babies)
- 2 sweaters or jackets
- 3 to 4 snap-crotch rompers
- Bibs (washable or disposable)
- A warm outer garment, bunting, or snowsuit that covers the hands and feet for cold-weather babies
- 1 or 2 hats (warm knit or fleece hats for winter babies; light, wide-brimmed hats for summer babies)

Blankets, Diapers, and So On

These are the basics that you will need to keep your newborn baby clean and dry:

- Diapers: 2 large packs of newborn disposable diapers, or 40 to 70 cloth diapers with 3 or 4 newborn-size diaper covers or plastic pants
- 3 hooded bath towels

- 3 baby washcloths
- 3 to 5 receiving blankets
- 4 to 6 washable crib or bassinet sheets
- 4 to 6 waterproof pads
- 6 to 12 cloth diapers (for protecting your clothing from spit-up)
- Three-gallon diaper pail with lid, lined with plastic bag
- Baby wipes

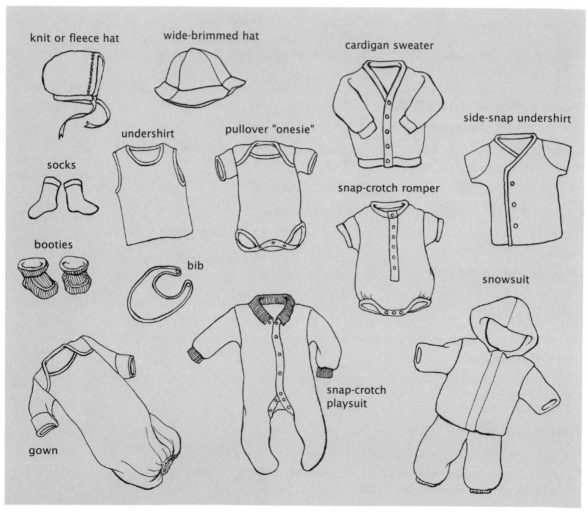

Baby clothes can be expensive, so it's best to decide on which items you really need.
Use the checklist of "must haves" above as a guide.

Beyond Diapers: Essential Gear for Newborns

Besides clothing and diapering needs, here are the remaining essentials for your newborn baby:

- Receiving blankets (for swaddling)
- Crib/bassinet blanket
- Changing table
- Petroleum jelly
- Diaper rash ointment (e.g., one containing vitamins A and D)
- Thermometer (a digital thermometer is easiest to use and read)
- Infant stroller (one that reclines to a lying-down position)
- Infant car seat (see p. 24 for safety information)
- Rubbing alcohol (for antiseptic cleaning purposes)
- Cotton balls
- Antibiotic ointment for cuts (e.g., one containing bacitracin)
- Rehydration, electrolyte fluids for infants (available in most drugstores and grocery stores)
- Calibrated dropper for measuring medicine doses
- Liquid children's acetaminophen (there are many formulations; be sure to get the "drops" for infants only)
- Infant bath
- Mild soap
- Baby shampoo
- Baby nail scissors or clippers

Bottles

In the excitement and anticipation of labor and delivery, don't forget this most basic piece of equipment. Your little one will need to start feeding right away. Even if you're planning to breast-feed, you may want to consider having at least one bottle, nipple, and some formula on hand in case of emergency or in case a supplemental bottle is desired once your breast-feeding is well established. On the other hand, some mothers who plan to breast-feed don't want their baby to experience the feel of any artificial nipples, so keep that in mind when considering supplemental bottles.

There is a wide choice of formulas. Your child's doctor can help you choose one, but for now, stock up on about a week's worth of a basic formula. If you plan to bottle-feed, make sure to have the items listed at right.

BOTTLE-FEEDING EQUIPMENT

Here are the basic items you will need if you plan to bottle-feed your baby:

- Four 4-ounce reusable bottles or bottles with disposable liners
- Ten 8-ounce reusable bottles or bottles with disposable liners
- 12 nipples and caps
- Large measuring pitcher marked in ounces
- Can opener
- Measuring cups
- Measuring spoons
- Long-handled mixing spoon
- Bottle brush
- Nipple brush

Practice

Even if you've read up on the basics of newborn baby care in advance, arriving home with a newborn can be a bit scary. After all, you may never have changed a diaper before, let alone fed, bathed, dressed, and comforted a newborn. To get the hands-on experience you need, practice in advance using a doll. This way, you will have at least gone through the motions of diapering, dressing, and bathing before you have to try it on the real thing. Of course, if someone you know has an infant and is willing to let you practice under her supervision, that's even better.

Practice diapering, dressing, and bathing, as well as breast-feeding positions or preparation of formula and bottles if you plan to bottle-feed (see Chapter 3 for step-by-step instructions). You'll find that the practice gives you confidence when you actually bring your newborn home.

Just remember, one big difference between a doll and a real baby is that the baby's neck will be weak and unstable: You must support your baby's head with your hand whenever you move her—another good thing to practice with your baby doll.

Choosing Baby Equipment

When purchasing or borrowing any baby equipment, the most important factor to consider is safety.

Infant Car Seat

A car seat is one of the first pieces of equipment you will use—you must have an infant car seat if you plan to take your baby home from the hospital in any vehicle. Many kinds of infant car seats exist: those that snap out to become a baby carrier, those that convert into a toddler seat, those that snap into a baby stroller. The choices can be confusing. Choose carefully and consult your doctor. Unless you don't use a car, you will be using this seat constantly. Safety comes first, and then ease of use and convenience. If you find that the straps and clips are difficult to use or come undone easily, your baby's safety will be compromised and your frustration level will be tested. It is most important that you install the seat correctly and securely and use it properly every time.

Ask around. Which car seat on the market do your friends or relatives like? Firsthand experience is often the best. Here are the safety considerations for an infant car seat:

▌ Choose a seat manufactured after 1981, when stricter safety standards went into effect.

▌ For small infants or low-birth-weight babies, a seat without a shield is the best choice for the first few months, because it provides the best fit.

▌ The safest seats for infants are rear-facing, reclining seats with a five-point harness.

■ Once you purchase a seat, send in the registration card so you can be notified if there is a recall.

■ The safest place for your infant's seat is in the center of the backseat facing the rear of the car.

■ Make sure the seat you choose installs easily in your car. You may be taking it in and out frequently.

■ When installing, make sure the seat is held snugly in place by your car's seat belts and that tether straps are fastened correctly, according to the seat manufacturer's instructions. A loose car seat will not protect your baby.

■ If your car has driver-side air bags, never place the infant seat in the front seat. Place the seat in the rear seat of the car facing backward.

■ Some types of side-impact air bags found in the rear seat pose a serious risk of injury to children. If you have side air bags, check with your car's manufacturer to see if they should be deactivated.

Infants should ride in rear-facing child safety seats, with a five-point harness, until they have reached both 20 pounds and 1 year of age. Never place a rear-facing child safety seat in the front seat of a car with air bags.

■ Make sure the infant car seat is in the reclining position for a newborn, to allow him to breathe freely.

■ When placing the child in the seat, make sure the straps are snug against his body.

See page 369 for a car seat safety checklist for children of all ages. The American Academy of Pediatrics has a listing of the different types and brand names of car seats available in pamphlet form or on its Web page (see Appendix: Parent Resources, You and Your Child's Doctor).

Baby's Crib

Your baby's crib should be the safest possible environment, because he will often be there without your direct supervision. The crib can double as a safe place to deposit your baby when you must turn your attention away for a few minutes. Some parents choose a bassinet for their baby's first few weeks of life, but these are not necessary. A secure, safe baby crib is a necessity, at least until your baby is tall enough to climb out—around 2 years old or 35 inches, whichever comes first.

If your crib was made after 1985, it probably meets federal safety standards. If you are using an older crib, make sure it meets these criteria. If not, you should borrow or buy a newer one. Follow these guidelines when preparing your baby's crib:

■ Slats should be no more than $2^3/8$ inches apart. No slats should be missing or cracked.

■ The headboard and footboard should be solid with no cutouts that might cause your baby's head to get stuck.

■ Be sure there are no corner posts over $1/16$ inch high on which your baby's clothing may catch.

■ Make sure screws and bolts are tightly secured.

■ The crib should not be painted or finished with a lead-based paint or finish. Have the paint on older cribs tested for lead content.

■ The crib mattress should be firm and fit securely into the crib (no more than two fingers' width between the mattress and the side of the crib).

■ Don't put pillows, quilts, comforters, or any toys in the crib.

■ Set the mattress in the lowest position as soon as the child can pull himself up.

■ The crib should not be placed within reach of blind or drapery cords.

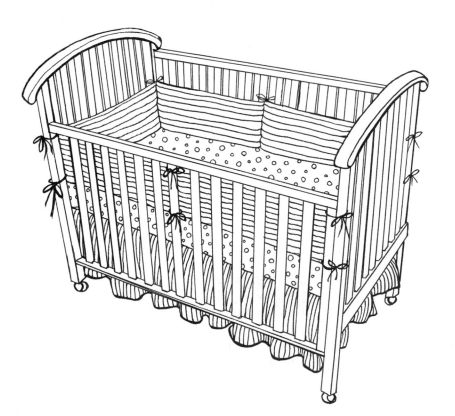

Be sure to choose a crib that meets the safety criteria described above.

- When fully lowered, the top of the side rail should be at least 4 inches above the mattress and the locking latch should lock securely.

- Any mobile above a baby's crib should be high enough that your baby can't reach it. Remove it when your baby begins sitting up or when he reaches 5 months, whichever comes first.

- Remove crib gyms when your baby is able to raise himself on all fours.

- Securely tie bumpers to the sides of the crib in at least six places to keep the bumpers from falling away from the sides. Be sure that the crib sheet is well tucked under all sides of the mattress.

Changing Table (or Place)

You need a safe place to change your baby's diapers and clothes. Many people buy a changing table, but you don't necessarily need one. The most important thing is to have a padded surface where you can always keep one hand on your baby while reaching nearby for the diapers, baby wipes, and clothing without letting go of your baby. A quilt on the floor is often a safer spot for your baby than a bed, because he can't roll off. If you use a changing table, follow these safety recommendations:

- Choose one of solid, stable construction with a railing at least 2 inches high on all four sides.

- A padded surface will make your baby more comfortable.

- Shelves below will make it easier to store diapers and clothing where you can reach them.

- Don't depend on a safety strap; keep a hand on your baby at all times.

- Store diapers out of the baby's reach. Like plastic bags, the plastic liners of diapers can cause suffocation.

- Place your diaper pail right next to the table.

Bathtub

Plastic bathtubs that elevate a newborn baby's head are available and can be set in a sink or the family bathtub while you wash. Make sure the faucet swings out of the way. Tap water should not flow directly onto the baby, because it might be too hot or cold. See page 75 for instructions on washing a newborn. Buy a removable sponge pad to put in the tub to support your baby's head. Never leave a baby unattended in a washtub. Keep one hand in contact with the baby at all times.

2 Meeting Your New Baby

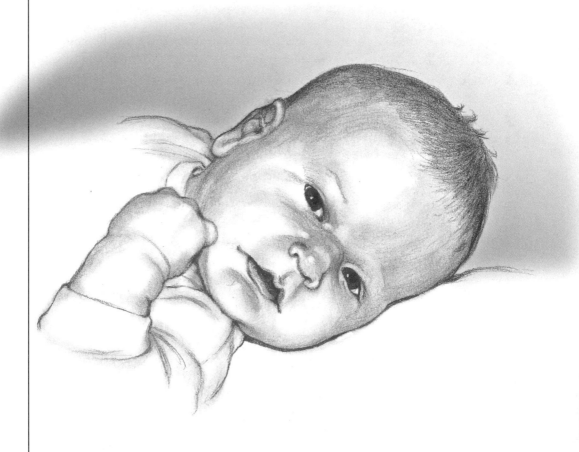

Nothing in life can quite compare with a parent's first few minutes and hours with a newborn baby. It is an exhilarating, confusing, and emotional time—a time when you begin the lifelong process of getting to know your child. This chapter will help you learn what to expect at the hospital after your baby is born, and how to begin to understand, care for, and bond with your new baby.

The Moments After Birth

A newborn baby is a surprise in more ways than one. A new human being has suddenly appeared in the world, appearing tiny and helpless, while at the same time using his powers (crying, sucking, sleeping) to communicate his needs. A newborn looks and acts differently from those plump, bright-eyed babies in the diaper commercials. For one thing, your baby has just squeezed through a tight birth canal, and he looks it. His skin has never felt air or seen the light of day, and he may be covered with a white, waxy paste. A newborn's eyes have never before gazed on the big, friendly faces of his parents and may be squeezed tightly shut. Your baby has a lot of living ahead of him—and so do you.

In the Delivery Room

It's a big change for your new baby—emerging into a new world of light, noise, and air. In a matter of seconds, your baby must begin to breathe air for the first time, regulate his own body temperature, and change the route his blood takes through the blood vessels. The hospital staff take several steps to help your baby accommodate during these first few moments.

Even before his body has fully emerged, while his head is protruding from the mother's birth canal, the obstetrician or nurse-midwife will help him start breathing by gently suctioning out any liquid from his mouth and airways. At this point, he may take his first breath. His body will quickly follow his head out into the world. Some newborns cry at this point—hospital staff often like to hear an infant's first cry as a reassurance that the infant is breathing strongly—but some babies begin breathing quietly; no slapping or crying is necessary. Babies born by cesarean delivery often look a little different from babies born vaginally because they have not passed through the birth canal (see p. 32).

Immediately after a vaginal birth, you will probably have the chance to hold your baby for the first time—wet and slippery—and spend a few moments with him before the staff completes the delivery room procedures. Savor these moments. In some cases, such as when the baby is covered by vernix (a white, waxy substance) or meconium (the dark, sticky substance expelled from the baby's bowels while still in the uterus), the staff may need to clean the baby, clear his airways, and complete the delivery procedures before you get to hold him. While you hold your baby for the first time, his umbilical cord may still be attached and pulsing, supplying him with blood and oxygen. Your doctor or midwife will clamp the cord and cut it at this time. Often the father is allowed to cut the cord if he chooses.

Delivery Room Procedures

After you have held your baby for a few moments, the staff will probably take the baby to complete a standard set of delivery procedures. A pediatrician may be present to examine your baby, but more often than not, the nursing staff will handle these procedures, which may be carried out right in the delivery room or sometimes in the nearby nursery. While all this is going on, you may be preoccupied with expelling the afterbirth (placenta) and possibly receiving some stitches if you have had an episiotomy (a cut made in the woman's tissues to help the baby emerge). During this time, the staff will be

A. making sure the baby is breathing.

B. giving him a few breaths of oxygen if he seems sluggish.

C. listening to his heart rate with a stethoscope.

D. looking at the color of his skin (a bluish color, which indicates lack of oxygen, should gradually turn pink in 30 to 60 seconds).

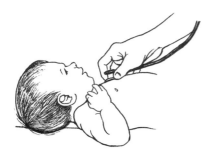

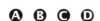

E. suctioning his mouth and nose more thoroughly.

F. placing the baby on a warming table to prevent heat loss.

G. drying the baby thoroughly with a towel.

H. positioning the baby on his back.

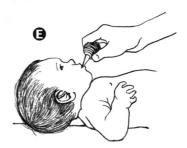

I. wrapping the baby in a blanket.

J. placing a name tag on the baby and a matching tag on the mother, and taking the baby's footprint for identification.

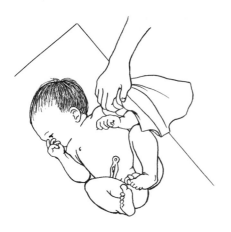

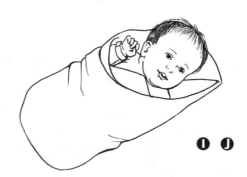

The Apgar Exam

Most parents know the name of this exam—it's the first standardized test your child will take! But don't worry if your baby doesn't get a perfect score. In fact, parents often place too much emphasis on their baby's Apgar score, which is really only an assessment of the child's health status during the minutes after birth. Studies show that a baby's Apgar score does not predict his future development in any way except if the score is extremely low, in which case it may indicate that the baby has a medical problem.

The Apgar score, named after creator Virginia Apgar, is a short exam performed twice—once at about 1 minute after birth and again at 5 minutes. To perform this exam, clinical staff observe the baby and give 0 to 2 points for each of five areas: heart rate, breathing, muscle tone, reflexes, and color. A total score of 7 to 10 is considered normal.

Very few babies score a perfect 10, because most babies' hands and feet have a bluish hue at birth. A score below 7 at 1 minute often improves at the 5-minute test. A completely normal, healthy baby may have a somewhat low score for several reasons. A baby who has been through a particularly long or difficult birth or who has endured such procedures as a forceps birth may not respond well, particularly at the 1-minute test. If the mother has had general anesthesia during childbirth, the baby may be somewhat sluggish, with slower reflexes and a lower score. Babies delivered prematurely are more likely to have a lower Apgar score. Some babies whose Apgar scores remain low after the 5-minute test will be treated in the special care nursery or watched over carefully in the nursery if the hospital has no special unit.

THE APGAR TEST
(A total score of 7 to 10 is considered normal)

Sign	Score		
	0	1	2
Heart rate	Absent	Below 100	Above 100
Respiratory effort	Absent	Slow, irregular	Good, crying
Muscle tone	Limp	Some flexing of limbs	Active motion
Color	Blue, pale	Body pink, hands or feet blue	Completely pink
Reflex irritability (responds to touch)	No response	Grimace	Cough or sneeze

Additional Procedures After Delivery

The staff may perform these procedures at delivery or sometime within the first 24 hours of life:

▌ *Protecting your baby's eyes:* Hospital staff will place antibiotic drops or ointment in your baby's eyes to protect them from gonorrhea infection. This procedure may cause some swelling or irritation of the eyes. This is a standard procedure to protect the baby from any chance of contracting the infection from the mother during childbirth.

▌ *Your baby's first shot:* Hospital staff will give the baby an injection of vitamin K to prevent excessive bleeding. All babies are born deficient in vitamin K, which aids in normal blood clotting. Excessive bleeding can be a life-threatening condition in newborns, so this injection is extremely important. In some cases, the vitamin K may be administered orally, but this is considered a less dependable method because it may not be well absorbed through the baby's immature digestive system. Hospital staff may give this injection at the time of delivery or may wait until later.

Before these procedures, you will be given your wrapped baby to hold for a good, long look. This is an excellent time to try breast-feeding for the first time.

Meeting Your Baby

Your first encounter with your newborn child is likely to be exciting despite the exhaustion you may feel after labor and delivery. This is a big moment. A newborn baby is often quiet and alert at this time, having just been pushed out of warm, calm surroundings into a place full of loud noises, bright lights, and air. He has taken his first breath and may be looking around for his first glimpse of the world—and his parents' faces.

Your baby is new to the world but not completely new to life. For 9 months, he has been growing steadily and developing inside his mother's body at a rate never to be equaled. He already knows how to suck, sleep, wake up, and move his body. He knows his mother's voice and possibly his father's. And he can see and hear. No two babies are alike, even at the moment after birth. He may be active or passive, crying or quiet. His body may be trembling or flailing.

What a Newborn Looks Like

A newborn baby has yet to develop the plump, wide-eyed look you may associate with babies. Instead, your infant is likely to be smaller, thinner, and less "pretty" than you might expect. He may be bald, with a pointy head. He may have birthmarks. Some babies are even born with a tooth. Nevertheless, most parents quickly develop an affection for the wrinkled little elf in their arms.

Skin   There's nothing quite like baby skin. Your infant's skin will be soft and wrinkled, and the hands and feet may be somewhat bluish. He may be covered with vernix, a white, greasy substance from the uterus. He may have various marks, rashes,

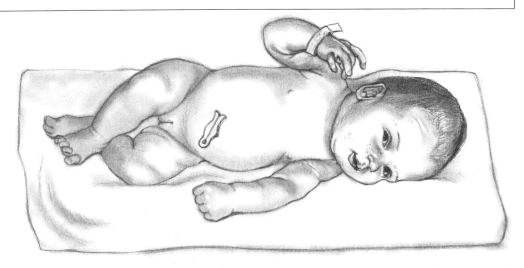

or spots on him from the trauma of birth or the irregular temperature control of his body. (For more information on birthmarks, see ***Birthmarks,*** Part 5.)

Head Your baby's head may be pointy—or at least less than round. But don't worry, the bones of a baby's skull are not yet fixed firmly together. During a vaginal birth, the head molds itself as it passes through the birth canal. Your baby's head may also be somewhat swollen on top. His head will gradually return to a rounded shape over the next 2 weeks. Babies born by cesarean section have a more rounded—or even square—shape to their heads at birth. All babies have two soft spots (fontanelles) on their heads, where bones of the skull have not yet grown together. Normal handling will not harm these spots.

Hair Some babies are born with dark hair on their heads. This hair begins to shed at about 1 month, to be replaced gradually by permanent hair, which may look completely different from the newborn hair. Some babies (particularly fair-skinned babies) are born bald and may stay that way for months. Younger babies, particularly those born prematurely, may have fine body hair called lanugo. It gradually rubs off in 1 to 2 weeks.

Eyes At birth, babies of darker-skinned ethnic and racial groups usually have dark brown eyes that will stay that color. White infants usually have dark blue or gray eyes at birth. The true color may not appear for as long as 6 months after birth. Your baby's eyes may appear slightly crossed—this is normal. His eyelids may appear somewhat swollen, either from the trauma of birth or from the antibiotics applied by the delivery staff. The puffiness should clear up in about 3 days. Notice that his eyes may open spontaneously if you tip his head back slightly. Watch his pupils grow smaller as they respond to light.

Hands and Feet Tiny and perfect, a newborn's hands and feet are fascinating. His nails may be long and need cutting soon (see p. 78). Occasionally, a baby may be born with extra fingers or toes or small skin tags on hands or feet—which can be removed with a simple surgical procedure. Hands and feet are often the bluest part of a newborn, because most of the blood is circulating to the vital organs at this time. Put your finger in your child's palm—he will grip it tightly.

Ears Soft and somewhat floppy, the ears of a newborn sometimes have an edge folded down or drooped over. Your baby's ears will attain their normal shape during the coming weeks.

Body Proportions Your baby's head may seem large in proportion to his body. He will not be able to hold up his head. That's not just because his neck muscles are weak but also because his head is large—about a quarter of his total body length compared with only an eighth for an adult. These proportions will change over time.

Breasts On some boy and girl babies, the breasts may be enlarged. This is caused by the passage of female hormones from the mother to the baby before birth. Breasts may stay swollen for 4 to 6 months, or even longer in breast-fed babies.

Genitals The genitals of boy and girl babies may seem large for such a tiny person. In girls, swollen labia (the outer lips of the genitals) will shrink in 2 to 4 weeks. Girls may have a clear or bloody vaginal discharge at first, caused by female hormones from the mother. It should discontinue after a week. In boys, a condition called hydrocele may occur—in which fluid accumulates around the testicles—and may take 6 to 12 months to recede. Erections are common in newborn baby boys.

BIRTHMARKS

Babies are born with various marks on their skin, some of which are permanent and some of which fade quickly. For more information on birthmarks and their treatments, see **Birthmarks**, Part 5. Here are some of the most common types:

- *Blue or gray spots:* These spots often appear on the backs and buttocks of darker-skinned babies, particularly those of African, Asian, Native American, or Hispanic ethnic groups. They may appear on other parts of the body as well. Most fade away after 2 to 3 years, but some persist into adulthood.

- *Milia:* Tiny white bumps appear on the faces of 40 percent of newborns. They are blocked skin pores, and they will disappear by about 2 months.

- *Port wine stains:* Patches of deep-red skin color caused by a surplus of blood vessels, port wine stains can appear anywhere on the body. They will not fade naturally but can be treated when the child is older.

- *Pustular melanosis:* This rash appears in the form of small blisters that dry and peel away, leaving dark spots that disappear in several weeks.

- *Stork bites:* These are pink birthmarks (also called salmon patches) that may occur on the bridge of the nose, the eyelids, or the back of the neck in about half of newborns. The stork bites on the nose and eyelids clear completely by ages 1 to 2 years. Those on the back of the neck may clear but also may persist into adulthood.

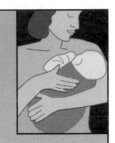

The first moments with my new baby girl were not as emotional as I expected. It was a big blur. I was up all night with labor pains and gave birth the next day. I had an epidural (regional anesthesia), and I think it made me a little groggy. When they first handed her to me, it was like an out-of-body experience. I was caught up in everything that was going on. I remember looking at her fingers and toes and marveling at her tiny fingernails. But I didn't feel that big surge of emotion that I expected. Instead, I feel like I'm bonding with her now, more every day. She's a year old now, and we're still bonding.

Bonding with Your Baby

Bonding is a gradual process—not something that happens instantly the moment after birth. Although many parents experience a surge of love and intense emotions upon holding their newborn infant for the first time, this is only the first step in bonding. And if you're too exhausted, overwhelmed, or simply too awed by the whole experience to feel an intense, intimate connection during the first few moments of life, don't worry about it. You'll have plenty of time to continue building that parent-child bond. Parents who have not had a chance to bond in these few minutes because of problems with labor and childbirth may feel unnecessarily worried that they have missed their one opportunity to bond. But more important than this moment are the many thousands of moments that will follow in the months and years to come.

This doesn't mean that the interaction with a parent in the early hours and days of life does not have an important and probably long-lasting effect on a child's development. Researchers say that mothers who spend more time with their infants in the first few days of life tend to be more attentive to their babies a month later. Keep your baby with you as much as possible during the time you are hospitalized. As a parent, you will feel your love for your baby grow over days and weeks ahead.

Making the Most of the First Hours of Life

When you hold your baby for the first time, cuddle him gently and notice his responses to you.

▐ Hold your face close to the baby's and exchange eye contact. You may notice some response or even a mirroring of your own facial expression: Open your mouth, and your baby may do the same—your baby is beginning a life of learning, and imitation is one important strategy.

▐ Cradle and stroke your baby softly, feeling his skin and hair and watching for signs of response.

▌ If both parents are present, make sure each has a chance to hold and interact with the child—this is part of the bonding process for father as well as mother.

▌ Many infants can try to breast-feed within the first hour of birth.

Newborn Behavior

Despite first impressions, a newborn is not entirely helpless. Your infant can see, hear, feel, and respond to things and people around him. An infant is born with a set of skills or reflexes designed to help him get the care and nurturing he needs. His brain, although not fully developed, is already a complicated network, controlling breathing, heartbeat, temperature regulation, and other body functions. Not only that, but the higher regions of your newborn's brain are ready for learning. Language, images, sounds, and facial expressions are an important part of your baby's experiences, helping to build the pathways of his brain. Working at approximately twice the energy level as an adult brain, an infant's brain is beginning a lifetime of learning and development that you, as a parent, will guide and shape.

Newborn Talents

Most first-time parents worry that they do not know how to take care of an infant correctly. If you share this concern, watch your infant's responses and behavior carefully as you hold, feed, and interact with your new baby. Notice that your infant is a unique person equipped with a set of tools he can use to signal you when he needs something. His signals include such things as crying and fussing, sleeping, waking, and calming. Prompt response to his signals and close attention to how he responds to your actions help you and your baby work together compatibly as a new family.

Seeing   Your baby can see you and can follow your face with his eyes. If you place your face within about 7 or 8 inches of his face (about the distance from a breast-feeding baby to his mother's face) and move in an arc past his face, he will follow your face as it moves. He will do the same thing if you move an object close to his face in the same way, but he is likely to be more active and engaged when he sees a human face. He may even imitate some of your expressions, such as opening his mouth or grimacing.

Hearing   Your baby can hear and will turn toward an interesting sound, particularly his mother's voice. Babies tend to respond to high-pitched female voices, but many newborns will also respond to their father's voice over that of a stranger—the doctor, for example.

Tasting and Smelling   Newborns are born with a sweet tooth—they prefer sweet foods like breast milk and refuse liquids with sour, bitter, or salty tastes. Babies are attracted to sweet smells and will grimace when they encounter an unpleasant smell. By 5 days old, they can tell the difference between the smell of their own mother's breasts compared with that of other breast-feeding mothers.

Touching Watching how your baby responds to touch is important. Many babies are most comfortable when held snugly or swaddled in a blanket—a position that mimics the tight, warm environment of the womb. Babies prefer to be touched in certain ways. For example, a slow, gentle pat soothes an infant, while more rapid patting causes agitation.

Your baby can feel pain. And in the first day of life, he may have more than one occasion to feel pain. The vitamin K injection (see p. 32) causes pain, as does the heel-prick blood test (see p. 42) and the circumcision procedure (see p. 45) for boys.

Sucking When awake, your baby will be actively looking for something to suck (see rooting reflex as listed under Reflexes below). Sucking not only provides nourishment to babies but also soothes and comforts them. Many babies like to suck for long periods, even after they have filled their tiny stomachs. Helping your baby find his hand to suck or giving him a pacifier can fill this need and calm your baby. A little extra suckling time at the breast, after he has eaten his fill, will also be welcome.

Reflexes

Infants are born with some remarkable reflexes that help them survive in their new world. Other reflexes are less clear in their purpose but are well known to doctors and indicate that the baby's nervous system is working as it should be. Among your baby's many reflex responses are the following:

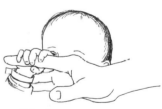

Rooting

▌ *Rooting:* Baby turns his head and opens his mouth when his cheek is stroked gently.

▌ *Gripping:* Baby grasps your finger when you stroke his palm.

▌ *Toe curling:* His toes curl when you stroke the inner side of his sole. The toes spread out when you stroke the outer side of his sole.

▌ *Walking or stepping:* Hold him upright with his feet on the bed, and he will take little "steps."

▌ *Sucking:* He begins to suck when you touch the roof of his mouth—feel that sucking power!

▌ *Startling:* Baby throws out his arms and arches his back when startled by a sudden noise or movement. This is also known as the Moro reflex.

▌ *Eye movement:* His eyes will follow an object (or your face) when moved past his face about 7 to 8 inches away.

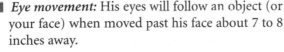

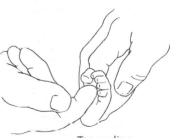

Gripping

Toe curling

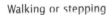

Walking or stepping

Normal Newborn Behavior

Parents often express concern about various normal newborn behavior. The following types of behavior are not signs of illness but are generally the harmless reflexes of an immature nervous system:

- Chin trembling
- Lower lip quivering
- Irregular breathing (without other signs of distress)
- Hiccups
- Sneezing
- Yawning
- Brief stiffening of the body after a loud noise or movement

Behavioral States

Your infant has six states of consciousness, including sleeping and waking. Most newborn babies will fall into a recurring pattern of wakefulness and sleep called behavioral states or states of consciousness. At times your baby will be alert, at other times he may be drowsy or sleeping, and at still other times he may be fussy or crying. But these states follow a predictable pattern—in other words, one state usually follows the next in a typical order. How long each state lasts varies from one baby to the next. And although most newborn babies will sleep 16 to 20 hours a day, sleep periods are short, only about 45 to 90 minutes at a stretch. Your baby may be up and down frequently throughout the day and night! Here are his six states of consciousness:

- *Active sleep:* His eyes are closed, but he is moving, making sounds, and is more likely to awaken if disturbed. His breathing may be faster than when he is fully asleep, and you may notice expressions on his face, including frowns and smiles.

- *Quiet sleep:* The infant's eyes are firmly closed, and he is not moving except for an occasional startle or a rhythmic sucking motion with his mouth.

- *Drowsy state:* His eyes may open and close but will appear dazed and unfocused. His breathing is steady but may be faster and shallower than when he sleeps. He probably will not respond to your attempts to play or interact with him.

- *Alert inactivity:* This is a time when you may be most successful in getting your baby to respond to you, because he is most attentive and ready to learn. His body and face are relatively quiet and inactive but alert, and his eyes appear shining and bright.

- *Fussing:* Eyes are open and alert, but he may seem mildly agitated, and he may cry briefly. This is a time when your baby may also be ready for your attention.

- *Crying:* Alert but moving around more and crying continuously. He may need feeding or cuddling, or he may simply need to sleep.

Every baby is different: Some sleep more than others and some cry more. This may be partially genetic or may be related to how long or difficult labor was. But you can do things to calm your baby—swaddling a baby snugly and letting him nurse when he seems fussy are two ways to calm your baby.

Babies use the behavior states to help them cope with their surroundings. They use crying and fussing to communicate that they need something: feeding, changing, or cuddling, for example. But sleep states are also useful to a baby. Studies show that babies use the drowsy or sleep states as a way of retreating from too much stimulation or excitement. Any new parent who has a room full of visiting relatives or friends may be surprised or even disappointed to see that the baby sleeps through the commotion. This is a good sign: It means your baby can protect himself from becoming overstimulated. This skill is known as habituation—a baby habituates to repeated stimuli (loud noises or bright lights) and goes to sleep to shut them out. A few babies have a hard time shutting out excessive stimulation. These babies are likely to cry and fuss more than others, because they can't simply tune out the noise by shutting down and going to sleep.

Babies born at full term tend to have sleep cycles of about 40 to 50 minutes. They don't know day from night, and it will be at least a few weeks before they will be sleeping mostly at night. Premature babies have shorter, less well defined sleep cycles and will take longer to develop a nighttime sleeping pattern.

The Brazelton Neonatal Behavioral Assessment Scale (BNBAS)

Various tests have been developed to assess the health of a newborn, but the one that assesses behavior, as well as physical and neurological health, is the Brazelton Neonatal Behavioral Assessment Scale, developed by T. Berry Brazelton, M.D., founder of the Child Development Unit at Children's Hospital Boston. This test, which takes 20 to 30 minutes for a health professional to perform, assesses various newborn behavior and reflexes, including the baby's ability to follow a moving object with his eyes and reactions to human voices and faces and nonhuman sounds and sights.

An interesting behavior assessed by this test is the infant's ability to habituate. If the doctor flashes a bright light in the newborn baby's eyes, the baby tends to startle. But if the light is flashed again and again, the baby gradually startles less and finally stops responding. This demonstrates the baby's ability to habituate to or shut out irritating sights and sounds. For example, many babies in a noisy, bright nursery appear quiet, drowsy, and slow to respond. Premature babies or babies born with developmental problems often have a more difficult time shutting out such stimulation and remain irritable and hard to calm.

The Newborn Exam

Usually sometime within the first 24 hours, a pediatrician will examine your baby while the parents look on. If you have chosen your pediatrician in advance, it may be your chosen doctor who comes to the hospital to examine your child. Or, it may be a pediatrician who is on staff at the hospital.

The pediatrician who examines your baby will not only perform a physical exam but will also ask you if you have any questions about your baby's health or about such topics as feeding, bathing, and caring for your infant. The doctor may also ask how you are feeling about being a new parent or whether you have other children and how they are reacting to the idea of a new brother or sister. She may also ask how you plan to get home, what kinds of help you will need at home, and whether you have an infant car seat (see p. 24).

Take advantage of this time. If you have any worries or concerns about your baby's health or your ability to care for your baby, say so now. You have probably spent hours with your baby already, and your doctor is seeing him for the first time. So if you have noticed anything unusual, by all means ask about it. If you are concerned about a lack of support in caring for the baby once you get home, tell the doctor. She may be able to refer you to support services and offer some helpful advice and suggestions.

During the exam, if the doctor notes anything unusual about your baby (rapid breathing, for example), the doctor and staff will carefully watch your baby over the next few hours until the problem is resolved or diagnosed. In some cases, such as if the baby has *jaundice,* a yellow color (see Part 5), or signs of infection, the baby— and possibly the mother as well—will stay in the hospital another day or so, so that the doctor can treat and observe the baby's condition. In other cases, you may need to bring your baby back the next day for further observation.

The Physical Exam

For the physical exam, the doctor will take the following steps:

▌ Check the baby's heart rate, which, at rest, should be about 140 to 150 beats per minute.

▌ Check the baby's breathing. Normal is about 30 to 50 breaths per minute, higher for babies born prematurely. A newborn's breathing may be less regular and more erratic than that of older children and adults. But signs of labored breathing could indicate respiratory distress, pneumonia, or other lung problems (see Fig. A).

▌ Check your baby's reflexes by noting his response to a human voice, holding him upright with his feet on the bed to see if he makes a reflexive stepping motion, and stroking his cheek to see if he turns his head, opens his mouth, and starts "rooting" to find a nipple to feed on (see Reflexes, p. 37).

▌ Place her hand on the baby's abdomen to make sure that the internal organs are the right size and to check for any unusual lumps or masses (see Fig. B).

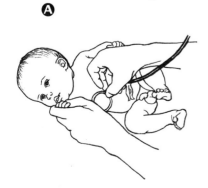

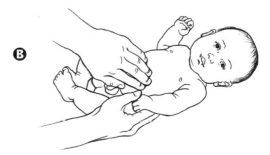

- Look in the baby's eyes for any sign of problems with the pupils, lens, or retina.

- Feel the baby's head to find the soft spots, both the front (anterior fontanelle) and the back (posterior fontanelle). These soft spots vary greatly in size at birth and may even grow larger over the coming weeks before the bony plates of the skull gradually close up.

- Check the baby's skin. She will look for any spots or birthmarks. She may press your baby's skin to look for a color change—normal blanching from white to pink. The doctor will also observe your baby's skin color. The bluish cast of the newborn should be fading to pink. Babies born earlier are pinker; babies closer to their due date or after are paler. A yellowish cast might indicate *jaundice* (see Part 5).

- Check the baby's nostrils to make sure they are open.

- Feel inside the baby's mouth for any clefts (splitting) or cysts in the palate or throat area.

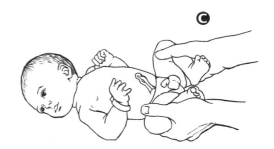

- Check the baby's neck for any masses or pits.

- Check for bone or joint problems. The doctor will feel the baby's collarbone for signs of fracture that may have occurred during birth. She will also check the baby's hips for dislocation (see Fig. C).

- Run her thumb down the baby's spine to make sure that the vertebrae are in place, and check for dimples or tufts of hair, which may indicate a problem with the spine (see Fig. D).

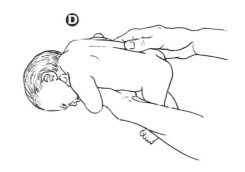

- Inspect the baby's genitals for abnormalities (see Fig. E). In boys, the doctor will check to see if both the baby's testicles have descended into the scrotum. Babies born before their due date are more likely to have one or both testicles undescended. Undescended testicles are not an immediate cause for concern and normally descend to their normal position within the first year. But the condition may require surgery if the testicles remain undescended after a year has passed. In girls, white vaginal discharge is normal in a newborn. The doctor will check to make sure the labial lips are properly separated.

- Inspect the umbilical stump for signs of bleeding or discharge.

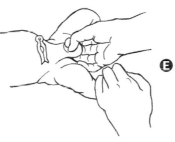

- Visually inspect the rest of the baby's body for any unusual or abnormal conditions.

Measuring Your Baby

Part of the newborn exam will be the careful weighing and measuring of your baby. These first measurements are important, because in the coming weeks and months, your doctor will be weighing and measuring your child regularly and comparing those measurements to those taken at birth to make sure that your child is growing at a healthy rate.

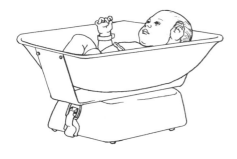

Weight   The doctor or nurse will place your naked baby on an infant scale. Full-term babies range widely in weight from about 6 to 10 pounds. The average baby weighs about 7 to 8 pounds at birth. Boys tend to weigh more than girls at birth.

Length   The doctor or nurse places your baby on his back on a flat measuring surface while one person holds his head and straightens his legs and turns his feet upward. The average newborn infant is about 20 inches long. Boys tend to be slightly longer than girls by about $1/2$ inch or 1.25 centimeters.

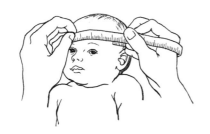

Head Circumference   The doctor or nurse will wrap a tape measure around the baby's head at eyebrow level and above the ears. The average newborn's head is about 14 inches, although boys' heads tend to be larger by about $1/4$ inch. The head circumference measurement will help your doctor monitor the normal growth of your child's brain over the coming months.

Tests, Vaccines, and Other Procedures

Before you and your baby leave the hospital, the staff will take a blood sample for laboratory analysis, perhaps test his hearing, and administer a vaccine to protect your baby against hepatitis B. If your child is a boy, you will need to decide whether he should be circumcised.

Blood Screening

Hospital personnel will take a blood sample by pricking your baby's heel. This is an important blood test given to every newborn baby to identify certain metabolic disorders, hormone disorders, blood disorders, and infectious diseases that may be present but have not yet caused any apparent problems. The blood sample is sent to a laboratory for analysis.

The hospital receives any abnormal results within 3 to 4 days, usually after you and your baby are home. If the test results are normal, you will not be notified. If a test result is abnormal, the hospital staff will notify your baby's doctor. An abnormal test result usually means that your baby must be retested. While this should not be ignored or put off, you needn't be alarmed. At least 90 percent of abnormal results are found to be normal when retested, indicating that your baby has no medical problems. Nevertheless, your baby should be tested again within 7 days. If the repeat test is abnormal, your pediatrician will probably refer you to a specialist to determine whether your baby has a disorder that requires special treatment.

The disorders identified through newborn screening are rare. However, any may be life-threatening or cause mental or physical impairment. Early identification is important so that treatment can begin and these problems can be prevented—many of the disorders do not produce visible symptoms until later, when it may be too late for effective preventative treatment. Some of the disorders for which infants are commonly tested are shown in the chart.

DISORDERS COMMONLY TESTED FOR IN INFANTS

Disorder	Cause	Treatment
Hypothyroidism	Insufficient production of thyroid hormone	Hormone therapy
Phenylketonuria (PKU)	A defect in the metabolism of the amino acid phenylalanine	Phenylalanine-free diet
Galactosemia	A defect in the metabolism of the milk sugar galactose	Galactose-free diet
Homocystinuria	A defect in the metabolism of the amino acid homocystine	Special diet
Maple syrup urine disease (MSUD)	A defect in the metabolism of the amino acid leucine (urine may have maple syrup odor)	Special diet
Biotinidase deficiency	The body's inability to recycle the vitamin biotin	Biotin supplements
Congenital adrenal hyperplasia	A defect in hormone metabolism	Hormone treatment
Sickle-cell disease	A disease of the blood caused by the presence of abnormal hemoglobin; fragile red blood cells cannot deliver adequate oxygen to the body	Penicillin to prevent infection
Congenital toxoplasmosis	An infection of the *Toxoplasma gondii* parasite transmitted to the baby from the mother during pregnancy (see p. 12)	Combination drug therapy

The law or public health policy in your state will determine which diseases your baby will be screened for. In all states, babies are screened for at least PKU and congenital hypothyroidism. Because most are genetic disorders, some ethnic or racial groups are more susceptible than others to certain disorders. For instance, sickle-cell disease is more frequent in African Americans, homocystinuria in people of Irish decent, and PKU in people with Northern European backgrounds. To be certain that no baby with a disorder is overlooked, however, all babies are screened for all disorders required by the state where the baby is born.

Newborn screening has nearly eliminated various newborn complications, including mental retardation from disorders like PKU and congenital hypothyroidism, and infant death from sickle-cell anemia and congenital adrenal hyperplasia. Although some parents are hesitant to subject their newborn infant to the discomfort of a heel-prick test, the long-term benefits far outweigh the momentary discomfort.

Hearing Screening

Many states now require that a newborn's hearing be screened before the baby leaves the hospital. This is an important screening test, because without it, hearing loss is often not detected until a year or two later, when the child begins to have problems learning to speak. Pediatricians' offices do not have the equipment necessary to test newborn hearing. In the hospital, a hearing screening may be conducted by an audiologist or another member of the hospital staff. It takes about 15 to 20 minutes. About 1 to 2 in every 1,000 newborn babies are found to have hearing loss. Detecting hearing loss early is important so that treatment can begin and delays in speech development and learning can be avoided. If hearing loss is detected in your child, you will be scheduled for follow-up services after you and your baby leave the hospital. Ask your child's doctor at the hospital if a hearing screening will be performed. Even after this testing, continue to be alert for signs that your child is not hearing the sounds around him (see p. 56).

Hepatitis B Vaccine

During his first few years, your baby will receive a series of injections (vaccinations or immunizations) to protect him from disease. The first will be a vaccine for hepatitis B—a liver disease that can lead to serious illness, cancer, and even death. Before you and your child leave the hospital, a nurse will inject your baby with the first of a series of three shots that constitute this vaccine. Your baby will receive the second and third shots in the pediatrician's office in the coming months (see our recommended Childhood Immunization Schedule, p. 110).

A baby can get hepatitis B from an infected mother during birth. Pregnant women are routinely screened for hepatitis B during pregnancy. Women more likely to have this disease and to pass it on to their babies are those who

▌ share needles for injecting drugs.

■ have unprotected sexual contact with an infected person.

■ live in the same household with someone who has hepatitis B (the virus can be spread through contact with an infected person's saliva, blood, or breast milk).

■ have a job that exposes them to human blood.

Babies who have a hepatitis B infection may not look or feel sick at first, but as they grow up, they may have serious liver damage. All babies should receive a hepatitis B vaccine to protect them from future exposure to the virus. For more information, see **Hepatitis,** Part 5.

Circumcision

If your baby is a boy, you will need to decide whether to have his penis circumcised. Circumcision is the surgical removal of the foreskin—the skin that covers the tip (glans) of the penis. It is usually performed by a doctor at the hospital during the first few days of life. Circumcision is one of the oldest-known surgical procedures and has been practiced for thousands of years for religious, cultural, and medical reasons. Although some studies have shown medical advantages to circumcision, such as a slightly lower rate of urinary tract infections during the first year of life, the advantages are not significant enough to recommend the procedure solely for medical reasons. If you do choose circumcision for your son, ask your doctor for pain relief for your baby during the procedure.

The choice of whether to circumcise a boy is a personal choice the parents must make. Some child development experts recommend that the father make the decision. A father may prefer, for example, that his son's penis look the same as his own. Some people have their sons circumcised for reasons of religious ritual. The rate of circumcision peaked in the United States during the mid-1960s at about 80 percent of males born in this country and has since declined to about 64 percent.

Circumcision is a safe and quick procedure, but like any surgical procedure, it carries some risks and causes some pain. Circumcision is best performed at the time of birth, so try to make a decision at or before the time of birth, and have the procedure done promptly if that is your choice.

Risks and Drawbacks Associated with Circumcision

■ Infection and bleeding

■ Rarely, the foreskin may be cut too short or too long or the incision may heal improperly

■ Unnecessary pain for the child

■ Financial cost

■ Rarely, if the child has a congenital malformation of the penis, known as hypospadias, circumcision may complicate the condition

Benefits Associated with Circumcision

▐ Reduces the risk of urinary tract infection during the first year of life

▐ Eliminates the chance of foreskin infection, which sometimes occurs at ages 3 to 5

▐ Prevents a condition called phimosis, a narrow opening that makes retracting the foreskin later in life impossible

▐ Eliminates the risk of cancer of the penis

QUESTIONS PARENTS ASK
Pain Relief for Circumcision

Q: We are planning to have our son circumcised. Will it be painful for him?

A: Newborn babies do feel pain. But there are several ways to reduce the pain of circumcision. Most babies will cry briefly in response to the procedure and will have an increased heart rate. A local anesthetic may be injected into the penis prior to the surgery to create a penile nerve block, or a topical anesthetic cream is sometimes used. Although the topical cream is less effective, it does eliminate the need for the injection and the risks associated with anesthesia. Research also shows that having an infant suck on a pacifier moistened with sugar water helps reduce pain during the procedure, although it is less effective than other methods. Ask the doctor or health professionals at your hospital which method of pain relief will be used.

The Procedure

The hospital staff swaddle or bind the baby to a board using straps around his arms and legs. A local anesthetic may be used (see Questions Parents Ask, above).

1. The doctor makes a small slit in the foreskin, which covers the glans (head) of the penis, and she separates the foreskin from the glans.

2. A clamp with a cap is placed over the glans, and the foreskin is tied with a string or ligature.

3. The doctor snips off the foreskin and removes the device (a plastic rim may remain in place, depending on which device is used).

4. In 5 to 10 days, the remaining plastic ring—if there is one—falls off.

5. You will need to keep the area clean and free of debris or particles of stool while it is healing.

Your Hospital Stay

Your hospital stay will probably be brief—often no more than 48 hours after delivery. That's the minimum required by federal law. You and your baby can leave earlier if you prefer and if your doctors approve. If you had a cesarean delivery, your stay will be longer—probably 4 or 5 days. Most new mothers take advantage of this time to recover, rest, and get to know their new baby. You can also learn about baby care basics from the expert nursing staff at the hospital.

Rooming In

After decades during which newborn babies were whisked away from their mothers to be cared for in hospital nurseries, hospitals now encourage rooming in—keeping your baby with you in your hospital room. Try to keep your baby with you as much as you can. Research shows that babies who spend the hours after birth with their mothers tend to cry less and secrete fewer stress hormones than babies cared for in a hospital nursery. And mothers who remain in close contact with their babies become more aware of their babies' needs more quickly. The benefits of rooming in to baby and mother are many—the more time you spend with your baby from the start, the closer to your baby you will feel, and the more confident you will feel about caring for your baby once you are home.

But every recuperating mother needs rest and recovery time. Many babies will fall asleep for several hours after an initial period of wakefulness. Take this time to rest. Don't make phone calls or fill your room with visitors. There will be plenty of time for that later. If you are having a difficult time getting any rest, by all means ask the nurses to care for your baby in the nursery for a few hours or overnight—an exhausted mother can't be an attentive mother.

WHEN TO CALL THE DOCTOR

Signs of Distress in Your Newborn

Now that more women are keeping their babies in their rooms rather than placing them in the nursery under the supervision of nurses, it's important for new parents to know the signs of newborn distress. Nurses will be checking on your baby regularly, but if you notice any of the following problems, talk to the nurse or doctor:

- Breathing problems

- Poor sucking or feeding

- Your baby changes color, looks blue

- Your baby doesn't move much, even when awake (seems quiet and listless)

- Your baby doesn't respond to loud noises

- Eyes don't focus on or follow an object held close to baby's face and moved from side to side

- Lower jaw trembles most of the time, or baby is jittery

- Irritability—baby is crying a lot and difficult to console

Feeding Your Baby

By the time you have given birth, you've probably decided whether you will feed your baby by breast or bottle. Breast-feeding is the recommended choice, unless you or your baby can't do so for some reason. If you do have a choice, consider that there are various medical, emotional, and developmental advantages to breast-feeding.

Advantages of Breast-Feeding for the Infant

▌ Breast milk contains antibodies that protect your baby from infection.

▌ Breast-fed babies have fewer ear infections, respiratory infections, rashes, and allergies than bottle-fed babies do.

▌ Breast-fed babies are less likely to develop asthma.

▌ The physical closeness and skin-to-skin contact provided by breast-feeding are valuable to infant development.

▌ Breast-feeding creates a physical interdependence between mother and child. The baby relies on the mother for food, while the mother relies on the baby's suckling to relieve the pressure of milk collecting in the breast.

Advantages of Breast-Feeding for the Mother

▌ Breast-feeding results in less postpartum bleeding.

▌ Uterus contracts to its normal size more quickly.

▌ Mothers who breast-feed their babies have lower rates of breast cancer later in life.

▌ Breast-feeding eliminates the need for preparing formula and washing bottles.

Truth be told, breast-feeding has a few disadvantages, including the fact that it is more difficult for the mother to leave the baby with someone else for more than a couple of hours. It also places the job of feeding the baby squarely on the mother, excluding the father from one of the most pleasurable early baby-care duties. But once breast-feeding is firmly established, you can express breast milk (see p. 68) and put it in a bottle to allow the father or a caregiver to feed the baby.

The ingredients in breast milk are many and not fully known. Because of this, breast milk cannot be duplicated by formula. Some studies suggest that breast milk may even boost a child's development. The American Academy of Pediatrics recommends breast-feeding your baby for the first 12 months, adding appropriate solid foods at about 4 to 6 months.

At the hospital, remind the nursing staff that you want to breast-feed your baby exclusively, and ask that bottles not be given to your baby except in the case of medical complications. Giving a baby a bottle at this early stage confuses some babies who are just learning to take their sustenance from the breast. Many hospitals now provide an experienced breast-feeding coach who can help you start breast-feeding your baby and give you advice and information about how to proceed.

Security and Identification

Hospital personnel will take several steps to ensure your baby's security and to make sure that you go home with your own baby and not somebody else's. The matching bracelets applied to your and your baby's wrists a moment after birth and checked by you in the delivery room are the most effective insurance that each baby is matched with his mother. Many hospitals also take a handprint, footprint, or photograph for added security, but the bracelets are the most effective form of identification. In addition, hospitals have security procedures to prevent uninvited strangers from entering a maternity ward and to restrict access to the babies. For example, many wards have color-coded badges given only to the family members authorized to have access to the baby. Ask your nurses about the security measures at your hospital if you have any concerns.

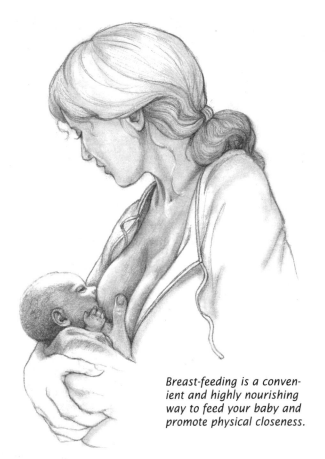

Breast-feeding is a convenient and highly nourishing way to feed your baby and promote physical closeness.

Taking Advantage of the Nurses' Expertise

The maternity nurses will help you get settled and give you some instructions for keeping your vaginal area clean and dry. When you are rested, take advantage of the nursing staff's expertise in baby care. Most likely, the nurses will tell you when they are about to demonstrate such things as bathing, diapering, and feeding your baby, and ask whether you want to watch. By all means go. These are the things that are best learned by observing firsthand.

One of the most important things you can learn in the hospital is breast-feeding technique. Nurses can advise you on how to help your baby to latch on and how to best position your baby while breast-feeding. For some women breast-feeding comes easily, but for many it takes time and practice. Always ask for advice if you're having problems.

Your Baby's Birth Certificate

One important form you'll need to fill out after your baby is born is the birth certificate. This form will be important in future years as a means of proving your child's identity in such situations as entering school, applying for a passport, and applying for a driver's license. Hospital staff will give you a form to fill out with the names, addresses, birth dates, and birth places for mother, father, and baby. This information will appear on the official form that will be kept on file at your state or county government offices. A copy will not be sent to you automatically. So a few weeks after the baby is born, you will need to contact your state or county health department to obtain a copy for a fee.

When filling out the form, make sure that your choice of the baby's name (first and last) is final. If you seek to change it later, you may need to get a court order or pay a fee. You will also be asked to fill out details concerning the baby's delivery and the mother's prenatal health. If you are unsure about answers to the medical questions, ask a hospital staff member for help. The information on this form is usually confidential. Most states will include a box you can check that allows the federal government to assign a Social Security number automatically to your baby. Checking this box will save you the time of applying for a Social Security card later, and the card will be sent automatically to your home address. Double-check your answers for accuracy and correct spelling before returning the form to the hospital staff.

Leaving the Hospital

It's time to go home. Many new parents are anxious about leaving the hospital with a new baby. You may be unsure about many things, including baby-care basics like feeding (pp. 62–73), dressing (p. 77), or calming (p. 80) your baby. Parents who have family or friends nearby to rely on often feel more secure about going home with a new baby. If you can arrange for someone to stay with you for a few days to help take care of some of the household responsibilities or to look after your older children, you can relax and concentrate on the baby. If not, make sure to have phone numbers ready for people you can rely on for help in a pinch. Accept the offers of family and friends to look after your older children. Don't try to do it all yourself. Concentrate on the baby. The cooking, cleaning, and other household responsibilities will have to wait a bit.

Make sure you have an infant car seat securely fastened in the backseat of the car or taxi you are taking home. Dress the baby in clothing that is appropriate for the weather. One extra layer is best for a newborn baby. (See p. 21 for more on baby clothes and equipment for a newborn.)

Before your baby leaves the hospital, the pediatrician will examine the baby one final time to ensure that he is healthy enough to go home. New parents can be reassured that they are ready to care for the baby at home as long as they are familiar with the following baby-care basics:

▌ Breast- or bottle-feeding (pp. 62 and 70)

▌ Burping the baby (p. 73)

▌ Bathing the baby (p. 75)

▌ Detecting some medical conditions that require a call to the doctor (p. 84)

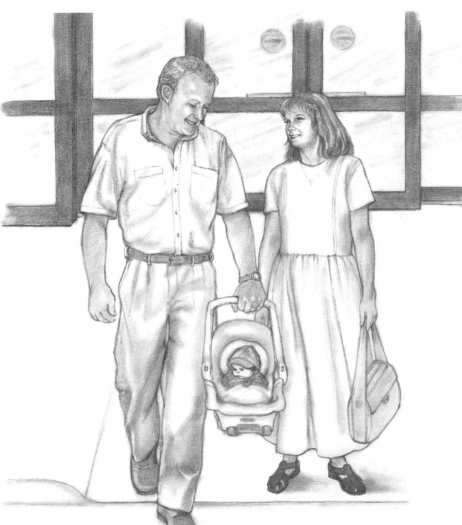

Leaving the hospital can bring on conflicting emotions, particularly for first-time parents. You may be thrilled to bring your baby home, yet be overwhelmed by your new responsibilities. Use this book as a guide during the weeks ahead, and rely on family and friends who offer to help.

Before leaving the hospital, a baby should

▌ complete at least two successful feedings.

▌ be able to suck and swallow and breathe while feeding.

▌ have urinated and passed one stool (within 24 hours of birth).

▌ be able to maintain a normal body temperature.

▌ show no excessive bleeding at the circumcision site or umbilical cord site.

▌ have no physical abnormalities that require continued hospitalization.

A woman who has had a cesarean delivery should be able to

▌ walk without excessive pain.

▌ eat solid foods.

▌ urinate normally.

▌ care for her stitches.

By the time you are ready to go home, you and your baby have already been through a lot together. You've already had a glimpse of your infant as a unique little person who will find his own ways to tell you when he is hungry, frightened, lonely, or bored. Now, get ready to step out into the world together. It's time to go home with your new family member.

PART TWO
YOUR CHILD AGE-BY-AGE

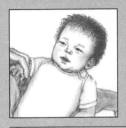

CHAPTER 3
YOUR BABY'S FIRST MONTH

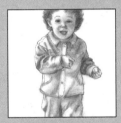

CHAPTER 4
YOUR BABY'S FIRST YEAR

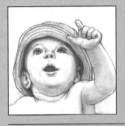

CHAPTER 5
YOUR TODDLER

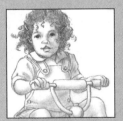

CHAPTER 6
YOUR PRESCHOOL CHILD

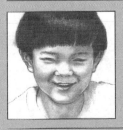

CHAPTER 7
YOUR SCHOOL-AGE CHILD

Your Baby's First Month

NEWBORN DEVELOPMENT

CARING FOR YOUR BABY

KEEPING YOUR BABY HEALTHY

A PARENT'S LIFE

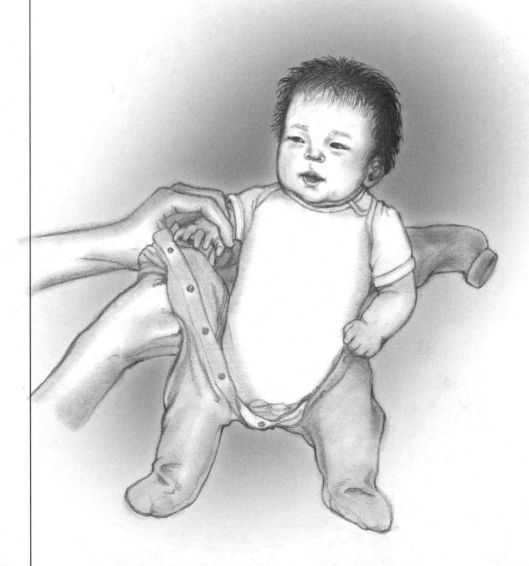

F or months, you have been awaiting the day when you bring your baby home. But no matter how much you know or have learned about babies ahead of time, you cannot anticipate what life will be like with your new family member. New parenthood is the ultimate on-the-job training.

Discovering the person behind the closed eyes and the tightly held arms and legs is what makes being a new parent one of the most thrilling adventures of a lifetime. In the weeks ahead, you will discover what upsets your baby and how to comfort her, learning the difference between a cry of hunger and a cry of boredom. You will see your baby grow, develop, and learn as rapidly in the first 4 weeks, perhaps, as in almost any other single month in her life.

Of course, this adventure isn't all thrills. New parents must learn to live without the security of predictable schedules and routines. You may feel exhausted or lose your patience. But sometime during the first few weeks, anxiety may give way to delight, and you will remember the reasons you wanted to be a parent in the first place.

Newborn Development

Many new parents are surprised by how little their baby can do at first. It's hard to imagine this dreamy newborn ever going to school, much less saying "Mommy" and "Daddy," taking her first steps, or even rolling over at will. But you may be surprised at how well a newborn makes her needs known simply by crying, fussing, and responding to her surroundings. Newborns grow and develop rapidly. Within the first few weeks, they learn many important skills.

DEVELOPMENTAL MILESTONES

Age	Most Babies
Newborn	Focus on a human face and follow it with their eyes
	Respond to parent's voice by turning head and searching with eyes
	Startle to sudden sound or movement
	Move limbs, hands, and feet
	Grasp tightly when something is placed in hand
	Make faces, sucking sounds, mouthing motions, or startle motions in their sleep

As you review this list of milestones, remember that children who are within the normal range will have some areas in which they excel and others in which they are slower. Not achieving a particular milestone at the designated time is not always a matter of concern. If you and your child's doctor are concerned about your child's overall development or any of your child's developmental skills, such as language, hearing, vision, or motor skills, seek the help of the appropriate specialist. For more information, see *Developmental Problems,* Part 5.

Vision and Hearing

An infant's senses are so well developed that she can use them moments after birth to begin making sense of her new world. At birth, your baby can tell a female voice from a male voice—most newborns show a preference for the female voice by turning toward it rather than a male voice. Babies can also recognize their mother's smell and, by 2 weeks, the sound of their mother's voice. And they can coordinate their senses to some degree. For example, babies can coordinate some sights and sounds: If your baby hears a voice, she will look for a face.

Newborns like to look at faces. Given a choice, a baby will spend more time gazing at a face or a pattern that resembles a face than at anything else. Hang a mobile with a black-and-white face on it above your baby's crib, and watch your baby follow it with her eyes. Newborns love to look at faces (real faces and pictures of faces), and researchers have discovered that babies are most likely to look at a high-contrast face. Black-and-white designs have the highest contrast, but other bright colors work well, too.

Color and Focus

Newborns can see in color and in three dimensions. But their vision is limited, so infants are more responsive to bright colors and distinct black-and-white contrast patterns than to softer pastel shades. Experts think it is no coincidence that a baby's depth of vision is the distance between the baby's face and the mother's face while nursing. In other words, infants seem to be ready to see what they need to see.

Looking Cross-Eyed

It's normal for a newborn's eyes to appear crossed or to move in different directions occasionally. This is because a baby cannot control her eye muscles enough to focus properly until she is 3 to 6 months old. But tell your doctor if these problems occur constantly during the newborn period or don't go away after 6 months (see *Amblyopia and/or Strabismus,* Part 5).

Checking Your Baby's Vision and Hearing

Checking your baby's vision and hearing informally is important, especially if anyone in the family has problems seeing or hearing. After all, a child learns primarily through these senses.

▌ *To check your baby's vision:* Hold a brightly colored toy or some other object about 12 inches away from her face, and move it in an arc in front of her. Most babies are able to follow the movement with their eyes.

▌ *To check your baby's hearing:* A simple test is to ring the doorbell, clap, or make another sudden noise. She should react in some way: startling, crying, or, if she's been crying, suddenly becoming quiet. If your baby responds, it's a good sign but not complete proof that your baby's hearing is normal.

❚ *What to do:* After you try these tests, or if you're unsure or concerned about your child's hearing or vision, talk with your child's doctor. Early detection of vision or hearing problems can help prevent developmental delays in the months ahead.

Growing and Moving

Many babies lose a few ounces of weight during their first few days of life. But by the time your baby is about 2 weeks old, she probably will have regained all the weight that she lost in the days following birth. For the rest of the month, her weight should increase by about 1 ounce each day or by about 1 pound total by the end of the first month.

It's not unusual for breast-fed babies to take up to 3 weeks to regain their birth weight. This doesn't mean that nursing isn't going well. More likely it reflects the fact that a mother's milk production increases gradually, in synchrony with the infant's appetite. As long as the doctor finds your baby healthy at the first checkup, rest assured that everything is fine. By the end of the first month, your baby may be about 1 to 1½ inches longer than the day she was born and markedly chubbier.

Tracking Growth and Weight

At each visit, the doctor will track your baby's length, weight, and head size and plot them on a growth chart (see Appendix: Growth Charts). There are different charts for boys and girls. The chart will show your baby's growth in relation to what is considered the normal range for babies of the same age and sex. For instance, if the doctor tells you that your baby is in the 40th percentile for weight and the 60th percentile for length, that means she's heavier than 40 percent of the girls her age and longer than 60 percent of them.

At this stage, there's no way of knowing whether a child who is above or below average in size or weight will stay that way over the long term. And there's no cause for concern if her percentiles change somewhat. But if either or both of the percentiles change significantly— weight drops, say, from the 60th to the 10th percentile— the doctor will probably want to know why. Is the baby getting enough to eat? Is infection or illness preventing weight gain? The doctor might also ask such questions if your baby's percentiles for weight and length move substantially farther apart— for example, if she is in the 60th percentile for length and the 5th percentile for weight.

Being "off the charts," meaning either below the 5th percentile or above the 95th percentile, can be a sign of either too little or too much growth or weight gain. Your child's doctor can help determine if your child has a problem or if she is simply following her natural pattern for growth and weight gain.

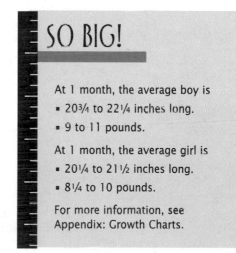

SO BIG!

At 1 month, the average boy is
- 20¾ to 22¼ inches long.
- 9 to 11 pounds.

At 1 month, the average girl is
- 20¼ to 21½ inches long.
- 8¼ to 10 pounds.

For more information, see Appendix: Growth Charts.

Tracking Head Size

In addition to height and weight, the doctor will pay close attention to your baby's head size. It will grow rapidly this month. In fact, it should grow faster during the first 4 months than at any other time in your child's life. The increase in head circumference (the measurement around the skull) reflects the growth of your baby's brain. A baby's head circumference is an average of 14 inches at birth for boys and 13¾ inches for girls. At 1 month, the average circumference is 15 inches for boys and 14½ inches for girls. The doctor or staff member will measure your baby's head circumference at each visit to make sure that your baby's brain is growing at a normal rate.

Tracking Movement

From a parent's perspective, the most dramatic evidence of your baby's development will be the increase in the number of things she can do. During the first several weeks, most of your baby's movements are involuntary, a function of the reflexes she was born with. If the baby is startled either by a sound or by the sudden movement of her own head, for example, she'll automatically extend her arms and legs as if she's trying to grab onto something. If you place your finger in the palm of her hand, she'll grasp it tightly.

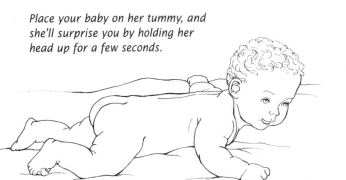

Place your baby on her tummy, and she'll surprise you by holding her head up for a few seconds.

One purposeful movement that most babies can manage by the end of the first month is lifting their head for a second or two when lying on their stomach on a firm surface. It's a good idea to put your baby in this position during her alert periods to give her a chance to exercise her head and strengthen the muscles in the back of her neck. But don't put her on her stomach at nap time or bedtime, since sleeping in this position has been associated with a higher risk of ***sudden infant death syndrome*** (SIDS) (see Part 5) than sleeping on the back.

Communicating

The bonding that occurs between you and your baby in the first month is the foundation for her lifelong ability to communicate. At this point, your baby's most obvious means of communication is crying, but it's not the only one. Babies also make their needs known through other sounds, like cooing to show pleasure, or body language, such as arching their backs, grimacing, and rubbing their mouths with their fists. Different cries have different meanings. A high-pitched cry often means hunger or pain, for example. To understand what your baby is trying to tell you, you'll have to become a keen observer and interpreter.

What Is Your Baby Trying to Say?

Learning your baby's language will take time. For now, it's enough just to recognize when your baby is trying to tell you something and to respond in some way. Pick her up, feed her, change her. Frequently what she needs is simply to be held or comforted. Try talking to her, singing to her, or picking her up. Your attempts to quiet your baby's cries are among the first signs that you and she are successfully communicating. Most importantly, watch for and reinforce her own ways of comforting herself. If she likes to suck on her hand, help her bring her hand to her mouth. Help her change position. Does she respond in a certain way to your voice or to gentle pressure on her abdomen?

Though it will be many months before your baby utters any sound resembling a word, it's not too early to encourage language development. To do this, talk to her as much as possible. Then pause occasionally to give your baby the chance to reply. You won't always get a response. But by punctuating your speech with silence, you will help your baby learn the give-and-take pattern of conversation. And in several weeks, she'll probably demonstrate what she's learned by responding to your words with her first smile.

When a Smile Is a Smile

Mothers and fathers eagerly await their baby's first smile. It's their reward for working around the clock to feed and care for her. Many parents take it as their baby's way of saying, "I love you."

But not all smiles are created equal. Soon after birth, babies smile when they're asleep, but this gesture probably has nothing to do with their feelings, or their desire to communicate. No one knows what causes it. By the time they're 6 to 8 weeks old, however, most babies make their first social smile in response to a friendly face or gesture. This is the one that parents, and your child's doctor, write down.

Though you know why your baby is smiling (she's happy, of course), researchers have been looking for more scientific explanations. For years they assumed that babies were imitating the people around them, but now they believe the capacity to smile socially is hardwired—it's not a learned response but a developmental ability. Evidence comes from studies showing that the first social smile coincides with a significant leap in brain

During the first months of life, which for you may be the most physically draining stage of parenthood, there's nothing more rewarding than seeing your baby look at you and smile.

development at about 6 to 8 weeks after birth. For premature babies, the first social smile comes at about 6 to 8 weeks after the date their mother was due to give birth.

Learning

Newborns are smarter than the experts long thought. Experts used to think, for example, that babies couldn't identify their mother's voice until they were 4 months old. Now we know that this recognition occurs within 2 weeks of birth, probably because their mother's voice is more familiar than anyone else's—it's the voice they heard in the womb. Babies are more likely to turn their head toward their mother's than their father's or a stranger's voice. But by the end of the first month, they may be able to recognize their father's voice, too. And babies know the difference between a parent's voice and a stranger's voice. For example, given the choice, a baby will turn her head toward the father's voice rather than the doctor's voice 80 percent of the time.

Newborns are fast learners. They can tell that a picture of a tree, for example, is different from a picture of a face. Babies' preference for looking at faces is probably a survival mechanism. Your baby gazes at your eyes, you gaze back at her, and the two of you become attached. Nothing is more essential to your baby's survival than this attachment.

Remembering

Babies remember what they've seen. If they are shown a picture that they've seen before and a different one that they have never seen, they'll spend more time gazing at the new one. By the same token, if your baby usually sees you without your glasses on, the first time she sees you wearing glasses she'll look at your face for an especially long time. And newborns quickly learn how to solve problems. Researchers have found that if they set up an arrangement in which a light goes on when the baby's head turns, the baby will learn, with a little practice, to put the light on by turning her head.

Nurturing Your Baby's Intelligence

There's a lot you can do to enhance your baby's capacity to learn. From birth onward, your baby's experiences shape the growth of her brain by stimulating brain cells to make connections. All kinds of things—the sound of your voice, the comfort of your arms, the sight of a mobile or crib toys—will help make this happen. The most stimulating experience in her life is your attention. Scientists have shown that loving contact between newborns and their parents actually increases the number of brain cell connections.

Certainly, much of a child's intelligence comes from "nature"—the intelligence she inherited from her parents. But it also comes partly from "nurture"—that is, her environment, experiences, and especially her relationships with her parents and other caregivers. No one knows how much of a child's intelligence is derived from nature and how much is nurtured. Responding when a baby cries, for example, seems to affect her intelligence. Research shows that very young babies who are responded to most promptly have the highest scores on tests of infant development and the highest IQs when they reach 4 years old.

Take these steps, and you'll be doing more than meeting your baby's basic physical and emotional survival needs. You'll be helping her learn.

▌ Go to your baby promptly when she cries.

▌ Feed your baby when she seems hungry.

▌ Talk to your baby frequently.

▌ Hold and soothe your baby frequently.

QUESTIONS PARENTS ASK
Spoiling a Baby

Q: Will carrying my baby around all the time make the baby dependent on constant attention or spoil the baby?

A: You can't spoil a newborn baby by holding or carrying her as much as she wants. Many new parents are surprised by the amount of time they need to spend holding their baby. Many babies cry whenever put in the crib or stroller and stop the instant they are picked up. So you may pass much of the day carrying your baby with you as you move about your home. It's not unusual or harmful for a newborn to be held most of the time she is awake.

Socializing

For now, your baby's social life revolves around the care you provide. Your being there for your baby builds her trust in you, and the capacity to trust will eventually help her form relationships with people. During the first month, your baby will acquire some social skills. When you look into her eyes and smile, she'll pay attention for progressively longer periods. When you come to feed her, she'll turn her head toward you. She may even stop crying and make contented sounds.

Your Baby's Temperament

Precisely how your baby socializes depends on her temperament—her way of reacting to the world. Chances are, you've seen infants lying in their strollers wide awake and looking around contentedly for 10 or 15 minutes. And you've probably seen other infants who cry the moment they awaken, impatient to be picked up. Both kinds of behavior are normal; they merely reflect different temperaments.

Wearing your baby in a front pack carrier often satisfies her need to be held and gives you the freedom to do household chores or a take peaceful walk. Be sure that the carrier you choose is sturdy and supports the baby's back and head. Leg holes should be small enough so that the baby can't slip through.

As with the color of her eyes and hair, much of your baby's temperament is inherited. Different temperaments can be seen at birth. Some babies cry more than others or are easier to console. But this doesn't mean that your baby's personality will be exactly like yours or her father's, any more than her face is a duplicate of either of your faces. It can be hard for parents when some aspect of their baby's nature is unlike their own. A mother who loves to hug and be hugged may be disappointed to find that hugging makes her newborn squirm and fuss. The baby isn't rejecting the mother; she's only trying to tell the mother to give her a little space or hold her differently.

Your baby's temperament isn't completely written in the genes. As with intelligence, a baby's temperament is partly shaped by nature (genetics) and partly by her environment (the world around her and the people in it), especially your relationship with her. That's why it's important for parents to listen to their baby's cues and respond to them quickly.

Caring for Your Baby

Newborn babies need a lot of care. They have to be fed and changed around the clock, as well as cleaned, carried, comforted, and protected. It's fair to say that for now, your entire life is focused on meeting your baby's basic needs. Whether you're breast-feeding or bottle-feeding, you'll be nourishing your baby in every sense of the word. Aside from providing the nutrients and calories she needs to thrive, feeding sessions are also prime times to socialize with your newborn. Talking to your baby, cuddling her, looking into her eyes, and smiling at her will help you get to know each other, even as you both fumble a little with the mechanics of these first meals.

Breast-Feeding

The benefits of breast-feeding your baby are many (see p. 48) and include boosting your child's immune system and protecting her from recurrent ear infections. But although breast-feeding is the ultimate natural experience, it doesn't always come naturally to mother or baby. It takes practice, and you may have some difficulties. Don't assume that because you're having trouble it's time to reach for the bottle. Many women quickly overcome early difficulties with advice from a nurse, friend, sister, mother, or breast-feeding expert (lactation consultant or breast-feeding coach).

Things You Can Do: How to Breast-Feed Your Baby

Here are the step-by-step basics of breast-feeding:

▌ Start right away, as soon as you both are ready. Many mothers make their first attempt in the delivery room. Your baby is born with a desire to suck. Let her try.

▌ Get comfortable, and use extra pillows to support your back and your baby.

▌ Make sure your baby is awake before you start feeding her.

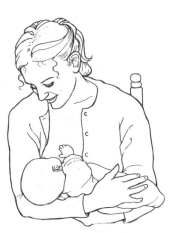

To breast-feed in the most common sitting-up position, cradle your baby in your arms with her tummy against yours. Use a pillow to help prop her up.

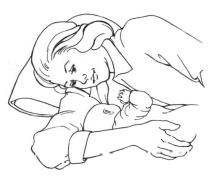

The side-lying position gives you an opportunity to rest while feeding your baby. Your baby's whole body should be facing you and aligned so that her mouth is directly in front of your nipple.

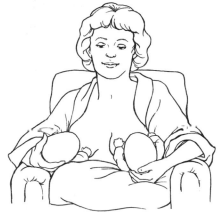

Many mothers, particularly those with twins, find that the football hold is the easiest way to support a nursing infant. Support your baby's body with your forearm, and hold her head in front of your breast so that she does not have to strain her neck to reach your nipple.

- Position your baby so that her whole body is facing yours, including her face.
- Lift her gently to breast level—don't lean down toward her.
- With your free hand, grasp your breast between thumb and forefinger, and gently stroke the baby's cheek with the nipple.
- When your baby opens her mouth and moves her head toward your nipple (the rooting reflex), place the nipple in her mouth, making sure she takes the whole areola into her mouth—this is known as latching on.
- If necessary, press gently on your breast so that it is not blocking the baby's nose.
- Let the baby nurse for 10 to 15 minutes on the first breast.
- To change breasts, gently break the suction of the baby's mouth on your breast with your finger or gently push down on her chin. Never pull the baby off the breast—it's too abrupt.
- Position the baby on the other breast, and repeat the above steps. Let the baby nurse for 10 to 15 minutes on the second breast. Encourage the baby to nurse on both breasts each time. The next time she nurses, start with the second breast first.
- Let your nipples air dry for about 15 minutes before covering them.
- Nurse your baby as often as every 1½ hours or as often as she wants it. She'll need to feed about 8 to 12 times in each 24-hour period.
- Don't try to put your newborn on a schedule. Nurse her when she seems to want it.

Getting Started

When you start breast-feeding, it may seem that the baby is not getting much milk. It's true. A new mother's milk takes a few days to "come in." In the meantime, your baby is getting small amounts of a yellowish white nutritious substance called colostrum. The baby's sucking action will cause your milk to come in. Because breast-feeding is a matter of supply and demand, the more the baby sucks, the more milk you will produce. Your milk should come in by about the fourth day after delivery. You'll know when this happens, because your breasts will become larger and harder between feedings, and they'll spontaneously leak or squirt milk.

Breast-feeding is comforting to a newborn baby. So if your baby is crying or fussing, and she hasn't had a feeding in more than an hour, try nursing her—it's usually what she wants. If she seems too sleepy to nurse the second breast, try waking her up by brushing her cheek with your finger or nipple to stimulate the rooting reflex. Or try changing her diaper or clothing to wake her sufficiently to feed on the other breast. Signs of hunger include increased alertness and activity and mouthing or rooting motions. If your baby tends to be sleepy and undemanding, wake her to feed if she hasn't fed in the past 4 hours.

Some babies want to stop nursing for a while to look around or socialize. When this happens, mothers are understandably eager to get them back on the breast. But it's best to be patient, to let her have a break. Research has shown that babies resume nursing sooner when their mothers don't hurry them. Ideally, by the end of the feeding, your baby will empty the second breast—at least partially.

Avoid giving your baby bottles of formula or water during the first 2 or 3 weeks of breast-feeding until your milk production is well established and your baby is nursing well. Infants generally get all the water they need from breast milk. If your baby is not getting sufficient fluids from breast milk, for whatever reason, your doctor may recommend bottles of sterile water or sugar water to avoid dehydration. Ordinarily, a breast-feeding baby won't need bottles at all. However, when breast-feeding is well established—usually in about 3 to 4 weeks—you can introduce a bottle of expressed milk or formula. Introducing it sooner runs the risk of the baby's preferring the bottle to the breast, since she doesn't have to work as hard to get milk from a bottle. The advantage of giving baby an occasional bottle of expressed milk is that the father or a caregiver can feed the baby and give the mother a break.

If your baby is feeding well after regaining her birth weight, she should gain about 1 ounce a day during the first month. If, in the first few days, your baby does not seem to be feeding well, talk to your child's doctor. He may want to see your baby to determine whether she's sucking well and feeding frequently enough. Or, a visiting nurse may come to your home to weigh your baby and assess her feeding. Either doctor or nurse may recommend a lactation consultant or breast-feeding coach for help. See Appendix: Parent Resources, Breast-Feeding/Lactation, for help in finding breast-feeding expertise.

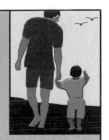

A FATHER'S STORY
Sidelined by Breast-Feeding

I was happy that my wife chose to breast-feed our son. But it wasn't until they returned from the hospital that I realized that there was a down side. There was nothing for *me* to do. Sure, I could change David's diapers and bathe him. But I could not feed him. And since feeding was the major part of his life in early weeks, he spent most of the time with my wife. I'd be there looking on, but I was out of the loop.

I did find ways to have some time alone with my son. When he was a newborn and he got up around 5 A.M. for a feeding, he wouldn't go back to sleep. My wife would be at her wit's end from having been up three or four times during the night to nurse him. So I'd take David into the living room and walk back and forth. Soon he'd fall asleep in my arms. It was so peaceful.

How Much Is Enough?

Unlike bottle-feeding, you can't see how much milk a baby is getting when you breast-feed. Instead, consider your breast-feeding successful if your baby

▌ seems content afterward.

▌ produces at least six wet diapers and several soft or liquid mustard-colored stools per day.

▌ wakes up at least every 4 hours around the clock to be fed.

▌ is gaining weight normally at regular doctor's checkups.

Mother's Diet

Most women can continue to eat their normal diet when breast-feeding. Some mothers report that their babies seem upset by certain foods, such as onion, garlic, cabbage, and chocolate, but many others experience no such problems. If your baby seems to react badly to some foods, try eliminating a food to see if the problem disappears. Otherwise, eat a healthy, well-balanced diet that includes iron and plenty of calcium to provide optimum nutrition for you and your baby.

Drugs and Harmful Substances

Just about any drug that you take will get into the breast milk and therefore can affect your baby. Other substances, such as alcohol, nicotine, and caffeine, also enter breast milk. Very little is known about the exact effect of these drugs and other substances, because few studies have been done. But one study showed that infants exposed to even small amounts of alcohol in breast milk slept less and for shorter times than other infants.

Drinking beverages containing caffeine or alcohol just before you nurse or at the same time that you're nursing is not a good idea, because each of these substances gets into the breast milk. It is safest to avoid these substances while you are breast-

■ BREAST-FEEDING PROBLEMS AND SOLUTIONS

Problem	Cause	Solution
Milk not coming in by fourth day after birth (breasts have not swelled, baby does not seem to be getting much milk when nursing, no signs of leaking or spurting breast milk)	Prior illness or complications from labor and delivery; baby not sucking properly; baby not feeding often enough	Rent an electric breast pump and express milk for 10 minutes after nursing to stimulate milk production. Make sure baby is latching onto breast properly, with the nipple and areola in her mouth. Make sure baby is feeding every 1½ to 2 hours.
Breast engorgement	Temporary condition caused by sudden onset of milk production following delivery	Compress nipple between index finger and thumb to help baby latch on; apply hot washcloth before nursing to stimulate letdown; apply cold compresses between feedings to reduce fullness.
Sore nipples	Baby not positioned properly	See illustration of breast-feeding positions on p. 63. Make sure baby is latching on properly.
Cracked nipples	Baby's vigorous sucking; your sensitive skin	Apply lotion containing lanolin, or coat nipples with breast milk after feedings.
Severe breast pain and flulike symptoms	Bacterial or yeast infection (mastitis) in breast	Call doctor. Breast infections must be treated with certain antibiotics known to be safe.
Baby not nursing enough	Nipple confusion (if the baby has had supplemental bottles); trouble latching on; sleepiness	Eliminate supplemental bottles on a trial basis. Tilt your nipple down to make it easier for the baby to latch on. Be patient. Many babies are sleepy in the first week. Try to rouse your child if she falls asleep at the breast after less than 10 minutes.

feeding, but if you do choose to have an occasional cup of coffee or alcoholic drink, drink it just after you've nursed, so that the caffeine or alcohol levels in your blood will have dropped by the next time your baby is hungry. Your body naturally eliminates these substances through liver metabolism and urination.

When you're nursing, avoid taking any medicines, even over-the-counter ones. If you can't avoid medication, check with your doctor first. The doctor may suggest a nondrug alternative, the safest drug for your condition, or times of day to take the medicine when it is least likely to reach the baby.

Whenever you take medicine, be on the lookout for changes in your baby's behavior or appearance. Such changes may indicate an adverse reaction. If a drug is affecting your baby, talk with your doctor about either not taking it or bottle-feeding until you no longer need the drug. The following are among the more common drugs that you should avoid during breast-feeding:

▌ Birth control pills containing estrogen (can decrease milk production)

▌ Nicotine, including antismoking aids containing nicotine (can cause many symptoms when it enters the baby's bloodstream through breast milk, including rapid heart rate, fussiness, vomiting, and diarrhea. Smoking can also decrease a nursing mother's milk production. Tobacco smoke, when breathed by your baby, can also cause allergies, asthma, and respiratory infections.)

▌ Tricyclic antidepressants

▌ Sedatives (e.g., benzodiazepines)

▌ Illegal drugs

The various substances found in illegal drugs pose a threat. For example, one study found that babies exposed to marijuana through breast milk during the first month of life were not able to move their muscles normally. Cocaine from breast milk can actually make an infant "high," causing such symptoms as tremors, irritability, and high blood pressure. Because an infant's body can't break down cocaine, it remains there and will accumulate with repeated exposure. Amphetamines can make your baby cranky and either overly tired or unable to sleep. Both cocaine and amphetamines depress a baby's appetite, which may prevent her from gaining weight at a healthy rate. Heroin can cause drowsiness, vomiting, and the inability to feed properly. A baby withdrawing from exposure to heroin will be irritable, restless, and tremulous.

Injecting street drugs is especially dangerous. In addition to the effects of the drugs themselves, sharing needles or using needles not properly sterilized increases the risk of infection with HIV, the virus that causes AIDS (see ***HIV/AIDS Infection,*** Part 5). HIV can be transmitted through breast milk.

QUESTIONS PARENTS ASK
Pacifiers

Q: If I give my baby a pacifier, will she be less likely to keep nursing?

A: One recent study found that babies who used pacifiers frequently nursed less often than other babies, and they were more likely to be weaned at 6 months. This doesn't mean that you shouldn't use a pacifier if you're nursing. But it suggests that you limit its use to only those times when you are sure your baby is not hungry.

Expressing Milk

Expressing milk with a breast pump to store for later use is essential if you're planning to return to work within a few weeks or months, but you still want your baby to have the benefits of breast milk. Another advantage is that your partner can share in the nurturing experience of feeding your baby.

There are many kinds of breast pumps sold and rented in drugstores. Some work manually; others are electric. Most women find electric pumps easiest to use. The most comfortable and efficient models allow you to express milk from both breasts at once.

The best time to express milk is when your breasts are full, but when you will not need to nurse soon—for example, at night when you expect your baby to sleep for 2 or more hours, or during the day, when your partner or a baby-sitter is giving the baby a bottle. Express as much milk as you can. If it will be given to your baby within 24 hours, it can be refrigerated in a bottle. If not, pour the expressed milk into a disposable plastic nurser bag, close it with a fastener, and freeze it. Breast milk can be frozen for 2 months in a freezer that is attached to a refrigerator and for up to 6 months in a sepa-

WHAT'S IN BREAST MILK AND FORMULA?[1]

Nutritional Characteristic	Breast Milk	Cow's Milk Formula	Soy Formula
Calories	100.0	100.0	100.0
Protein (grams)	1.5	2.07	3.0
Fat (grams)	5.7	5.49	5.3
Vitamin A (IU)	330.0	300.0	300.0
Vitamin D (IU)	2.9	60.0	60.0
Vitamin E (IU)	0.34	3.0	2.0
Vitamin K (mcg)	0.31	8.0	8.0
Vitamin B_1 (mcg)	31.0	100.0	80.0
Vitamin B_2 (mcg)	51.8	150.0	90.0
Vitamin B_6 (mg)	30.3	60.0	60.0
Vitamin B_{12} (mcg)	0.07	0.25	0.3
Niacin (mcg)	227.5	1050.0	1000.0
Folic acid (mcg)	7.4	15.0	16.0
Vitamin C (mg)	5.9	9.0	12.0
Calcium (mg)	41.4	78.0	105.0
Iron (mg)	0.04	1.8	1.8

1. Amounts are per 5-ounce serving. *Abbreviations:* IU (international units), mcg (micrograms, one-millionth of a gram), mg (milligrams, one-thousandth of a gram).

rate freezer. (A separate freezer maintains a more consistent temperature than a freezer attached to a refrigerator, which you open and close frequently.)

To thaw milk for a feeding, place the closed plastic nurser bag in a pan of warm water until the milk is warm. Don't microwave breast milk; microwaves destroy some of the ingredients that enhance the baby's immune system, thereby defeating one of the main purposes for nursing in the first place.

Ingredients in Breast Milk and Formula

Although formula has more of some nutrients than does breast milk, breast milk doesn't need such high levels, because babies can absorb nutrients more easily from it. Breast milk is superior to formula, because it has many substances that benefit a baby's immune system. The only ingredient that breast milk lacks in adequate amounts is vitamin D. However, since the skin produces vitamin D when exposed to sunlight, many breast-fed babies can get all the vitamin D they need simply by being outdoors—a mere 15 minutes a week is sufficient for light-skinned babies. Dark-skinned babies, whose pigment screens the sunlight, as well as light-skinned babies who don't go out in the sun enough, may need vitamin D drops in addition to what they get naturally during the cold winter months.

SOME BENEFICIAL INGREDIENTS FOUND ONLY IN BREAST MILK

Substance	Benefit
B lymphocytes	Produce antibodies to fight infection
Macrophages	Kill germs in a newborn's digestive tract and activate other immune system chemicals
Neutrophils	Fight off bacteria in a baby's digestive tract
T lymphocytes	Kill infected cells and stimulate the immune system
Bifidus factor	Promotes growth of beneficial bacteria in digestive tract that fight harmful bacteria
Fatty acids	Attack some viruses and bacteria
Fibronectin	Boosts immune system activity against germs
Gamma interferon	Boosts immune system activity against germs
Hormones and growth factors	Help baby's digestive tract mature
Lysozyme	Kills bacteria
Mucins	Prevent bacteria and viruses from attaching to mucous membranes

Bottle-Feeding

For mothers who can't breast-feed or decide not to, it is important to know that formula contains all the nutrients that babies need for normal growth. During the 1950s and 1960s, mothers abandoned breast-feeding in droves. No long-term problems are apparent among that generation of babies, now in their 30s, 40s, and 50s. As for the bonding that breast-feeding fosters, you can get it by lovingly feeding your baby a bottle, too. And fathers can share equally in the bonding experience this way.

The formula you choose is largely a matter of personal preference—yours, your baby's, and your doctor's. Most formulas are made from cow's milk that has been processed so that infants can digest it. Some formulas are made from soybeans. Your baby's doctor may also recommend some specialized formulas for infants with health problems.

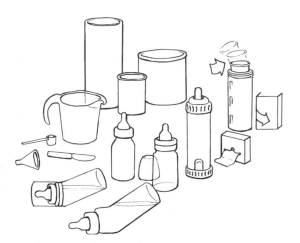

There is no shortage in variety when it comes to bottle-feeding equipment on the market. Bottles, which usually come in 4- or 8-ounce sizes, come upright, angled, or with presterilized liners. Nipples are flat, round, wide, or long. Before investing in one type, you may want to sample a few to see what works best for you and your baby.

Cow's milk formulas are more nutritious than soy formulas, because babies can absorb more calcium and phosphorus from them. For this reason, soy formulas are not recommended for premature babies, whose nutritional needs are greater than those of full-term babies. If you decide to put your full-term baby on soy formula, the doctor might recommend that you give her vitamin and mineral supplements.

Some babies are allergic to cow's milk. For these babies, soy formula may be a solution. But about a third of these babies are also allergic to soy formula. Your child's doctor can recommend special formulas for these babies. For a small number of babies with lactose intolerance (problems with carbohydrate absorption), lactose-free cow's milk formula or a lactose-free soy formula may be the right choice. These lactose-free formulas are not recommended for babies with a different, short-term form of lactose intolerance known as temporary lactose intolerance (caused mainly by infectious diarrhea), which is common in infants. True lactose intolerance is rare in infants.

Formula Safety

When preparing formula from a powder or liquid concentrate, use sterilized water. You can sterilize tap water or bottled spring water yourself by boiling it for 5 minutes, or you can buy sterile bottled water made especially for baby formula. Use a standard U.S.-made pot or kettle for sterilizing water; some imported kettles contain high levels of lead, which can leach into the water and cause lead poisoning. Sterilized water should be kept in the refrigerator for no more than 48 hours. Unrefrigerated, it can be kept for several hours.

Be sure to follow the instructions on the formula container's label. Adding too much water will prevent your baby from getting the nutrients and calories she needs. Adding too little water can cause diarrhea or dehydration.

A can of powdered formula that's been opened can be stored, covered, in a cupboard for 1 month. A can of opened liquid formula must be covered and refrigerated, and it will keep for only 48 hours. A prepared bottle of formula can be left at room temperature for only half an hour. If you'll be out for longer than that with your baby and know she'll need a feeding, you can stretch a bottle's shelf life by storing it in an insulated container with an ice pack until you're ready to use it.

If you're using tap water, have your water tested for lead by your local health department. Should your tap water have more than 15 parts per billion of lead, get a water purifier that filters out lead, or use commercially prepared lead-free sterilized water for your baby's formula.

How Much Formula?

During the first week, your newborn will probably drink 2 or 3 ounces at each feeding. By the end of the month, she may need 4 ounces at each feeding. The larger your baby, the more she'll consume. A general rule is that, during the first few months of life, babies need about 2½ ounces a day for each pound of body weight.

Bottle-Feeding Basics

You can either prepare one bottle at a time or make a day's worth of bottles at once and leave them in the refrigerator. Prepared bottles should be refrigerated for no more than 24 hours. Most babies prefer to have their formula warm. Don't microwave it, since this heats liquid unevenly and can make some areas of the formula too hot. It's better to warm formula either with a bottle warmer or by placing the bottle in a pan of water and gently heating it on the stove. Test the temperature by shaking a few drops onto your wrist—it should feel warm, not hot. For nighttime feedings, many parents keep ready-made bottles of formula in a cooler in their bedroom and then quickly heat them in a bottle warmer.

Whenever the baby is fed, she should be cradled in someone's arms, not left in her crib with a bottle. Putting a baby to bed with a bottle can increase her risk of ear infections and, later, may cause decay in her developing teeth by allowing milk to pool around her gums. See *Cavities,* Part 5, for more information on tooth decay in babies. And don't leave your baby in an infant seat with a bottle propped against her chest. Feeding times are not just for filling your baby with food, but for cuddling and communicating with her as well.

As with breast-feeding, bottle-feeding should be done when the baby's hungry, not on a predetermined schedule. This isn't to say that you must feed your baby whenever she cries. If you do, you risk overfeeding her. If she has recently fed, check other things first. She may need to be changed, or she may simply want to be held. When a bottle is half finished, take a break and burp your baby. Then go back to feeding until she doesn't want any more. Leftover formula should be discarded to prevent contamination.

Six Steps to Bottle-Feeding

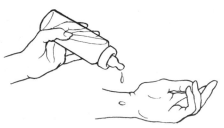

1 Put a drop on the inside of your wrist to test the temperature.

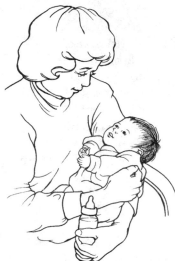

2 Get your baby into a semi-upright position, and settle yourself comfortably before letting her know the bottle is near.

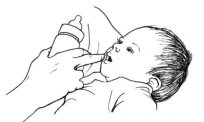

3 Use one finger of your bottle-holding hand to stroke the baby's cheek.

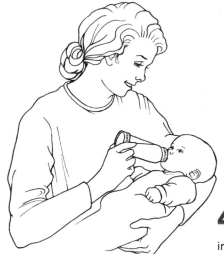

4 When your baby turns toward the bottle, allow her to take the nipple deeply into her mouth to begin sucking.

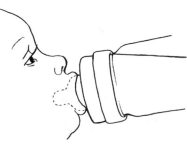

5 Make sure that the tip of the nipple is well back in baby's mouth.

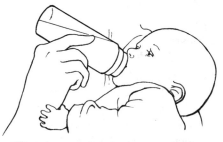

6 Make sure that the bottom of the bottle is tilted up so that no air is sucked in by the baby. Hold the bottle firmly so that baby's sucking efforts pull against your pressure.

QUESTIONS PARENTS ASK

Sterilizing Bottles

Q: Do you have to sterilize the bottles and nipples as well as the water you use to prepare formula?

A: You do not have to boil bottles, nipples, nipple rings, or breast pump paraphernalia or put them in a sterilizer to keep them from growing harmful germs. Scrubbing them thoroughly with warm, soapy water and rinsing them thoroughly or putting them in the dishwasher is sufficient. Make sure that they go through the hot-heat drying cycle in the dishwasher, because this step kills bacteria. And follow these steps to further assure cleanliness:

▌ Use a bottle brush to scrub bottles. Pay special attention to necks and screw threads.

▌ Dislodge caked-on formula by rubbing salt into nipples. Rinse thoroughly.

▌ In a dishwasher, place nipples pointing up so that they don't hold water.

Vitamin Supplements

Babies do not need to take vitamins if they're healthy and full-term. Breast milk and formula contain all the vitamins and minerals they need. But babies who were born prematurely or have certain medical problems may need multivitamin drops. Some breast-fed babies, such as very dark-skinned babies who don't go outside much, may not get enough vitamin D from their mother's milk (see p. 69). In addition, doctors often recommend a B-complex supplement for breast-fed babies whose mothers are vegetarians, since a meat-free diet may be lacking in vitamin B12.

Burping Your Baby

After your baby has fed, burping her will help release any air that she may have swallowed and that can cause her to be uncomfortable and fussy. You can burp your baby after she feeds on each breast or wait until she has finished feeding on both. A baby who hasn't finished her bottle may need to be burped before she continues feeding. Some babies need burping more than others. If your infant falls asleep after feeding or is content and peaceful, you don't need to wake her or disturb her.

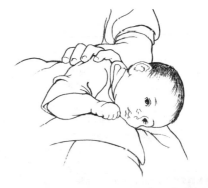

Two ways to burp your baby: Hold her so her head rests on your shoulder, and pat or rub her back gently, or, lay your baby on her stomach across your lap, and turn her head sideways. You may need to support her head with your hand. Pat or rub her back gently.

Fluoride

Babies under 6 months old should not have fluoride supplements, because they get sufficient amounts of this tooth-strengthening mineral from formula or breast milk. Babies run the risk of getting too much fluoride if their powdered or liquid-concentrate formula (which comes fortified) is mixed with water that has more fluoride than 1 part per million. Extra fluoride can affect a baby's developing teeth, causing brown spots to form. To avoid the problem, use water that has little or no fluoride, such as low-fluoride distilled water or tap water that has had most of the fluoride removed by a water filter.

Umbilical Cord Care

It generally takes from 1 to 3 weeks for the umbilical cord stump to fall off. Until then, you can take several preventative measures to avoid infection.

▮ Swab the area with rubbing alcohol three times a day: in the morning, afternoon, and night.

▮ Keep diapers from irritating the stump. You can fold down the top of the diaper to keep it away from the stump.

▮ To hasten the healing process, avoid wetting the area when you bathe your baby until the umbilical cord falls off.

▮ Call the doctor if you see any signs of an umbilical cord infection (see *Umbilical Cord Bleeding/Infection,* Part 5), such as pus or redness at the base of the cord, or if the navel appears wet and swollen after the stump falls off.

Circumcision Care

If your infant son has been circumcised, you need to take several steps to keep the wound free of infection until it heals.

▮ Until the area heals, cover it with a dab of petroleum jelly whenever you change the baby's diaper.

▮ Some doctors also advise covering the petroleum jelly with gauze.

▮ Avoid immersing the penis in bath water until it has healed, but wash it gently with soap and water if it gets soiled with the baby's stool.

▮ While the circumcision is healing, it's normal for the tip of the penis to look red and secrete a yellowish liquid. Infections are rare, but call the baby's doctor if you see the following warning signs:
  • Redness that lasts longer than about 10 days
  • Swelling
  • Crusted sores

Bathing

Just because your newborn has recently emerged from the secure, watery world in utero doesn't mean she'll love to bathe. Many parents are surprised to find that rather than relax peacefully in their infant tubs, their babies howl in agony. Being naked may make newborns overstimulated and upset. They seem to prefer being wrapped closely with their arms and legs held in. The chill caused by any slight draft may compound their discomfort. Fortunately, infants don't need a bath every day. And on the days when they do, you can do certain things to make the experience more tolerable.

Giving a Sponge Bath

Your baby should have only sponge baths until the umbilical cord stump falls off. If the baby was circumcised, continue with sponge baths until the circumcision has healed. Here are some sponge bath suggestions (also, see the illustration on p. 76):

▌ Find a place that's warm enough for your baby and comfortable for you. You might spread a towel on a counter in the bathroom or kitchen for your baby to lie on, or sit with the baby in your lap.

▌ Hold the baby securely with one hand to keep her from falling.

▌ Have your materials within reach—washcloths, warm water, and a mild soap.

▌ If your baby is uncomfortable being naked, or if the room is cool, wrap her in a towel during the sponge bath, uncover the parts that you are washing, and then cover them as soon as you are finished.

▌ Wash your baby's face first to prevent irritation and contamination. Using a washcloth moistened with warm water, wipe around the eyes, nose, mouth, and the rest of the face. Don't use soap, which can irritate the eyes, on the face.

▌ Using a mild soap on a cloth, wipe the rest of the baby's body. Pay special attention to the folds of skin where grime tends to accumulate, for instance, around the neck and behind the knees and elbows.

▌ Wash the dirtiest part of the body—the diaper area—last.

Giving a Tub Bath

When the time comes to give your newborn a tub bath, most parents find it easiest to use either a portable infant tub or a small sink. Most infants need bathing only two or three times a week. More than that can deprive the skin of its natural oils and even cause a rash.

▌ Fill the tub or sink with about 2 inches of warm water.

▌ Test the temperature with your elbow to make sure it is warm but not hot.

▌ Ease the baby into the water and hold her securely at all times, keeping her head well above the water.

Six Steps to a Sponge Bath

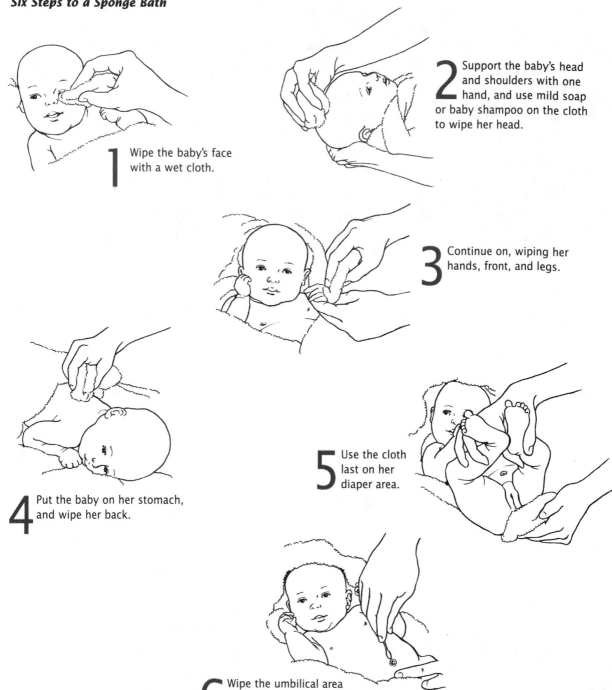

1 Wipe the baby's face with a wet cloth.

2 Support the baby's head and shoulders with one hand, and use mild soap or baby shampoo on the cloth to wipe her head.

3 Continue on, wiping her hands, front, and legs.

4 Put the baby on her stomach, and wipe her back.

5 Use the cloth last on her diaper area.

6 Wipe the umbilical area with a cotton swab.

- Position her against your left arm (if you're right-handed), and hold her firmly with your hand beneath her left arm (see Fig. A).

- Wash her in the same order you did when giving her a sponge bath (see Fig. B).

- Pour water on her often to keep her from feeling chilled (see Fig. C).

- If she has hair, clean it with a baby shampoo (see Fig. D). You don't have to do this more than twice a week, unless your baby develops *cradle cap* (see Part 5), a red rash covered with white flakes on her scalp. Cradle cap is common in the first weeks of life and, although it may look worrisome, it's not harmful. Most parents can control the condition by shampooing the baby's hair every few days and brushing it with a baby brush.

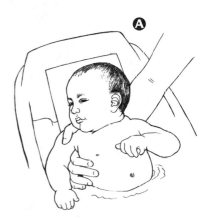

- After the bath, don't bother using moisturizing baby lotions, unless your baby's skin is dry.

Avoid using powder of any kind (including baby powder) on your baby. Inhaling powder can be dangerous for a baby.

Dressing Your Baby

Infants can't regulate their body temperatures very well. They lose heat more easily than adults, so they're more easily chilled. But they're also more sensitive to heat. To keep your baby comfortable, put a cotton undershirt underneath her pajamas or other clothes on all but the hottest days. You don't need to bundle up your baby; in general, dress her in one more layer than you are wearing. On very hot days, your baby doesn't need to wear anything but a diaper and a T-shirt, and she may perspire and become cranky if you put anything more on her. There is also evidence that overdressing a baby at night can increase a baby's risk of *sudden infant death syndrome* (SIDS) (see Part 5).

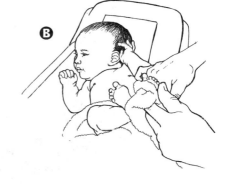

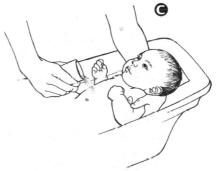

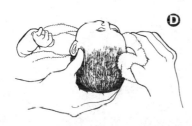

SAFETY ALERT

Sun Exposure

On outings during seasonably warm weather, remember that your baby needs protection from the sun's harmful rays. It's best to keep baby in the shade, dress her in a wide-brimmed hat, sunglasses, lightweight long pants, and a long-sleeved shirt. If it's simply too hot for long sleeves and shade isn't available, apply PABA-free sunscreen to the exposed areas, but use it sparingly during the first 6 months of life, when skin is especially sensitive.

Clipping Nails

Many infants are born with surprisingly long nails. And their fingernails grow so quickly that they may need to be clipped as often as twice a week. Be sure to keep your baby's nails short so that she doesn't scratch herself in her uncoordinated early attempts to rub her eyes and suck her thumb.

Because newborns' nails are more supple than those of older children or adults, they tend to bend when you try to cut them with nail clippers designed for babies. Many parents find blunt-edged nail scissors easier to use. The best time to do the job is when your baby is lying quietly. You and your partner can work together, with one of you holding the baby while the other clips her nails. If you're afraid that she'll squirm and you'll cut her skin, you're not alone. Many parents prefer to wait until their babies are asleep to trim their nails.

Sleeping

Maybe you know of some lucky parents whose newborn started sleeping through the night from day one. Or maybe other people's babies just seem to sleep more than yours does. But the fact is, the only sleeping that most newborns and their parents can manage is short naps. Though newborns sleep an average of 16 hours a day, many parents lament that they are the "wrong" 16 hours. Your baby may wake up every 2 hours through the night and then snooze for 4 hours in the afternoon.

Doctors used to think that newborns' sleeping and waking cycles were governed almost exclusively by their stomachs. In other words, they would wake up when they were hungry and sleep when they were full. But hunger isn't the only factor. Babies also wake up because they're no longer tired. You may notice that your baby sometimes lies in her crib or bassinet, looking around or moving without crying to be fed.

Your Baby's Biological Clock

Your baby's sleep is out of step with yours (or what you'd like yours to be once again) for two main reasons. First, she cannot yet sleep for 8- to 10-hour stretches without waking and feeding. Second, her biological clock is not yet synchronized with the rising and setting of the sun, so she may not sleep more at night than during the day.

There is little you can do in the first month to help your baby sleep more. She's too immature to adhere to a regular schedule. Every day and night may be different. One night your baby may sleep for 4 hours straight, but the next night she may be up every 1½ hours. The best thing you can do is make the frequent nighttime awakenings as easy as possible on yourself. Many parents prefer to have their baby in their room for the first several weeks, either in a bassinet next to their bed or in bed with them. But make sure the baby is sleeping on her back on a firm surface, not on a soft surface like a pillow or comforter. Don't worry that having your newborn in bed with you will later on make sleeping in a crib hard for her. Nothing you do now will influence her sleep habits in the weeks and months to come.

Some parents take turns comforting and feeding a newborn at night in order to give the other parent a chance to sleep. This works well if the baby is bottle-feeding.

SAFETY ALERT
Sleep Safety

Most infants should be put down to sleep on their backs. Research has shown that **sudden infant death syndrome** (SIDS) (see Part 5) is much less common among babies who sleep in this position than on their stomach. And the problem with putting infants on their side is that they often roll onto their stomach. No one knows why the stomach position is related to SIDS (just as the cause of SIDS is unknown).

These recommendations don't apply to all infants, however. The face-down position is still considered better for premature babies with respiratory problems and for infants with certain health conditions, such as **gastroesophageal reflux** (see Part 5).

Several other measures are essential to ensure that your baby sleeps safely. If you're offered a hand-me-down crib, make sure the slats are no wider than 2 inches apart. Otherwise, a baby can fit her head through the slats and possibly choke. And make sure it is not painted with lead paint. Don't furnish the crib with pillows or fleece blankets. You might want to consider using a blanket sleeper or sleep clothing with no other covering as an alternative to blankets. If your child sleeps with you, be careful of the bedding on your mattress. Newborns can easily smother if their faces become buried in soft materials. And make sure there's nothing in the crib small enough for a baby to choke on. (For more on crib safety, see p. 26.)

Finally, try to choose pajamas labeled "flame resistant" for your infant and older children as well. Cotton and cotton-blend clothing is more flammable in case of a fire. Flame-resistant sleepwear can save your baby's life. If there's a fire, cotton will burn, whereas flame-resistant pajamas will resist burning.

Thumb or Pacifier?

Whether you encourage your baby to suck her thumb or a pacifier is a matter of personal preference. Contrary to many parents' fears, neither thumb sucking nor pacifier sucking, during the first few years, harms the development of a baby's teeth by causing an overbite. Over the long term (after about 3 years old), however, both thumb sucking and pacifier use can contribute to an overbite.

The advantage of thumb sucking over a pacifier at this age is that your baby's thumb can't get lost in the middle of the night the way a pacifier might. The advantage of a pacifier comes in later months, when you can remove it when you want your child to stop using it. But most children kick the thumb or a pacifier habit long before it becomes a social, or a dental, issue anyway. Don't use a pacifier until your baby's breast-feeding is well established; it may cause nipple confusion and interfere with her breast-feeding at first.

If you decide to use a pacifier, choose one made for babies under 6 months old. Look for one that has material from the nipple knotted around the back of the handle. This type of construction prevents the nipple from coming off and causing the baby to choke. You can attach the pacifier to the baby's clothing using a clip with a cord or ribbon that is too short to wrap around the baby's neck, but never put the baby to sleep with this cord. And never hang a pacifier around a baby's neck like a necklace, since the cord can strangle the baby. The best way to get around the problem of babies' losing their pacifiers is to have several on hand. Wash them once a day with warm, soapy water to reduce the chance of infection.

Coping with Crying

Babies cry. Usually there's a reason: They're hungry, tired, or uncomfortable, or they want to be held. It's the crying for no apparent reason that drives parents to tears. Most babies do a lot of crying. Studies show that babies cry for an average of 1 hour and 45 minutes a day when they're 2 weeks old, and 3 hours a day when they're 6 weeks old.

Why do babies cry so much? That question is as old as parenthood. Doctors think that at least part of the blame lies with their immature nervous system. It can't selectively shut out stimuli, so their senses get overloaded. For them, crying is like turning off a circuit breaker.

Time of Day

Most babies have a fussy period each day from the time they're 3 weeks old until they are about 12 weeks old. More often than not, it begins just before dinnertime and can last for hours. Doctors think that babies fall apart at this time as a result of the accumulated stimulation of the day. The one good thing that can be said about these intense crying sessions is that they usually make the baby so tired that she falls into a deep sleep afterward.

Calming Down

Another reason newborns cry a lot is that they haven't yet developed ways to soothe themselves. There's nothing more comforting to a baby than sucking, but newborns lack the coordination to suck their thumbs. You can help by putting your baby's thumb or hand in her mouth, giving her a pacifier, or putting her to the breast.

TOUCHPOINT

Consoling a Crying Baby

T. Berry Brazelton, M.D., founder of the Child Development Unit at Children's Hospital, Boston, uses the term "touchpoints" to describe the predictable moments that occur just before a period of rapid growth in development, when, for a short time, a child's behavior falls apart.

During the newborn period, whenever your baby cries, go to her and assure her that you hear her and are there to help. Research shows that infants whose cries are promptly responded to in the first 6 months cry less in the second 6 months.

But you don't have to offer your breast or a bottle. There are many other ways to comfort a crying baby, and they are more appropriate to try first if your baby had a full feeding less than an hour earlier. Check if your baby's diaper is soiled or wet. If not, try the following techniques in this order:

1. Put your face right in front of her face, or talk to your baby. Seeing you or hearing your voice may be enough to soothe her.
2. Do both of these things at the same time. Seeing you close up and hearing your voice together can have a more powerful effect than either one alone.
3. Place your hand gently on your baby's stomach.
4. Hold your baby's hands and arms gently against your baby's body as she lies down. Many babies are comforted when restrained this way.
5. Pick up your baby.
6. Rock your baby.
7. Swaddle her (see p. 83).
8. Give her something to suck (a pacifier or her thumb), and hold it in her mouth so that it doesn't slip out.

Source: Touchpoints Project (see Appendix: Parent Resources, Child Development).

SAFETY ALERT

Never Shake a Baby

It can happen innocently enough. You try everything you can think of to quiet your crying baby, but nothing works. In a moment of frustration, you shake her or handle her roughly. Both activities are hazardous. They can cause fatal brain or spinal injuries in newborns because babies' neck muscles are too weak to withstand abrupt movement.

Each year, thousands of babies go blind, experience brain damage, or are killed as a result of being shaken. Never shake your baby. Whenever you are holding a baby, always support the head and neck. For tips on how to control your anger, see page 213.

TOUCHPOINT

What Different Cries Mean

The rhythm, pitch, and other qualities of a baby's cry can tell parents a lot about what's bothering her. As you get to know your baby, you will become familiar with the different kinds of cries and what they mean. Here are several kind of cries and what they often mean.

Cry	Meaning	Try This
High-pitched, abrupt	She's in pain.	Look for a minor cause, like a finger caught in a buttonhole, or a scratchy clothing tag or diaper. If you can't find a cause, call the doctor.
High-pitched, intense, and prolonged	She's in pain, is ill, or, rarely, may have been born with a neurological problem.	If efforts to calm her fail, call the doctor.
Rhythmic and urgent	She's hungry.	Feed her.
Rhythmic but not urgent	She's tired.	Lay her down to sleep.
Hollow-sounding	She's bored.	Talk to her; play with her.
Irritable, fussy	She's overstimulated and needs to let off steam.	Eliminate sources of stimulation: Dim the lights, turn down music or television, speak softly.

Source: Touchpoints Project (see p. 81).

Colic

All babies cry, but some babies cry more than most and keep on crying no matter how you try to comfort them. These babies have *colic* (see Part 5)—one of the most stressful challenges of new parenthood. Colic is sometimes defined by the "rule of three." That is, an infant who cries more than 3 hours a day for more than 3 days a week for more than 3 weeks is considered to have colic. About 20 percent of infants fall into this category. Instead of being confined largely to one fussy period at the end of the day, the crying goes on through much of the day and night. During these crying periods, the baby may look as though she's in pain. She may clench her fists and pull her arms and legs in toward her chest and then thrust them out straight. Responses that usually quiet a baby, like carrying or feeding her, don't work.

Managing Colic

Colic isn't caused by an illness. Doctors don't know what does cause colic. They used to think intestinal gas was to blame, since babies often pass gas when they're colicky. Many doctors recommended an over-the-counter remedy to reduce gas. But that theory was cast in doubt when research found that medication doesn't relieve colic.

Many parents think that colic is caused by something their babies ate, but this is rarely the cause. Switching formulas or having a nursing mother eliminate certain foods from her diet usually has little or no effect.

The latest thinking is that colicky babies may be more sensitive to overstimulation than average. A few techniques may help:

▌ Keep your baby's surroundings calm and quiet. Turn the lights low, talk to her in a gentle voice, and limit activity around her.

▌ Swaddle your baby in a receiving blanket to prevent her from startling.

▌ Carry your baby in an infant carrier or sling that fits across your chest.

Swaddling Your Baby

To swaddle your baby, follow these tips:

1. Spread a receiving blanket out on a bed, and fold down the top corner; lay the baby down on the blanket with the top of his head slightly above the fold; fold one side of the blanket across the front of your baby, and tuck the end under his back.

2. Pull the bottom corner of the blanket up over the folded side of the blanket.

3. Bring the unfolded side of your baby's blanket across his front, and tuck it behind his back.

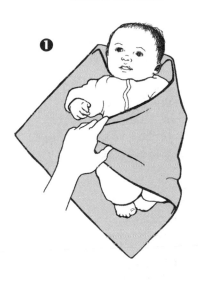
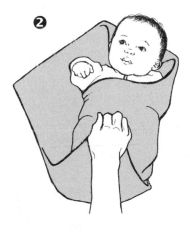
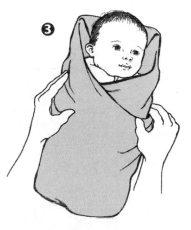

How I Survived Colic

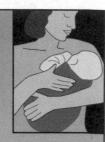

Don and I were going crazy. We never knew when Anna would explode. All we knew was that when she did, she would cry for hours and nothing we did would make her stop. It got to where we were afraid to go out with her because we couldn't stand to hear one more person ask us, "What's wrong with the baby?" or "Why's the baby crying?" We had all these expectations about having a happy baby to care for, and we couldn't help but feel disappointed that our baby seemed to be crying all the time.

The pediatrician tried to help. He suggested that I stop eating garlic and onions, just on the chance that they were getting into my milk and upsetting the baby's stomach. This didn't stop Anna's fussing. Then he told us to give the baby an ounce of warm chamomile tea a day because it's supposed to settle the stomach. This didn't work either.

The doctor was out of suggestions. All he said was, "No one knows why this is, but colicky babies aren't colicky forever. It usually doesn't last more than 3 months." His words helped us more than any colic remedy did, because they gave us hope at a time when we'd completely run out. We recruited my parents and Don's to occasionally help out with the baby for a couple of hours to give us a break. That made all the difference for me. And as things turned out, the doctor was right about our daughter. Now we brag about her sweet disposition.

Keeping Your Baby Healthy

Newborns look so helpless that it's easy to understand why many new parents worry about every strange sound their baby makes and every blemish that appears on her skin. But you can avoid most potential problems with proper preventative care. That means taking her to the doctor for regular checkups, making sure she gets the recommended immunizations on schedule (see Childhood Immunization Schedule, p. 110), and taking safety measures.

WHEN TO CALL THE DOCTOR

When Your Newborn Is Sick

Now that you are home with your new baby, you are on the front line of her health care. You must notice when your baby is ill, and take the appropriate steps—usually calling your doctor. There are a variety of signs that your newborn may be ill, and you can learn to recognize them. In the first few days and weeks after your baby's birth, be on the lookout for the following symptoms. They can signal underlying medical problems and should be checked out immediately. (For specific conditions, see Part 5, Guide to Common Childhood Illness, Injury, and Conditions.)

CALL FOR EMERGENCY HELP IF YOUR BABY HAS TROUBLE BREATHING.

For first aid information, see page 380 if your child is less than 1 year old and page 383 if your child is 1 year of age or older.

CALL YOUR DOCTOR TODAY IF YOU NOTICE THE FOLLOWING SYMPTOMS:

▌ Failure to eat

▌ Fewer than three stools a day or six wet diapers a day

▌ A fever higher than 100.2°F (see *Fever*, Part 5). Never place a glass (mercury) thermometer in a baby's mouth. See Taking Your Child's Temperature, page 352.

▌ Unremitting crankiness

▌ Excessive sleepiness (more than 16½ hours of sleep per day)

▌ Coughing or choking regularly during feedings

▌ Vomiting regularly after feedings

▌ A blue cast to the baby's skin

▌ A yellow cast to the whites of the eyes and a suntanned appearance on the face

▌ Redness or pus around the umbilical cord stump

▌ Bloody diarrhea

▌ A bright red rash, or one with blisters or fluid

▌ Consistent lack of response to sounds around her

Checkups

Your infant's regular checkups are your opportunity to talk with your doctor about your favorite subject—your baby. This is the time to discuss even the most minute details of newborn care—the doctor is concerned to know that your baby is off to a good start in every way. Jot down your questions ahead of time about baby care, immunizations, and any aspect of your child's health and behavior you can think of, so that you don't forget to ask anything that's been on your mind.

Your Baby's First Checkup

Your baby should have a checkup with the doctor once during the first month. The doctor may want to see your baby earlier for some reason, such as if she was under 6 pounds at birth or if her weight dropped below that mark in the days afterward.

Your baby's first checkup will be a new experience for both of you. Sitting in the waiting room is no longer a quiet time to read magazines. Instead, you may spend the time rocking, feeding, and arranging your baby's clothes to make her comfortable and calm. When it's your turn, don't be surprised if your baby cries through much of the exam, no matter how pleasant the doctor and nurse are. Newborns usually don't like to be undressed, and yet the nurse or doctor must remove babies' clothes to weigh them accurately and examine them carefully. And the bright lights, new voices, and general commotion may unsettle her for the entire visit.

Measuring and weighing your infant will be the first order of the day. First, the nurse will weigh her by laying her on a scale. By about 2 weeks your baby should have regained her birth weight, although many babies regain any lost weight earlier. Then, the nurse will measure your baby by laying her on an examining table covered with paper, holding her legs straight, and then marking the paper at the top of her head and the bottoms of her feet. The nurse will also measure her head circumference with a type of tape measure. Next, the doctor will examine your baby. Many doctors conduct as much of the exam as possible with the baby in a parent's arms to minimize the baby's discomfort.

At the first visit, the doctor or nurse will take the following steps:

▌ Weigh and measure the baby.

▌ Look at your baby's skin for signs of *jaundice* (see Part 5), *birthmarks* (see Part 5), and *rashes* (see Part 5).

▌ Observe the neck, hands, feet, arms, and legs for normal movement.

▌ Rotate the baby's legs to check for hip dislocation.

▌ Listen to the baby's chest for signs of abnormal breathing and heart functioning, particularly for signs of a *heart murmur* (see Part 5).

▌ Check the baby's underarms and neck for swollen glands.

▌ Examine all visible body parts for abnormalities.

▌ Ask whether your baby is feeding well.

▌ Ask how you and your partner are coping with new parenthood.

▌ Discuss your concerns and questions.

▌ Administer the first hepatitis (Hep B-1) vaccine if it was not given in the hospital (see Childhood Immunization Schedule, p. 110).

Preventing Infections

Gone are the days when doctors ordered new parents to keep their newborns indoors for weeks to shield them from germs that their immature immune systems would have trouble fighting off. You can safely take your baby for a walk in the park or to Grandma and Grandpa's home for an adoring visit. But doctors still recommend avoiding crowded indoor places, like cramped stores, for the first 4 weeks. In addition, don't let people visit if they have colds or other infectious illnesses. If you are sick, wash your hands before holding the baby and try not to cough on her. And don't let anyone smoke around the baby. Exposure to secondhand smoke increases the risk of colds, ear infections, allergies, and asthma.

Call the doctor if your baby has any symptoms of an infection, such as a fever, runny nose, cough, or marked change in behavior, like decreased appetite, increased sleepiness, or excessive crankiness. Illnesses that are minor in older children and adults can be serious in a newborn.

Keeping Your Newborn Baby Safe

When traveling as well as staying at home, you'll need to take several precautions to protect your newborn from injuries.

At Home

Though it will be many months before you'll have to childproof your home against an adventurous crawler, you'll need to guard against the safety hazards in the chart below as soon as your baby comes home.

On the Road

In cars and planes, babies must be in a car seat that is suitable for infants. It should be in the rear-facing position until your baby weighs 20 pounds and is 1 year of age.

▬ NEWBORN SAFETY

Potential Danger	Preventative Measures
Burns	Don't drink coffee, soup, or anything else hot while holding your baby. Always test the temperature of the bottle and the bath water with your wrist or elbow before exposing your baby to them. Don't ever let anyone smoke around your baby. Have your baby sleep in flame-retardant pajamas.
Fire	Keep smoke detectors on every floor of your home, and test them monthly to make sure they work. Reduce the risk of a fire by making sure no one smokes in bed. Discard frayed wires, don't overload electrical outlets, and don't use space heaters.
Older siblings	Children shouldn't be left alone with a baby. The risk isn't so much that older children will intentionally hurt the baby (although the possibility exists), but that they may accidentally harm her, for instance, by trying to pick her up, hug her, or hold her.
Pets	Don't let the dog or cat in the same room with your baby unless an adult is there. This includes familiar pets with no history of unusual behavior.
Falls	Never leave your baby unattended on a changing table, couch, bed, or any other surface above the floor unless it is designed to safely contain a baby (crib, bassinet, playpen). Whenever she is in the crib, keep the sides raised. Be careful when climbing stairs while carrying your baby.
Drowning	Stay with your baby the entire time she's in the bath. Don't answer the phone or doorbell. Bathe her in a small container like an infant bath or a small sink to prevent her from sliding into the water.
Choking	Keep tiny objects, like older children's toys, out of the crib. Don't put anything, such as a necklace or a pacifier attached to a string, around a baby's neck.
Shaking	Don't shake your baby. Vigorous shaking can cause brain damage and fatal spine injuries in newborns.

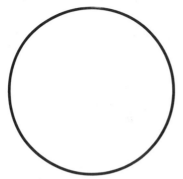

Measure small toys: *Toys should have a diameter greater than 1 3/4 inches. Hold a toy up to this circle. Unless it covers the circle, it should be thrown away or stored in a safe place until your child is at least 3 years old.*

According to the American Academy of Pediatrics, the safest car seats are five-point harnesses, with two straps at the shoulders, two at the hips, and one at the crotch. You can choose from infant car seats designed for babies under 20 pounds or convertible car seats designed to accommodate older babies as well. But for premature infants and small full-term babies, infant car seats are safer because they hold the babies more securely. Whichever kind of car seat you choose, put it in the backseat, since this is the safest place for a baby. Never put an infant or a child in a front seat, especially one equipped with air bags. For more on choosing a car seat, see page 24.

SAFE TOYS FOR NEWBORN BABIES

Toys for Newborns	Safety Check
Small soft, washable animals, dolls, or balls	Make sure eyes, noses, and other small parts are attached securely to avoid choking. Remove ribbons. Avoid toys stuffed with pellets or other small objects that the baby can choke on if the toy breaks. While the baby is sleeping, keep soft toys away from her (either at the foot of the crib or out of the crib) to avoid having them fall across her face and restrict her oxygen supply.
Mirror	Read the label to make sure it's unbreakable. Make sure it has no sharp edges.
Rattles	Check that seams are secure, so that the pieces inside can't fall out and present a choking hazard.
Squeeze toys	Look for sturdy construction. Avoid toys with loose parts or weak seams.
Busy boards	Don't attach them to the crib with strings longer than 12 inches. Once your baby can move around, long strings are a choking hazard.
Mobiles	To prevent any chances of strangulation, it's best to remove mobiles or crib gyms when baby turns 3 months, before she is able to get up on her hands and reach for her hanging toys.

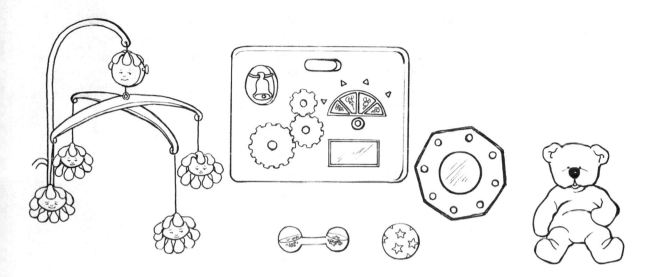

A Parent's Life

When you look at your baby, it's natural to feel tremendous pride. Whatever your past glories, they may pale compared to the creation of life. But it's also natural for there to be times when you can't help but wish for your old life back. Suddenly, you and your partner have no time for each other, much less for doing things you used to enjoy. Few people realize what a luxury it is to go out on the spur of the moment until it becomes impossible to do so without first lining up a baby-sitter. You're a parent and life has changed.

The New Mom

What matters just as much as taking good care of your baby is taking good care of yourself. Mothers need to recover from childbirth. If you had a long, difficult labor, you may feel exhausted for weeks. If you had an episiotomy or a tear while your baby was being born, that area may sting for several days. If you had a cesarean, it may be a few weeks before you can lift the baby without pain.

Whether you delivered vaginally or by cesarean, expect to have vaginal bleeding for about a month. But if the bleeding is exceptionally heavy, or if you have symptoms of illness, like a fever or pain and swelling in the legs, call the doctor. These could be signs of complications from childbirth.

Along with good food and regular support from loved ones, the thing your body needs most during this postpartum period is plenty of rest. This may seem like a joke, given that your baby wakes up four times a night. But getting enough sleep is a serious matter. It both helps you feel better and is important for successful nursing.

Sleep increases your level of prolactin, the hormone responsible for milk production. Also, since lack of sleep can make you more susceptible to stress, insufficient sleep may also make you more sensitive to stress-related difficulties, like problems releasing (letting down) the milk that your breasts produce.

So, as your friends and family have probably told you, sleep when the baby sleeps. Unplug the phone, delay writing thank-you notes for those adorable baby gifts. Ask for help from family, friends, and neighbors, or hire some help if you need to and can afford it.

Baby Blues and Postpartum Depression

You longed to have a baby, and now you have one. She's healthy and beautiful. You expected to feel like the luckiest person alive, but you keep bursting into tears and blowing up at your loved ones. About 70 percent of new mothers experience the baby blues, sadness, or mood swings that start a few days after delivery and last for about a week. About 20 percent to 25 percent of women become clinically depressed after childbirth. Their symptoms are more severe than those with brief postpartum blues and can last for many weeks.

Many people assume that postpartum blues and depression are a new mother's reaction to the enormous demands of parenthood. But there is a biological explanation. In the 6 weeks following childbirth, women have lower than normal levels of a stress hormone called corticotropin. Low levels of this hormone, which acts as a buffer against stress, are associated with several forms of depression. New mothers with the lowest levels feel the most depressed.

Even though postpartum depression is usually temporary, it's important to get help, for your sake and your baby's. For one thing, a mother who's depressed may have trouble giving her baby proper care. Her low tolerance for stress also increases the chance that she could harm her own baby. In addition, a mother's depression can reduce her baby's brain activity, possibly because the baby isn't getting enough nurturing and attention, which foster brain growth. Tell your obstetrician or midwife if you have the following symptoms of depression:

▌ Insomnia or excess sleeping

▌ Lack of appetite

▌ Loss of interest in friends and activities you once enjoyed

▌ Feelings of helplessness or hopelessness

▌ Feeling out of control

▌ Thoughts of suicide

▌ Thoughts of harming the baby

Chances are, your health practitioner can refer you to a therapist for counseling or to a postpartum depression support group.

The New Dad

Fathers don't experience the physical trauma of childbirth, but they share the emotional experience, the lack of sleep, and the general disruption in lifestyle that a newborn brings to a household. Because they don't have to recover physically from their baby's birth, fathers may be expected to do whatever new mothers are unable to do during the postpartum period—run errands, field phone calls, fix meals, make sure their older child doesn't feel left out, walk with the screaming newborn at 4 A.M., and, of course, go to work. What many people don't realize—least of all many men themselves—is that new fathers are often thrown into an emotional tailspin.

Some men may worry about how to connect with their new baby. Despite their profound love, many fathers don't quite know how to show it. If the baby is breastfeeding, she spends most of her time with her mother. A father may wonder what he can do. And when he does have a chance to hold the baby, he may be afraid of dropping her. His wife, without meaning to, may make him feel inadequate by correcting him when he handles the baby. If he holds the baby, she may tell him to support the head better. If he dresses the baby, she may question whether the clothes are warm enough, and so on.

It's important for fathers and mothers to understand that fathers need a postpartum recovery period, too. It helps for a couple to discuss these feelings when the baby's asleep and they are not too tired.

The best way for dads to feel comfortable being dads is to care for the baby as much as possible. The more involved a father is with his baby, the more attached he and the baby become. Children whose fathers regularly care for them and play with them during the first month of life score much higher on developmental tests of motor skills and problem-solving when they reach a year old. Even a diaper change is an opportunity for loving interaction—it gives you a chance to dress and handle your baby in a gentle, caring way. As with other aspects of parenting, being a father gets easier with practice.

QUESTIONS PARENTS ASK

Time Management

Q: I don't understand why I get nothing done when I'm busy every second of the day. I used to be a highly organized, efficient person. What's happened to me?

A: You're accomplishing more than you think. After all, you're feeding your baby eight or more times a day, changing her diaper at least as often, and giving a lot of other care besides. What bothers a lot of new mothers and fathers is that they think they have nothing to show for all this effort—the place is a mess, the newspapers are piling up unread. You're not disorganized or inefficient. You're simply too busy. Do yourself a favor, and don't expect to get everything done. At least not now.

New Parenthood

In the storybook version of new parenthood, having a new baby brings a couple closer together. Their love grows as they gaze at their angelic creation. Certainly new parents have their share of picture-perfect moments. But in reality, a couple's relationship may be less than idyllic during the first month.

One reason is the temporary loss of intimacy. New mothers are generally advised not to have sexual relations for the first 6 weeks in order to give the vagina and surrounding tissue (or, after a cesarean, the abdominal incision) time to heal. Many women find intercourse painful for several months. Even if pain isn't an issue, parents may not feel like having sex. Sleep loss, and the new demands of parenthood, may make sex the last thing on your mind.

New parents may feel estranged from each other emotionally. With all that needs to be done for the baby, a couple may sometimes see each other as little more than another pair of hands. A woman who's home all day with the baby may envy her husband's freedom when he goes off to work. A man may feel left out of the special relationship that his wife has the time to cultivate with their baby.

Keeping Communication Open

Take steps to keep communication open. Most important, talk. Tell your partner how you're feeling—whether you're scared, confused, lonely, ecstatic, or a combination of all these things on any given day, and encourage your partner to do the same. Criticism, however gentle, is best left for a time when you're both better able to handle it. Use the following test as a guide: If your partner were to say that you put the diaper on too tight, would you feel hurt or angry? If the answer is yes, hold your tongue the next time you think that your partner's skills are less than perfect, unless you're concerned for your baby's health or safety.

Your Older Child

No matter how much you wanted to have another child, you may feel that you've slighted—even betrayed—your first one. Rest assured, you haven't done anything terrible to your older child by bringing a new baby into your home. But there's plenty that you can do to make him know that he's loved as much as before. Spend time with him, and don't be discouraged if, despite your best efforts, your child still has a hard time. From his point of view, all the time you spend with him is still not enough.

Anger Is Normal

It's normal for older siblings to become angry and to throw more tantrums than usual during the first several months after a new baby is born. In addition, a toilet-trained toddler or preschooler may start having accidents or show some anger or aggression toward you or the new baby. This is one reason to make sure not to leave an older sibling in the room with an infant. When you're nursing or giving the baby a bottle, your older child may wedge himself into your lap as if to stake his claim to territory he considers rightfully his. Take a deep breath, and try to be patient. This will pass.

Here are some ideas for keeping an older child happy when you come home with a new baby:

▪ Tell him with words and actions that he is an important member of the family.

▪ Find jobs that he can do to help you with the baby—for example, handing you baby wipes when you're changing a diaper. Tell him he's a great helper.

▪ Tell him you love him, again and again.

▪ Do things with the baby and her older sibling together, like taking walks, reading stories, or playing a board game with the baby on your lap.

▪ Encourage other family members to spend extra time with your older child.

▪ Make a point of setting up "special times" to do things with your older child, even if this is simply reading a bedtime story.

Allow your older child to cradle her new sibling carefully on her lap while you remain close by. Finding creative ways for her to participate in your baby's care will help her adjust to the new situation.

▪ If family members bring a gift for the baby, have them bring a little gift, or something special, for the older child too. It doesn't have to be expensive—just an acknowledgment that he's still special.

QUESTIONS PARENTS ASK

Friction from an Older Child

Q: Our 3½-year-old son is running around the apartment saying that he wants to cut his baby sister's head off. We know that sibling rivalry is common, but is our son's behavior abnormal?

A: Older siblings often say things like, "I hate the baby," "Send the baby back," and worse. Though these words are extremely upsetting for parents to hear, they're only words. The feelings behind them are normal, and it's healthy for your child to be able to express them. Still, never leave him alone in a room with the baby. It's unlikely that he'd intentionally harm her, but accidents happen, and kids are unpredictable. Let your child know that you understand his feelings by acknowledging that "it's hard to learn to share" or "it sure is noisier around here now." Remind him that he is loved just as much as always and that he is important to the family as a big brother.

4 Your Baby's First Year

GROWTH AND DEVELOPMENT

CARING FOR YOUR BABY

KEEPING YOUR BABY HEALTHY

KEEPING YOUR BABY SAFE

A PARENT'S LIFE

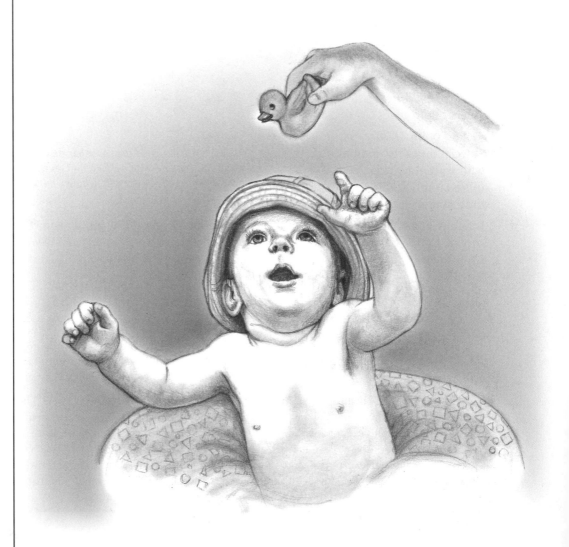

Your child's first year is a time of change and excitement. It's hard to imagine that the tiny infant in your arms today may be walking, laughing, playing, throwing a ball, and possibly saying some first words by year's end. The challenges of the first year are many, not the least of which is adjusting to life with a dynamic and often demanding new family member.

Because change comes so rapidly during your baby's first year, this chapter is divided into three sections: 1 to 3 months, 4 to 7 months, and 8 to 12 months. For information on caring for a newborn, see Chapter 3.

Watching your child grow and develop is both thrilling and reassuring, but keep in mind that children acquire skills at different rates. Your early walker, for example, may turn out to be a later talker. Or a child who is good with his hands may have a tougher time walking up steps or riding a tricycle. You may also notice that the progress your child makes is not always steady. At times, your child's development may look like one step forward and two steps back, as he boldly explores new behavior and activities for a while and then retreats to more familiar, and comfortable, ground. A child who takes his first few steps may then choose to go back to crawling for a few days before stepping out boldly again.

It is important to remember that you can do only so much to nurture the development process. You can't *teach* your child to sit up, walk, or develop memory. But looking for signs of readiness, creating an environment filled with opportunities for learning, and supporting your child's efforts will give your child the best possible start in life.

YOUR BABY AT 1 TO 3 MONTHS

Growth and Development

By the end of the first month, your baby doesn't look so helpless anymore. He's bigger, plumper, more wide-eyed. He kicks vigorously and reaches out to explore. More and more, when he expresses himself, you understand.

By the time your infant is 2 to 3 months old, he smiles back at you and talks to you in cooing sounds. He's even settled into enough of a feeding and sleeping schedule that you can plan when to do things for yourself, like take a shower, make a phone call, or read the newspaper— at least some of the time. Of course, you're still exhausted because your days are busy and you're still feeding your baby at night. But you know how to care for your baby now. Being a parent may feel less overwhelming and more fun.

Listed on the next page are the milestones that most babies reach at this stage. If your baby can't do everything on the list, chances are that your baby's doctor will suggest that you test him again in another week or two. Babies born prematurely will reach these milestones later than average—at about the age they would have had they been born at full term.

As your baby reaches 3 months of age, you'll notice that his hands become his favorite toy.

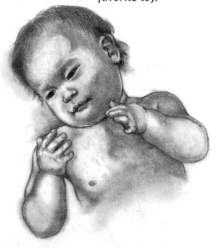

DEVELOPMENTAL MILESTONES

Age	Most Babies	Some Babies
1 month	Lift head slightly for a second or two when lying on stomach	Follow a toy or another object moved in an arc 6 inches away from face
	Hold head steady when held upright against parent's shoulder	Make several vowel sounds, like "ah-ah" or "ooo"
	Startle, cry, quiet, or respond in another way to a loud noise	Sleep for 3 or 4 hours at a time, and stay awake for 1 hour or longer
	React to parent's face or voice	Communicate with sounds in response to a parent's voice
	Quiet or calm down most of the time when being spoken to or held	
	Follow a familiar face (10 inches to 3 feet away) with their eyes	
2 months	Smile a real social smile (not just reflex)	Look at their hands
	Coo (sounds like "ooo-aah," or another vowel sound combination)	Squeal with pleasure
	Communicate with sounds in response to a parent's voice	Laugh
	Show interest in sights and sounds	Keep head steady when held upright or in a sitting position
	Show pleasure	
	Lift head to a 45-degree angle when lying on stomach	
	Follow object moved in an arc 6 inches from face	
3 months	Squeal with pleasure	Grasp a rattle
	Laugh	Look at a small object
	Keep head steady when held upright or in a sitting position	Turn head in direction of a rattling sound
	Bring their hands together	Hold head upright when pulled into a sitting position
	Look at their hands or feet	Roll over
	Lift heads to a 90-degree angle when lying on stomach	Raise body on hands when lying on stomach
		Follow an object that moves 180 degrees from one side of the face to the other
		Bear weight on legs when held in a standing position

As you review this list of milestones, remember that children who are within the normal range will have some areas in which they excel and others in which they are slower. Not achieving a particular milestone at the designated time is not always a matter of concern. If you and your child's doctor are concerned about your child's overall development or any of your child's developmental skills, such as language, hearing, vision, or motor skills, seek the help of the appropriate specialist. For more information, see *Developmental Problems*, Part 5.

Vision and Hearing

If you watch, you can't miss it. Your baby is seeing, hearing, and just plain noticing more each day.

Looking and Seeing

As your baby's brain grows and eye muscles strengthen, his visual world expands. As a newborn, he could see only about 12 inches away, but by about 3 months, he can see things in greater detail, up to several feet away. He can tell a smile from a frown, a square from an oval, his bottle from a vase. He'll look at your face as if he's studying it. He'll react when you stick out your tongue. He may enjoy looking at his face in a mirror.

Your baby's improved vision becomes apparent in various everyday circumstances. Show your baby a new toy, and watch his eyes widen—he knows he hasn't seen it before. Hold the new toy in one hand and a familiar toy in the other, and he'll probably spend more time looking at the new one. Because his eyes focus better now, he can shift his gaze from the mobile 2 feet above him to the teddy bear beside him and then to you at the door. With the ability to see at various depths, he can also watch things move. He can follow you with his eyes as you enter and exit the room.

You may notice that your baby's eyes still appear slightly crossed or that one eye turns out intermittently. This condition will gradually improve on its own during the first 3 months or so. If it is still apparent after 4 months, tell your child's doctor, who will determine whether your child has strabismus (see ***Amblyopia and/or Strabismus,*** Part 5) and needs referral to a pediatric ophthalmologist. The earlier this condition is treated, the better.

Hearing and Listening

Your baby is hearing new sounds every day and may even make sounds that seem to imitate your own. During these months, he'll gradually be able to hear clearly enough to react to your voice and even distinguish among the sounds that you make. Change your tone of voice, and watch his reaction. A certain tone might make your baby turn to look at you or smile. If he's been crying, it may make him stop.

By the time they're 2 or 3 months old, babies turn their heads, not just to a parent's voice, but toward an ever-greater variety of sounds, showing that they're more interested in and aware of these sounds and better able to locate where the sounds are coming from. Your baby may turn his head when the phone rings or when you stand behind him shaking a rattle.

Checking Your Baby's Vision and Hearing

Be sure to assess your baby's vision and hearing early on. Some vision problems that aren't corrected within the first several months of life may become permanent, because the brain areas responsible for vision may not develop properly. What's more, untreated hearing difficulties can interfere with your baby's ability to understand and develop language.

Here are some informal ways to test your baby's eyes and ears. These methods are not a substitute for professional hearing and vision screenings. If your baby does not respond to these methods, or if you suspect that he is having some hearing or visual difficulty, consult your child's doctor—or seek a referral to a pediatric ophthalmologist (for vision) or audiologist or otolaryngologist (for hearing). Here's what to do to check your child's vision:

1. To check your child's ability to see objects at a distance, stand about 2 to 6 feet in front of him. He should look at you and smile or react in some other way by the time he's 3 months old.

2. To test his ability to track a moving object, hold your face about 2 feet away and move your face from one side of your baby's head to the other. Your face is a better choice than, say, a toy, because babies are more likely to look at a face. His eyes should follow the movement of your face.

3. While you're performing these tests, notice whether his eyes move in conjunction with each other. If one wanders to the side, up or down, tell your child's doctor about this condition. Strabismus must be treated early for vision to develop normally in the affected eye.

Follow these steps to check your child's hearing:

1. Stand about 10 feet behind your baby, and clap your hands. He should startle or turn his head to look for the sound.

2. Standing in the same place, call to your baby to see if he reacts. He may not turn in your direction—babies under 6 months old sometimes have trouble figuring out where a sound is coming from. He'll probably look around randomly to try to locate the sound. But if he doesn't react at all, he may have a hearing problem.

3. Compare the results from this informal assessment with your everyday observations about how he responds to sound in general. Does he respond to sounds during the normal course of the day? Does he respond to loud sounds (not your voice)? If you have any concerns, ask your baby's doctor about a hearing test.

Growing and Moving

Already, those adorable newborn clothes no longer fit. Your baby is growing by leaps and bounds! If your child is formula-fed, his growth rate should stay the same as during the first month, about 1 to 1½ inches and 1 to 1½ pounds each month. But if your baby is breast-feeding, his growth rate may decrease after the second month. Standard growth charts don't accurately reflect the growth rate of breast-fed babies. Compared with the charts, breast-fed babies grow faster during the first 2 months and more slowly from the third through the twelfth month. But whether breast-fed or bottle-fed, by the time they reach 3 months, most babies look fairly chubby.

Remarkably, by the end of the first year, a child's head size reaches 90 percent of its adult size. Not only that, but by 12 months, a child's height is about 43 percent of what his adult height will be. By 2 years, many children reach about half their full adult height.

On the Move

In terms of motor development (movement), babies are often said to develop from the head down. Evidence of this top-down development can be seen in the way your baby moves. At 2 months old, when placed on his stomach, your child will probably lift his head for a few seconds, then put it down and lift it again. This exercise strengthens his back and neck muscles so that when he's 3 months old, he'll probably be able to hold his neck steady when you prop him against your shoulder. And several months later, he'll be able to keep his back straight enough to sit up.

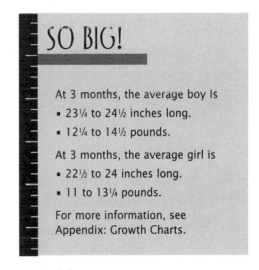

During these months, a baby's newborn reflexes gradually give way to more purposeful movements. For example, when your baby is placed on his back, his head no longer automatically turns to one side, but instead faces straight ahead. Now he can see more of his surroundings and focus on things that interest him. The ability to look forward is the foundation for other important achievements. In this position, your baby can more easily see both of his hands and put them in his mouth, helping him develop hand-eye coordination.

During this period, your baby will gradually relax his arms and legs. By the second month, his legs will be markedly straighter, and by the third month, he'll probably be able to extend them and flex them at will. When he gets excited, he may rotate his arms and legs like tiny windmills. If you look closely, you'll see that these movements are part of a master plan for crawling and walking. Put your baby on his stomach, and watch him rotate his arms and legs as if he's trying to crawl. Hold him upright with his feet on your lap, and watch him straighten his legs and try to stand.

His ability to reach and grab is awakening, too. The two tight fists of his newborn days are gradually unclenching. By the third month, he should be able to open and close his fingers at will. If you put a rattle in his palm, he may grasp it for a few seconds. If you dangle a toy above him while he's on his back, he may try to bat it with his arms and legs.

Stimulating Hand-Eye Coordination

Help your baby practice his hand-eye coordination by holding a small toy, or even your face, in front of him while he's lying down or sitting in your lap. Move the toy or your face from side to side and then back and forth in front of his face. By the end of the third month or soon after, he'll try to reach for the toy or you.

Communicating

When your baby's about 2 months old, he may begin to converse with you in a language that's part gesture and part wordless sounds. He knows that smiling makes you react, so he smiles at you a lot. Then you smile back. He smiles again. Then you

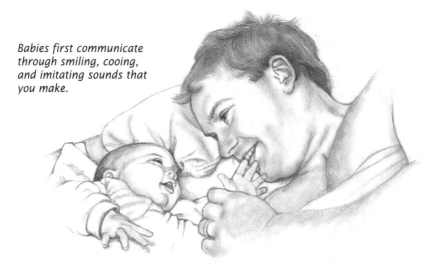

Babies first communicate through smiling, cooing, and imitating sounds that you make.

change the subject by sticking out your tongue. He sticks out his tongue. You open your eyes wide and say, "Oooo." He imitates your expression and your sound. And so it goes.

Your baby is imitating you and learning that one of the foundations of communication is taking turns. The more you talk to him, the more he's apt to repeat the sounds and rhythms of your speech. Because you say words with inflections, he coos with inflections, saying things like "aaa-ooo."

Learning Language

Babies don't learn language by imitation alone. One of the most remarkable characteristics of babies under 6 months old worldwide is that they all make the same array of cooing sounds, regardless of the language spoken in the home and regardless of whether the sounds they make actually occur in that language. What this suggests is that babies are born with the capacity to learn any language, and the one they actually learn becomes shaped over time as they interact with people speaking it to them. They'll learn this language as long as their parents talk to them. The more their parents talk to them and respond to them with words, the better and faster they will learn to understand and speak.

Body Language

Your baby is also learning to read your mood from the look on your face—an important part of social interaction between any two people. If he's smiling and you look sad, he may then look sad. He's expressing his moods with body language and facial expressions. He may convey happiness by widening his eyes and smiling and then maybe puckering his lips. If he's excited, he may open and close his hands, kick, and open his eyes wide. He's come a long way from his first weeks of life, when the most reliable cue that he was happy was that he wasn't crying.

Learning

Like all of us, babies learn by trial and error. A 1-month-old reaches in front of him and encounters something soft. It feels good, so he reaches again and again. By 2 months or so, babies bring their hands together, accidentally at first and then purposefully. They like the warmth and movement of their hands, so they keep touching them. As babies hold their hands and shake them in front of their face, their fingers somehow wind up in their mouth. They suck their fist or thumb. Enjoying how that feels, they keep putting their hands in their mouth and trying to suck on them. After doing something by accident, babies repeat the action on purpose. When they succeed, they realize that they can make things happen. It's a powerful feeling.

Building Memory

In addition to learning the basics of cause and effect, your baby is also building his memory. A 3-month-old can remember faces and events for about a week or longer. In one set of experiments, researchers tested infants' memories by watching how they behaved when one end of a string was tied to a mobile above their crib and the other was tied to their leg. The babies figured out that by kicking they could make the mobiles jerk and dance. When the string was untied and the mobiles were removed and then returned up to 10 days later, the babies remembered what to do to make the mobiles move.

Your baby's most vivid memories will be of daily rituals. When you bring him a bottle or hold him in a nursing position, he knows he's about to be fed. He may pucker or smack his lips with anticipation. When you hold him face to face, he knows that you're going to talk with him or play with him. He may smile, kick excitedly, and coo, as if preparing himself for a fun time.

Playtime

You can help your baby learn through play. Clap his hands together when he's sitting in your lap. Though he can't clap at will yet, getting him used to what clapping feels like will help him learn to do it on his own. You can also create games or songs that include a rhythmic pattern and then a change: Rock your baby back and forth saying, "Baby says hello. Baby says hello. Baby says hello." Then lift him up high saying, "Baby says good-bye!" Your baby will begin to anticipate the change at the end and laugh or even "ask" for more if your words don't change.

Try to gently pull your baby's arms to a sitting position. By 4 months, he should be able to hold his head almost in line with his body.

A FATHER'S STORY
Ben and Me

For the first month or so after Ben was born, I didn't really know what to do with him. Basically, he either slept or nursed. I was nothing special to him. When I picked him up, I could have been anybody. Now that he's 3 months old, Ben knows that I'm his daddy. When I walk in the room, he gets excited. He does this little dance lying in his crib or in his bouncy seat. He knows we're going to have fun. I tickle his belly, and he laughs. Then I put him on the rug to exercise. I move his legs as if he's riding a bike. I hold his hands, and he pulls himself up to sit. He looks at me as if to say, "Aren't you proud of what I just did?" And I tell him that I am.

He doesn't take his eyes off me. He adores me. It's the most incredible feeling to be loved by your kid. If something bad happens during the day, I think, "I'm Ben's dad." That means I'm the most important man in the world.

Socializing

Now that you and your baby are smiling at each other, interacting, and communicating with sounds and gestures, your baby is more responsive to your voice. You'll see the strongest evidence of this responsiveness when he's crying. To get him to stop crying when he was 1 month old, you probably needed to pat his back or pick him up much of the time. By 3 months, all it may take to stop him from crying is to talk or sing to him in a comforting voice.

A baby this age may act differently with his mother, his father, and others whom he knows less well. It may seem like a stereotype, but researchers have found that fathers really do tend to be somewhat rougher and more physically playful than mothers. When they come to get their babies from their cribs, fathers are likely to pick them up and do things like bounce them and tickle them. Mothers are more soothing. Their impulse is to wrap the babies in their arms and hug, kiss, and whisper to them. Both parents play with and nurture their babies, but mothers tend to do so with a softer voice and a gentler touch. Both methods are natural, normal ways of interacting, and babies benefit from them.

Babies at this age are delighted to be around people, be they parents or strangers. They're likely to smile at anyone who smiles at them. They're not scared of strangers, as they will be in several months. But they may put up their guard. At first the baby will smile or widen his eyes with interest in a new person. But then he's likely to look away or stare just beyond her, as if to limit the social encounter.

Caring for Your Baby

You've got the hang of it now. Feeding, bathing, and other baby-care details are probably becoming routine. But during these months, you'll need to adjust your routine to meet your baby's ever-changing needs, as well as his emerging likes and dislikes.

Feeding

Breast milk or iron-fortified formula is the only food your baby needs now. He's not ready for cereal or other solid foods, which, if introduced too early, can lead to allergies and interfere with growth, because babies this age cannot digest these foods fully. Neither is your baby ready for fruit juice. For one thing, juice doesn't contain any nutrients that he's not already getting from milk or formula. In addition, juice has lots of sugar. (See p. 131 for more discussion of juice.)

At 1 to 3 months old, your baby will need to be fed every 1 to 3 hours if breast-fed, and about every 3 to 4 hours if bottle-fed. At 1 month, he'll probably drink 3 to 4 ounces at each feeding, but by the time he's 3 months old, he may be hungry enough to consume 4 to 5 ounces. Overall he should not need more than 30 to 36 ounces of breast milk or formula per day.

Don't give your baby water in a bottle unless your doctor advises you to do so, for example, as a treatment for constipation. Most babies get the fluids they need from breast milk or formula. And plain water in large amounts can be harmful to babies under age 6 months.

Also, adding extra water to formula is not a good idea unless your baby's doctor directs it. Excess water dilutes the formula and may prevent your baby from getting the calories and nutrients he needs. Although formula is expensive, most states give financial assistance for it. Call your state public health department for assistance. Or contact the Women, Infants and Children Program (WIC), which supplies formula and food to women and children who qualify (see Appendix: Parent Resources, Medical/Financial Assistance).

QUESTIONS PARENTS ASK
Is My Baby Constipated?

Q: Sometimes several days go by without my 2-month-old's having a bowel movement. Is he constipated?

A: It's not unusual and not harmful for breast-fed babies over 1 month old to go a few days without a bowel movement. That's because breast milk, being the ideal food, is so completely absorbed that little waste is left after digestion. As long as your baby is growing at a normal rate, he's getting enough nourishment. Still, whether you feed your baby formula or breast milk, he will usually have at least one bowel movement every day or so. If he doesn't, or if his stools are hard, he might be constipated. Discuss this with your doctor (see **Constipation,** Part 5).

QUESTIONS PARENTS ASK

Spitting Up

Q: My baby girl spits up after almost every feeding. I wonder if she's getting enough food.

A: If your daughter frequently spits up after a meal, you may think she's losing important nutrients and calories. But this usually isn't the case. Most babies spit up occasionally, either shortly after they're picked up or right after a feeding or burping. The reason is that the valve at the top of the stomach, which is supposed to keep fluids from backing up, is still relatively weak. Some babies will spit up because they are being overfed. Young infants rarely need more than 4 or 5 ounces of milk in a single feeding. You should call the doctor, however, if your baby is spitting up large amounts or not just spitting up, but **vomiting** (see Part 5) forcefully, or if your baby is not gaining weight properly.

Unlike spitting up, vomiting is serious because it can dehydrate your baby. You can tell the difference between spitting up and vomiting because spit-up trickles out of the baby's mouth, and vomit shoots out and appears in greater quantities. Babies often cry after they vomit because their stomachs are upset, but they don't usually react after spitting up. If the vomiting lasts for only about a day or so and is accompanied by fever, the likely cause is a stomach flu. But if a baby vomits daily after most feedings, the cause may be **gastroesophageal reflux** (see Part 5), an exceptional weakness or malfunctioning of the valve at the top of the stomach. Check with your child's doctor.

If your baby spits up frequently, you can reduce the problem by keeping the baby propped up at a 30-degree angle during and after a meal. That way, gravity will help keep the meal where it belongs. Be sure to elevate your baby's whole body, not just the head and upper torso. Don't prop your baby up in a sitting position—bending at the waist can worsen reflux by putting pressure on the abdomen.

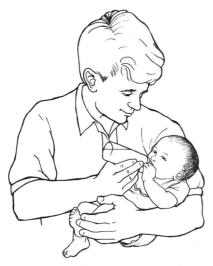

Propping your baby up at a 30-degree angle during feedings will help prevent him from spitting up.

Introducing Baby to Bottle

Many women, particularly those returning to work within several weeks after delivery, will need to introduce a bottle after breast-feeding is well established, before 4 to 6 weeks of age. The American Academy of Pediatrics recommends breast-feeding for at least 1 year, and many working mothers choose to follow that advice by expressing breast milk. If you plan to do this, start before you return to work by offering your baby 1 or 2 ounces of breast milk in a bottle. You don't have to do this every day, but you can give your baby a bottle a few times a week to get him used to it. Another option is to give your baby some breast milk or formula in an infant sipping cup. The baby won't take much, but it may help him get used to the idea of drinking from a source other than the breast.

Despite your efforts, your breast-fed infant may refuse to take a bottle. The longer you wait, the more likely this will happen. His reluctance is understandable, given that he's used to the loving experience of being fed while cuddling with mom. But you can cuddle a bottle-fed baby during feeding times as well. Here are some tips to help your baby make the transition from breast to bottle:

■ *Offer your baby expressed breast milk at first.* Some babies don't like the taste of formula once they're used to breast milk.

■ *Mix formula with breast milk* if you're planning to use formula eventually. This will help your baby get used to the taste.

■ *Use a long nipple* (either conventional or orthodontic). Some mothers have more success with this kind than the short nipples, even if short ones appear more "natural."

■ *Have someone other than the mother give the baby his bottle at first.* Many babies associate their mothers with the pleasure of nursing so strongly that they refuse to take a bottle from them. You may even have to leave the house while someone else tries bottle-feeding the baby.

■ *Hold your baby in a position other than the "nursing position."* Try holding him so that he faces away from you with his head against your chest. Walking with him as you feed him the bottle in this position may further distract him from the breast.

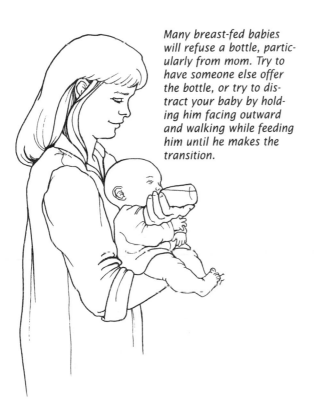

Many breast-fed babies will refuse a bottle, particularly from mom. Try to have someone else offer the bottle, or try to distract your baby by holding him facing outward and walking while feeding him until he makes the transition.

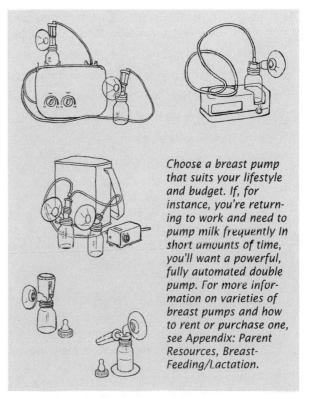

Choose a breast pump that suits your lifestyle and budget. If, for instance, you're returning to work and need to pump milk frequently in short amounts of time, you'll want a powerful, fully automated double pump. For more information on varieties of breast pumps and how to rent or purchase one, see Appendix: Parent Resources, Breast-Feeding/Lactation.

Crying

If your baby had a predictable fussy period each day when he was 1 month old, chances are he still has it, and it's gotten worse. But rest assured, it will likely get better soon. Every baby is different, but the amount of time that babies cry peaks when they're about 6 weeks old, at up to 3 hours a day. After that, things gradually improve. By the time babies are 3 months old, their crying has usually decreased to about an hour a day. Of course, this crying doesn't happen all at one time during the day, and your baby may seem to be crying much more than he did when he was younger.

Coping with Crying

Your baby may be crying more now than he was a month ago, but you now have the advantage of experience. Use your understanding of his body language, facial expressions, and tones of voice to figure out why he's crying, and respond in ways that have worked before. Check to see whether he is hungry or uncomfortable or needs a diaper change or some playtime. For information on *colic,* see Part 5.

TOUCHPOINT

Responding to Fussiness

With experience, parents gain confidence in learning to quiet a crying baby. Watch your baby's response carefully while trying the following techniques:

▌ Talk to your baby in a soothing voice.

▌ Rub your baby's back or stomach gently and rhythmically.

▌ Hold your baby in different positions.

▌ Walk with your baby, taking gentle, rhythmic strides.

▌ Give your baby something to suck.

▌ Dim the lights, turn off the television, and close the door to create a quiet, soothing environment.

▌ Rock your baby in a cradle or infant seat, or in your arms in a rocking chair or glider.

▌ Create "white noise" with the sound of a washing machine or vacuum cleaner.

Source: Touchpoints Project (see p. 81).

Sleeping

Much to your relief, your baby's sleep schedule is probably becoming more like yours. He's sleeping for longer stretches at night than during the day. Though some babies sleep through the night by the time they're 3 months old, most still need at least one nighttime feeding. By the time your baby is about 2½ months old, you can encourage him to sleep for longer stretches at night with the following techniques:

■ *Keep nighttime feedings brief.* Make nighttime feedings and diaper changes as brief and businesslike as possible. Save the socializing and play for daytime.

■ *Space out the times between feedings.* Space them gradually by about 30 minutes a night.

■ *Hold or rock your baby.* If necessary, do this before nursing or giving him a bottle each night until your baby is fed only once every 4 to 6 hours. In addition, make sure that your baby is eating enough during the day.

■ *Decrease daytime sleep.* If your baby is still sleeping more during the day than at night, decrease the length and frequency of his daytime sleep periods. Rather than put him right back in his crib after a feeding, play with him for as long as he can stay alert. If he's regularly sleeping for more than 3 hours at a time during the day, consider waking him up earlier.

■ *Feed your baby before you go to sleep.* If your baby goes to sleep several hours before you do, try scheduling a feeding just before you go to bed to increase the length of time he sleeps before he needs his first middle-of-the-night feeding.

■ *Don't rush in.* When your baby cries in the middle of the night, make sure that he's awake before going to him. Babies often cry in their sleep or wake briefly from a dream. Rushing in too quickly may interfere with their sleep or their ability to fall back to sleep by themselves.

■ *Don't let him cry for long.* When your baby does wake up fully, always go to him. Don't let him cry himself back to sleep. You have nothing to gain from doing so. You can't "train" a baby at this age to sleep through the night yet, and you may be denying him a feeding, and possibly a diaper change, that he needs. Later, when he's a few months older, you can take steps to help your baby learn to fall back to sleep on his own.

Where Should Your Baby Sleep?

For many years, parents were strongly advised not to let their babies sleep in their beds with them. The prevailing view was that the practice was fundamentally unhealthy for the family: It interfered with the parents' sexual relationship and prevented babies from learning how to fall asleep on their own.

But many parents want to have their baby in bed with them. This desire, or necessity, is more common in some cultures than in others. But for some parents, it's a practical matter. If the baby is breast-feeding, a mother may find it convenient to have the baby in bed with her. In fact, bed-sharing tends to encourage breast-feeding, according to a recent statement from the American Academy of Pediatrics. Some parents feel that having their baby sleep between them helps them bond as a family. So "co-sleeping" is not a problem as long as it is what both parents want, it is working well, and the family is happy.

There is no evidence that bed-sharing reduces the risk of sudden infant death syndrome (SIDS). In fact, bed-sharing under certain circumstances, such as when the baby is placed on top of a soft surface like a quilt or a blanket to sleep, may actually increase the risk of SIDS (see ***Sudden Infant Death Syndrome,*** Part 5). If you choose to have your baby sleep in your bed, follow these recommendations from the American Academy of Pediatrics:

▌ Have your baby sleep on his back unless your baby's doctor tells you otherwise.

▌ Avoid placing soft surfaces, such as quilts, blankets, pillows, or comforters, under your baby.

▌ Do not smoke or use alcohol or any drugs that may prevent you from waking.

One thing to think about if your baby is sleeping with you now is when you want him to move to his own crib or bed. Make a plan. Don't just wait to see what happens. Moving your baby out of your bed before he's 9 months old is easiest. After this age, many babies have trouble separating from their parents, whether they've been sleeping together or not. But if your baby is still in your room when he's 9 months old, don't think that you've missed your opportunity to make the transition. Babies can learn to sleep on their own at any age.

Is Your Child Getting Enough Sleep?

Do you ever wonder if your child is getting enough sleep? Or whether he is sleeping too much? As they age, infants and children gradually require less sleep. Newborns sleep up to 16 hours a day. But they don't sleep for long stretches. Instead they sleep on and off throughout the day and night. By 4 to 6 months, an infant will be sleeping longer stretches at night and napping about three times during the day, for a total of 12 to 14 hours. After 12 months, however, most children nap only once a day and

HOW MUCH SLEEP DOES THE TYPICAL CHILD NEED?

Age	Total Sleep Hours	Number of Naps
0–1 month	15–16	4–5
2–3 months	14½–15½	3–4
4–6 months	12–14	3
7–12 months	11½–12½	2–3
1–3 years	11–12	1
4–6 years	10–11¼	0
7–9 years	9½–10¾	0
10–13 years	9–10½	0
14–18 years	8½–9¾	0

Source: Richard A. Ferber, M.D., clinical director, Center for Pediatric Sleep Disorders, Children's Hospital Boston.

sleep a total of 11 to 12 hours. And by their late preschool years, most children stop napping altogether, sleeping only 10 to 11 hours—leaving you less time to do all those things you used to do when your child was sleeping.

Keeping Your Baby Healthy

You are the most important person on your child's health care team. You must watch for signs of illness, take your baby for regular checkups and immunizations, and care for your baby when illness occurs. So work with your child's doctor or nurse practitioner to give your baby the best possible health care in his first few months.

Checkups

You'll be seeing your baby's doctor once a month at this age. Your baby should have a checkup before the end of his first month and again when he's 2 months old. During each visit, the doctor or nurse will measure your baby's length, weight, and head circumference and plot them on a growth curve to determine how well he is growing. Your doctor will make sure that your child gains about 20 to 30 grams a day (or about ¾ ounce a day) during this phase of rapid growth. For information on percentiles, see page 57.

The doctor will thoroughly examine your baby to make sure that his appearance and movements are normal.

Immunizations

Vaccines give a child's immune system exposure to a common virus, killed bacterium, or some of an organism's identifying protein or carbohydrate, so that when the child is exposed to the actual disease, he can fight the infection more easily. Each state requires that children receive certain vaccines before they attend day care, school, or camp. But waiting until a child is ready to enter school is too late, because many diseases are more prevalent or more dangerous in infants and young children.

Without question, vaccines save lives. Polio, measles, whooping cough, diphtheria, and tetanus once killed hundreds of thousands of people a year, but these diseases have been nearly eliminated (only smallpox has been completely eliminated), thanks to immunization. Immunizing a child against illnesses that are now uncommon may seem unnecessary, but the shots are needed because these illnesses can return if widespread immunization stops. Measles had been almost vaccinated out of existence by 1983, when it hit a record low of 1,497 cases in the United States. But a measles epidemic occurred between 1989 and 1991, with 55,000 cases and 132 reported deaths. The main reason for the epidemic was an increase in the number of children who weren't vaccinated on time, or at all.

Not all vaccines are for deadly illnesses. Some of these illnesses, such as rubella, icken pox, and mumps, are not life-threatening to most children, but they are hly contagious. They can also be uncomfortable for a child and inconvenient for

the parent who needs to miss work to care for a sick child. They may also have serious complications, such as hearing loss or sterility with mumps or hearing loss or birth defects with rubella, that can be avoided if the disease is prevented.

All routine childhood vaccines are now given in the form of shots. The oral version of the polio vaccine is no longer recommended (see p. 114). Though more vaccines exist today than ever before, children will soon be getting fewer injections, because many vaccines are now being combined into single shots. Combining vaccines is considered just as safe and effective as giving them separately, which used to be the norm.

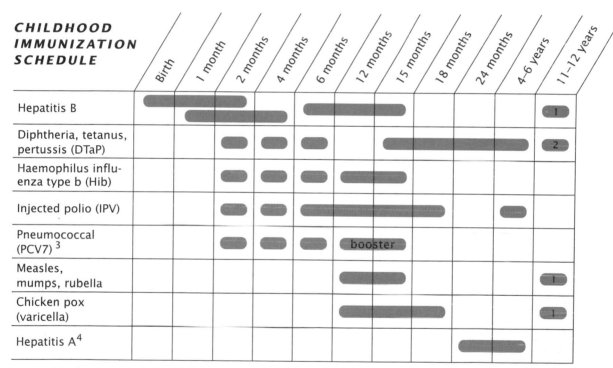

CHILDHOOD IMMUNIZATION SCHEDULE

	Birth	1 month	2 months	4 months	6 months	12 months	15 months	18 months	24 months	4–6 years	11–12 years
Hepatitis B	███	███			███						1
Diphtheria, tetanus, pertussis (DTaP)			██	██	██	████					2
Haemophilus influenza type b (Hib)			██	██	██						
Injected polio (IPV)			██	██	████					██	
Pneumococcal (PCV7) [3]			██	██	██	booster					
Measles, mumps, rubella						██					1
Chicken pox (varicella)						████					1
Hepatitis A [4]									████		

Approved by the American Academy of Pediatrics, the Advisory Committee on Immunization Practice, and the American Academy of Family Physicians.

Note: A band represents the range of time during which each immunization should be given once.

1. Vaccines should be administered to children at this age if needed. For example, Hep B is given to children 11 to 12 years old who were not previously vaccinated.
2. Tetanus and diphtheria only.
3. Catch-up immunizations for children who haven't received this new vaccine include two doses 8 weeks apart f̶ dren 7 to 12 months old, with a booster at 12 to 15 months (at least 6 weeks after the second dose); and ↗ 8 weeks apart for children 12 to 23 months of age, with no booster required. Children 12 to 23 months previously immunized should receive two doses at least 6 to 8 weeks apart. The vaccine is also reco↗ children 24 to 59 months of age who are at especially high risk for invasive pneumococcal infecti↗ includes children with *sickle-cell disease* (see Part 5), *HIV/AIDS Infection* (see Part 5), and other↗ immune systems.
4. Hepatitis A is administered only in select areas of the United States.

Are Vaccines Safe?

Rest assured, the vaccines in the United States have undergone rigorous safety testing by the federal Food and Drug Administration. They are safe. Some offer complete protection against an illness, whereas others protect most immunized children from getting sick and the rest from getting as sick as they would have otherwise. Some vaccines require more than one dosage to take effect, which is why they're given in a series of two or more. For some vaccines, booster shots are needed every decade or so to strengthen the immune system defenses.

Vaccines can cause side effects. Most are minor, such as fever or soreness or swelling at the injection site. But in rare cases, reactions can be severe. New vaccines reduce or eliminate the chance of these severe side effects. On balance, the benefits of vaccines far outweigh the risks.

PREVENTABLE CHILDHOOD DISEASES

Infection	Description	How the Vaccine Helps
Hepatitis B	A liver disease caused by a virus. Symptoms include jaundice, joint pain, and abdominal pain. Illness is spread by infected blood through cuts, blood transfusions, intravenous drug use, and sexual intercourse. An infected mother can pass the disease to her baby during birth.	Prevents transmission of the disease through exposure to the hepatitis B virus and also prevents the chronic consequences of the disease, including cirrhosis and liver cancer. Among women of childbearing age, the vaccine prevents transmission of the disease from mother to child during pregnancy and later, and protects against exposure to the disease through sexual contact or intravenous drug use.
Haemophilus influenza type b	An illness in which bacteria that infect the throat can cause two other, life-threatening illnesses: meningitis, an infection of tissues covering the brain and spinal cord, and epiglottitis, an inflammation of the epiglottis (the valve over the voice box). Hearing loss, mental retardation, and seizures are long-term complications. Although infants and young children have the highest risk of contracting these infections, the infections can occur at any age.	Reduces the risk of infection by up to 99 percent. Has substantially reduced the incidence of meningitis.
Diphtheria	A serious bacterial respiratory infection that causes a cough and difficulty breathing. It can cause life-threatening airway obstruction and respiratory failure.	The disease has been eradicated in the U.S. because of immunization. But it is still common in some parts of the world because of inadequate immunization.

Continued on p. 112

■■■ *PREVENTABLE CHILDHOOD DISEASES* (continued)

Infection	Description	How the Vaccine Helps
Pertussis (whooping cough)	Bacterial infection of the respiratory tract that can come and go for many months, causing serious breathing problems and pneumonia, leading to death, particularly in an infant up to 4 months old. The main symptom is a severe cough that may have a whooping sound when the child inhales. Pertussis is often transmitted to children by mildly infected adults who don't know they have it.	The DTaP is up to 80 percent effective in preventing infections. Booster shots are needed between 4 and 6 years of age.
Tetanus	This bacterial infection releases a toxin that affects the nerves. The bacteria, which live in soil that contains animal feces, can enter the body through a wound, especially a puncture wound or a burn. Symptoms include muscle stiffness and spasms, including lockjaw. Tetanus can be fatal, especially in young children.	Highly effective. The vaccine has nearly eradicated tetanus in the United States. Boosters are required both between 4 and 6 years and 11 and 12 years.
Polio	A highly contagious viral infection of the central nervous system (brain and spinal cord) that can cause temporary or permanent paralysis.	The polio vaccine has eliminated the disease in the United States. But the disease is still present in other parts of the world.
Pneumococcal disease	Invasive pneumococcal disease includes bacteremia, an infection of the bloodstream, and bacterial *meningitis* (see Part 5), a potentially fatal infection of the brain and spinal cord. The pneumococcus bacterium is also a major cause of bacterial *pneumonia* (see Part 5), *sinusitis* (see Part 5), and ear infections (see *Earache/Ear Infection,* Part 5).	The vaccine is more than 90 percent effective in infants after three doses. In clinical trials, the vaccine decreased invasive infections by more than 93 percent and pneumonia by 73 percent. It was associated with a 7 percent decrease in middle ear infections (see *Earache/Ear Infection,* Part 5) and a 20 percent decrease in ear tube placement.
Measles	A viral infection characterized initially by a fever and a hacking cough, as well as cold-like symptoms and a bright red rash that spreads across the body. Measles can be fatal, especially in previously ill children or those whose immune systems are already depressed by other health problems. Measles can cause encephalitis, hearing loss, and retardation.	The vaccine is 90 to 98 percent effective and will prevent infection even after someone has been exposed to the virus.

■ PREVENTABLE CHILDHOOD DISEASES *(continued)*

Infection	Description	How the Vaccine Helps
Mumps	A very contagious viral infection that causes fever, headache, loss of appetite, and painful swelling of the salivary glands below the ears and sometimes also those under the jaw. Uncomfortable but usually not serious, mumps can cause encephalitis or, after puberty, orchitis, an inflammation of the testicles.	The vaccine is 90 to 98 percent effective.
Rubella (German measles)	A mild viral disease that often causes an itchy red rash on the face and behind the ears, which spreads down the body. About 25 percent of cases cause no symptoms. Rubella is most dangerous during pregnancy, when it can cause birth defects or miscarriage. Before the advent of the vaccine, rubella during pregnancy was a leading cause of congenital deafness, mental retardation, congenital heart disease, and cataracts.	Immunization is 90 to 98 percent effective and offers lifelong immunity.
Chicken pox (varicella)	A viral infection that can cause fever and flulike symptoms followed by a rash. The rash begins as red spots, which quickly become raised and fluid-filled. These gradually crust over and heal. Complications include skin infection or, rarely, *pneumonia* (see Part 5) or encephalitis.	Immunization is 70 to 90 percent effective. Those who get chicken pox after immunization have mild cases.
Hepatitis A	A viral infection of the liver caused by the hepatitis A virus. Some children display no symptoms, while others exhibit fever, tiredness, loss of appetite, nausea, joint pain, abdominal discomfort, and jaundice. Most children make a full recovery after a few months.	Immunization is 97 to 100 percent effective 1 month after it is given. It is recommended for select groups considered at risk for contracting the disease, including children living in communities that have high rates of hepatitis A. Check with your doctor.

Immunization Side Effects

Most vaccines cause minor side effects, including slight fevers, soreness, and occasional allergic reactions. Some are due to the viruses or bacteria they contain, while others are allergic reactions to inactive ingredients, like proteins, that are used to make the vaccine. What follows is a list of the most common side effects. Call your doctor if the reaction seems severe or the child is experiencing pain, a fever over 100.2°F, or lethargy.

DTaP   DTaP is now the most commonly used vaccine to prevent diphtheria, tetanus, and pertussis. Side effects are soreness or redness at the injection site, drowsiness, and irritability the day following immunization. These side effects are less common than those associated with the DTP vaccine, which preceded DTaP as the vaccine of choice, but is no longer recommended.

There is an ongoing controversy in the role of the pertussis part of the DTP and DTaP vaccines in causing serious neurological damage and seizures. The problem, however, is exceedingly rare and the connection is unproven.

Hib   The most common side effects of the Hib vaccine are pain at the injection site in up to 29 percent of babies and fever in up to 6 percent.

IPV   Side effects of IPV are pain at the injection site, redness, and warmth. No other complications have been noted. IPV replaces the oral polio vaccine (OPV). OPV is no longer recommended, because in rare instances (about 1 case for every 2.4 million doses administered), the vaccine, which is made from a weakened live polio virus, caused vaccine-associated polio paralysis. IPV is made from an inactive form of the virus.

OPV may still be used in special circumstances. It may, for example, be given to a child of parents who do not accept the number of injections recommended. It may also be given to children who will be traveling to areas where polio is widespread, since, in this circumstance, the vaccine is more effective than IPV.

PCV7 (Pneumococcal)   Reactions to the PCV7 immunization are mild and may include localized redness or swelling at the injection site, irritability, drowsiness, low fever, and decreased appetite.

MMR   From 5 to 15 percent of 1-year-olds may develop a high fever (103°F or higher) from 5 to 12 days after immunization. About 5 percent develop mild rashes. More serious reactions can occur in babies who have severe allergies to eggs or to the antibiotic neomycin, because both are ingredients in the vaccine.

Varicella   Reactions are mild. Occasionally, small chicken-pox lesions will appear a week or two after the vaccine is given.

Hep A   The most frequently reported side effect of the hepatitis A injection is soreness at the injection site.

Easing Immunization Pain

Chances are, your baby will cry when he gets a shot. You probably won't be able to prevent him from crying, but you can comfort him and relieve his pain. First of all, hold him when he gets the shot if your doctor allows it. He'll feel better being in your arms than lying on an examining table. Bringing along a favorite toy or security blanket may also help. If your baby gets the DTaP shot, give him a dose of acetaminophen (available over the counter) before or immediately afterward. This vaccine is more likely than the others to cause discomfort. There are several ways that a doctor can help make immunization shots less painful. One method is for the doctor to put pressure on or even vibrate the skin near the injection site. The pressure interferes or competes with the pain of the shot, thereby reducing the sensation of pain. Another method is a painkilling cream that you can apply to your child's arm about one hour before the shot. For pain and swelling at the site of the shot afterward, apply a warm washcloth to relieve the discomfort.

QUESTIONS PARENTS ASK
Vaccinating a Sick Child

Q: My baby has a bad cold. Is it safe for him to get an immunization while he is sick?

A: Colds, respiratory allergies, mild stomach flu, and even low-grade fever don't reduce the effectiveness of any vaccine. Nor do such minor illnesses increase the likelihood that your baby will have an adverse reaction. But if your child has a more severe illness, such as a high fever, your doctor might postpone a scheduled immunization until your child is better. Side effects from the shot, like fever or drowsiness, could make your baby feel worse. Also, you may have trouble telling the difference between the symptoms of your child's illness and the signs of potential adverse reactions to the immunization, which should be reported to your doctor. So if your child is already sick, ask your doctor whether he should receive a shot. The doctor will take several factors into account, such as the side effects of the immunizations in question (some immunizations, such as those for MMR, Hib, and hepatitis B, are less likely than others to cause side effects), whether your child is behind on his immunization schedule, and how common a particular disease is in the community.

Your Baby's First Illness

At some point during these months, there's a fair chance that your baby will get his first cold or some other minor illness. Initially, you may not realize that he's sick. But signs that something is wrong include unusual crankiness, diarrhea, and fever. Here are some infections that often occur early on, how to spot them, and what to do. For more information about treating common childhood illness, see Part 5, Guide to Common Childhood Illness, Injury, and Conditions.

Colds

Babies may have the same cold symptoms as do adults: sneezing, runny nose, and coughing. They also sometimes run a low-grade fever of about 100°F. Babies of this age often have trouble breathing through their noses even when they're well, but having a cold increases the problem. They may have trouble sleeping because of their nasal congestion. And they may have a hard time nursing or taking a bottle, because they can't suck and breathe at the same time.

To help relieve your baby's congestion while he's sleeping, put a humidifier in his room. Raise his head slightly by propping up the mattress on one end of the crib or bassinet or elevating one end of the crib. Do this by stuffing a blanket or book underneath the mattress. Don't give your baby a pillow, because it can cause suffocation. See *Colds/Flu,* Part 5. Call your baby's doctor if you have any concerns.

Diarrhea

The first signs of a viral infection are likely to be increased spitting up accompanied by diarrhea. Your baby may also have a low-grade fever. Diarrhea is usually caused by an intestinal virus that will go away on its own. Still, you should call the doctor to rule out a more serious illness. If your baby has a virus with mild symptoms, the doctor will probably recommend that you do nothing except make sure your baby has plenty of formula or breast milk to prevent dehydration. But if your baby drinks cow's milk formula and seems bloated or gassy afterward, the doctor might recommend temporarily using an oral rehydration solution (not water or juice). Don't give your baby antidiarrheal medicine. Upsetting as vomiting and diarrhea are, they are the body's way of getting rid of the infection. See *Diarrhea,* Part 5.

Rashes

After the first month, some infants develop a dry, scaly, itchy rash that appears as red patches on the face, in the folds of the elbows, and behind the knees. The rash is eczema, also called *atopic dermatitis.* Some babies get it because they have very sensitive skin. Others get it from repeated contact with a substance that can cause irritation or allergy, like wool or other rough fabrics or perfumed soaps. You can control eczema by limiting your baby's baths to three times a week, using a mild soap, and dressing him in cotton clothes. Avoid those foods, fabrics, soaps, or shampoos that seem to cause a rash. The rash isn't harmful, but mention it to your child's doctor because she might want to prescribe some cream or ointment to treat it. Call the doctor if the rash has signs of infection, like blisters or pus. See *Rashes,* Part 5.

Keeping Your Baby Safe

Now that your baby is kicking and reaching and possibly even trying to roll over, he's also more likely to have an accident. You can protect your child by learning about safety precautions and procedures (see Chapter 11, Preparing for and Handling Emergencies) and by taking various measures around the home.

Ten Steps to Infant Safety

Prevent falls and other mishaps by taking the following precautions:

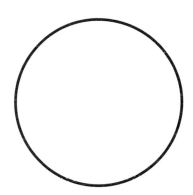

1. *Changing table:* Never leave your baby alone on a changing table, not even just to dash across the room to get a diaper. Keep your supplies within reach, and either stand in front of the changing table to block him from falling or keep a hand on him.

2. *Beds and couches:* Don't leave your child alone on any surface above the floor. See page 26 for information on crib safety.

3. *Infant seat:* Always strap your baby in. Don't put the infant seat on a table unless you're there to guard it. An active baby can make the seat tip over and fall off.

4. *Infant swing:* Strap your baby in so that he won't fall out. Never leave him unattended in a swing.

5. *Mobiles:* If you have one, put it high enough that your baby can't touch it. A curious 3-month-old practicing his hand-eye coordination can get tangled in a mobile and risk strangulation.

6. *Small objects:* Keep anything $1^3/4$ inches or less in diameter out of your baby's reach, because he could choke if he tries to put it in his mouth. That includes loose change, rings, hair ornaments, barrettes and hair beads, nuts, grapes, and small toys belonging to older siblings.

7. *Baby powder:* Avoid using any kind of powder (including baby powder) with your infant. Breathing powder can lead to respiratory problems. An infant may grab the bottle of powder and turn it over on his head, causing him to breathe in large amounts and suffocate.

8. *Water:* Always keep one hand on your baby while he is in the bath or in any water.

9. *Pets and siblings:* Never leave your baby unsupervised with pets or siblings.

10. *Hot stuff:* Don't hold your baby while drinking hot drinks or while cooking over a hot stove or oven.

Measure small toys: Toys should have a diameter greater than $1^3/4$ inches. Hold a toy up to this circle. Unless it covers the circle, it should be thrown away or stored in a safe place until your child is at least 3 years old.

SAFETY ALERT
First Aid Courses

Take a course in emergency first aid at a local hospital or through a health or parenting organization. Such a course should include such lifesaving techniques as cardiopulmonary resuscitation (CPR), maneuvers to open an obstructed airway in infants, and how to stop external bleeding. For more information on first aid, see Chapter 11, Preparing for and Handling Emergencies.

YOUR BABY AT 4 TO 7 MONTHS

In many ways, this is an exhilarating stage of life. Your baby's personality is emerging. You may find your baby more fun to play with now. She can do more, and she reacts to just about everything you do. Children at this stage tend to sleep longer at night, and that makes everyone feel better. By the end of this period, your baby will probably be sitting up. Many babies can get around by crawling or creeping now. Don't blink. Your baby is changing fast.

Growth and Development

The development milestones that your baby reaches during these months will be grand gestures, the kind that will send you running for the camera—so keep it ready! Most babies can now reach out and grab toys, and many can crawl across the room to get them. During this period, they eat their first real solid food and might get their first tooth. Babies in this age range usually begin to babble in sounds that resemble words. Many also begin to recognize some spoken words, like their names. Just about every week something new and exciting happens.

Chances are that your baby's attention span is now long enough that she can concentrate when you read her a book. Instead of merely biting the pages, she'll begin to look at them, and when you point to particular pictures, she'll follow your finger with her eyes. The same is true when you go for a walk. If you point to the red car or the noisy helicopter, she may well look at them. And you might sense that the nature of your relationship is shifting. She's no longer just a baby. She's a pal.

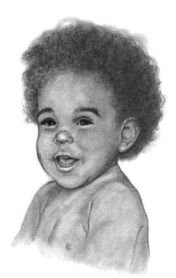

Sometime during the first year, usually the second half, your baby's first tooth will emerge.

Vision and Hearing

Suddenly, "seeing the world through a baby's eyes" is more than just an expression. Babies are now absorbed in observing and listening to the people and things around them.

Looking and Seeing

It's probably no coincidence that at the same time that your baby is learning to move around, she's also becoming interested in the objects she sees moving around her. By the time infants are 5 months old, they love watching their parents and older siblings walking around a room. Their heads often turn from side to side to keep track of darting brothers and sisters, as if they're watching a Ping-Pong match.

Just as babies enjoy watching things that move, they are also drawn to certain colors. If you have an activity bar across the infant seat or stroller, you may notice that your baby reaches for

DEVELOPMENTAL MILESTONES

Age	Most Babies	Some Babies
4 months	Hold head up and keep it steady when on stomach	Sleep for at least 6 hours at a time
	Raise body on hands when lying on stomach	Imitate the sounds of some words
	Roll over from front to back	Turn to a voice
	Hold own hands	Sit alone
	Grasp rattle	Grab feet with hands
	Bear weight on legs when held in a standing position	Look for a fallen spoon
	Reach for and bat at toys	
	Look at and may react to a mobile	
	Recognize parent's voice and touch	
	Smile at parent's approach or mimic parent's expression	
	Comfort themselves (by sucking the thumb or falling asleep without the breast or bottle)	
5 months	Reach for a toy	Bring food to mouth with hand
	Look at a raisin or another small object	Imitate some sounds
	Turn head in direction of a rattling sound	
	Hold head upright when pulled into a sitting position	
6 months	Bring food to mouth with hand	Bang two blocks together
	Imitate some sounds	Pick up a small object using raking motion with fingers
	Turn to a voice	Say "mama" or "dada" without meaning mommy and daddy
	Pass a block from one hand to another	
	Make buzzing or razzing noise	Sit without support
	Get their first tooth	
7 months	Stand when held in place	Stand while holding onto something
	Take two blocks or other small objects	Use thumb and finger to pick up small object (pincer grasp)
	Pick up a small object using raking motion with fingers	Play patty-cake
	Look for a toy that has dropped out of sight	Wave good-bye
	Respond to each parent in unique ways	Begin to show stranger awareness
	Say "mama" or "dada" without meaning mommy or daddy	

As you review this list of milestones, remember that children who are within the normal range will have some areas in which they excel and others in which they are slower. Not achieving a particular milestone at the designated time is not always a matter of concern. If you and your child's doctor are concerned about your child's overall development or any of your child's developmental skills, such as language, hearing, vision, or motor skills, seek the help of the appropriate specialist. For more information, see *Developmental Problems*, Part 5.

the red or the blue toy more often than the yellow one. Infants this age might like red and blue best. At the least, it means that they can tell these colors apart.

Checking Your Baby's Vision

You can informally test your baby's vision by showing her interesting pictures or objects of different colors and shapes held about 2 or 3 feet away. She should show special interest when she sees something new. If she doesn't, she may not be seeing as well as she should; be sure to tell your doctor.

Other indications that your child is seeing well include these two signs:

▌ An ability to reach for and grasp objects that she sees

▌ An ability to distinguish strangers from family members without hearing their voices

Hearing and Listening

Your baby's hearing is becoming sharper. She knows her parents by their voices. In fact, a baby can hear the difference between a man's voice and a woman's voice before she can tell the difference between their faces.

Does your child turn to look at you when you speak to her? Does she respond to your speech with her own sounds? These are good indications that she hears you. Talking to your baby is crucial at this age. This is when babies are taking in everything they hear to help in language development later. Hearing other sounds, like music, will help, too, because it enriches the sound range that your child can recognize and make.

Growing and Moving

"Is your baby rolling over yet?"
"My sister's baby is crawling."
"Mine is sitting up."
"Mine is standing."

The playground Olympics are on. By 4 months many babies are rolling over, and by 6 months many are crawling. Naturally, their proud parents want to spread the news. But some babies aren't moving around much at all, and their parents are getting anxious. Is there something wrong?

Probably not. Though babies progress at a fairly similar pace during the first month or two, now they are progressing in different areas at different rates. Some babies are more active than others by nature. There's a wide range of normal. Some babies never crawl. Some babies start rolling over as early as 2 months old, whereas others don't do it until they're 4 to 5 months old. Not only do children have different strengths and weaknesses, they also progress in fits and starts. A baby a little ahead in motor skills may lag a bit behind on language. Your baby may make big strides one week and then settle in for a few weeks or months when nothing seems to change.

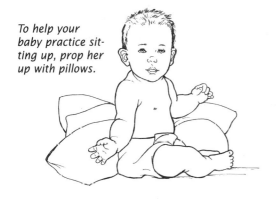

To help your baby practice sitting up, prop her up with pillows.

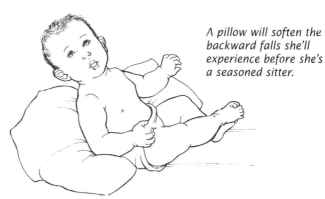

A pillow will soften the backward falls she'll experience before she's a seasoned sitter.

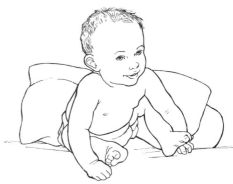

Once she gets the hang of it, she'll learn to lean forward and use her hands for stability.

More important than rolling over or crawling is the baby's ability to keep her head steady when held in a sitting position, something virtually all 4-month-olds can do. It may be less exciting, but it is a more crucial building block in gross motor development. A baby must keep her head steady in order to sit up. She must sit up before she can stand. And, of course, she must stand before she can walk.

A baby as young as 6 months old may be able to sit by herself if placed in a sitting position. But her back will be rounded, and she'll support herself with her hands, looking something like a tripod. By the time she's 7 months, she'll probably be able to sit up straight on her own. But if she keels over, she might not be able to return to a sitting position. At 7 months old, some babies begin pulling themselves up to a standing position while holding onto something. They often do this in their crib, starting out on their hands and knees, and then gradually pulling themselves up to stand while grasping the bars.

Using Hands

Your baby is also making great strides in working with her hands (fine motor development). At 4 months old, most babies can grasp a rattle or some other small toy. They hold it between their thumb and their other four fingers, as if they're wearing mittens. Their fine motor

SO BIG!

At 7 months, the average boy is
- 26¼ to 27¾ inches long.
- 17 to 20 pounds.

At 7 months, the average girl is
- 25½ to 27 inches long.
- 15½ to 18¼ pounds.

For more information, see Appendix: Growth Charts.

skills are not refined enough for them to use only the thumb and index finger for grasping. To pick up a small object, like a raisin, babies use their four fingertips to rake it into their palm and then scoop it up. Be careful: Small objects like raisins, beads, and buttons can be choking hazards.

Everything in the Mouth

Aside from her growing brain, your baby's major learning center is her mouth. Now that her hand-eye coordination is good enough for her to put objects in her mouth, she keeps on doing it. By sucking and biting down on rattles, soft blocks, stuffed animals, her fists, her blanket, pacifiers, bottles, and whatever else she can get into her mouth, she learns about their shapes, textures, temperature, and tastes. And by sucking on her fist or pacifier in particular, she also learns that she can comfort herself.

Don't think of mouthing objects as a dirty habit that you must discourage. Your baby needs to explore the world this way. If you deny her the experience by pulling toys or her hands out of her mouth, you will deny her an important part of her development, as well as a great source of comfort. Make her oral explorations safe by putting only clean, safe items within reach.

Encouraging Movement

Here are some activities to help your baby's motor development:

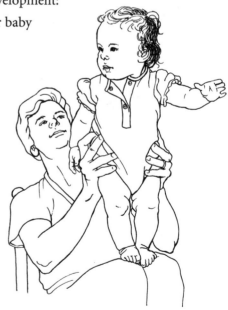

- Put several interesting toys on the floor around your baby to encourage her to reach for and grab things.

- Sit in a chair, and let your baby stand on your lap while you support her under the arms. She'll push her feet into your legs and bounce, exercising muscles she'll need for standing.

- Help your baby practice sitting up. With her lying on her back on your lap or on a bed, have her grab hold of your hands and pull herself up to a sitting position.

- Place your baby on her stomach, and let her practice pushing herself up.

- Give your baby a lot of time—and space— to practice rolling and crawling.

Playpens: Pros and Cons

Once a baby starts moving about, playpens can be useful, but they also have their downside. On the positive side, a playpen can be a relatively safe place to put the baby when you need to make dinner or talk on the phone or do something else

As your baby is able to bear more weight on her legs, you can let her practice standing on your lap by supporting her with your hands.

that prevents you from watching your baby carefully. On the negative side, by limiting the baby's range of movement, a playpen can also inhibit her curiosity.

You can strike a balance. Use the playpen only when you can't watch your baby. If a baby-sitter comes to your home, make sure that she understands this ground rule. Even if you fill the playpen with toys, it's no substitute for letting your baby explore. Looking at toys in a distant corner of the room and figuring out how to get there is how she learns. Baby-proof your home, and make that her playground.

Just because a playpen is padded doesn't mean it's safe. Here are some features to look for and precautions to follow:

▌ If the sides are mesh, make sure there are no tears or loose threads. Small openings can become large enough to trap your baby's head. Also make sure that the mesh is securely attached to the top rail and the floor plate.

▌ Old-style wooden playpens should have slats spaced no more than 2 inches apart to prevent the baby's head from becoming trapped.

▌ Check that any staples used in the playpen's construction are firmly in place and that none are missing or loose.

▌ If your playpen doubles as a portable crib and can collapse, never leave the drop side, or sides, in the down position when your baby is inside. Otherwise, an infant can roll into the loose pocket formed at the side and suffocate.

QUESTIONS PARENTS ASK
Shoes

Q: Does my daughter need shoes now that she's crawling and beginning to pull herself up?

A: Infants don't need shoes until they're ready to walk outside, when their feet have to be protected from the hard, cold ground and the dirty or dangerous objects that litter it. Indoors, babies do just fine barefoot. In fact, they can learn to balance better barefoot than in shoes because their toes can more easily grip the ground. Don't bother with shoes at this point. If it's chilly, put booties or socks on your baby's feet. Look for socks with gripper soles, which provide traction on slippery floors.

Sometime between 6 and 12 months, consider beginning to accustom your child to wearing shoes. Once she's walking, she'll need to wear them outside, and she is less likely to resist wearing them if they are already familiar. When you do choose shoes, the flexible sneakerlike footwear is a better choice than more rigid shoe styles. Pick up the shoe, and see if it bends easily.

Communicating

Newborns exercise their lungs with hearty cries. Babies from 4 to 7 months old typically exercise their mouths and throats with vocal gymnastics. They delight in making new sounds. Some as young as 4 months old begin to make wordlike sounds, repeating combinations of vowels and consonants, like "ah-goo" and "da-da." But babies also like to make nonverbal sounds, like coughing, gurgling, gagging, and squealing.

All the time you've spent talking to your baby since her birth is now beginning to have an effect. At first, her babbling will seem meaningless. But with time, she'll come to learn that some sounds get certain reactions. It often starts by accident. She says "em-em," and Mom comes. She says "da-da," and Dad smiles. At some point she'll use sounds like these to mean mommy and daddy, although this does not usually happen until the end of the first year. Meanwhile, she repeats many of the sounds that get a reaction. If her parents stop what they're doing and rush over to her when she coughs, she'll keep coughing to get their attention.

Your baby is sharpening her nonverbal communication, too. By about 6 months old, she may try to "ask" for something she wants using her eyes or her hands. For example, if she's sitting in her father's lap and she wants the car keys that her father is holding, she may look at her father's face, then look at the keys, and then grab for the keys.

Talking to Your Baby

To encourage your baby to babble, expose her to language continuously. Read her baby books. Play and sing songs. Keep talking to her while dressing, bathing, and feeding her; playing with her; and doing almost anything else.

Learning

Your baby is still learning about objects by putting them in her mouth, but now she's learning about them in other ways, too. She shakes, bangs, and drops them. She rakes small toys and bits of food in one hand and passes them to the other. These activities teach her about the sizes of different objects, their textures, and the sounds that they make when they hit the floor. She also learns that her mother or father come running when she drops things; that makes her happy. This becomes a game: She drops, you fetch. Of course, this can easily wear you out, and when it does, you can teach her something else: that you won't fetch, at least not right away.

Another thing that many babies begin to learn at about 7 months old is that an object still exists even if they can't see it. Before, anything that dropped from their hand and was out of sight was out of mind. But when 7-month-olds drop something, they usually look for it. At roughly 6 months, many babies begin to understand some words, like their names, "mommy," "daddy," and the names of brothers and sisters, as well as "bye-bye" and "no." But just because she understands the word "no,"

don't expect her to obey when you say it. That won't happen for many months—
or even decades—later.

TOUCHPOINT

Let Your Baby Get Frustrated

When you see your baby cry in frustration as she tries to do something new, like crawl or sit
up on her own, try to resist the temptation to rush over and help her. Frustration is a powerful learning tool. When the baby keeps trying to do something and then finally succeeds, she'll
beam with satisfaction. If her frustration builds to the point that she gets upset, offer some
assistance, like putting your foot behind her feet so that she can push off and crawl forward or
helping her go through the motions needed to sit up.

Source: Touchpoints Project (see p. 81).

Socializing

As the months pass, your baby will become increasingly sociable with you and other
people she knows well. If you walk into the room, she'll probably smile and she
might raise her arms as if to say, "Pick me up." She craves your attention. She'll use
every device she has to get your attention, including—frequently—crying. Often as

---

A MOTHER'S PERSPECTIVE

Attention-Getting Techniques?

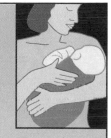

When Corey was about 6 months old, I
noticed that he was doing certain things to
get my attention. He'd make coughing sounds or
cry, or throw his pacifier on the floor over and
over so I'd have to pick it up.

Then one day, my sister-in-law came over. She
has four kids, so she's an experienced mom. We
were sitting in the living room trying to talk after
I put Corey in his crib for his nap. But we couldn't
talk because Corey kept throwing his pacifier on
the floor, and I kept jumping up to retrieve it.

After about the sixth time, my sister-in-law
looked at me as if I was nuts. "You're letting that
child make you crazy," she said. "You know he's
dropping those pacifiers on pur-
pose. If you don't keep picking
them up, he'll stop throwing
them."

I decided to try her suggestion. If he threw his
pacifier I'd wait until later to pick it up. If he
made one of those fake coughing sounds, I'd look
at him and say, "What's the matter?" But I would
not rush over and act like there was a crisis. I
think he stopped doing quite so many things to
make me hop. Maybe I was training him to be less
manipulative. Or maybe I was training myself to
be less easily manipulated.

soon as you go to her, she'll stop. Your loving attention is what she needs. There are lots of fun ways to interact with your child now: Playing, singing, talking, and reading to her are all good activities.

Aside from your baby's smile, perhaps her greatest social skill is imitation. She'll attempt to repeat your sounds and activities. If you bang your hand on the table, she'll bang her hand. This is a good age for playing interactive games that invite imitation, like peekaboo and patty-cake. Your baby won't be able to follow all the movements of patty-cake just yet, but she'll love being included in the game.

Showing Likes and Dislikes

A lot of fun can be had at this age, but this isn't to say life's always a party. Babies at this age have various ways of showing unhappiness, anger, and other negative emotions. If you offer your baby a spoonful of food that she doesn't like, for example, she may shut her mouth tight and turn her head away—although this could also mean she's full. If you take away something that she's grabbed, she may scowl at you. Sometimes her lower lip quivers, and she looks as if her feelings have been hurt. And, of course, she may protest loudly by crying.

Caring for Your Baby

As your baby grows and acquires new skills, you, too, must quickly adapt your baby care methods. You will need to learn new things, such as how to feed your baby solid foods, and new safety precautions to take, as when bathing a larger, more active baby in the tub. As your baby learns, you do, too.

Feeding

At about age 4 to 6 months, your child's doctor may recommend introducing solid food. You may be surprised to discover that what is commonly referred to as "solid food" for babies is anything but solid. It's soft, mushy food such as soupy rice cereals or pureed bananas—perfect for your toothless wonder. Now is the time to get ready for a major photo opportunity: your baby's first real meal—of baby food, that is. You've probably been looking forward to this event for weeks, eyeing the baby cereals and baby food jars in the supermarket, admiring the adorable infant bowl and spoons.

Rice cereal is usually the first solid food a baby eats. Babies should also continue taking breast milk or formula. Talk to your pediatrician about when your baby is ready for solids. Doctors often recommend that a larger baby start on solids sooner than a small baby, although this is not always the case.

Introducing solids earlier than 4 months is unnecessary. Your baby doesn't need foods other than breast milk or formula, and her stomach can't digest them well. Giving solid foods earlier can increase the risk of food allergies, because the baby's digestive system isn't mature enough to break down and absorb the food completely.

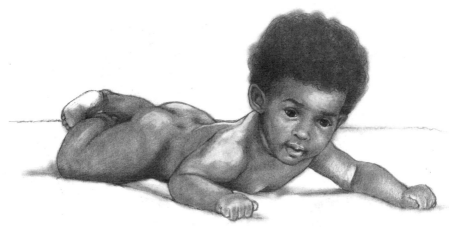

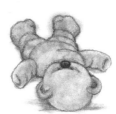

By about 7 months, before she learns to get up on all fours and crawl, your baby will creep around on her belly, often motivated by objects she wants to grab.

QUESTIONS PARENTS ASK

Is My Baby Ready for Solid Foods?

You can tell when your baby is ready by looking for any of the following signs:

▌ She is at least 4 months old.

▌ She can hold her head and neck steady while sitting up either in your lap or in an infant seat.

▌ She puts her hands, as well as handheld toys, in her mouth.

▌ When you put a spoon in her mouth, she doesn't keep pushing it away with her tongue.

▌ She shows an interest in what you are eating by looking at your food or possibly trying to grab it.

▌ She demands to be fed more frequently, say, every 2 hours, for more than a couple of days (a sign that she's no longer satisfied by breast milk or formula alone).

How to Feed Your Baby Solid Foods

It's a big change. Suddenly, your doctor says to start solid foods, and your comfortable feeding routine with breast or bottle has to make way for baby foods, baby spoons, cups, bowls, high chairs, and splat mats. Life is about to get messy.

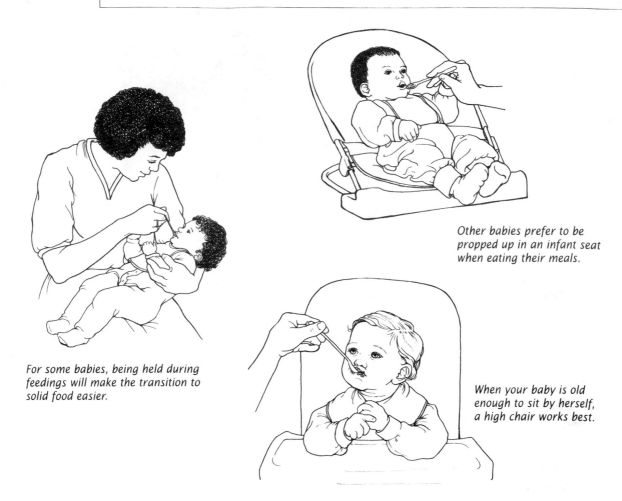

Other babies prefer to be propped up in an infant seat when eating their meals.

For some babies, being held during feedings will make the transition to solid food easier.

When your baby is old enough to sit by herself, a high chair works best.

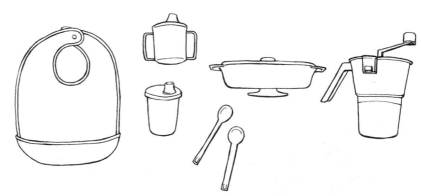

Bibs that fasten with a snap or Velcro, baby spoons with soft tips, plastic cups with nonspill sipper lids, a flip-proof suction-based bowl, and a baby-food grinder are some basic feeding tools you'll want on hand for your little one's solid food debut.

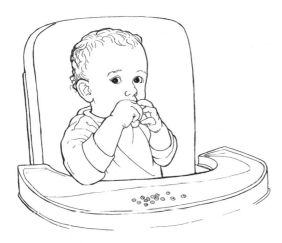

Once your baby develops a raking grasp, usually by 7 months, she'll be able to feed herself small O-shaped oat cereal, which makes a great finger food for babies.

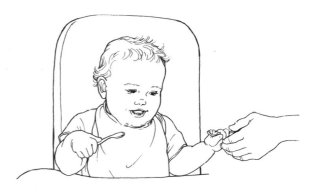

If your increasingly independent baby's habit of grabbing the spoon out of your hand prevents any food from reaching her mouth, give baby her own spoon so she can practice feeding herself, and your loaded spoon can reach its target.

Start with one of the iron-fortified infant cereals, whichever your doctor recommends. Baby cereals made of rice, oats, or barley are suitable first foods because they don't usually cause allergies. Follow these steps:

▌ Mix the cereal with either breast milk or formula, as directed on the package, for a soupy consistency.

▌ At first, make 1 tablespoon of cereal.

▌ With your baby sitting in your lap or in an infant seat, put a small dab of cereal in an infant spoon, and gently put the spoon in her mouth.

▌ Have fun. Smile and smack your lips and say, "Mmmm," to let your baby know this is something good to eat—and that mealtime is a fun, joyous, social occasion.

▌ If she pushes the food out with her tongue, scoop the cereal off her lips and chin, and try again.

▌ She may continue to thrust her tongue out as soon as the spoon goes in for the next week or so. She will take a while to get used to this new way of eating. Don't assume she doesn't like it. Try putting the food a little farther into her mouth. Many babies lack the muscle control to guide the food into their mouths if it is only placed on the tip of the tongue. Help her by doing some of the work for her.

▌ If she continues to refuse the food and doesn't swallow any for the first day or two, or if she fusses and turns her head away whenever you try to feed her, she's probably not ready for solids. Try again in a few days, but don't force her. Wait until she is ready.

Do not "thicken formula" by putting cereal in the bottle unless your child's doctor so directs. It confuses the baby and accustoms her to eating solids from a bottle rather than a spoon. It may also tempt the baby to overfeed.

Unless your doctor tells you otherwise, plan on serving your baby about 1 tablespoon of cereal once or twice a day at first, once for breakfast and again for dinner. Watch for signs of allergy, like a rash, diarrhea, or increased spitting up. If you notice these symptoms, stop feeding that food for now and try something else. If all goes well, after about 4 to 7 days you can add another food, such as a strained fruit (mashing your own bananas is easy) or vegetable, or another type of cereal grain. Introduce meats last. Although the risk of food allergies is real, it is also rare. Fewer than 8 percent of babies have even mild food allergies, and fewer than 2 percent have severe food allergies.

Feed your baby either commercially prepared baby food or pureed fruits and vegetables that you prepare yourself (see p. 133). Some good books available in stores have recipes for making your own baby foods. When choosing prepared baby foods, read the ingredients on the label. Avoid foods with additives such as sugar and salt. Refrigerate opened jars of baby food. Throw away any prepared cereal that your infant doesn't eat.

 QUESTIONS PARENTS ASK
High Chairs

Q: When can I feed my baby in a high chair?

A: Your baby is ready for a high chair when she can sit up without support. Until then, feed her either in an infant seat or on your lap.

Balancing Solids and Breast Milk or Formula

For now, your baby will still get most of her nutrients and calories from breast milk or formula. Continue giving formula or breast milk on demand, about four or five times a day. Most babies at this age will take between 24 and 32 ounces of formula or breast milk per day, depending on how much solid food they are also eating.

Offer solid food twice a day on a schedule. Time these meals so that they don't interfere with nursing or bottle-feeding. Try nursing or giving your baby a bottle when she first wakes up, and an hour or two later, give her some cereal and fruit. Give her more cereal and some vegetables at dinnertime, about an hour or two before her last milk or formula feeding of the day. Once your baby is enthusiastically eating about 4 ounces of solids twice a day, you can add a third meal sometime between the other two. Gradually, your child will eat more solid food and need less breast milk or formula:

▮ Newborn to 4 months: breast milk or formula only

▮ 8 months: half solid food, half formula or breast milk

▌ 12 months: mostly solid foods (baby should drink only for thirst, eat for hunger)

Breast milk or formula has about 20 calories of energy-producing nutrition per ounce. A baby needs about 100 to 110 calories for each kilogram (2.2 pounds) of weight to grow at the proper rate.

To determine how many total calories your baby needs per day from breast milk or formula and solid foods, divide your baby's weight in pounds by 2.2 then multiply by 100. To determine how many ounces of breast milk or formula she needs, divide the total calories by 20.

For example, a 9-pound (4-kilogram) baby needs about 400 calories, or about 20 ounces of milk or formula, each day to grow. Most larger babies need no more than 36 ounces of formula each day.

QUESTIONS PARENTS ASK
Should Babies Drink Juice?

You may have heard that fruit juice is bad for babies and young children. Recent research has shown that drinking too much juice can cause problems such as stunted growth, chronic diarrhea, and even malnutrition. The reason is that the juices children tend to drink the most, like apple juice, are relatively low in nutrients—even those that are 100 percent juice. The calories are primarily from sugar and leave the baby feeling satisfied and less hungry for more nutritious food. Apple juice, in particular, is a problem because it contains large amounts of the sugar sorbitol, a common cause of food intolerance, which can cause diarrhea (but is sometimes used to treat constipation). Another problem with juice is that it promotes cavities when babies drink it from a bottle, particularly if the baby falls asleep with the juice in her mouth, leaving it to pool around the teeth (see *Cavities,* Part 5).

You can prevent these problems by not giving your baby any juice until she's about 6 months old, and then by giving it to her only in a cup, not a bottle. That way, she'll never fall asleep drinking juice from a bottle.

If you choose to give your baby juice after she's 6 months old, give her only 1 or 2 ounces a day diluted with an equal amount of water in a cup. Your baby is ready to drink from a cup when she's able to sit without support. Start with pear juice or white grape juice, since these are less likely to cause allergies or diarrhea. Hold off on orange juice at first, because it often causes rashes in younger babies.

Hand It Over: Giving Finger Foods

Once your baby can sit without support, she's ready to eat finger foods—that is, small bits of food that she can pick up in her fingers and feed herself. Choose a variety of foods, including these tried-and-true offerings:

▌ Ripe bananas

▌ Well-cooked vegetables, like green beans, yams, or potatoes

▌ Small, O-shaped oat cereals, which don't need to be chewed

Even if your baby has gotten her first tooth by now, she can't chew yet. Other than bananas, cook all fruits and vegetables until soft, and cut them into small pieces to prevent choking. Preparing the fruits and vegetables yourself is best. If you buy them in cans, check the labels to make sure that no salt, sugar, or other seasonings or chemicals have been added—babies do not need these additives.

Place a few pieces of finger food on the high chair tray. At first, your baby probably won't know what to do. Even if you demonstrate, she'll probably approach the food as she would a new toy, picking it up and throwing it down. Or she may mash it with her palm. At first, don't put the finger food in a bowl, because she'll be tempted to dump it over. After a day or so, she'll understand that the food is supposed to go in her mouth, although most of it probably will still land on her lap and on the floor. So, plan on spoon-feeding her baby food, too, for now. Don't push, some babies adapt to finger food more quickly than others.

Expect your baby to make a mess. That's part of her fun. To you, food is nourishment. But to your baby, it's both food and another toy to be picked up and dropped, squeezed and thrown. At this point your baby will gain more from "exploring" her food than from eating all of it. She's still getting most of her calories and nutrients from milk or formula.

What to Feed Your Baby

Start your baby off with soft foods that don't require chewing and are unlikely to cause allergies. The following foods are suitable for babies:

▌ *Good foods for a 4- to 6-month old:*
  Single-grain, iron-fortified infant cereals made of rice, oats, or barley
  Multigrain infant cereals
  Strained fruits, such as pears, apples, apricots, peaches, and prunes
  Strained vegetables, such as squash, sweet potatoes, carrots, peas, and green beans
  Strained cooked meats, such as chicken, turkey, beef, and pork

▌ *Good foods for a 6- to 7-month old* (or when she can sit up):
  Ripe bananas cut into small pieces
  Cooked fruit, such as apples and pears cut into small pieces
  Cooked vegetables, such as peas, green beans, yams, and white potatoes
  Small, O-shaped oat cereals

What NOT to Feed Your Baby

Some foods, though nutritious and enjoyable for adults and older children, can cause problems with young babies. The following list shows foods to avoid while your baby is still exploring the new world of solid food.

▌ *Citrus fruits:* Oranges, grapefruit, and other citrus fruits can cause allergic rashes in infants under 1 year old.

▌ *Corn:* Hard to digest for babies under 6 months old.

▌ *Honey:* Can cause botulism, a life-threatening food poisoning. Honey is sometimes tainted with spores of the bacteria that cause botulism. Children under 1 year old are most vulnerable to the illness.

▌ *Egg whites:* Can cause allergies in babies under 1 year old.

▌ *Peanut butter:* Wait until child is age 2 years or older, because peanut butter can cause choking in younger children. Also, if your child or your family tends to have allergies, delay giving peanut butter until after age 3 years, because of high risk of allergies. Withhold chunky-style peanut butter until after age 3 years for all children.

▌ *Shellfish:* Shrimp and lobster are among the most allergy-provoking foods.

▌ *Other foods:* Small, round, or hard foods, including grapes, raw carrots, hot dogs and hot dog rounds, and raisins, can cause choking.

Making Your Own Baby Food

If you have the time and the desire, you can make your own strained fruits and vegetables for your baby. The easiest baby food to prepare at home is mashed bananas. Simply mash enough banana for one feeding (about a half a banana) through a strainer. Other fruits and all vegetables must be cooked ahead of time and then pureed. Don't add sugar, salt, or other seasonings.

Although one reason for preparing food at home is to give your baby the purest, safest food possible, four vegetables are actually safer for your baby when bought in jars. They are carrots, collard greens, beets, and turnips. Depending on where they're grown, these vegetables may contain a lot of nitrates, a chemical that can cause anemia in babies. Baby food manufacturers test vegetables before processing them and avoid using any that are high in nitrates.

Storing Leftovers

When you feed your baby homemade baby food, you may wonder what to do with the leftovers. Don't automatically throw them away. Whatever isn't served right away can be refrigerated or frozen for future meals. You may find it convenient to store the food in ice cube trays in the freezer, then warm a cube or two in a pot on the stove or in a microwave. If you use a microwave, stir the food thoroughly to eliminate spots that are too hot. Always test food to make sure it is not hot before giving it to your baby.

Lack of Interest in Breast-Feeding

Q: When I try to breast-feed my 4-month-old, she'll nurse for a few minutes, then look around or even pull at my breast with her fingers. Does this mean she's weaning herself?

A: What it means is that breast-feeding is no longer the center of your baby's universe. But it doesn't indicate she wants to be weaned. She's grown so interested in everything there is to look at and listen to that she has trouble concentrating on breast-feeding. Also, babies naturally cut back on breast-feeding once they begin eating solid foods. She's not giving you a cue to switch her to a bottle, or rejecting you. Think of her behavior as the normal, 4-month-old equivalent of a schoolchild who's so eager to run outside and play that she can't finish her peanut butter and jelly sandwich.

Your baby's loss of interest in breast-feeding may be short-lived. In another week or so, she may approach nursing with the familiar gusto, at least for a while. If you want to continue breast-feeding—the American Academy of Pediatrics recommends breast-feeding your baby for the first year—you may need to make a few adjustments.

▌ Feed your baby in a quiet room away from others.

▌ Dim the lights if that seems to calm her.

▌ Make the most of the feedings that take place first thing in the morning and just before bedtime, the times of day when your baby is least likely to be distracted.

▌ Once you introduce solid food, breast-feed before a meal so your baby won't be too full of solid food to take the breast.

Into the Tub

Once your baby can sit up, she can have her bath in the family bathtub. You'll need either to hold her at all times or to put her in a bath seat designed to keep infants this age from falling over. Of course, these products are not a substitute for your attention. Never leave your baby alone in the bath. An active baby can tip over in a bath seat, and she can drown in as little as 2 inches of water.

Now that your baby's in the grown-up tub, you can make bath time even more fun. You can introduce bath toys, like rubber ducks, boats, and plastic bath books that are easy for her to grab. Use this time, too, as an opportunity to encourage language by talking brightly to your baby about what you are doing. Don't use bubbles in the bath. The detergents that make up the bubble ingredients can dry your baby's skin and cause rashes. In girls, they can promote vaginal infections. They tend to break down the mucus in the vagina that normally fights bacteria.

How to Bathe Your Baby—and Have Fun, Too!

You don't have to bathe your baby every day—two or three times a week is enough.

▌ Using a cloth, wash her face and ears first, when the water is still clean and relatively soap-free and therefore least likely to irritate her eyes.

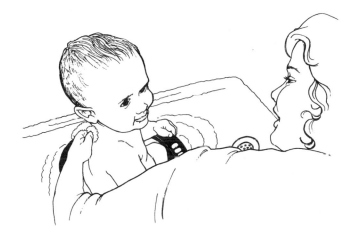

Even if your baby sits up well, she's likely to slip in the tub. To help support her, place her in a sturdy tub seat with a strong suction base while you wash her. But remember, babies can still easily slip down in a bath seat, so you don't leave her side, even for a second.

- Next, move down to her torso, arms, legs, and diaper area.
- Shampoo your baby's hair using a mild baby shampoo.
- Place a washcloth across the baby's forehead, and tilt her head back slightly while rinsing her hair to prevent water and shampoo from running into her eyes.
- Make sure to play and have fun while bathing—that way she'll look forward to her next bath.

Sleeping

By the time they are 6 months old, most babies fall into a routine of napping just twice a day, once in the morning and once in the afternoon. These naps probably shouldn't last more than about $1\frac{1}{2}$ or 2 hours, or they may start to cut into the amount of time a baby sleeps at night. If that's happening, waking your baby is OK.

At 5 months old, most babies can go 9 hours between nighttime feedings, which means they don't need to be fed in the middle of the night. And by 5 or 6 months of age, most babies are sleeping through the night, at least sometimes. If they wake up hungry in the middle of the night, it's because they are used to having a feeding at that time, not because they need to be fed then.

Encouraging Your Baby to Sleep Through the Night

Often babies wake up in the middle of the night for reasons other than hunger. As with adults, their sleep pattern includes cycles of deep and light sleep. When they enter a light sleep cycle, they're likely to wake up briefly. Adults and older children usually go back to sleep without even realizing that they've awakened. But babies can't do this yet, so they cry. If they usually get rocked, held, or fed when they cry in the middle of the night, they come to expect it and can't get back to sleep without it.

One of the best ways to encourage your baby to fall back to sleep on her own at this age is to wait a few minutes before you respond when your baby wakes up crying in the middle of the night. Listening to your baby cry in the middle of the night is one of the hardest things you'll do as a parent, because you think that your little baby needs you and because you want a good night's sleep. But research has shown that when parents stick to a routine of waiting a few minutes before going in and comforting their babies, most babies learn within a matter of days to fall back to sleep on their own.

Some parents choose not to let their babies cry at this stage. You may feel you must respond to your baby immediately and rock or nurse her back to sleep. This is fine, so long as you and your partner can tolerate the lack of sleep that your activity is encouraging. A tired, irritable, sleep-deprived parent may find it more difficult to be attentive to and patient with a child during the daytime than one who has had a good night's sleep.

Eight Steps to a Good Night's Sleep

You can help your baby learn how to settle down when she goes to sleep and also when she wakes up in the middle of the night. This method was developed by Children's Hospital Boston Clinical Director of Pediatric Sleep Disorders, Richard A. Ferber, M.D. Beginning at about 5 months of age, try these steps:

1. Maintain a regular sleep schedule each day.

2. Follow a bedtime ritual with your child in the room where she sleeps.

3. Before putting your baby to bed, feed her, but try not to let her fall asleep in your arms.

4. Lay your baby down awake at the time she usually goes to sleep, and wait for her to fall asleep. She may whimper or cry for a while.

5. If the whimper builds to a cry, comfort your baby briefly by talking to her in a soothing voice. It is usually not necessary to pick her up. Don't talk a lot because you might stimulate the baby. The last thing you want to do is let her think that you're there to play at bedtime. (This advice also applies if your baby wakes up in the middle of the night.)

6. If your baby cries when you leave the room, wait at least 5 minutes before returning to comfort her briefly—picking her up is usually not necessary. Check the clock. Otherwise you may think your baby is crying for a longer period than she really is.

7. After you comfort her briefly, leave again.

8. If your baby keeps crying, wait a few minutes longer before you go to her again. There's no magic number of minutes—the key is to keep stretching out the intervals by a few minutes each time between your visits. Over a period of time, she should gradually learn to comfort herself enough to fall back to sleep.

If, despite your efforts, your baby continues to wake up crying at night, there may be a problem other than your baby's associating waking up with your coming to her. For example, your baby might be napping too much or going to bed too early in the evening. If your baby won't settle down even when you pick her up or feed her, call your doctor, who may want to check to make sure she doesn't have a painful condition such as *gastroesophageal reflux* (see Part 5) or an ear infection (see *Earache/Ear Infection,* Part 5) that may be keeping her up at night.

TOUCHPOINT

Solving Your Baby's Sleep Problems

Some babies who have been sleeping through the night for several weeks may wake up again during the night when they're about 6 months old. They may also have trouble settling down for bedtime and naps. Sleep problems tend to crop up at this time for several reasons. One is that babies' repertoire of activities is expanding rapidly. Naturally, they practice rolling over and creeping in their cribs, and this activity can make it hard to settle down. And the frustration that builds during a day of struggling to master new skills like sitting up and crawling can make for restless nights. Other problems, like a cold or another illness, a change in routine, or going on vacation and having to sleep in a strange room, can also interfere with sleep.

The best way to overcome these setbacks is to maintain a predictable schedule during the day and a set routine at bedtime. Babies are comforted by routine. And it may help them sleep for longer stretches. A recent study found that 6-month-old Dutch babies sleep for an average of 10 hours a night, whereas American babies sleep 8 to 9 hours. The researchers believe that cultural differences are a crucial factor: American babies have less predictable routines. They are often on the go, napping in their cribs one day and their car seat the next, spending one afternoon at home and the next at an older sibling's soccer practice. Dutch babies, on the other hand, spend more time at home.

The point here isn't that you should plan all of your errands and appointments around your baby's schedule. But try to stick to a schedule as much as possible, and if you work, tell your caregiver to do the same. Source: Touchpoints Project (see p. 81).

PACIFIERS

Many babies show less interest in their pacifier at around 4 months old. They spit it out or don't suck on it as much as they used to. If this happens with your baby, consider it your opportunity to gradually get rid of the pacifier. Don't put it in your baby's mouth whenever she cries or spits it out. Breaking the pacifier habit now is easier than it may be later. But don't worry if your baby won't part with it just yet.

The need to suck is normal for an infant. Sucking a pacifier has its advantages and disadvantages. One advantage is that you can take it away (unlike a thumb or a finger). But don't remove it so soon or abruptly that your child will substitute another undesirable behavior, such as thumb sucking or hair pulling (see *Behavioral Problems,* Part 5). Many babies lose interest in the pacifier on their own. Dental experts advise that children be weaned off either pacifier or finger sucking before permanent teeth erupt to prevent interference with their development. But most children drop the pacifier long before this.

Another good time to consider eliminating the pacifier is around a child's second birthday. A child's memory is short at this age. If the pacifier gets "lost" one day, it may be only a few days before your child forgets she ever had one. Plus, a 2-year-old is much less likely than a younger child to revert to thumb sucking when you take the pacifier away.

Make Way for That Toothy Smile!

You'll probably notice when your baby starts teething (the process by which tiny teeth gradually break through the gums). If your baby is 4 months or older and seems to be unusually fussy or irritable, look in her mouth for signs of emerging teeth. Most babies begin teething when they're 4 to 8 months old. The average age when the first tooth appears is 6 months, although a wide range of ages is normal. The exact timetable depends on family history. Some babies get their first tooth when they're only 3 or 4 months old. Indeed, in rare cases a baby is even born with a tooth. And then there are babies whose first tooth doesn't poke through until around their first birthday.

Common Signs of Teething

The signs of teething vary from one child to the next. Some babies sail through with barely a fussy spell, while others show all these symptoms. Almost all babies at this time will want to chew on whatever they can put in their mouths.

▌ Crankiness

▌ Drooling

▌ Red or inflamed gums

▌ A rash around the mouth from drooling

▌ A tendency to chew on rubber toys or their fingers or even on the edges of objects like tables and blankets

▌ Waking more often at night

▌ Fussiness during meals

Soothing Your Baby's Teething Pain

Teething pain is caused by the tooth's growing into the jawbone and periodically hitting nerves. One of the best ways to relieve your baby's teething pain is to give her something to chew on. The pressure of chewing reduces the discomfort, and the act of chewing itself helps the emerging tooth break through by wearing down the gum in front of it. Try an assortment of teething rings and rubber toys to see which one works best for your baby. Some babies like soft rubber or plastic, and others prefer hard objects, such as a metal teething ring or even a frozen bagel.

The colder the object, the more effectively it will numb your baby's pain. So keep some teething rings in the refrigerator. As an alternative to teething rings, wet some

washcloths, fold or twist them into a long. th⌐
shape, and then put them in the fr⌐
your baby is in pain. gi⌐
frozen washcl⌐

    There ma⌐
strategies w⌐
about trying⌐
as infant ibup⌐
from the over⌐
babies. These ⌐
work for such a⌐
the baby an ove⌐
gic to them and ⌐
shortness of brea⌐

Tooth Care

Schedule your child⌐
within 6 months of⌐
tooth or by 1 year of⌐
baby has a few teeth,⌐
an infant-sized toothb⌐
toothbrush will do the⌐
that contains fluoride. ⌐
low the toothpaste (and⌐
ride, which can cause flu⌐
the teeth. For this reason,⌐
babies under 6 months old⌐
drinks fluoridated water or⌐
water). For children over 6 ⌐
ments if local drinking wate⌐
Part 5).

⌐'s teeth are likely to emerge in the
⌐n.

Incisors

3   2   2   3   Canine

7

5   Molars

TOP TEETH   10

⌐TOM ⌐TH   9

6   Molars

8   4

Canine

Keeping Your Baby He⌐

Now that your baby is putting her hands and toys in her mouth more often, she's bound to come in contact with more germs. Children in child care with other children also tend to pick up more infections. You can reduce the chance of infection by washing her hands (and yours) several times throughout the day and encouraging your child care providers to do the same. One way to practice good hygiene is to put your baby's pacifiers, teething rings, toys, and any other things she likes to put in her mouth into the dishwasher at night. The hot water and dry heat will sterilize them. Make sure to put them on the top rack to avoid the possibility of their melting from being too close to the heating elements.

Checkups

Your baby should have checkups when she's 4 months old and 6 months old. As with the previous well-baby visits, the doctor or nurse will weigh the baby and measure her length and her head circumference, then plot the numbers on a growth curve (see Appendix: Growth Charts). The doctor will also completely examine your baby, including checking her eyes and ears, listening to her heart, and watching her arms and legs move.

Your doctor will also ask you about your baby's development, eating habits, and temperament. Remember that your regular checkups are a good time to ask your doctor about any health or child care concerns you may have. Are you thinking of putting your child in child care for the first time? Tell your doctor. Is your baby not taking solid foods? Speak up now.

See Childhood Immunization Schedule, page 110.

QUESTIONS PARENTS ASK

Flat Feet

Q: My baby has flat feet. Is this a problem?

A: All babies have flat feet. The reason there's no pronounced arch is that there's a layer of fat on the bottoms of the feet. But as babies spend more time on their feet walking, running, and climbing, the fat gives way to muscle and an arch develops, usually by 3 years of age. If an arch does not develop, consult your child's doctor.

When Your Baby Is Sick

Between 4 and 7 months of age, many babies experience the following common childhood infections.

Ear Infections

One recent study found that by the time they're 6 months old, 70 percent of infants have had their first dose of antibiotics, most of them for middle ear infections. Babies often get ear infections after a cold, because the cold spreads to the eustachian tube connecting the nasal passages to the middle ear. Drinking a bottle while lying down can promote infection: The fluid can back up because of a poorly draining eustachian tube, allowing germs to thrive. Exposure to secondhand tobacco smoke also increases your baby's chances of getting an ear infection. Symptoms of an ear infection include fever, fussiness, decreased appetite, refusal of the bottle or breast, and a cold that lingers longer than usual. Ear infections must be treated by a doctor, so if you notice any or all of these symptoms, call your child's doctor. For more information, see *Earache/Ear Infection,* Part 5.

Croup

Another common complication of an ordinary cold is croup, an inflammation of the area just below the vocal cords. The symptoms are unmistakable: a persistent, low-pitched cough that sounds like a seal barking. The cough may last for only a few hours, or it may continue off and on for up to a week. If the coughing doesn't stop after about 15 minutes, or if the baby seems to be having trouble breathing or has a fever, call the doctor. For more information, see *Croup,* Part 5.

SAFETY ALERT
Secondhand Smoke

Small children who breathe secondhand smoke (sidestream smoke) are more likely to develop respiratory infections, ear infections, and asthma than other children and may be at higher risk of developing heart disease and high blood pressure later in life.

Protect your baby from secondhand smoke. Don't smoke in your home or in the car when your baby is with you. Don't allow other people to smoke around your baby. Traces of tobacco smoke can linger in a room for more than a week.

Keeping Your Baby Safe

It's the moment you've been anticipating—or worrying about: the time when your baby begins to move about on her own. She no longer stays where you put her on that comfy baby blanket on the floor. Once a baby begins to move about—even slightly—it's time to baby-proof your home and take other precautions to prevent accidents.

For emergency procedures, including what to do if your child is choking, is drowning, has stopped breathing, or has lost consciousness, see Chapter 11, Preparing for and Handling Emergencies.

Baby-Proofing Your Home

Don't wait until your baby starts crawling toward the electrical outlets and opening the kitchen cabinets to make sure your home is safe. The time to baby-proof your home is before she's mobile. Baby-proofing isn't just a matter of putting safety plugs in outlets and a gate at the top of the stairs, although those are essential steps to take. It's a matter of looking at your home in a whole new way. Unless you have spent a lot of time with babies and toddlers, you may not be able to imagine how seemingly harmless fixtures and accessories, such as tablecloths and doors, lamps and coffee tables, can be hazards to a curious, roaming baby. Even if you got down on the floor and tried to see the world through your baby's eyes, you probably couldn't dream up all the ways that she can get into trouble.

Making your home safe for infants and children involves three steps in this order:

1. *Supervision:* This is the front line in child safety; close supervision by a responsible adult is the most important step you can take.

2. *Hazard removal:* Remove all hazardous objects, substances, and opportunities from your child's surroundings. For more information on poison control, see page 211.

3. *Child safety devices:* Baby gates, cabinet locks, electrical outlet plugs, and other baby-proofing devices are valuable tools in making your home safe. But supervision and hazard removal come first.

Baby-proofing isn't terribly expensive, but it takes some effort to do and to live with. Home won't feel quite as comfortable as it used to when you have to unlock a gate to go downstairs and release a safety latch to get the silverware. But the inconvenience is worth it once you've created a safe environment where you can relax with your baby. Accidents are the main cause of death in children. Each day, nearly 39,000 children in the United States are injured seriously enough to require medical treatment. Baby-proofing your house can save your child's life.

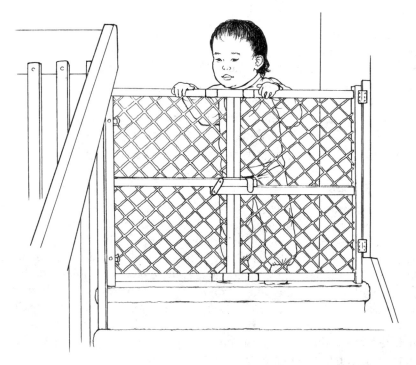

Never use an accordion-style gate anywhere in your home. Rather, choose a gate with a straight wooden or plastic top edge. At the top of the stairs, use only a gate that can be secured safely with screws and appropriate hardware rather than a pressure-mounted gate.

Baby-Proofing Checklist

Here's what you need to do and how to do it (see illustrations on the next few pages):

1. *Stairs:* Put a safety gate at the top and bottom of the stairs to prevent your baby from falling. Use gates that are screwed into the wall. Removable gates cannot be secured firmly enough to keep a baby from pulling them down. Choose a gate with a straight top edge and rigid mesh screen.

2. *Stair or upper floor hallway railings:* Prevent children from falling through wide banisters that you may have along your stairway or upstairs hallway by attaching acrylic, plastic, or netting specifically designed to cover these openings. These types of coverings are available through most child safety product vendors.

3. *Electrical wires and outlets:* Fasten wires from the television, VCR, and other equipment to baseboards with electrical tape or electrical safety staples. Cover unused electrical outlets with plastic safety plugs.

4. *Cabinets:* Install safety latches or locks on lower cabinets so that your baby can't open the doors. The main purpose is to keep your baby from getting to the objects inside. But another purpose is to prevent your baby from squeezing her fingers in the cabinet doors. Store dangerous items like cleaning fluid and dishwasher soap on a high shelf, out of a child's reach and sight.

5. *Doors:* Fasten hook and eyes to doors at adult eye level or attach doorknob guards, which spin freely unless side buttons are squeezed, to keep babies and young children from opening the doors.

6. *Radiators:* Shield them with wood or metal radiator covers to prevent your baby from being burned.

7. *Fireplaces, wood stoves, space heaters:* Surround them with a fireproof safety grate or screen that locks into place. If the hearth is raised, cover it and the area around it with fireproof padding to protect your baby if she falls. Chimneys and flues should be checked regularly for blockages, corrosion, or loose connections that could lead to the escape of carbon monoxide gas. Keep matches and lighters out of your baby's reach. If possible, don't use a wood stove while your child is too young to recognize the hazard it poses.

8. *Windows:* Screens aren't strong enough to keep children from falling out of windows. Use window guards that prevent windows from opening more than 3 inches. In addition, move couches, chairs, tables, and other furniture away from windows to discourage your child from trying to climb out.

9. *Blinds and shades:* Cut looped cords to prevent strangulation. If you have older miniblinds, test them to make sure they don't contain lead by using a lead-testing kit, available in hardware stores. For more information on preventing **lead poisoning,** see Part 5.

10. *House plants:* Keep house plants out of your baby's reach. Some house plants, such as philodendrons, and forced spring bulbs, such as narcissus, are poisonous. But other dangers exist, such as heavy flower pots that may topple onto the baby and the baby's eating dirt from flower pots.

11. *Dining tables:* Don't use tablecloths. Your baby will only try to pull them down, at the risk of bringing plates, bowls, glasses, knives, and other dangerous objects from the table down on herself.

12. *Bookcases:* Screw freestanding bookcases into a wall. Babies often try to pull themselves up by holding onto shelves, but doing so can cause a bookcase to topple over if it's not secured. Pack the books tightly to prevent your baby from pulling them out.

First Floor

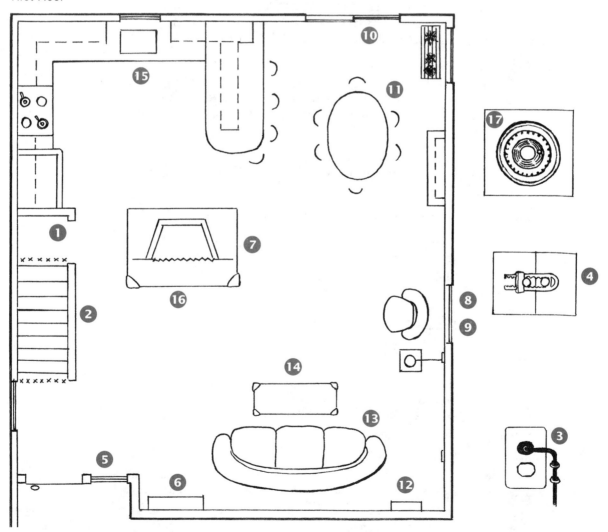

13. *Purses:* If you own a purse, keep it and any purses belonging to visitors out of your child's reach.

14. *Coffee tables:* More than 70,000 babies and young children in the United States are rushed to emergency rooms each year with injuries from the sharp corners and edges of coffee tables. You can reduce the risk of injuries by covering the corners with plastic corner guards.

15. *Kitchen:* Put latches on drawers that contain knives, forks, corkscrews, pizza cutters, and other sharp objects. If your baby will be able to reach the stove knobs once she starts pulling herself up to stand, use plastic stove knob covers or a special stove shield to keep her from turning on the stove. When cooking, turn pot handles away from the front of the stove so that your baby can't pull them down and get burned by hot food. Store small electrical appliances like food processors and toasters out of your child's reach.

16. *Toy chest:* If you have an old wooden toy chest with a heavy lid, remove the lid—a child can suffer serious head injury if the lid comes down on her head.

17. *Throughout home:* Install smoke detectors on each floor, especially near sleeping areas, and be sure to change batteries annually. Since carbon monoxide gases can spread throughout the home, install on the wall or ceiling just outside sleeping areas a carbon monoxide detector that has been approved by Underwriters Laboratories. To prevent carbon monoxide from accumulating in your home, be sure that any appliance fueled with gas, oil, kerosene, or wood is installed, maintained, and used properly.

18. *Balloons and plastic bags:* Babies and young children can choke on latex balloons and plastic bags. Keep them out of your child's reach, whether they're inflated or not.

19. *Bathroom:* Keep hair dryers, curling irons, electric shavers, and other appliances unplugged when not in use. When curling irons are cooling off, put them out of the baby's reach. Keep medicine and vitamins in medicine cabinets out of a child's reach. If possible, lock the cabinets. Install no-skid strips or mats on the bathtub floor to prevent falls, and install new circuit-breaker electrical outlets.

20. *Prescription medication:* Make sure that medications are in containers with child-resistant tops. These tops have reduced the death rate from poisoning by 90 percent. Store medicines in locked cabinets, and be alert to your baby's whereabouts when medications are in use.

21. *Hot water:* To prevent scalding, turn the temperature on your water heater below 120°F. A baby's skin is more sensitive and scalds more easily than adult skin.

22. *Bathtub/pool/water buckets:* To avoid the risk of drowning, never leave your child alone in the bathtub or near any water. Keep children away from all standing water, including water in toilets, 5-gallon buckets, and pools.

23. *Gun safety:* Guns are one of the most common causes of accidental death in children. The best way to prevent accidents is not to have a gun. But if you have one, keep it unloaded, equipped with a childproof safety lock, and locked out of sight. Store ammunition in a separate location.

24. *Bedrooms:* Keep rings, earrings, and other small jewelry that a baby can choke on, as well as nail files, clippers, pen knives, and other sharp objects, out of her reach. Lock cosmetics and personal care items away or keep them in childproof containers to prevent poisoning.

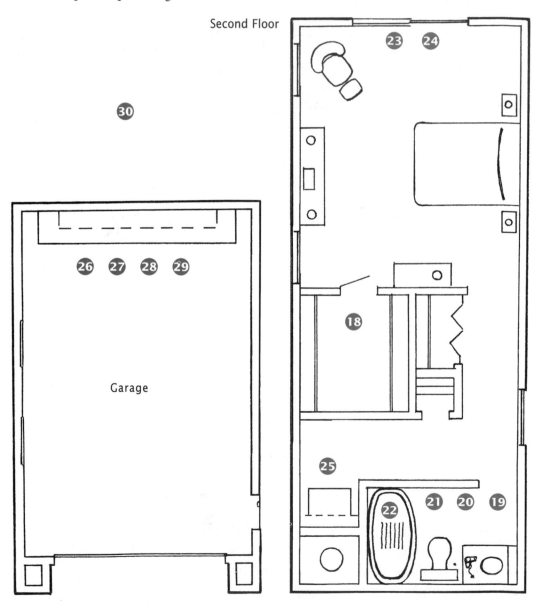

Second Floor

Garage

25. *Laundry room:* Keep detergents and household cleaners on high shelves. Keep washer and dryer doors closed to prevent your child from crawling in and getting trapped.

26. *Workshop:* Although this area should be kept off-limits, be sure to store tools, paints, and other such equipment out of your baby's reach. Dispose of old paints, varnishes, and solvents.

27. *Garage:* If you have an electric garage door opener, make sure that it stops or reverses upon hitting an object. Place a large roll of paper towels under the door to test it. Don't let children play in the garage. Store rakes, mowers, shovels, leaf blowers, and other equipment out of the reach of children. Keep children away from pesticides, fertilizers, antifreeze, gasoline, and road salt.

28. *Refrigerators:* The door to any unused old-style refrigerator should be completely removed, or the latch should be disabled so that the door will no longer stick when closed. Refrigerators built before the mid-fifties cannot be opened up from the inside, and many of these refrigerators are still used or stored in basements or garages. This is a serious entrapment and suffocation hazard for a child who may, while playing, climb inside the old abandoned or carelessly stored refrigerator. If you decide to dispose of an old refrigerator, many local jurisdictions require you to take the door off first.

29. *Exercise equipment:* Don't exercise when your baby is in the room unless she is contained in a playpen or another safe place. More than 6,000 children in the United States are injured each year by exercise equipment. Their tiny fingers get trapped in the spokes of the spinning wheels of exercise bikes or crushed by weights in weight machines. If possible, lock up home exercise equipment away from the baby.

30. *Yard:* If you have a swing set, check it periodically to make sure that it is sturdy and won't topple over or break under your child's weight. Also, make sure that it's located over grass or another soft, energy-absorbing surface, like mulch. Keep children away from outdoor sheds. Lawns newly treated with fertilizers, pesticides, and herbicides should be off-limits for 48 hours. Don't let children play on a recently treated lawn or in the area when anyone is operating a lawn mower or snowblower. Don't give rides on a riding mower.

Grandparents' House (or Others Often Visited)

Expecting your parents and in-laws to childproof their homes as thoroughly as you do yours is unrealistic. But once your baby begins to move about and if your baby will be visiting them regularly, encourage them to take as many safety measures as they can. At the least, they can make the following accommodations:

- Put safety plugs in unused outlets.
- Move breakable or dangerous objects and house plants out of your baby's reach on the days when the baby visits.

▌ Cut looped cords to blinds and shades, or at least tie them up high enough so that the baby can't touch them.

▌ Put a removable lock on the kitchen cabinet beneath the sink if that's where dishwasher soap and other cleaning fluids and chemicals are kept.

▌ Move vitamins and medication, including prescription medication, out of reach.

▌ Have prescriptions filled in child-resistant containers.

▌ Install a permanent fence with a locked gate around the pool, if they have one.

▌ Avoid using old baby cribs and other equipment that doesn't meet current safety standards (see p. 26).

▌ Put simple, adult-eye-level latches on doors of rooms that are off-limits (workshops, laundry rooms, offices, etc.).

▌ Keep a first-aid kit on hand containing the items recommended on page 350.

SAFETY ALERT
Avoid Baby Walkers

Walkers injure more children than any other baby equipment. Since 1974, walkers with wheels have been responsible for the deaths of 34 children. Most injuries are caused when babies fall downstairs, tip over, or get their fingers trapped in the X-shaped joints on the sides of older models. Using a baby walker also increases the chance of poisoning and choking in an infant, because the walker allows the baby to reach more places more quickly than infants who don't use walkers.

The best way to prevent such accidents is not to use walkers. They do not benefit a baby's development and may actually discourage crawling. Several alternatives to conventional walkers are available in baby equipment stores. Stationary activity centers that do not have wheels, jumper chairs, and bouncer seats without wheels are safer choices.

A Parent's Life

You've been totally involved in caring for your new baby for several months now. But you also have your own life to live. Gradually, parents must learn how to do both—care for their babies and live their own lives. Returning to work is a big issue for many parents. The decision of how long to wait before returning to a job or starting a new job after a baby's birth varies according to the individual parent's preferences and financial situation. For those who decide to return to work after the birth of a child, several steps can ease the transition.

Going Back to Work

Returning to work after the birth of a child isn't easy. No matter how much you need or want to work, you may be surprised to find yourself wondering whether you're doing the right thing. More than half of mothers of infants work outside the home. Even though more fathers are choosing to stay home to care for their children, many families find that having one parent stay home full-time is not an option. As you prepare to go back to work, be prepared to encounter many stumbling blocks.

Arranging child care is often the first concern. If you feel that leaving your baby with someone other than immediate family is one of the hardest things you've ever done, you're not alone. Finding good child care is difficult enough (see Chapter 9, Leaving Your Child in the Care of Others), but parting with your precious baby at day care or even at home with a baby-sitter can be emotionally wrenching.

Of course, balancing the demands of family and work falls on both parents. If a mother decides to stop working, the father may feel pressure to increase his salary to make up for the family's lost income. The opposite may be true if the father decides to stay home full-time while the mother works. Single parents may be particularly hard-pressed to provide both the financial and the emotional support for their children. In each case, there are trade-offs. All working parents at times feel out of touch with the baby. But a stay-at-home parent may feel isolated from the company of adults and overwhelmed with the constant demands of child care.

The solution to these work-family dilemmas isn't necessarily all or nothing—work or stay home. Some parents compromise, with one or both of them working less than full-time or sharing a job with a colleague, doing more work from home, or taking fewer business trips than before the baby was born. The workplace may not be as family-friendly as parents would like, but it's more flexible than it once was.

A MOTHER'S PERSPECTIVE
The Rush-Hour Meltdown

What bothered me most about working full-time was that my baby-sitter got to see my daughter at her best, and I saw her at her worst. When I'd leave in the morning she'd be cooing and smiling. But every night when I came home, she'd be fussing and crying and carrying on.

What turned things around for me was a lunchtime lecture that my company held on family and work issues. A child psychologist spoke. She began by asking, "Have any of you experienced the rush-hour meltdown? Does your child save her bad mood just for you when you walk in the door at night?" Everyone nodded. Then she said, "It's not because your child hates you. It's because your child loves you more than anyone. When you come home, she feels comfortable enough to have a breakdown. Take it as a compliment." I laughed, and then I cried.

The psychologist suggested just letting the meltdown happen. Don't expect anything different, she said. Then set aside 5 or 10 minutes just for the child. Don't make dinner. Don't look through the mail. Don't answer the phone. Take your child in your arms, and tell her about your day, and then let her coo and babble and tell you about hers.

I took her advice. It didn't prevent my daughter from crying when I came home most nights. But it gave me something to look forward to when the crying stopped. And I felt more comfortable being a working mom.

YOUR BABY AT 8 TO 12 MONTHS

Growth and Development

Your baby is growing more independent. But at the same time, he's still firmly attached to you. One minute he's crawling or cruising away from you; the next minute he's clinging to you. He may love to hand you things, but he may sometimes be afraid that you'll take them away. He may act jealous or possessive if he sees you playing with another child.

During these months, parenting enters a new phase. As your child becomes more independent, you will need to set limits when he is doing something unsafe or troublesome. Your baby's increasing mobility and willfulness may get him into trouble, and sometimes you'll have to say no. But you may be pleasantly surprised at how easily you can distract him or redirect his attention at this stage by handing him a toy or a teething biscuit.

Vision and Hearing

During this period, babies are setting their sights on things far away. They enjoy looking at objects and people across the room and even across the street. With their improved distance vision, babies can use their eyes to communicate more often. If your baby wants something that he can't reach from his high chair—a cracker from a box that's on the counter several feet away, for example—he's likely to look at it and then at you, as if to say, "Could you bring me a cracker, please?"

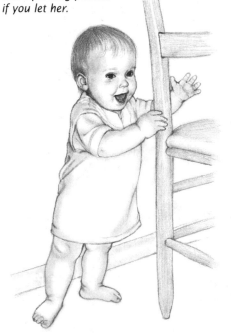

An 8- to 12-month-old baby is eager to stand and will try to pull herself up using just about any piece of furniture in her path. As if wanting to fully take in the view from this new vantage point on her world, she'll probably stand there for long periods if you let her.

You might also notice your baby looking at you for cues on how to behave. For example, he may crawl over to your slippers on the floor beside your bed, then stop and look at you across the room. If you smile, he will understand that it's OK for him to pick up one of the slippers. (He may pick it up even if you frown disapprovingly; just because he's looking at you doesn't mean he'll obey you.)

At the same time, babies become increasingly engrossed in tiny objects up close, like the O-shaped cereal and cut-up apple on the tray of their high chair. Now that your baby can see such small things well and can pick one up and put it in his mouth, watch out! All sorts of small objects will catch your baby's eye, and most will not be safe for him to eat. So make sure to keep things like loose change and your older child's small toy pieces out of your baby's reach.

■ DEVELOPMENTAL MILESTONES

Age	Most Babies	Some Babies
8 months	Stand holding onto something or someone Bang two blocks together, one held in each hand Use thumb and forefinger to pick up a small object (pincer grasp) Wave good-bye Sit without support	Say "mama" and "dada," meaning mommy and daddy Pull up to stand
9 months	Respond to their own name Understand a few words, like "no" and "bye" Imitate some sounds you make Crawl, creep, or move forward by scooting on their bottom or stomach Poke with index finger Play interactive games like patty-cake or peekaboo Feed themselves with fingers	Drink from a cup Get into a sitting position by themselves
10 months	Get into a sitting position by themselves Indicate what they want by gesture or sounds Put a block in a cup Say "mama" or "dada," meaning mommy and daddy	Say one word other than "mama" or "dada" Stand alone Roll a ball back to someone who has rolled it to them Imitate a parent's motions (So big! Holding arms wide)
11 months	Stand alone Bang two blocks held in hands	Say two words other than "mama" or "dada" Walk alone
12 months	Walk alone Have precise pincer grasp using finger and thumb Try to imitate some words Drink from a cup Look for hidden objects Wave good-bye Feed themselves most of a meal Throw a ball in play	Scribble Say three words other than "mama" and "dada" Point to named pictures ("Where's the dog?") Show own shoe or other clothing when asked Point to doll's eyes, nose, hair when asked

As you review this list of milestones, remember that children who are within the normal range will have some areas in which they excel and others in which they are slower. Not achieving a particular milestone at the designated time is not always a matter of concern. If you and your child's doctor are concerned about your child's overall development or any of your child's developmental skills, such as language, hearing, vision, or motor skills, seek the help of the appropriate specialist. For more information, see *Developmental Problems*, Part 5.

Recognizing Shapes

You may also notice that your baby is beginning to recognize some shapes. If he has blocks in different shapes and a shape sorter, you can watch him try to fit the shapes into the right hole. At first, he'll try putting any block through any opening—a square block in a round hole, for example. But by the end of the first year, he's likely to figure out that the round block is supposed to go through the round opening, and the square through the square opening. For some reason, babies recognize circles and squares long before they recognize triangles.

Checking Your Baby's Hearing

You can get a general idea of whether your child is hearing well by observing whether your child

▌ seems to understand simple phrases like "bye-bye" and "no."

▌ begins to imitate some speech sounds.

▌ enjoys and responds to toys that make sounds, such as rattles and squeaking or beeping toys.

▌ responds to sounds like a doorbell, a siren, and an airplane.

If you don't think your baby is reacting to your voice or other sounds the way he should, talk to your doctor and have his hearing tested (see ***Hearing Loss,*** Part 5). Even mild hearing loss can interfere with a baby's ability to learn to speak and understand speech.

Growing and Moving

By the end of the first year, a baby's weight has about tripled. You'll notice that your baby's head no longer looks so large in relation to the rest of his body. The rate of his head growth slows down slightly now. These proportions make it easier for your baby to sit up, stand, and walk. By 8 months, most babies can sit without support and may even start reaching for toys from a sitting position without toppling over. By about 9 or 10 months, if your baby does fall over, he'll probably be able to get back into a sitting position by himself.

During these months, your baby is constantly in motion. Put him on the floor to change him, and he's likely to flip over and crawl away. Changing such an active baby on a changing table becomes nearly impossible. Many parents diaper their babies while they're standing, just to avoid a struggle. Even this may not be so easy as your baby's first birthday approaches, and he's more likely to struggle or walk away.

SO BIG!

At 12 months, the average boy is
- 29 to 30½ inches long.
- 21 to 24½ pounds.

At 12 months, the average girl is
- 28¼ to 29¾ inches long.
- 19½ to 22½ pounds.

For more information, see Appendix: Growth Charts.

When Will My Baby Walk?

Many parents expect their babies to walk by their first birthday. Most babies begin to walk between 9 and 16 months, but a few start as early as 6 months. The exact moment when your baby takes his first steps will depend on many things, including his genes and his personality. Some babies are more active or more fearful than others, characteristics that can affect their interest in walking.

Before your baby walks by himself, he'll cruise, which means he'll walk while holding on to furniture or on to your hands. Sometimes he'll just stand for several seconds or minutes, and you'll stare at him, waiting for him to take that memorable first step. This may go on for weeks. One day, possibly when you're not expecting it, he'll take a step or two on his own. Then he'll drop to the floor and crawl again.

Many parents wonder why their babies don't just keep on walking once they've taken their first baby steps. That's because walking is hard work. For now, getting around the way he's been doing, by crawling or scooting, is easier. Eventually, of course, he'll spend most of his time walking.

As soon as she can hold her body upright while moving her legs, your baby will start cruising and she'll use anything in her path for support: a coffee table, couches, the wall, or an encouraging hand.

Eventually your baby will dare to take his first steps. They won't be graceful, and he may not do it again as soon as you'd like.

It will take practice and a good deal of energy, but eventually your baby will fine-tune her new skill

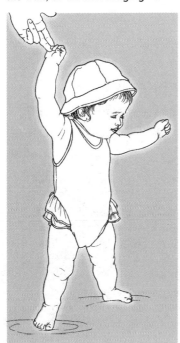

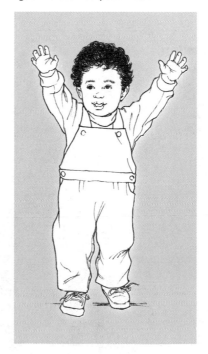

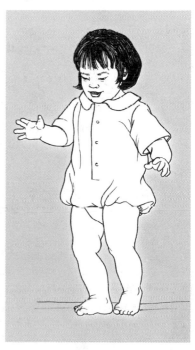

When standing or walking, babies have a unique posture: stomach and backside sticking out, back swaying, legs wide apart, feet pointing out, arms extended. Babies stand this way because the ligaments in their hips are so loose that keeping their balance is hard. The hips rotate out, forcing the legs apart and the feet to point out. A wide-based stance is more stable. Walking tightens these ligaments, thus improving a baby's balance.

QUESTIONS PARENTS ASK
Crawling, Scooting, and Other Ways of Getting Around

Q: My 10-month-old son isn't crawling, but he gets around by pulling himself across the floor in a sitting position. He looks so odd—is this normal?

A: Babies are pretty resourceful. They come up with all sorts of ways to move. Some look like soldiers on a commando raid, pulling themselves along with their arms and dragging their legs. Others adopt a spiderlike crawl by putting their hands and feet on the floor with their rear ends sticking up. Some babies never crawl. Unless you notice other signs of delay or physical problems, you needn't worry that anything's wrong. Pulling up, standing, and cruising—the activities that lead to walking—are more important.

A MOTHER'S PERSPECTIVE
My Early Walker

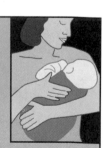

Everyone told me how lucky I was that Rose started walking early. She was only 8½ months old. When I'd take her to the playground, she was by far the smallest child walking around. I have to admit, she looked adorable.

But I felt a little sad. Rose didn't seem like a baby anymore, and I wasn't ready to give up her babyhood. She was my only child. None of her friends in our apartment building were walking yet. They sat in their mothers' arms, some of them nursing. I missed that. Seeing mothers holding their babies made me feel like crying. Rose didn't want to be held. She just wanted to walk.

I have a friend with two older children whom I talked with about it. We both realized that although we work hard to help our kids do things by themselves, when they do something new, like walk or talk, or go to school, it feels like something is lost.

Once I realized that feeling a bit sad when your child does something new is normal, I felt a little better. I went home, and as soon as I opened the door, Rose toddled over to me. I picked her up and hugged her. Of course she was still my baby! Then she wriggled out of my arms and practically swaggered into the living room. I had to laugh at the sight of this tiny person acting so grown up.

Hand It Over!

Though walking is the highlight of this period, your baby's fine motor skills are making great strides, too. With his pincer grasp, he can use his fingers skillfully to do many things. He can pick up tiny objects and move them from hand to hand. He can give objects to you. He can stick his fingers through openings, press the buttons on the telephone, and point his finger at things that catch his eye. At times, your baby may seem like a little king, sitting in his high chair throne and pointing at things that he wants you to get for him.

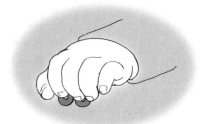

You may notice that your baby favors one hand. He uses it more often than the other one to reach for toys or feed himself. This preference doesn't necessarily mean that your baby will be right-handed or left-handed. It can change between now and the time he starts school. However, if you notice a strong preference for one hand as your baby approaches 1 year, tell your doctor. It could indicate a possible weakness on his opposite side or a neuromuscular problem.

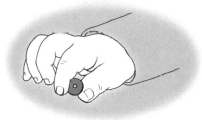

Up to this point, your child has picked up objects using a raking motion (top) with his fingers. Now, his raking grasp will give way to use of his thumb and forefinger in a more efficient pincer grasp that will enable him to pick up small objects (bottom).

Communicating

If your baby's life were a movie, he'd say his first words on or around his first birthday. But your baby's development doesn't unfold quite so neatly. Don't be alarmed if he hasn't spoken his first word by the end of his first year. Though some babies begin to talk before they're 10 months old, others wait until they're 15 months old. Most babies utter their first recognizable word when they're 12 to 15 months old. Research has found that talking to a baby can accelerate his ability to talk and understand words.

A baby's first word may be something less than endearing, like "no." Many babies find this to be an extremely useful first word and use it frequently. Or they choose something practical, like "keys" if they frequently like playing with Daddy's keys.

Naming Things

Months before your baby can say any words, he'll be able to understand some, like "bye-bye" and "Give me the ball." You can help him understand new words by pointing to objects as you name them. Tell him the word for everything that is part of his world: teddy bear, ball, truck, car, banana, juice, bottle, cup. When reading to him, point out and label the people and objects in the illustrations: girl, boy, swing, dog, cat. Use adjectives while pointing, such as "big dog" and "yellow chick." He's not ready for a story with a plot yet, but he does want to know the name of everything he sees.

Before they actually say any words, babies use certain sounds to mean certain things. All babies do this differently, but some might say "bah" for bottle or "cah" for cat. Or they might use one sound to mean a lot of things. For instance, they might say "cah" for cat, dog, and rabbit, or "duh" every time they point to or hand you something. Don't use your baby's sounds when talking to him, even if you think they're cute. Keep saying "bottle," "cat," and "car," and eventually he'll learn how to say the words himself.

During this period babies also use more gestures to communicate. They may nod or shake their heads yes or no, wave good-bye, and point to things they want. These nonverbal gestures are no less important than speaking. Gesturing is a crucial milestone that reflects your baby's desire and ability to tell you what's on his mind.

QUESTIONS PARENTS ASK
Baby Talk

Q: When I talk to my baby, I usually find myself talking in baby talk. But I feel foolish, and I don't want to teach my baby to talk like a baby. Should I stop doing this?

A: If by "baby talk" you mean that singsong, high-pitched speech that parents often use when talking to babies (called parentese), keep it up. Research shows that babies prefer listening to high-pitched voices. Using parentese may even enhance your baby's language development. In one study, the more high-pitched speech that was used when babies were 9 months old, the greater their understanding of language at 18 months, regardless of other important factors in language development, such as how well the babies communicated at 9 months and how stimulating their homes were. No one knows how parentese promotes language development. One possibility is that it effectively captures the baby's attention. The more your baby pays attention, the more he will understand. Still, you're better off using your own words rather than baby talk words when naming things. This way your baby will learn the correct names for things.

Learning

A combination of new developmental skills are working together now to enable your baby to learn new things, from tossing a ball to working a light switch. For one thing, his attention span is increasing. At 8 months old, he may have spent no more than a few minutes playing with any one toy, but at 12 months, he can probably concentrate for many minutes doing something that fascinates him. The greater his attention span, the more he learns. At the same time, the more he learns, the longer his attention span becomes, because he wants to discover more and more about how things work, feel, look, and sound. Learning breeds learning.

Babies learn by moving around, picking up whatever toys, pots, pans, or other household objects they can reach, and then handling them in different ways. They grab their parents' keys and then throw them down. They open the kitchen cabinets, take out pots, and bang them on the floor. They love making things move, pressing buttons, turning dials. They're learning about size and shape by fitting small cups into bigger cups. They're learning about cause and effect by pushing the toy car on the floor and seeing it move.

TOUCHPOINT

Don't Just Say No

Crawling and cruising babies are "into everything," and your job is to keep the dangerous things out of their reach. But try not to go overboard by saying no to everything. Babies need to explore in order to learn, and if you keep telling your baby not to touch, you risk inhibiting his curiosity. You also risk making him more determined to get the forbidden objects.

So, save your no's for immediately harmful things (matches, knives). If your baby is reaching for something that's potentially dangerous (a pen, a flashlight, the television remote control, a coin), let him handle it for a few minutes—with your close supervision. He may soon lose interest. But even if he doesn't, and he cries when you take it away, you'll be able to substitute a toy and distract him more easily if he's been allowed to get to know the object that you're removing from his grasp.   Source: Touchpoints Project (see p. 81).

Playing Memory Games

Another change that's expanding your baby's capacity to learn is his growing memory. A 9-month-old will remember that you put his toy trains in a box. He may even open the lid of the box to find them. A 12-month-old will also remember a sequence of events—for example, that you put his trains in a box, then put the box on a shelf. He might go to the shelf and point at the box when he wants to play with the train.

During these months, your baby will learn to recognize his face in the mirror, and he will love looking at it. Your baby's grasp of the concept called object permanence is also becoming more sophisticated. Now he can figure out that there's food behind the closed cabinet doors, crackers in a box, clothing in his drawers, and scores of other things tucked away out of view. It also means that he can hold an image of you in his mind when you're away from him. You can come up with fun games to entertain your baby and to test his memory at the same time. Hide a favorite toy under a blanket or put it behind you, and ask, "Where's the toy?" If he can say where it is, put a toy in a box, and then put the box in a basket. You and he can have lots of fun finding things all over the house.

Having Fun with Language

Here are several things you can do to encourage language development at this stage:

- When your baby grabs your nose, say, "nose." Do the same when he touches your ears, chin, fingers, and so on. After a while, his hand will go right to your nose when you ask, "Where's Daddy's nose?"

WHICH TOYS TO CHOOSE?

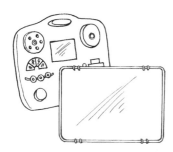

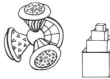

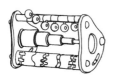

Toy	Educational Value
Unbreakable mirror	Helps babies recognize themselves
Nesting cups, stacking rings	Develop dexterity and the ability to sort objects by size and shape
Blocks	Develop dexterity; encourage crawling (babies like to crawl over to stacked blocks in order to knock them over)
Cushions or soft blow-up pillows on floor	Encourage crawling and other movement by making the baby want to explore them; promote game-playing (like playing peekaboo behind a pillow)
Bath toys like rubber ducks, jack-in-the-boxes, spinning tops, busy boxes, squeeze toys	Help children learn about cause and effect
Puzzles with knobs, boards, books, balls	Encourage fine and gross motor development
Sturdy pushcart or wagon	Helps with walking

▮ Help him see and identify his own features by giving him an unbreakable mirror to play with.

▮ Start the reading habit early using books and pointing to and naming the pictures on the page.

▮ Play turn-taking games like peekaboo or find the bunny (under the blanket).

Toys to Learn With

Gone are the days when toys were just toys. Now, they have a higher calling. Some toys are designed to develop hand-eye coordination, strengthen gross motor skills, or benefit your child's development in other ways.

But what makes a toy educational? It doesn't have to be labeled as such, and it doesn't have to cost a lot of money. Above are some toys for babies up to 1 year old that challenge their minds and bodies, in addition to being lots of fun.

Socializing

Even if you used to have no trouble leaving your baby with someone else when you went out, you may now find him clinging to you and crying. He probably has separation anxiety (see *Anxiety Disorders,* Part 5), which means that he's distressed to part from you. This distress doesn't mean that your baby is high-strung. All babies experience this problem to some degree. In fact, it's a normal development stage. Although his personality may influence how much separation anxiety he feels and how intensely he expresses it, personality is less important than his development stage. What gives rise to this anxiety is your baby's new ability to understand that when you're not with him, you're somewhere else. He misses you, and he doesn't know when he'll see you again. The moment when you leave is hardest for him. Caregivers often report that a baby cries for about 5 minutes after a parent leaves, then calms down.

Along with separation anxiety comes what is known as stranger awareness. Babies of this age are wary of strangers and other people outside their familiar circle of family and caregivers. Very young babies often don't mind if someone new picks them up, but by 8 to 12 months, babies are more likely to cry. Their discomfort around strangers is the result of their increased awareness of the world around them. The experience of meeting new people jars their senses, making them feel overwhelmed.

Dealing with Stranger Awareness

Stranger awareness can begin anytime in the second half of the first year, but it often becomes most pronounced at around 8 or 9 months. Try to avoid introducing a new caregiver at this time. But if you can't, here are some steps to pave the way:

▌ Have the caregiver get to know your baby slowly.

▌ Ask her not to rush over to your baby, but allow your child to become familiar with the new sitter from the safety of your arms or lap as you talk and listen to the sitter talk back. Your baby will see that "this is someone Mommy smiles at, who smiles back and doesn't lunge at or loom over me."

▌ Stay with the caregiver and your baby at first, then go out for short periods and gradually increase the amount of time you spend away.

▌ Schedule one or two visits with the child care person before the day you will actually be leaving your child.

▌ When it comes time for you to leave, prepare to hear your child crying. When it happens, take a deep breath and leave anyway. Expect that this flood of tears may happen again and again, even when your child is in child care. For some children (and parents), this process is easier than for others.

Striving for Independence

It may puzzle you that at the same time that babies become more clingy, they also become more independent. They show their independence in various ways: crawling away from you when you try to diaper or dress them, throwing tantrums when it's time to stop playing, and sometimes by saying the word "no." A baby who has recently learned to walk often becomes even more difficult to control. Seeing the world from a higher vantage point and being able to walk wherever he likes is exhilarating. Don't listen to people who tell you that this negative behavior is a sign that

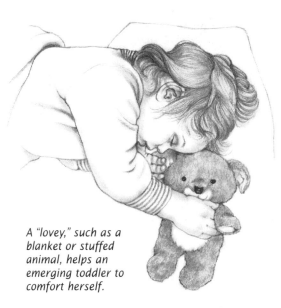

A "lovey," such as a blanket or stuffed animal, helps an emerging toddler to comfort herself.

your baby is spoiled. On the contrary, it's a sign that your baby's social and emotional development is normal.

Reading Facial Expressions

Not only is your baby more emotional, he's also more aware of other people's emotions. By about 9 months old, he can tell whether you're happy, sad, or frightened from the look on your face. And he'll "read" your face for clues on how he should behave. Parents often say they've noticed their baby glancing at them to see how they'll react when he's about to do something that he's not supposed to, like press the buttons on the television or pull books out of the bookcase. The baby wants to know what a parent thinks. A stern look is sometimes enough to stop him.

Just as you can use facial expressions to tell your baby not to do something, you can use them to tell your baby that something or someone is OK. If someone new comes to the house, for example, your baby will probably be somewhat reserved or even fearful at first. But you can help him overcome his reticence by smiling and acting upbeat.

Now that your child is beginning to understand other people's feelings, he's developing empathy. If he sees another child or someone close to him cry, he probably won't react the way an adult or an older child might, by going over and comforting the person. But he may react in another way. In one study, 12-month-olds responded to another person's distress about half the time, usually by crying, frowning, or looking at their mothers.

BINKIES, BLANKIES, AND LOVEYS

As a child, you probably had a special blanket or stuffed animal that you slept with, clutched when you were afraid, and dragged around the house. Most children have one, sometimes beginning when they are about a year old, and they may go on loving it for years, often until it falls apart. You can't pick out a so-called transitional object for your baby. But you can give him the chance to pick one for himself by leaving an assortment of stuffed animals and even receiving blankets around for him to play with. He'll find comfort in his transitional object during rough times, like when you leave for work or when he needs an immunization at the doctor's office. And when he wakes up in the middle of the night, having it near him will help him fall back to sleep on his own. You'll find he'll want it with him wherever he goes. So don't forget it, particularly when going on a trip.

For some babies, the bottle becomes their transitional object, which creates problems when you are trying to wean the child off the bottle. To avoid this, try to wean your baby from the bottle to a cup by the time he is 1 year old.

Caring for Your Baby

As your child creeps, crawls, or begins to walk his way into many new situations, your parenting skills will need to change as well. You will need to develop strategies to restrict or redirect him when he gets into trouble. Other things change at this time, too. You can offer your baby a wider array of foods, especially those that he can pick up with his fingers and feed himself. This is also the time to introduce a cup and begin weaning your baby from the bottle.

Feeding

By the time your baby is 8 to 10 months old, milk or formula will be less important in his diet than solid foods. He'll need about three meals and two snacks a day, although you'll have to be flexible about this, letting your baby determine how much he will eat and when. To encourage him to eat solids, feed him when he's hungry. In other words, don't put him in his high chair right after you've breast-fed him or given him a bottle. When your baby is about 12 months old, you can switch him to whole cow's milk rather than formula or breast milk, although there is no need to wean your baby off the breast if you and the baby want to continue breast-feeding.

Finger Foods

Toward the end of the first year, your baby should be feeding himself most of his solid food meals. You can offer him firmer, chunkier finger foods. And you can encourage him to use a spoon by giving him creamy or pureed foods that aren't too runny and stick to the spoon, like yogurt, cottage cheese, applesauce, and oatmeal. At this age, the spoon may seem like just another toy to your baby, but by 18 months he should recognize it as a tool with a purpose.

Like other facets of your baby's life, mealtime becomes less under your control and more controlled by your baby as he asserts his independence. He'll refuse to eat foods that he loved last week. Offer him well-balanced meals consisting of protein, grains, and fruits or vegetables, but don't expect him to eat something from each food group at each meal. As long as he eats well at least some of the time, he shouldn't need vitamin and mineral supplements. But if you're concerned, consult your child's doctor.

You can increase the variety of finger foods that you offer your baby. Now he can handle firm food that is chopped into small pieces. He'll eat best if you feed him when he's hungry. Put just a few things on his tray at a time so as not to overwhelm him. As in

FINGER FOODS FOR 8- TO 12-MONTH-OLDS

Fruits and Vegetables	Cereals and Grains	Protein
Cooked carrots, zucchini, potatoes, broccoli, and other vegetables cut into strips that are easy to grasp; soft fruit, like banana, apple, and pear, peeled and cut into small chunks	Macaroni, whole-grain bread cut into small pieces, crackers	Well-cooked hamburger, pieces of soft cheese, fish (avoid shellfish), chicken, tofu

the past, introduce new foods one at a time and wait about a week between each new food to watch for rashes or other allergic reactions. Offer some foods from each group at each meal (see chart).

Avoiding Unsafe Foods

Though your baby is getting better at chewing, he can still choke easily on foods that are too hard, slippery, or chewy. Never give your baby round foods like grapes and hot dogs without first cutting them into irregular shapes. Round foods can easily roll down a baby's or a toddler's throat and make him choke. Don't feed these foods yet:

- Nuts
- Raw vegetables
- Chips
- Lollipops and other hard candy
- Popcorn
- Raisins and other dried fruit
- Tough meats
- Whole grapes
- Whole hot dogs or round hot dog slices

SAFETY ALERT
Preventing Peanut Allergies

The number of children with food allergies and sensitivities has been rising, and recent research lays the blame partly on the increasing number of foods containing peanut oil and other peanut products that are fed to infants and toddlers. Peanuts are among the foods most likely to cause allergic reactions, ranging from rashes to life-threatening shortness of breath or rapid heartbeat. And although infants and toddlers outgrow most food allergies as their immune systems mature, peanut allergies sometimes remain for life. The best way to prevent peanut allergies is to avoid giving your child peanut butter until about 3 years of age, particularly if your child already has allergies or if your family has a tendency toward allergies.

Introducing a Cup

Once your baby starts feeding himself finger food, he's ready to drink from a cup. Look for a sipping cup with handles and a screw-on top with a spout. Some cups have tops that snap on, but your curious infant may pull them off and pour the contents all over himself. Begin by offering your baby a small amount of water, juice, formula, or breast milk in a cup. You might even try showing him how to drink from the cup by pretending to take a sip from it and then handing it to him.

Don't expect him to drink much, if anything, at first. To your baby, the cup is just another plaything to be shaken, banged, and tossed. It can take many months before he drinks enough formula or milk from a cup to be completely weaned from a bottle or the breast. The important thing is to stick with the cup. Offer it to your baby at mealtime, and he'll gradually get used to it.

Weaning Your Breast-Fed Baby

As your baby approaches his first birthday, you may hear comments from relatives and acquaintances like, "You're still nursing!" or "Now that your baby's walking, isn't he too old to nurse?" But the American Academy of Pediatrics recommends that babies breast-feed for at least a year, if possible. The time for weaning is when you and your baby are ready.

In a perfect world, mothers and babies would be ready to give up breast-feeding at the same time. But things often don't work out that way. A mother may want to wean earlier because she needs to return to work and doesn't want to use a breast pump. Or a baby who's been breast-feeding and bottle-feeding may prefer bottles, because he can hold his own bottle now and bottles make it easier to drink and look around at the same time. Babies often send signals that they are ready—mainly by squirming or turning away or repeatedly biting on the breast.

It'll be easiest on you and probably on your baby if you wean gradually. Your breasts will become less engorged if you stop nursing over a period of weeks and give your body a chance to decrease milk production. To start weaning, follow these steps:

▌ Replace one breast-feeding every few days with formula (or whole milk if your baby is at least a year old).

▌ Offer your child milk or formula in a cup rather than a bottle so that you won't have to wean your baby later on from the bottle. If using a bottle, feed it to your baby by hand.

▌ Continue your morning and bedtime nursing for a while if these are the most special or relaxed times for you and your child.

▌ Relieve breast engorgement, if it is painful, by wearing a support bra and applying ice packs to the breasts to reduce the swelling.

QUESTIONS PARENTS ASK
Weaning from the Bottle

Q: I've heard that babies shouldn't drink from a bottle after 1 year old, but my son seems so attached to his bottle that I don't like the thought of taking it away until he seems ready.

A: There are good reasons for weaning your baby off the bottle by 12 months. Babies over 1 year old are more likely to consider their bottle a security object, demanding to carry it around when they play or have it when they sleep. These habits can lead to health problems. For one thing, a baby may consume too much milk or juice, and not enough solid foods. In addition, a child is likely to fall asleep while drinking, a practice that can lead to tooth decay and possibly to ear infections.

Your best course is to gradually wean your baby off the bottle by his first birthday. At this age, children have short memories, and within a few days he will forget about it. Encourage him to find other ways to comfort himself—by choosing a favorite toy or blanket to have with him, for example.

Food Fights

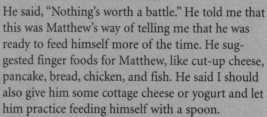

Matthew started out as a great eater. He loved every baby food I gave him. He loved yogurt, cottage cheese, and bananas. He'd smile and make little windmill motions with his arms to show his enthusiasm whenever I put him in the high chair. We'd eat together and have conversations. Mealtime was a special time for us.

But things started to change when Matthew was around 9 months old. Sometimes when I put him in the high chair, he'd arch his back and fuss. When I tried to put a spoonful of food in his mouth, he'd grab the spoon and wave it around. Food splattered on the floor, on the walls, and all over him. I didn't mind the mess so much, but I was getting worried that he wasn't eating enough. He wasn't coordinated enough to spoon-feed himself, but he resisted when I tried to feed him.

I called our pediatrician. I said, "I have so much trouble getting Matthew to eat when I feed him. Is it worth the battle?" He said, "Nothing's worth a battle." He told me that this was Matthew's way of telling me that he was ready to feed himself more of the time. He suggested finger foods for Matthew, like cut-up cheese, pancake, bread, chicken, and fish. He said I should also give him some cottage cheese or yogurt and let him practice feeding himself with a spoon.

To my surprise, Matthew ate more finger food than I thought he would. I wasn't worried that he'd starve. He still tossed the foods he didn't like, and when he used the spoon more food landed in his hair than in his mouth. But I could see that he was just being a baby, not an angry baby.

Sleeping

By 8 to 12 months, most babies can sleep for 9 to 10 hours at a stretch without a feeding. So some parents are enjoying a full night's sleep by now. But just when you were getting used to feeling well rested, your baby starts waking up at 2 A.M. again. What's going on? Is something the matter with him? Did you do something wrong?

It's nobody's fault. Your baby's nighttime awakenings at around 9 months old are as normal a part of his development as his new ability to understand that an object (or a parent) still exists even when he can't see it. He will naturally want to see you when he wakes up in the middle of the night and you're not there. He knows you're somewhere in the house, and he knows how to bring you to him—by crying.

Responding to Nighttime Crying

Just how you handle his nighttime separation anxiety is up to you. You may feel that it's your responsibility as a loving parent to comfort him when he awakens. Just realize that the more you go to him in the middle of night, the more he's going to demand that you be with him then. So you may not have a good night's sleep for a while.

Another option is not to go to him right away. Let him cry for several minutes to give him a chance to comfort himself. He'll have the easiest time settling down if he has a special doll or a security blanket to cuddle up with. If he doesn't, encourage him to find one by putting a choice of stuffed animals, dolls, or receiving blankets in his crib. Many babies will cry for a few minutes, grope around for their "blankie," then hug it, suck their thumb, and go back to sleep. For a step-by-step method of helping your child learn to fall back to sleep by himself, see page 136.

If your baby doesn't stop crying, or if the crying grows louder and more urgent, don't overlook the possibility that he's getting sick. If your baby is sick, you'll see other signs, such as fever, runny nose, congestion, cough, or diarrhea. Ear infections, a common illness in babies in this age group, often cause nighttime awakenings. When your baby is not feeling well and can't sleep, he can't help but cry. Take his temperature to see if he has a *fever* (see Part 5). Do whatever you can to comfort him, and call your baby's doctor for advice.

TOUCHPOINT

Up at Night

When babies are on the brink of doing something new, like standing or walking, they often become crankier than usual and wake up more often at night. The effort of trying to do something new may be creating inner turmoil that makes babies restless, frustrated, or just out of sorts. Rest assured that these setbacks are temporary, and once your baby is comfortable with his new skill, he'll sleep better and have a sunnier disposition.

Source: Touchpoints Project (see p. 81).

Setting Limits

On the one hand, your baby is still so small and innocent. On the other hand, he can be quite a terror. He may hit or bite you when he gets angry. He may put dirt in his mouth. He may dart into the street. How do you get the upper hand without being heavy-handed? First of all, praise him and reward him for good behavior. Next, stop him when he does something wrong.

It is important for parents to set clear, consistent limits for their children, which form the basis of discipline. Although an infant under 1 year old is not ready for regular discipline techniques, the use of simple commands and an authoritative tone of voice can be effective when your child is doing something that may harm him, another child, or the upholstery on your new sofa. When he misbehaves, pull him aside immediately and say, "No biting," or "Stop!" Or, if he puts something from the floor into his mouth, say, "Yuck! No!" Keep it brief. Your baby can't follow elaborate explanations, like "Biting is really bad, because it hurts and spreads germs." He has only the vaguest concept of cause and effect. But he does understand the word "no," even though he doesn't always obey you when you say it.

There is never a good reason to spank a child. The American Academy of Pediatrics recommends that parents of children of all ages choose other methods of disciplining their children.

No One Likes to Be the Bad Guy

Being the one who has to say no is hard. But if you set consistent, loving limits for your child, he can learn, gradually, to set limits for himself. That is, he can learn self-control. To do this, he needs to know where the boundaries are, and within those boundaries, he needs freedom to make his own choices. It may surprise you to know that children want to have clear limits set by adults. These limits make them feel secure because they fear unpredictable situations where the rules are not clear. So set your limits, and let him go. If he exceeds those limits, it's time to step in.

One way to control your child's problem behavior at this age while allowing him as much freedom as possible is to take certain measures to prevent problem behavior. You can't prevent all bad behavior, of course, but you can reduce the number of times it occurs by avoiding the situations that make it happen. Here are some examples:

▌ If your baby bites, give him a teething ring or a soft plastic toy to bite instead.

▌ Cover or remove fragile or valuable items. If he keeps banging his toys on the good furniture, remove or cover the furniture to protect it. Put anything you don't want him to touch out of reach.

▌ Child-proof your home. Though you may not have thought of it as a disciplining tool, childproofing is one of the most effective ways to keep young children in line—or at least to reduce the opportunities to misbehave. If your baby delights in throwing things in the toilet, for instance, get a lid lock that holds the toilet seat down. See the section on baby-proofing that begins on page 141.

Your baby is too young to be punished. Don't hit or spank him. You may lose control and seriously hurt him. And don't give him a time-out yet; he won't understand the connection between the time he spends alone in a chair and what he did wrong. Time-outs often become effective after about age 12 months.

Catch Him Being Good

Discipline isn't just a matter of correcting bad behavior. Make sure to praise your child when he does something good. After crossing the street you might say, "Great job holding hands." Or if you see him crawl over to the VCR and not put his hand inside, give him a hug for exercising self-control. Your baby craves your attention, and pretty soon he'll understand that he will get it when he behaves well.

Other effective discipline strategies are substitution and distraction. If your 12-month-old is trying to grab a toy away from another child, hand him another toy. He'll probably become fascinated with the new toy and forget about the other one. If he's fussing while sitting in a waiting room, take him to look out a window or in a mirror or take him outdoors. Distraction is a handy trick to use now, because the baby is so easy to distract. As he gets older and more headstrong, he'll be less willing to change his focus or accept substitutes for the things he really wants.

In a baby's mind, any attention from you—even if it's a firm "No!"—is better than no attention at all. So be selective when you correct him. Besides, if you react whenever he does something that annoys you, your firm tone of voice and stern look will lose their power. Correct only the behavior that's dangerous to your baby, to another person, or to your property, then grit your teeth and ignore the rest. Ignoring behavior that you want to discourage can be a powerful tool if your child is doing it to gain your attention. Disciplining your baby often means disciplining yourself.

Keeping Your Baby Healthy

More and more, your baby is out in the world. He may be attending a play group or child care. The more people your child comes in contact with, the more likely he is to pick up infections. That makes your job as the front-line health caregiver all the more important. Take him for regular checkups. Keep him up-to-date on immunizations, watch for signs of illness, practice good hygiene, and keep your home and car safe.

Checkups

Your baby should have a checkup at 9 months and 12 months. As usual, the doctor or nurse will weigh your baby, measure his length and head circumference, and plot them on the growth chart (see Appendix: Growth Charts) to be sure he is growing at a normal rate. The doctor will examine your child and then ask questions about language development, learning, behavior, and health concerns. Be prepared with your own questions.

At 12 months, if your baby is walking, the doctor will examine his feet and observe his gait to make sure the bones in his legs and feet appear normal. The doctor will probably also ask whether your baby is saying any words—she will have to rely on your report, because your baby probably won't speak in her office. If your baby isn't saying any words yet, discuss the sorts of babbling sounds that he's making and mention his use of nonverbal communication, such as pointing, and whether he seems to understand some of what you are saying.

Finally, at the 12-month visit, many doctors take a few moments to acknowledge the milestone of the baby's first birthday. It's a time for the doctor and parents to reflect just how far the child has come.

See Childhood Immunization Schedule, page 110.

Screening Tests

At the 12-month checkup, your baby may have the following tests:

Tuberculosis: This skin test indicates whether your baby has been exposed to the bacteria that cause *tuberculosis* (see Part 5), a chronic infectious disease that usually affects the lungs, yet can affect almost any part of the body. The test detects the presence of antibodies—immune system chemicals that are produced to fight bacteria—and is given only to children in high-risk groups.

Hemoglobin screening: This finger-prick blood test measures the concentration of hemoglobin in red blood cells. A hemoglobin deficiency is a sign of anemia. The test is usually done at the same time as the lead screening (see below), usually at 9 or 12 months of age.

Blood lead: A finger-prick or venous (blood taken from the vein) blood test measures the amount of lead in your child's blood. Ask your doctor about getting the venous test, which is sometimes more accurate than the finger-prick. For information on test results, see **Lead Poisoning,** Part 5.

Lead is a toxic metal that can cause lowered intelligence, **attention-deficit disorder** (see Part 5), or other neuro-developmental problems. After getting into the bloodstream, lead is stored permanently in the brain, bone, liver, kidneys, and other organs, where it can cause symptoms including irritability, fatigue, weakness, and clumsiness. Lead can get into a child's body from various sources, such as deteriorating lead paint, lead-containing dust around the house, and drinking water contaminated by lead pipes in your house or town. For information on taking steps to make your home safe, see **Lead Poisoning,** Part 5.

The Centers for Disease Control and Prevention considers an infant or a young child to be at high risk of lead poisoning under the following circumstances:

■ He lives in, regularly visits, or attends day care in a house built before 1978 that either has peeling paint or is undergoing a renovation. (Lead paint was banned in 1977.)

■ He has a brother, sister, or playmate with lead poisoning.

■ He lives with an adult exposed to lead through a job or hobby.

■ He lives near an active lead smelter, a battery recycling plant, or another industry likely to release lead into the environment.

Keeping Your Baby Safe

Around this time many parents find that their babies have acquired certain skills that are not listed among the milestones—the skills of an escape artist. They include climbing out of the high chair, standing up in the stroller, and dashing into the street. It's time to take some new steps to keep your child from harming himself, while still allowing him to explore his world.

To prevent accidents, make sure that your baby is always strapped securely into the high chair or the stroller. If your baby is walking, carry him when crossing the street or walking in a busy parking lot or insist that he hold your hand. Once your baby can stand, remove the bumpers from his crib and move the mattress to the lowest level to prevent him from climbing out.

Other hazards for your increasingly mobile baby are your older child's toys. Even if you're careful to store toys with tiny pieces on a high shelf, your baby can still reach them when your older child is playing with them.

Your child's car seat shouldn't be changed to the forward-facing position until he has reached at least 1 year of age and weighs at least 20 pounds. If your infant's weight exceeds the seat's weight limit before the end of his first year, the American Academy of Pediatrics recommends switching to a convertible seat with a higher weight limit and that can be used facing the rear or front. Be sure to check the instructions on your convertible seat. For more information on car seat safety, see page 369.

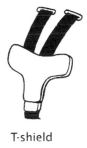

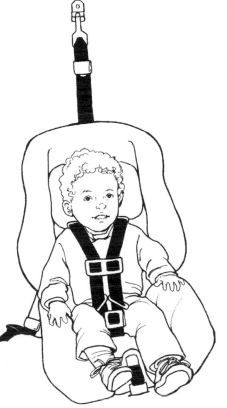

Convertible seats have three types of harnesses. If you are using a convertible seat for a small infant, the American Academy of Pediatrics recommends using the five-point harness for a more secure fit. Whatever seat you choose, follow your car seat instructions to be sure that the harness is adjusted to fit your baby and that the seat is buckled into your vehicle correctly. If your car seat has a tether strap, be sure it is properly secured to its anchor.

Overhead shield

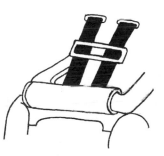

T-shield

Five-point harness

A Parent's Life

Each stage of your baby's life presents new parenting challenges. For example, though you may feel more comfortable leaving your baby with a sitter for a night out now than when he was younger, your baby may actually protest more when you leave. In addition, he's probably interacting and interfering more with his older siblings—another challenge for your parenting skills.

Going Out

Unless you're fortunate enough to have relatives who can watch your baby whenever you go out, you'll have to find some baby-sitters (see Guide to Selecting the Occasional Baby-Sitter, p. 336). When and how often you go out is up to you. Some parents find it important to have a night out once a week. Others avoid going out entirely during their baby's early months because they're worried about the things that can go wrong if they do—their nursing baby won't take a bottle, the baby won't go to sleep, the sitter won't be able to stop him from crying. Working parents who think that they don't spend enough time with their babies may feel guilty about spending more time away. But it is important for parents to have some stress-free time away from their children, to pay attention to their own needs, and, if married, to have time to maintain their relationship with their spouse. Taking some time for yourself will make you a better parent to your baby.

Your baby will probably find it easier to get used to you going out regularly if you begin before he's 9 months old, the age when separation anxiety usually begins. Your baby may cry when he's first held by a baby-sitter, but that's more a reaction to the strangeness of a new experience than to sorrow that you're leaving. The crying probably won't last for more than a few minutes.

If you're happy spending most of your time with the baby, that's fine. But if the daily routine of either being housebound with your baby or taking him with you wherever you go is wearing on you, you'll do your baby and yourself a favor by getting out of the house on your own now and then. Some time apart can be the best thing for both of you.

Parent as Referee

Many parents find that their older child's competitive feelings intensify when the baby starts to crawl or walk. At first, the only thing that the baby could take away was your attention. Now he's grabbing the older child's toys. He's a double threat. Your older child may start behaving more aggressively toward the baby, treating him roughly, grabbing toys away, or deliberately pushing him down when he walks.

By the end of the first year, sibling rivalry begins to cut both ways. Suddenly, your baby no longer sits placidly as you listen to your 4-year-old tell a long story or help her do a jigsaw puzzle. The baby whimpers and puts his arms up for you to carry him. He's competing for your attention.

Helping Your Older Child Cope

Here are some suggestions for making your older child feel less threatened:

▍ Store her toys in a place where the baby can't get them, for example, in a closet or in boxes with lids that he can't open. Aside from the rivalry issue, keeping these toys out of the baby's reach is necessary for safety if they are small enough to choke on.

▍ When your older child is playing with her toys, distract the baby with his own toys, preferably in another room.

Preventing the baby from vying for your attention when you're with your older child is more difficult. Perhaps the best you can do is put his whining in the same category as his throwing food and throwing tantrums. It's something babies do, and you'll have to live with it. Some parents become skilled at dividing their time between two or more children at once—picking up the baby and handing him a rattle while reading to an older child. Your children will come to realize that each one can't have the spotlight all the time. Each one, however, is entitled to have some of your undivided attention. Spend time alone with your older child when the baby naps, and let the baby have you to himself when the older one's at school or playing with a friend.

Meeting Other Parents

If you have friends with babies who are close in age to yours, consider yourself lucky. You can call people other than your immediate family when your baby does something new, delightful, disturbing, funny, or amazing. Other parents also give you someone to ask for the kind of advice that you can only get from a friend.

Knowing other parents has additional benefits. New parents can feel isolated and alone at home with a baby. Joining friends or participating in activities with other parents can stave off feelings of depression and loneliness. So connect with a play group or parent group in your area. You may find these groups through churches, libraries, and other local community organizations. Even attending infant exercise classes or other classes geared toward babies can help you meet other parents with children the same age as yours.

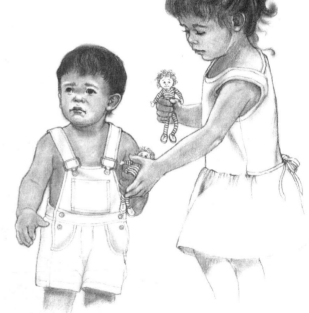

In your older child's eyes, one of the worst offenses an emerging toddler can commit is taking one of her toys. She may launch into a tantrum or rip the toy out of the baby's hand. One way to help avoid sibling conflict is to store her toys out of your baby's reach.

5 Your Toddler

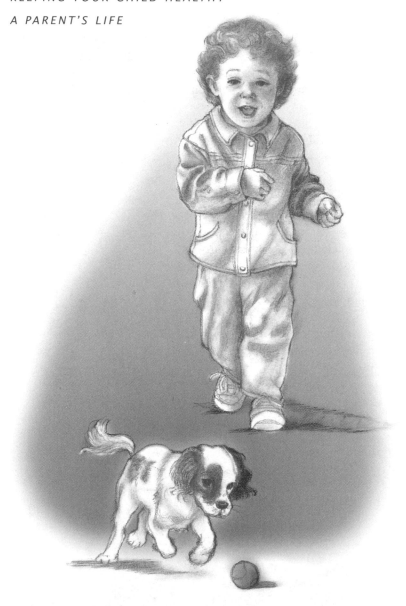

172

S tand back. The toddler years are here. But don't back off too far, because although your child is seeking independence at every turn, he'll need your constant attention and vigilance to feel safe and well loved and on the road to learning.

Because children change so rapidly from ages 1 to 3, the growth and development part of this chapter is divided into two sections: Your 1-Year-Old and Your 2-Year-Old. The later sections on health care and parenting in this chapter address the needs of both 1- and 2-year-old children.

Your 1-Year-Old

One-year-old children are exuberant. They walk into a room as if they own it. They think everything is theirs to explore. There's no cabinet door they won't open, no button they won't press, no knob they won't turn. Nothing can stop them. Fear? Danger? Self-control? These don't exist in the mind of a 1-year-old child.

Of course, these perils and concerns are uppermost in your mind. You may feel that you spend most of your time shadowing your child to make sure that he doesn't get into trouble. Turn your back to get groceries out of the car, and your child is tumbling down the front steps. Answer the phone, and he's heading for the bathroom to unroll the toilet paper. More than infancy, toddlerhood is a time of contrasts: On the one hand is your child's growing ability to walk and talk, on the other is his lack of coordination and limited vocabulary. Toddlers don't know that they can't do everything, and when they bump up against their limitations—or limitations imposed by you—they may cry in frustration or scream, "NO!"

Don't take this personally. A child's "no" is a declaration of independence, an all-purpose expression for complicated thoughts that he doesn't know how to express, like, "I want to do it my way!" A child's love affair with the word "no" is actually a sign of normal development.

Growing and Moving

A 1-year-old child grows more slowly than he did in the first year. Between the first and second birthday, a child gains roughly 3 to 5 pounds, about the same amount that he gained during only 4 months last year. The average child grows about 4 inches during this year. Head circumference may increase by about 1 to $1\frac{1}{2}$ inches. Although growth is slower, your child's appearance will change significantly between 1 and 2 years old. At 12 months his arms and legs, his face, and his middle will still be round and soft. But as he spends his days in perpetual motion, he'll slim down. By 15 months, a noticeable amount of baby fat will have disappeared.

Learning to walk (a gross motor skill) ushers in a new development phase of almost every kind of physical ability. Your child's first steps are shaky, with feet apart and arms extended for balance. But with time and confidence, his legs will move closer together and he'll no longer need to hold his arms out to keep from falling.

DEVELOPMENTAL MILESTONES

Age	Most Children	Some Children
15 months	Walk well, stoop	Say more than six words
	Climb stairs with help	Remove some clothing
	Say three to six words	Use words to make wants known
	Understand simple commands, like "Go and get your shoes"	Walk upstairs with help
		Stack two blocks
	Stack two blocks	
	Drink from a cup	
	Use a spoon or fork	
	Listen to a brief story	
18 months	Walk backward	Stack four blocks
	Throw a ball (but not overhand)	Brush teeth with help
	Say 10 words	Wash and dry hands
	Use a pull toy	Put on some clothing
	Stack two blocks	Combine words ("Go car" or "More juice")
	Name some objects in a book while listening to a story	Throw ball overhand
	Point to several body parts	Point to pictures in a book
	Scribble with a crayon, and copy a vertical line drawn by parent	

As you review this list of milestones, remember that children who are within the normal range will have some areas in which they excel and others in which they are slower. Not achieving a particular milestone at the designated time is not always a matter of concern. If you and your child's doctor are concerned about your child's overall development or any of your child's developmental skills, such as language, hearing, vision, or motor skills, seek the help of the appropriate specialist. For more information, see *Developmental Problems*, Part 5.

Note: The 1-year (12-month) milestones appear in Chapter 4, Your Baby's First Year, page 151.

This frees his hands to do other things while he walks, like carry a toy, or stoop to grab something. He'll also be free to grasp railings and rungs, which allows him to climb stairs and playground ladders.

The more children use their hands (a fine motor skill), the more things they learn to do with them. Their growing dexterity will be especially apparent at mealtime. At first, self-feeding skills will be limited to picking up pieces of food with their fingers. At 12 months, their use of the thumb and forefinger together to grasp things is usually quite refined. By 12 to 15 months, many children can drink from a sipping cup. And by 15 to 18 months, they often begin using a spoon. Children this age also have some success using a fork for easy-to-stab foods, like sticky bits of cake.

Your baby's maturing fine motor skills open up new possibilities for play. Look, for example, at the way your child handles building blocks. At 12 months, chances are he won't do much more than knock down the towers that you build. But by about 15 months, he may be able to build two-block towers of his own, and at 18 months, his towers may be three or four blocks tall.

Making Physical Activity Fun

You can encourage your child's motor development by providing opportunities like these:

▌Find something your child can climb on safely (foam cushions, for example) and encourage him to do so. Some parents place a baby gate across the second step of a carpeted stairway to let their toddler practice going up and down two steps safely.

▌Provide stacking toys and lots of bulky, brightly colored toys so that your child can handle a variety of things.

▌Encourage hand skills with cloth or board books that have doors to open and textures to feel.

During the initial stages of toddlerhood, fine motor skills become more refined.
(A) *Toddlers grow increasingly keen on imitating what you do. Show your little one how to stack blocks, and he'll follow your lead. By the time he's 18 months old, he may be able to build a four-block-high tower.*
(B) *With spoon in fist, your independence-seeking 15- to 18-month-old will insist on feeding himself. Expect the learning experience to be a messy one.*
(C) *During this stage, your toddler may discover that crayons really aren't meant to be chewed on. She'll grasp a crayon in the same fisted fashion she does a spoon and will scribble her first masterpieces fit for your baby book.*

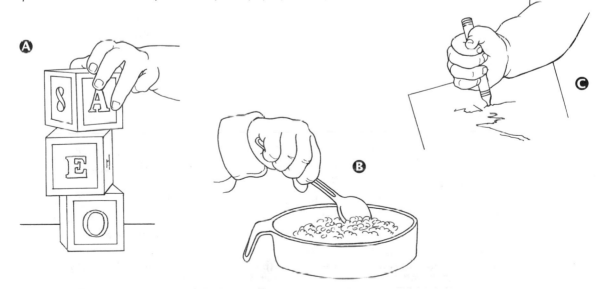

Communicating

Learning to communicate with words is one of the most remarkable achievements of the second year. At the beginning of the year, children may just babble or may say a few words and communicate mostly with gestures, like pointing. But by the end of the second year, at age 2, they usually show signs of being able to hold a rudimentary conversation. They may link words into short sentences, such as "Go out!" And in between they'll be adding to their vocabulary day by day. Parents tend to get most excited about the words their children say (expressive language), but just as important are the words children understand (receptive language). Receptive language tends to develop more rapidly than expressive language. An 18-month-old may say few words but understand a great deal more, including two-step instructions like, "Hold your doll and feed her." Language skills mirror more closely the growth of a child's brain than any other aspect of development.

Remember that the development rate of both of these language skills varies widely. It depends on many things, including family history, gender, and how much a child is spoken and read to. In general, girls learn to speak sooner than boys. At 15 months, most children are saying at least three words, but children this age have astonishing variation in vocabulary. Keep a record in your baby book.

Labeling Things

One reason that language development gains momentum from roughly 18 to 24 months is that children come to understand a concept that most adults take for granted: that there's a word for everything. So, now they go around pointing at objects and asking, "What's this?" Another possible reason, new research suggests, is that toddlers this age can learn new words by watching someone who's talking. If you say, "I'm going to close the window," for example, a 12-month-old baby may simply glance around the room and focus on the most interesting object. But gradually, as the months pass, your child may be able to figure out what "window" is by following your gaze and gestures while hearing the label spoken. When a toddler says "car," he may mean car, bus, or truck. Toddlers this age commonly use one word for many related things, like "car" for all wheeled vehicles.

Pronouncing Words

Regardless of how many words your child is saying, he probably isn't pronouncing them all clearly. You may have a lot of trouble understanding what he's saying. You may wonder, for example, what your 15-month-old means when he says, "cah": Is it "car" or "cat"? Your child's pronunciation may improve as he nears 2 years, but you'll still have to guess at what he's trying to say on occasion.

It will be years before your child can pronounce everything flawlessly. Some sounds are difficult for many toddlers to pronounce, such as the consonant sounds of *s, sh,* and the combination *th.* But even when they can pronounce a sound, toddlers still tend to simplify or shorten words by repeating the first consonant and vowel sound and not saying the sounds that follow. So, "noodle" becomes "noo-noo"

...your child's mispronunciation. But if you ...ld may hear the difference and improve his ...king baby talk. You may think it's cute when ...example by calling noodles by their proper ...hat you say and imitating the sounds you

...y string together sounds and made-up words ...of language development, and by about 2 ...ctual speech.

...ent, talk to your toddler in simple sentences and ask ...s and repeat them in words. Say, "Play with teddy?" ...ed animal. Expand things he says. For example, if ...r bunny book," or "Do you want Daddy to read ...e a sentence by guessing what he wants to say and ...ere are some more suggestions:

- Look at picture books together, naming what you see.
- Don't use baby talk; use the correct word, and eventually your child will catch on.
- Sing to your child.
- Play audio tapes of children's songs.
- Try talking books and toys.

Learning

Toddlers learn by doing. They learn best where they have the freedom to wander around and pick up, pull, push, hold, sit, and move with various toys. For example, hands-on experience playing with blocks helps children understand that squares are different from triangles. Pointing at pictures of animals in books teaches children that although dogs come in various shapes, colors, and sizes, they're all dogs and they're all different from, say, ducks. Children at 15 months may show that they understand these concepts by grouping squares separately from triangles and dogs separately from ducks. Through play, toddlers also learn that their actions can make things happen. Turning the crank on the jack-in-the-box makes the clown pop up, for example, and leaning forward on the rocking horse makes it move.

Symbolic Play

Another important concept that children understand at this age is that toys are symbols for things in real life. In the course of playing with a doll and a doll's bottle, your child will see that the doll's bottle is like his own, and he'll probably put the bottle in his own mouth. He'll soon build on the association by using the bottle to feed the doll. Or he may put the doll on the miniature bed or push a car as if he were driving

Symbolic play is the basis for a broad range of learning, such as understanding what is real and what is imaginary and, in years to come, how to add and subtract, read and write. Letters and numbers, after all, are just symbols representing other things.

Learning Through Ideas

As with language development, 18 months is a turning point in the development of your child's mind. He used to learn exclusively from his senses—how things looked and smelled, how they felt when he put them in his mouth. Now he can learn from ideas. Some toddlers begin to develop a sense of past, present, and future, for example, looking forward to when Mommy or Daddy comes home late in the day.

Developing Memory

Your child's memory is also becoming keener. You may see evidence of this when you take him to someone's home that he visited a few weeks before. He may look for certain toys that he played with before or point to the location on the kitchen counter where the cookie jar sat last time.

Solving Problems

Between 1½ and 2 years, children start to solve problems creatively. If a ball rolls under the couch beyond your child's reach, for instance, he might try to get it out by prodding it with something long and thin, like a ruler. If he wants something in the kitchen that's too high for him to reach, he might figure out that one solution is to carry the step stool from the bathroom and stand on it.

Stimulate Learning

You have many opportunities to encourage your child's learning at this time:

▌ Allow your child to try new things, and don't assume he can't do something because he couldn't do it a few weeks ago.

▌ Let your child "help" with the housework. Give him a dust cloth to buff the chair rungs. Give him a sponge to help wash the car's hubcaps.

▌ Provide puzzles with large pieces or with handles.

▌ Encourage your child to dance to music.

▌ Go to the playground, and let your child try out the equipment.

▌ Show him a mirror; children this age can now recognize themselves.

Social and Emotional Development

Your child's most important social relationship is still with you, the parent. You are his anchor in a sea of wonderful things to explore. He is more independent but still clings to you—he wants to know you're there when he sets out across the play area, and what's more important, that you will be there when he returns. Take him to a birthday party, and he'll probably be excited by the sight of children playing. But he may not leave your lap. If he does, it might be just to make short forays into the group and then to return. You are his home base. Knowing that you are there for him and feeling securely attached to you gives him the confidence to leave your lap for those brief periods and explore the world.

Your child's love for you spurs another facet of social and emotional development during this period: empathy, or feeling for others. Many 12-month-old children can recognize, based on a person's expression and behavior, whether someone is upset. They may respond by crying, frowning, or looking at their parents. In one study, children this age responded to another person's distress about half the time. By the time they're 18 months, many children try to comfort a distressed person by touching or patting her. But it isn't until they're 2 years old that children actually try to help, for example, by saying comforting words. Children are most likely to be empathic if they are treated with empathy themselves.

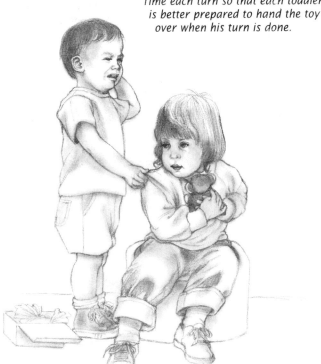

When toddlers play side by side, they often imitate each other and, as a result, usually compete aggressively for the same toy. Try teaching the young playmates to take turns. Time each turn so that each toddler is better prepared to hand the toy over when his turn is done.

TOUCHPOINT

Playing with Other Children

As your child's second year progresses, you may have serious concerns about his social graces. He'll play alongside other children without a smile to acknowledge their presence—a style of playing often called parallel play. But when he does interact with peers, it may be to grab toys out of their hands or shout, "Mine!" At some point, you might even catch your little angel hitting or biting another child. Sandbox encounters frequently turn into screaming matches.

It may not seem that much good is happening when two possessive toddlers get together, but there is. By 18 months, your child can benefit from spending time with other children regularly, whether in a play group, at the park, in day care, or with play dates. Children learn from one another as well as from adults and siblings. They learn new words and gestures by copying what other children say and do. They learn about social relations by giggling when a playmate giggles, scooping sand alongside another child or, of course, clutching their possessions or seizing other children's toys and then seeing what happens. So let your child spend time with other children his age—even if all they seem to do is fight or ignore each other— he's taking the first steps toward making friends.   Source: Touchpoints Project (see p. 81).

Gender Differences

Are girls by nature partial to dolls and boys to trucks and trains? No one knows. Some parents try to counter these stereotypes by buying their girls train sets and making sure their boys have at least one doll. But despite these efforts, many parents treat their sons and daughters differently—even if they do so unconsciously. For example, researchers have observed that parents tend to show more sympathy when their daughters are in pain than when their sons are. Their response to their children's anger is a different story. Mothers tend to become angry when their daughters express anger, but show concern and sympathy when their sons are angry. How do these cues shape a child's behavior? They may encourage boys to hide their pain and vent their anger. And they might be telling girls that showing pain is OK, but revealing anger isn't.

Attachment and Working Parents

As your child grows more independent and yet continues to need your constant attention, you may wonder whether working outside the home will make him less attached to you. But research shows that this is not the case. Toddlers whose mothers work are no less attached to them than toddlers whose mothers stay home are attached to their mothers. In one study, researchers measured attachment by observing a child's reaction when his mother returned after having been away. The amount of time mothers spent at work mattered less than how well they interacted with their children when they were with them. Mothers who were sensitive to their children's needs, who listened and talked to them, and who were generally cheerful had strongly attached children. Mothers who were depressed or indifferent had children not as strongly attached. This study suggests that parents needn't feel guilty about working. Instead, when you are home, make sure to be attentive to your child, playing and interacting with him in a positive and focused way.

QUESTIONS PARENTS ASK
Masturbation

Q: Our 15-month-old son has started handling his penis every chance he gets. What should we do?

A: Toddlers are fascinated by their ears, noses, and other body parts, so it's natural for them to touch their genitals. This is normal exploration, and it probably feels good to him. Don't pull your son's hands away or scold him. The behavior is not bad or harmful, and the best response is no response. If he seems to be doing this out of boredom, you can try to distract him by engaging him in a game or offering him an interesting toy. If your child is touching his genitals very often or persistently, consult your doctor just to make sure there is no health condition that may be causing him discomfort.

Your 2-Year-Old

Just how terrible are the twos? Many parents approach their child's second birthday in trepidation because of the horror stories they've heard: the temper tantrums, the defiance, the nightmares. They're all true. Two-year-old children throw tantrums, disobey their parents, and wake up in the middle of the night crying.

But there's a flip side that makes the twos, in many ways, terrific. The rapid brain growth and development at this time causes an astonishing leap in maturity, which most parents find far outweighs the difficult behavior. You may notice that your child might be less clingy and more talkative and may begin to show the first signs of readiness for toilet training. Turn around, and you may see your child copying your movements as you set the table or brush your teeth or engage in other daily rituals. Imitation reaches new heights. You'll hear your own words coming out of your child's mouth. So watch what you say—children imitate the bad as well as the good.

Growing and Moving

Two-year-olds don't look so much like toddlers anymore. Gone is the wide stance with the feet pointing outward. Now that their balance has matured, they stand with their feet pointing straight, like an older child or an adult.

Toddlers this age also act more like big kids. The change in their posture enables them to run faster than before and walk up and down stairs without clutching an

■ DEVELOPMENTAL MILESTONES

Age	Most Children	Some Children
2 years	Go up and down stairs one step at a time	Jump
	Kick a ball	Stack eight blocks
	Throw overhand	Brush their teeth with help
	Stack five or six blocks	Ask questions
	Wash and dry hands	Count to 3
	Say at least 20 words	Name or comment on pictures in a book
	Put two words together ("Go car," "More juice")	Put on some clothing
	Follow two-part instructions, like "Get your socks, and put them in the bag"	
	Imitate what adults say and do	
	Match items of the same color	

As you review this list of milestones, remember that children who are within the normal range will have some areas in which they excel and others in which they are slower. Not achieving a particular milestone at the designated time is not always a matter of concern. If you and your child's doctor are concerned about your child's overall development or any of your child's developmental skills, such as language, hearing, vision, or motor skills, seek the help of the appropriate specialist. For more information, see *Developmental Problems*, Part 5.

adult's hand. They're well coordinated enough to kick a ball or throw a ball overhand using the whole arm, rather than just the wrist. And their dexterity has improved to the point that they can begin to undress themselves by unzipping their jackets or pulling off their shoes. But their exploration and curiosity can get them into trouble. They'll be climbing on countertops or standing up in their strollers and getting lots of bumps and bruises in the process.

QUESTIONS PARENTS ASK
Left or Right?

Q: My son consistently favors his left hand. He uses it to draw, to hold a spoon or fork, and to pick up toys. Does this mean he's going to stay left-handed?

A: Many children stay left-handed or right-handed from age 2 on. But it's not unusual for a child to show a preference for one hand and then the other off and on even into the preschool years. You needn't be concerned about this switch-hitting unless it seems to interfere with your child's ability to do things. Use the following list as a guide. By 2 years old, most children can hold a spoon or fork well enough to feed themselves, handle small objects skillfully (for example, place pea-sized items into a narrow jar), and hold a piece of paper in place when drawing.

Communicating

During the year between 2 and 3 years of age, most children are not only naming things and people, but they're beginning to talk about what people and objects do: "Mommy go work," "Man throw ball." They also start to say pronouns, especially "me" and "you," although most children don't refer to themselves as "I" until close to their third birthday. And 2-year-olds may confuse pronouns when using them together in a sentence, saying things like "carry you," when they mean, "I want you to carry me."

A 2-year-old's speech is far from perfect. Chances are, your child still doesn't use words like "the" and "a," for instance. He'll say, "Open door," rather than "Open the door." And, in addition to being rife with mispronunciations, many of his sentences appear to defy grammar rules—or he may follow them too consistently. He may say, "I runned outside," rather than "I ran outside." Subjects and verbs don't agree; plurals are not always correct. Because of these limitations, it may be hard for people other than you and his regular caregivers to understand him much of the time. But don't worry; over the next year, his language skills should improve so much that even strangers will be able to understand most of what he says.

SO BIG!

At 2 years, the average boy is
- 33½ to 35¼ inches tall.
- 26 to 30 pounds.

At 2 years, the average girl is
- 32¾ to 34¾ inches tall.
- 24½ to 28½ pounds.

For more information, see Appendix: Growth Charts.

For now, what's important is what your child says, not how he says it. Here are some things to look for in your child's language development:

▌ Descriptions of events or things that he just saw ("plane in sky")

▌ Using time concepts such as "now" or "before" and "after"

▌ Categorizing ("little stick, big stick")

▌ Understanding cause and effect ("If I push my cup over, the milk spills out")

The 2-year-old milestones are important in terms of speech development. Check them carefully. Two years of age is when most pediatricians and child development experts recommend a hearing test and a speech assessment if the child appears to be having problems understanding or expressing language. Consult your child's doctor or a speech-language pathologist if you have concerns about your child's speech at this stage. Speech difficulties often go hand-in-hand with developmental problems or may be a symptom of hearing impairment.

Talking and Intelligence

Many people assume that children who talk a lot are smarter than quieter children. But this isn't necessarily the case. Just because a child doesn't talk much doesn't mean that he can't talk well—or that his development lags behind that of more talkative children. He may simply be more selective about what he wants to say, and to whom. He may be more of a listener than a talker by nature.

As long as your child talks, his vocabulary is growing, and he's communicating thoughts and descriptions of increasing complexity, you needn't doubt his language development or his intelligence. But if he lags behind the developmental milestones on page 181, consult your child's doctor or ask to see a speech-language pathologist.

TOUCHPOINT

Playing Language Games

Two-year-olds are learning language rapidly. Along the way, they make lots of mistakes: "Daddy goed out!" You may be tempted to correct the error or fill in the "right" word. Instead, when you speak, use the correct word. More importantly, play a supporting role in your child's language development with games like the following that encourage learning through singing, repetition, and pretend play:

▌ Sing songs with your child. Listen to children's songs and repeat them with your child.

▌ Have your child fill in the last word of each phrase when you sing a song or repeat a rhyme.

▌ Take turns. Have your child repeat each phrase when you sing a song or say a rhyme.

▌ Use rhythm sticks. Have your child bang, roll, or swing the sticks while you say, "Bang, bang, bang. We're banging our sticks." Repeat this several times, then add, "Then we stop!" Have everyone stop and say, "Shhh!" before the next person has a turn saying the phrases.

■ Pretend play. You and your child can pretend to be eating, going to bed, going shopping. Use dolls or stuffed animals. Have your child imitate some simple phrases like, "Time to eat."

As you play these games, let your child take the lead and even encourage him to change the rules. He'll enjoy being in charge.   Source: Touchpoints Project (see p. 81).

Stuttering

Once they're old enough to speak in sentences, virtually all children occasionally stumble over their words. They repeat the sounds: the beginning of words (b-b-b-bottle), entire syllables (unc-unc-uncle), or short words in sentences. And when they're at a loss for words, they may use sounds like "uh" and "um" to fill in the gaps. These sorts of problems, known as dysfluencies, are most common in children from 2 to 4 years old. The cause is not fully understood. One possible explanation is that the muscles used for speech aren't yet coordinated well enough to always produce words smoothly and clearly. Another is that young children are still relatively emotional, so when they're frustrated, angry, or excited they may have trouble getting words out.

A difference exists between normal dysfluencies and the dysfluencies that over time become more pronounced and represent what is known as stuttering. Normal dysfluencies generally go away by themselves as a child matures. But how do you know if dysfluencies are normal or if your child is stuttering and needs help? Here are some things to look for—these are normal for any small child:

■ Your child repeats sounds in the beginning of a word or sentence, but no more often than once every 10 sentences.

■ Your child pauses, fumbles for the right word, or says, "uh," "eh," or "um" when he doesn't know what to say.

■ Your child doesn't act upset or bothered when he makes mistakes.

Most children overcome these normal dysfluencies on their own, but parents can help by ignoring them. Listen to your child calmly and patiently. Do not correct your child or draw attention to the "bumps," which will only make him more anxious.

WHEN TO CALL THE DOCTOR
Speech Problems

If your child's stuttering or dysfluencies seem to be increasing or if he shows the following symptoms, ask your doctor about consulting a speech-language pathologist to discuss when and how to address these difficulties.

■ The child does not speak at all, or words are few.

■ His speech cannot be understood, especially by caregivers.

▌ His speech seems stuck in his throat.

▌ Other physical symptoms, such as facial tics or grimaces, develop when he makes speaking mistakes.

▌ He seems frustrated or embarrassed by his errors.

QUESTIONS PARENTS ASK
Repetition

Q: My daughter wants me to read her the same book over and over again, and this is driving me crazy. She has lots of other books; why doesn't she want them?

A: Toddlers love to hear the same story, song, or poem over and over again. They learn from it, and they also find security and a sense of mastery in it. Grit your teeth, and keep reading her the book. Eventually, she'll get as tired of it as you are and she'll ask you to read something else—over and over again.

Learning

Every moment, your child is learning new things, soaking up everything he sees and making use of it. Children this age have a general sense of time and quantities. They may understand the concepts of today and tomorrow. They know that "2" is more than "1." But their understanding of numbers usually stops there. As far as most 2-year-olds are concerned, two can be 2 or 200. Toward the end of this year, toddlers commonly become fixed on the number 3, as they look forward to their third birthday. In fact, by then many can count to 3, or even higher.

Despite this new learning, it is a mistake for parents to talk to 2-year-olds as though they were adults. Two-year-old children do not understand long explanations or lots of details about future events. Keep your explanations simple and short.

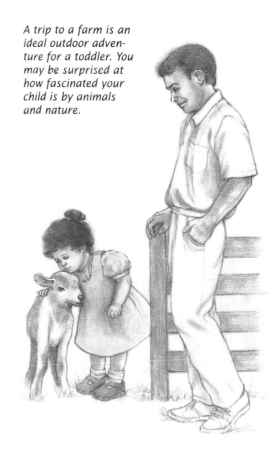

A trip to a farm is an ideal outdoor adventure for a toddler. You may be surprised at how fascinated your child is by animals and nature.

Routines and Rituals

Along with learning about time ("now," "before," "after"), 2-year-olds also have a near obsession with order. When you say, "It's time for a bath," your 2-year-old may imagine the entire bath time ritual in a particular sequence: having his bath, getting into his pajamas, brushing his teeth, and then combing his hair. If you comb his hair before brushing his teeth, he may get upset and correct your mistake, not just because you have done something "wrong," but because he needs the security of having rituals unfold in their usual sequence.

Another aspect of toddlers' love of order is their need to categorize things. For example, many children this age know whose seat is where at the table and won't approve if you sit in the "wrong" seat. They recognize the difference between an object that looks normal and one that is broken. And they're beginning to understand the distinction between "real" and "pretend."

This understanding gives rise to more complex pretend play. Whereas in the past, your child might have fed a doll a toy bottle or a slice of toy pizza, now he can pretend that a pine cone is an ice cream cone and "feed" it to the doll, and then follow the usual sequence of routines in his own life—after feeding the doll, he may carry it to the couch, cover it with a "blanket" that is really a towel, and put the doll to bed.

QUESTIONS PARENTS ASK
When Travel Disrupts Your Child's Routines

Q: Our daughter was sleeping through the night until we took her on her first plane ride to spend a week with relatives. She cried the whole time on the plane, and while we were away, woke us up several times a night. What happened?

A: Young children do not like change, and 2-year-olds are especially upset by it. Traveling to a new place, changing baby-sitters, or having a new a sibling can throw a toddler into a tailspin. Perhaps the most obvious sign is that the child's sleep is disturbed. Having to get up in the middle of the night to comfort your toddler is frustrating, but it won't last forever. Once her routine returns to normal, so will she—although it might take her a few nights to get back to her usual routine. In the meantime, make the best of the situation by bringing your child's favorite blanket or stuffed animal, as well as taking some new toys for the plane and repeating some of her familiar rituals, such as reading at bedtime, even while you are traveling.

Solving Problems

Those scissors you placed on an upper shelf are suddenly in your child's hands. How did that happen? Your child is learning problem-solving. He figured out that by pushing a chair over to the bookshelves he can reach things higher up. You may notice him using the handle of a toy broom to get something out from under the bed or turning the doorknob to get out of the house. Your child can now analyze a situation and figure out new ways to get what he wants. He is also becoming more interested in how things work.

Social and Emotional Development

Two-year-olds are copycats. For them, imitation is a wonderful way to play with another child—or an adult. Children this age are beginning to play together for brief

---

A FATHER'S STORY

A Trip to the Farm

Iknew that Allison loved animals. She enjoyed playing with her stuffed animals, looking at pictures of different animals in books, and, of course, singing songs like "Old MacDonald Had a Farm." But I had no idea how much she could really learn about them until I took her to my brother's farm.

It was spring. We showed her the calves and chicks. My brother explained the different ways that they're born. He told her that the calves grew inside their mothers' bellies, just like she grew inside her mother's belly, and that chicks hatched from eggs that their mothers sat on to keep warm. She paid attention to everything he said.

I couldn't believe how much of this Allie remembered. For months after we got back home to the city, she was talking about the similarities and differences among the animals: which ones drank milk from their mothers and which ones could eat right away, the shapes of their tails, and the sounds they made. I was amazed. It had never occurred to me to explain anything more complicated to Allison than that horses go "neigh" and cows go "moo." Now I know better.

---

periods. A common way for one child to get another's attention is by imitating him. If two children meet in the park, they may first look at each other. Then if one starts to giggle, the other will giggle. If one starts to run, the other will run after him. By doing what another child is doing, a toddler is saying, in effect, "I understand you, and I like you."

Toddlers also spend a lot of time imitating adults, in particular their parents. Many enjoy sweeping or vacuuming with their toy brooms and vacuums, pounding pretend nails with their toy hammers, driving their toy cars, and talking on toy telephones.

Tantrums

Though tantrums are considered the hallmark of the "terrible twos," in reality most children don't throw as many of them now as they did when they were 18 months old, because they've got more self-control and can communicate better. But tantrums are still a centerpiece of their social and emotional lives. Contrary to what you may think, your child doesn't throw tantrums because of something you said or did; he throws tantrums because he is trying to work through his inner turmoil. Your child will throw tantrums when he's least able to control his emotions: for example, when he's tired, hungry, scared, or frustrated; when he can't get his way; or when he wants two incompatible things.

You can reduce the number of tantrums to some degree, but you may not be able to eliminate them. Nor would you really want to. If there's anything positive to say about tantrums, it's that they're normal for toddlers. And toddlers learn from them that they can come through such rage and survive it. With time, they will accept help in avoiding tantrums and eventually learn how to do this themselves.

How to Handle a Tantrum

If your child is throwing a tantrum in a store or some other public place, silently pick him up and leave. Once you're alone with your child, ignore him until the tantrum is over. Paying too much attention to him is likely to teach him to throw more tantrums for two reasons. One is that your attention is a kind of reward. In addition, by asking or ordering your child to stop screaming, you're attempting to control him, something that tends to make children angry in the first place. If your child is in such a rage that you fear that he might harm himself or something else, hold him securely until the tantrum passes.

There are two things to avoid when your child throws a tantrum. First, don't lose your temper. Shouting will fan the flames, making the tantrum worse by scaring your child or making him think that he's "bad" (which, of course, he's not). Shouting or getting angry will also teach your child to do the same. Second, don't give in to your child's demand. Doing so will let him know that throwing tantrums is a good way to get his way. For more information on persistent or severe temper tantrums, see *Behavioral Problems,* Part 5.

Dealing with Fears

Is your child afraid of the dark? Does he think monsters are hiding in the closet? As your child becomes more aware of his world and his emotional responses to it, he may also become more fearful. Fear of the dark, loud noises, barking dogs, and monsters are common fears for 2-year-olds. Many children refuse to enter a room unless it's well lighted. Your child will sometimes cry hysterically while pointing at something, but you can't figure out what is scary or why. Sometimes a book illustration that's not intended to look threatening is so terrifying that he refuses to look at the book again.

Don't bother trying to convince your child that there is nothing to fear. His feelings are real to him. And don't be alarmed by his behavior—it's part of being 2. Instead, acknowledge his feelings by saying, "That's scary, isn't it?" or "You're feeling scared, aren't you?" Tell him you understand, and reassure him that he doesn't have to see anything that scares him. If he's frightened by a picture in a book, don't read it and avoid ones you think might scare him. Turn off videos that scare him. If he's scared of the dark, leave a night-light on in his room. If he's scared of the darkness outside his window, block his view of it by pulling down the window shades or closing the curtains at night. Ask your child what would make him less afraid. This is also a good time to think about whether your child has been exposed to any television shows or commercials, movies, or scary stories that might be frightening him.

Power Struggles

At this age, children normally begin to want some control over their lives. This can be frustrating for a parent who struggles with an uncooperative child in order to accomplish basic things like getting dressed in the morning, eating meals, or getting ready for bed at night. Your child's favorite response may be to run away, hide, or even hit or kick you. To deal with this, consider ways to give a limited number of choices. Say, "Do you like the red shirt or the green one?" But don't open the closet and ask, "What do you want to wear?" That will overwhelm him, and he won't be able to choose. Phrases such as "your choice" or "you decide" or "Which would you like to do first?" can turn an uncooperative toddler enthusiastic.

Also allow for lots of lead time when you make a transition from one activity to the next. Say, "We're going to go for a car ride soon—get ready to ride in your car seat." A 2-year-old needs time to adjust. But these techniques won't always work. So be prepared, and know that your child is behaving this way because it is part of being 2. Be ready to remove your child from a situation by using time-outs for unacceptable behavior until he can regain some emotional control. For more information on discipline, see page 201.

QUESTIONS PARENTS ASK
Going Naked

Q: Our 2½-year-old likes to take her clothes off and run around the house naked. Should we make her stop?

A: Not unless she's doing it in front of strangers or in public. She's probably undressing to show off her ability to do it or to get a reaction from you. It may give her a sense of control both because it is something she can do herself, and because it is something that you did that she can undo. Some children simply like the feel of being naked. Ignoring her behavior will take the fun out of it, and she'll probably stop. Don't worry about this behavior, and don't pay too much attention to it.

Caring for Your Toddler

In a way, your life is easier. Many toddlers can feed themselves; some are even toilet trained before their third year. Now that your child can do some things by himself, you don't have to do as much for him. But your job has also gotten more complex. Caring for your child now means not only providing for his physical needs and protecting his safety but also nurturing his need for independence. Often these needs clash, and you must decide which is most important and which to let slide.

What does this mean for everyday life? It means taking a lot of deep breaths and learning to pick your battles. You might let your toddler's vegetables go uneaten to avoid a food fight. You might let him wash himself because he really wants to, even though he can't get himself perfectly clean. But insist on doing the important things, like using his car seat whenever he is in the car. Whenever you can, give your toddler some limited choices to empower him, like giving him a choice of shirts to wear or foods to eat.

Feeding

Though your child is growing, his appetite may not be. Many parents become concerned because their toddlers don't seem to eat much. A typical day may go something like this. Your child eats part of a waffle or a bowl of cereal for breakfast. Two hours later he's hungry again, so you give him some pretzels or cut-up fruit for a snack. At lunchtime he takes two bites out of his grilled cheese sandwich. In mid-afternoon he has some yogurt and a cup of juice. At dinner he squirms in his chair, picks up his food and plays with it, perhaps pounding it with his open hand, then fusses until you let him out of his high chair or excuse him from his booster seat. Then he points to the cookie cabinet.

Two things are going on here. First, he's not as hungry as he used to be, because his growth has slowed down. Second, he's asserting his independence. One of his favorite situations for saying no and for struggling to get his way is at mealtime. Expect your child to eat one good meal a day—on a good day. Don't take it personally when he refuses much of what you offer. He's just being a toddler.

Keep on Trying

This isn't to say that you should give up trying to get your child to eat well. Never give up. Keep offering nutritious food in frequent small meals throughout the day. Rather than eating three large meals a day, most toddlers eat small meals every 2 to 3 hours (breakfast, snack, lunch, snack, dinner, snack). Set a good example by eating good food yourself. Good toddler nutrition begins with your choices in the supermarket. If you don't buy sugary, high-fat junk foods, your child will learn to like the more nutritious choices you make available.

Don't push. Pressuring children to eat predisposes them to eating disorders and behavior problems. Don't reward a child for eating or punish him if he doesn't. One study found that children who were rewarded for tasting a new food were less likely to eat the food again than children who were left to try the food when they were ready. At this point, your job is to provide a selection of healthy foods, and your child's job is to decide what he wants to eat and how much.

Things You Can Do: Making Food Fun

Here are ways to increase the odds that your toddler will eat well:

▮ Offer finger foods, like cut-up fruits and cooked vegetables, chicken, fish, macaroni, or cereal without milk. Make sure the pieces are small

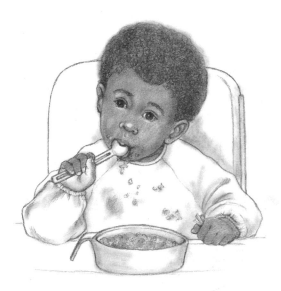

Toddlers are notoriously picky when it comes to eating. If the traditional three meals a day don't seem to suit him, offer him a selection of nutritious food throughout the day and let him decide when he wants to eat.

enough so that your child won't choke. And don't give hard foods like raw carrots or nuts.

▌ Offer small amounts of several foods, rather than a lot of one or two foods. Given a broad choice, he's bound to find something that he likes.

▌ Limit high-sugar foods such as fruit juices and cookies, which will dampen your child's appetite for more nutritious food.

How Much Fat?

Children need enough fat in their diet for proper brain growth and development, which is occurring especially rapidly up until age 2. Some debate exists over precisely how much fat toddlers need, but the standard recommendation has long been to give whole milk, yogurt, cheese, and meat until age 2. After age 2, once brain growth slows, children can have lower-fat milk and foods as part of an overall plan to restrict fat intake. At this point, the fat in your child's diet should be the same as yours: It should make up no more than 30 percent of his total calories each day. As with adults, the long-term goal is to prevent high cholesterol and obesity, risk factors for life-threatening illnesses like heart disease, diabetes, and cancer. For more on overweight children, see *Overweight,* Part 5.

Cutting fat out of your child's meals doesn't mean putting him on a diet. Restricting his calories is dangerous because it can interfere with his growth. Instead, let him choose from low-fat healthy foods, like grains, fruits, vegetables, lean meats, and eggs, and keep high-fat snack foods to a minimum. You don't have to ban ice cream and cookies from your home, but try to get your child accustomed to healthier snacks.

Is Meat Necessary?

Meat is not a necessary component of a child's diet. A vegetarian diet can be healthy and nutritious. But for children who like meat, there's no reason for them not to eat it at this age.

During the first year, introduce different kinds of meat one at a time so that you can notice food allergy symptoms, like rashes or diarrhea. Cut the meat into small, easy-to-chew pieces. Meat in general is a good source of protein and minerals, and red meat in particular is a good source of iron. But since meat also tends to be higher in fat and calories than fruits, vegetables, breads, and cereals, it shouldn't be the mainstay of a child's diet. Also, choose meats that are lower in fat—poultry with no skin, and lean cuts of beef, pork, and lamb with the fat cut off. Cook meat thoroughly, avoiding raw or rare meat, which can cause illness from bacterial contamination, and refrigerate leftover cooked meat immediately to avoid the same problem. The intestinal upset and illnesses that many parents assume are caused by flu can be a case of *food poisoning* (see Part 5).

Food Safety

Even though children have most of their teeth by about 3 years old, they are still at relatively high risk for choking. One reason is that their windpipe (trachea) is so

▬ *MEAL PLANNING FOR 1-YEAR-OLD CHILDREN*

Food Group	Daily Servings	Foods	Serving Size
Grains	6	Whole-grain cereal, pasta, rice (cooked) Whole-grain cereal (dry) Whole-grain bread Whole-grain crackers	¼ cup Up to 4 tablespoons ¼–½ slice 1 to 2
Fruits	2	Cut-up raw fruit	½ piece
Vegetables	3	Cooked vegetables	1 tablespoon
Milk, yogurt, cheese	2–3	Whole milk, yogurt Hard cheese Cottage cheese	½ cup ½ oz. ¼ cup
Meat, eggs, legumes, tofu	2	Beef, chicken, fish, pork, turkey Beans, peas (cooked), tofu Egg	1 oz. ¼ cup ½

▬ *MEAL PLANNING FOR 2-YEAR-OLD CHILDREN*

Food Group	Daily Servings	Foods	Serving Size
Grains	6	Whole-grain cereal Whole-grain bread Rice or pasta	⅔ oz. ½–1 slice 4 tablespoons
Vegetables	3	Leafy greens Cooked vegetables Raw vegetables	½ cup 2 tablespoons ½ cup
Fruits	2	Apple, orange, banana, or other fruit Fruit juice Cooked fruit (applesauce) Melon pieces or other cut-up fruit	½ piece ⅓ cup ⅓–½ cup ⅓–½ cup
Milk, yogurt, cheese	2	Low-fat or nonfat milk Yogurt Cheese	1 cup 1 cup 1½ oz
Meat, eggs, legumes, tofu	2–3	Cooked, lean meat Eggs Beans, peas (cooked), tofu	1 oz. 1 ½ cup

narrow that a piece of food can easily block it. Another reason is that toddlers don't always chew their food well. They talk, walk, giggle, and horse around while they eat—activities that can lead to choking.

Children are most likely to choke on small and round or sticky food, like grapes, hot dogs, nuts, and spoonfuls of peanut butter. After age 2, you can mix peanut butter with jelly or melt peanut butter on toast to make it less likely to cause choking. Grapes and hot dogs can be made safe if they're cut up into small (not round) pieces. Slice grapes in half lengthwise and cut hot dogs lengthwise and then across into bite-sized pieces.

The following foods are not safe for toddlers. Do not offer these foods to children age 3 years and younger:

- Celery
- Cherries with pits
- Grapes with seeds
- Hard candies, gum balls
- Nuts
- Raw carrots
- Spoonfuls of peanut butter
- Raisins
- Round hot dog slices
- Watermelon with seeds

For more information on choking, see Chapter 11, Preparing for and Handling Emergencies, page 397.

QUESTIONS PARENTS ASK
Eating Sweets

Q: Will sweets make my child hyperactive?

A: There is no scientific evidence that sugar causes children to be hyperactive. In experiments, researchers have *not* found that children's behavior changes after they eat sweets. With that said, it is still important to limit the amount of sugar your child eats (including fruit juices), because sugar contains empty calories with no vitamins or minerals and will dampen your child's appetite for more nutritious foods. Sugar also promotes tooth decay.

SAFETY ALERT
Hold the Chewing Gum

Two-year-old children have a mouth full of teeth, but hold off on giving children chewing gum until they are old enough to understand that it must not be swallowed. Repeatedly swallowing chewing gum can obstruct a child's digestive tract, causing constipation and other blockages. Until they are about 4 or 5, it is difficult for young children to understand that they may chew but not swallow gum.

QUESTIONS PARENTS ASK
Vegetables

Q: I've read that kids should have a green vegetable and a yellow vegetable every day, but my daughter won't touch vegetables. What should I do?

A: Even if she doesn't like vegetables, she may be willing to eat fruit. Offer fruits high in vitamins A and C, which are also found in green and yellow vegetables. Good choices are oranges, strawberries, cantaloupe, and kiwis.

Don't give up on vegetables, however. Keep giving your child vegetables, and make sure to show and tell her how much you enjoy them. The more she sees vegetables at the table, the more likely she is to accept them eventually. But be alert to signs of tomato or other food allergies.

Here are some hints for making vegetables more appealing to your child:

■ *Offer different vegetables.* Just because she doesn't like yellow squash doesn't mean she won't eat green beans.

■ *Prepare vegetables in different ways.* Cut them in different shapes or sprinkle them with cheese. Make the presentation fun. Try arranging vegetable pieces on her plate in the shape of a face. It may sound corny, but it often works.

■ *Think finger food.* Many toddlers prefer eating food with their fingers than with a spoon or fork. So cut cooked vegetables into strips that kids can pick up and put in their mouths.

■ *Try vegetable soup.* Soup is one kind of food that toddlers tend to like because they can pick and spoon up the vegetables as they float around the bowl.

■ *Remember tomato sauce.* It counts as an orange vegetable. And you can include other vegetables when you make it. Puree some kale, parsley, or cooked carrots into your sauce and pour it over noodles.

■ *Sneak vegetables in.* When making homemade pizza, try tucking small pieces of squash, broccoli, or other vegetables under the cheese. Bake zucchini bread.

Giving Up the Bottle

Getting a toddler to stop drinking from a bottle is often easier said than done. Why do it? For one thing, toddlers don't need bottles once they can drink from a cup. For another, those who drink from a bottle often drink too much milk or juice and therefore don't have enough room for important foods like fruits, vegetables, and grains. Also, as teeth come in, frequent bottle sucking can change the natural position of the emerging teeth.

Try phasing the bottle out gradually. First, stop letting your child walk around with it. Toddlers who do this tend to use the bottle less as a thirst quencher than as an oversized pacifier. If your child still craves the security of having a bottle of milk before nap time and bedtime, let him have it as long as he drinks it before he gets into the crib. As with infants, putting toddlers to bed with a bottle can cause cavities and may contribute to ear infections (see *Earache/Ear Infection,* Part 5).

To further encourage your child to give up the bottle, don't put anything in it other than milk. Offer him juice and water only in a cup. How will you know when to get rid of the bottles entirely? You'll see signs. Your child will drink less milk from the bottle, a cue for you to fill it less. Eventually the bottle will become unimportant to the bedtime and nap time rituals. At that point, try not giving your child a bottle one day and see what happens.

QUESTIONS PARENTS ASK
Refusing Milk

Q: My 15-month-old doesn't miss her bottle, but she won't drink more than a few ounces of milk from a cup. How can I make sure she gets the calcium she needs?

A: Try other good calcium sources, such as yogurt and cheese. A cup of yogurt has nearly as much calcium as a cup of milk. Other high-calcium foods include tofu, soy milk, sardines, and calcium-fortified orange juice. Also try mixing powdered milk into casseroles, muffins, cookies, puddings, and other foods. Another good technique is to offer only milk at meals. No water, juice, or other beverages should be allowed at mealtime. Ask your preschool or child care providers to do the same. You can even send shelf-stable milk boxes (find them in the supermarket next to the juice boxes) in her lunch to preschool or child care.

Dressing

By about 2 years old, many toddlers want to undress themselves—often in the strangest places (at the park, in the grocery store, in church). So encourage your child to undress himself at the appropriate time and place, such as before bath and bedtime.

Around age 3, children start being able to dress themselves. Don't be surprised if one morning your child enters his room only to emerge many minutes later fully dressed. Never mind that the shoes are on the wrong feet and the plaid shirt and striped pants are not the combination you'd have selected. This is a real accomplishment. Be proud of your little person. Give him a smile and a hug and lots of praise for his effort, and put his shoes on the right feet without making a big deal about it.

Choosing New Shoes

One article of clothing to pay special attention to is shoes. It's less obvious when your child has outgrown a pair of shoes than a shirt or a pair of pants. Chances are, he won't tell you when his sneakers are too tight. You can check by pressing the front of each shoe while your child is standing. If you can fit a finger's width between the tip of your child's longest toe and the front edge of the shoe, the shoe fits. If not, it's time for new shoes. Check every 2 or 3 months. If a child's shoes are too tight, they may cause blisters or make him trip or fall.

Sleeping

During the toddler years, several changes affect your child's sleep. For one thing, within several months of his first birthday, he'll be ready to give up his morning nap, taking only one nap in the afternoon. A typical sign that the time has come is that your child simply won't settle down or fall asleep twice during the day. See How Much Sleep Does the Typical Child Need? on page 108. Toddlers also make another big change in their sleep habits: They move from crib to bed.

Moving from Crib to Bed

Usually children are ready to switch from a crib to a bed at around 3 or 4 years of age. However, the age for this transition varies in different families, and no set rules exist. The classic sign that a child is ready for a bed is that he climbs out of his crib. Because he can fall and hurt himself while trying to do this, it's safer for him to be in a bed. But some toddlers indicate their desire for a bed in other ways, like crying when they're put in their crib but not when put down on your bed or on the guest room bed. Other toddlers ask to have their own bed. And many others move to a bed because their crib is needed for a new baby.

Whatever the circumstances, you can do several things to ease the transition. First, tell your child that he's going to get a bed. Talk about the event for several weeks before it happens to get him used to the idea. Ask him to help choose sheets and blankets. When the new bed arrives, put the new sheets and blankets on, and decorate it with stuffed animals. Put one side of the bed against a wall, and put a bed rail on the other side to keep your child from rolling off. Let your child jump on the bed, lie on it, or do whatever makes him feel comfortable with it. Alternatives to a full-size bed include toddler beds or even a mattress or futon on the floor.

Wandering out of Bed

Unlike a crib, a bed has no barrier keeping your child in it. Some toddlers stay put, but others get up and wander. If this happens with your child, put him back in his bed and tell him to stay there. The warning may do the trick, but if it doesn't, your child, like many toddlers, probably lacks the self-control to stay in his room on his own. If so, you can make his room into one large, baby-proof space by putting a gate at the door that he can't remove or climb over (some parents mount a screen door instead). Your child may cry at first, but he will gradually grow accustomed to the new situation.

Nighttime Visits

Many toddlers—even those who usually stay put at bedtime—surprise their parents by crawling into bed with them in the middle of the night. How you choose to handle this is up to you. If you don't mind your child's 5 A.M. visits, then they're not a problem and you needn't do anything. If your sleep is disrupted, you could try putting a sleeping bag on the floor in your bedroom and telling him to use that if he wakes up during the night. Otherwise, simply take your child back to his bed, explaining that this is where he is supposed to sleep. Make sure that he has his special blanket or other transitional object for comfort (see p. 160). If he says that he's scared or that he had a bad dream, stay with him until he's settled down. It's also a good idea to put a night-light in his room or leave the hall light on.

If, despite your best efforts, your child keeps coming to your bed at night, consider putting a gate at his door. Tell your child that he can call to you if he wakes up at night and needs you.

Nightmares and Night Terrors

Nightmares and night terrors are not the same, although toddlers are prone to both. Nightmares are bad dreams. If your child has had a nightmare, he'll wake up crying, although he may not know why he's crying. He may just say that he's scared. As he gets older, he'll be more apt to tell you about the dream. Like adults, children are most likely to have nightmares if they've had a rough day—if they've just started day care, for example, or if a parent is out of town—although the dream itself may have nothing to do with a particular event of the day.

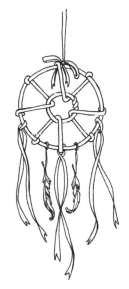

A "dream catcher" that your child makes helps to provide the feeling of security she needs to overcome her nighttime fears. Use a variety of craft materials, such as yarn, feathers, or pipe cleaners, and hang it up to catch all bad dreams.

When your child has a nightmare, he needs you. Comfort him by telling him that it was just a bad dream and that it's over. Toddlers commonly dream about monsters and are afraid that these monsters are lurking in their rooms. In that case, you may have to "chase" the monster away. Some parents do this by squirting "magic" water under the bed and inside the closet with a plant sprayer. Others find that a night-light helps. Some children make dream catchers in preschool. You can hang these near the bed to "catch" any bad dreams.

Night terrors may seem more mysterious than nightmares. They are partial arousals from deep, nondreaming sleep. Unlike nightmares, which tend to occur in the second half of the night, night terrors happen within the first 4 hours of sleep. A child screams out suddenly. He may sit or stand up, but he's not fully awake. When he talks, he makes no sense. If you try to hold him, he may push you away or not respond at all. Though children may be afraid to go back to sleep following a nightmare, they usually fall right back to sleep after having a night terror. Night terrors are not usually associated with stresses in a child's life. They tend to be most common in children who are on an irregular schedule or who are overly tired when they go to bed. If your child has a night terror, don't panic. Just let it run its course, realizing that this can take anywhere from 5 to 45 minutes.

Sleep and Day Care

Many day care centers schedule a nap every day so that the children can rest and the staff can take a break. But for a child who no longer needs to sleep during the day, an enforced nap can cause such problems as preventing him from going to bed at a decent hour at night. Staying up late, in turn, can make waking up early in the morning for day care difficult. This is a common source of friction between parents and day care providers. But sleep experts now believe that requiring a child to lie down on a mat for an hour or more when he's not tired is counterproductive and unnecessary.

Once your child gives up his nap, ask the day care center to let him get up after 15 minutes and spend the rest of the nap time looking through books or engaging in quiet play.

QUESTIONS PARENTS ASK
Nap Time

Q: My 2$\frac{1}{2}$-year-old refuses to nap, but she's extremely cranky at the end of the day. What should I do?

A: You can't make a child nap, but you can make her have a period of quiet time in place of a nap. Take her to her room, and tell her that she can look at books or play quietly by herself. If she protests, let her have her quiet time elsewhere in the house for 20 to 30 minutes, which is long enough for her to fall asleep if she's going to do so. Don't force her to go to her room when she doesn't want to; she may come to feel unhappy there and have trouble going to bed at night.

THREE STEPS TO A BETTER NIGHT'S SLEEP

Even though most toddlers can sleep through the night, they're bound to wake up sometimes. But if he's waking up regularly in the middle of the night, you may need to take steps to help your child sleep through the night. Here are the most common reasons toddlers habitually wake up at night and what you can do to break the habit:

- *The child is still nursing or getting a bottle when he wakes.* Toddlers don't need a middle-of-the-night feeding. Eliminate the nighttime bottle so that your child will eat more during the day and sleep longer at night.

- *The child's sleep schedule is inappropriate or chaotic.* Your child may be napping too long during the day, going to bed too early, waking up too late in the morning, or going to bed at different times each day. If so, adjust your child's sleep schedule to make sure he goes to bed at the same time each night and doesn't sleep too long during the day.

- *Toddlers often appear for "curtain calls"*—popping out of bed three or four times to find their parents after having been put to bed. Deal with this patiently but firmly, returning the child to bed consistently with words of reassurance. If you want your child to stay in bed, don't play with him or allow him to stay up with you when he gets up at night.

Toilet Teaching

Somewhere between their second and third birthdays, most children have at least started learning how to use the potty or toilet. Toilet teaching can be stressful for parents who are anxious to get their children out of diapers and for children who may or may not be ready. Friends and family members may tell stories of their own children who were trained by 2 years old. Preschools may not accept a child who is not toilet trained.

The key to toilet teaching is readiness. Your child will show a number of signs when he is ready to learn.

Signs of Readiness

Consider toilet teaching when your child

The more signs of readiness your child shows, the quicker his transition from diapers to the potty.

▌ has regular bowel movements at relatively predictable times of day.

▌ indicates through words, grimaces, or posture that he's urinating or making a bowel movement in his diaper.

▌ complains or appears uncomfortable when his diaper is wet or dirty.

▌ begins to pull his pants up and down.

▌ asks to use the toilet or a potty.

▌ asks to wear underpants.

▌ wants to please you and can follow simple instructions.

▌ stays dry for much of the day.

▌ shows an interest in hand washing and keeping clean.

Step-by-Step: Using the Potty

When you first get a potty, don't put it in the bathroom. Instead, place it in your child's bedroom or in whichever room he plays, so that he can get used to it without feeling pressured to use it. Then follow these steps:

▌ Encourage your child to sit on the potty with his clothes on at first to see what it feels like.

▌ After several days or weeks, whenever he seems open to the idea, suggest that he sit on the potty without his pants or diaper, but don't expect him to do anything in it yet.

▌ For boys it's easier to start off sitting on the potty to urinate, although you can tell your son that he'll do this standing up when he gets bigger.

▌ Look for cues that your child needs to go to the bathroom, and then ask him if he'd like to use the potty. If he doesn't want to, don't push. If he wants to use the potty, be patient. You might try reading him some books to pass the time and relax him. It can take a long time for your child to urinate or have a bowel movement, but when he does he'll be thrilled with himself. Show him that you're happy, too.

- If your child leaves the potty without doing anything in it, don't act disappointed. Just say something like, "We'll try again next time."

- If your child won't sit on the potty for more than a few moments, try giving him incentives to sit there, such as letting him play with a toy or eat a snack. But if he won't, he won't. Don't push too hard.

- Celebrate any success, but don't overdo it, which might make him feel pressured.

- Make sure you take his potty with you when traveling—to grandparents' house, for example, or on vacation.

WHEN TO CALL THE DOCTOR
Toilet Teaching

Talk with your child's doctor if your child

- complains of discomfort in the pelvic region or has other symptoms of illness.

- unexpectedly loses a previously established pattern of using the toilet and starts wetting or soiling again.

- is having tantrums, smearing feces, or being willful or disruptive in regard to potty training.

How Long Does Toilet Teaching Take?

That depends. Some children sail through in just a few days or weeks, whereas others take a year or more. One study found that 22 percent of children are out of diapers by age $2^{1}/_{2}$, 60 percent by age 3, and 88 percent by age $3^{1}/_{2}$. In general, girls learn faster than boys, and second children learn earlier than firstborns. Daytime bowel control usually comes before urine control, although with some children the opposite is true. Even once your child is regularly using the potty, it may be many months before he stops needing diapers. It can be even longer before he stays dry at night (see **Bed-Wetting,** Part 5). New events in the family, such as the birth of a sibling, may cause a child to regress and ask for diapers again if he is recently trained.

Toddler Discipline

What can you do when your child misbehaves? What do you do when he doesn't listen? Is spanking an acceptable way to punish your child? Parents start asking these questions the first time their toddler hits another child, throws a tantrum when he can't have a cookie, or does something else dangerous, disrespectful, or annoying. And parents keep asking these questions until their children are grown.

First, it helps to keep in mind that discipline and punishment are not the same. Discipline is what you do to prevent your child from behaving badly. For example, you hold your child's hand while crossing the street so that he won't run into the street, and you set clear, consistent limits and rules for him to follow. Punishment is what you do when your child behaves badly. A firm "No!" and a time-out are forms of punishment. The better you are at disciplining your child, the less you'll need to punish him.

Of course, no matter how well you discipline your child, he'll still act up sometimes. And most discipline strategies don't work right away. The goal with discipline is not so much a quick fix as a long-term gain. The discipline you use now will prevent behavior problems weeks, months, and years down the road.

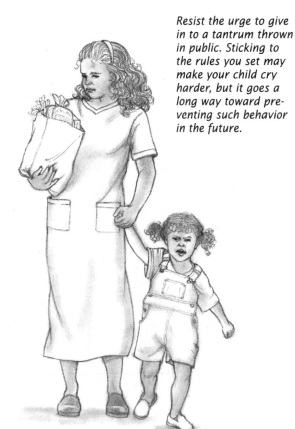

Resist the urge to give in to a tantrum thrown in public. Sticking to the rules you set may make your child cry harder, but it goes a long way toward preventing such behavior in the future.

Toddler Discipline Survival Guide

The key to disciplining a toddler is anticipating how and when he's likely to misbehave and preventing him from doing so. Every child has his own particular ways of acting up, depending on personality, daily schedule, and countless other factors. But certain categories of misbehavior are common to most toddlers. Use the following chart as a guide. And be consistent: These strategies won't work unless you use them every time.

Pick a Few Rules and Enforce Them Consistently

Probably the biggest favor you can do yourself and your child is to be consistent with your discipline.

Decide on a few rules and stick to them—every time. If you tell your child not to climb on the table once and then let him do it the next time because you're too tired or busy to enforce it, you will defeat your own efforts. Pick a few important restrictions—and enforce them.

Also, act quickly and decisively. If you tell your child to stop doing something and he doesn't stop, don't just keep nagging. Step in right away to stop the behavior. Walk over, put a firm hand on his shoulder, and guide him away or distract him.

Scolding, Punishing, and Spanking

Don't scold or punish your child every time he makes a mistake. Do so only when he does something dangerous to himself, to someone else, or to someone's property. If he hits another child, for example, take him aside and say something like, "You may not hit," in a sharp tone of voice. When scolding your child, make it clear that you're punishing him because his behavior was bad, not because he is bad. One way to do this is to say, "I love you, but I don't like it when you hit" (or run in the street, etc.).

TODDLER DISCIPLINE STRATEGIES

Misbehavior	How to Prevent It
Cries or goes limp when it's time to leave the park, a friend's house, day care, etc.	Give advance notice. Say, "In two minutes, we have to go."
Runs down the block or into the street	Hold his hand whenever crossing or standing near the street. Repeat clearly, "Don't go in the street."
Grabs toys from other children	Prevent this common behavior from causing a tantrum by having other toys on hand to offer as replacements when you remove the toys that have been grabbed.
Insists on doing/having certain things and fusses or throws a tantrum when he doesn't get his way	Give your child limited choices: Do you want to wear the blue shirt or the green shirt? Would you like to go to the park or the petting zoo?
Scatters the newspaper, unravels the toilet paper, or gets into other mischief	Redirect the behavior. When you see your child heading for the toilet paper, offer a toy or suggest a game instead.
Fusses to be picked up when you're making dinner; whines for attention when you're on the telephone	Give your child plenty of attention before times when you know you'll be busy. This will temporarily decrease his need for attention when you can't give it. If he carries on anyway, ignore him. Giving him any attention at these times, be it yelling at him or giving in to his demands, will encourage him to fuss more.

If the child misbehaves again, consider giving him a time-out, which means having him sit by himself. Keep time-outs brief, no more than a minute for each year of your child's age. When the time-out is over, remind him briefly why he was punished. Then hug him to reassure him that you love him.

Don't hit your child. Spanking or slapping sends your child the message that it's OK to hit at a time when you're trying to teach him the opposite. The American Academy of Pediatrics recommends finding other ways than spanking to discipline a child, including time-outs and rewards and consequences. Not only is spanking less effective than these methods, but if you hit your child in anger—which is when parents are most inclined to hit—you risk doing physical harm. Children who are punished by being hit can grow up to be angry, insecure adults who punish their own children by hitting, thereby passing on this mistake to the next generation.

SIX DISCIPLINE MISTAKES

When their child misbehaves, parents say and do a lot of things in the heat of the moment that they later regret. Here are six common parental reactions to avoid because they can make a child's behavior worse.

1. Ignoring a child until he does something bad, then scolding him. This teaches him that he'll get attention if he's bad.

2. Shouting or arguing with your child over his behavior. This, too, rewards his negative behavior with attention.

3. Turning your child's misbehavior into a game or being playful when reprimanding him. Your child will be confused about whether you're disciplining him or playing with him.

4. Threatening your child ("If you do that once more . . ."). The child will see your threat as a dare and misbehave more.

5. Making threats you can't or won't deliver: "If you don't stop, you can't come on vacation next week" teaches your child that your threats are meaningless.

6. Using time-out whenever your child misbehaves. It will lose its effectiveness, and you'll feel as if all you do is fight with your child. Use time-out as a last resort, when other techniques, like distracting your child, don't work.

When Your Child Bites

One out of 10 toddlers occasionally bites other children, parents, or caregivers. Though the behavior is disturbing, it doesn't mean that a child is abnormal. But it can be harmful, so you must discourage it. Sternly tell the child not to bite, because it hurts. Other discipline strategies can also help. To decide which ones to use, look at the situations in which your child bites and figure out why he's doing it.

Is he climbing into your lap playfully and then nipping your shoulder? In that case, he may simply be biting to see what it feels like or what you'll do. Offer him something safe to bite on, like a soft toy.

Does your child bite when he wants something, like another child's toy or your attention? If so, he's biting out of frustration because he doesn't know what to say or do to get what he wants. Suggest words that he can use when he wants something.

Does your child bite in self-defense, for example, when another child grabs a toy away from him? Tell him how to ask for his toy back and suggest that he ask a parent or caregiver for help.

Does your child bite for no apparent reason? It could be that he's looking for a reaction—any reaction. He may have noticed that biting has provoked strong responses from children and caregivers in the past. Do two things. First, channel his behavior by giving him choices: Do you want to paint or play ball? Do you want to sit in the red chair or the green chair? Second, praise him when he behaves well—for example, when he shares a toy or says please and thank you. If he gets attention when he's not biting, he'll stop.

Other things you can do if your child is biting, hitting, or otherwise acting aggressively toward other children include the following:

- Keep your child away from other children or people who act aggressively.
- Do not roughhouse too wildly with or act aggressively toward your child. To do so only encourages aggressive behavior.
- Do not use physical punishment, such as biting your child back, to teach him a lesson. This only reinforces the behavior.
- Refrain from angry verbal reprimands. Try to maintain a calm, but firm approach.
- Give your child frequent brief, gentle touches: a hug or a pat on the back.

Playing with Your Child

It's often said that play is a child's work. That's because play is as vital to a child's well-being as work is to an adult's. Children learn practically everything through play, from how to tell a triangle from a square to how to take turns. Toddlers need to play with other toddlers, but they also need to play with their parents. Play is your opportunity to connect with your child in a way that you can't when you're feeding him or bathing him or doing many other chores.

Playing with your child isn't always easy. Shifting gears and sitting down to stack blocks after a day at work or when you have things on your mind, such as planning dinner or having your car repaired, can be difficult. And playing with your child can seem like work when your child frequently demands, "Play with me."

Setting Aside Time for Play

No matter how busy you are, you owe it to your child and to yourself to set aside time each day to play together. Go outside and bounce balls back and forth. Sit on

BEST TOYS FOR TODDLERS AGES 1–2 YEARS

Toy	Benefit
Toys to pull, push, ride, and climb on	Develop gross motor skills
Balls	Provide exercise and develop hand-eye coordination
Puzzles with knobs, shape sorters, toys to take apart and put back together	Develop fine motor skills, teach different shapes
Shopping cart, doll stroller, toy kitchen, toy telephone, toy hammer, and Peg-Board	Teach toddlers to imitate, something they love to do
Fat crayons and paper	Help toddlers learn to draw and prepare them to learn to write
Music (tapes to listen to and toy drums, whistles, xylophones, and other instruments to play)	Encourages toddlers to enjoy music by singing songs and dancing to music
Stuffed animals and dolls	Toddlers like to hug and hold them
Sets of similar toys, cars, animals	Encourage sorting and categorizing objects by color, type, size

the floor to do a puzzle or sort toys of different shapes. Playtime doesn't have to be structured or elaborate. It can be as simple as lying down on the couch together, pointing to your nose, eyes, and ears, and asking your 18-month-old to name them. Or, with a 2½-year-old, make up a story, taking turns thinking up what happens next. The important thing is to give your child your undivided attention and to enjoy each other's company.

Playing Alone

What if your child wants to play and you don't? It's OK to say no, even if you have nothing better to do than sit and read the newspaper. It's not your job to constantly entertain your child. In fact, it's good for your child to learn how to play on his own. If he can't figure out what to do, put out some crayons and paper or some modeling clay or dough to get him started. If you are craving some time to yourself—take it. Either enlist a sitter or simply give yourself a short break after making sure your child is in a safe spot nearby.

As your child grows older, he'll be resourceful enough to use his alone time to engage in pretend play, concocting stories involving stuffed animals and toy figures. Don't even think about trying to join in—if you do, he'll stop. This kind of play is between your child and his imagination. No parents allowed.

BEST TOYS FOR TODDLERS AGES 2–3 YEARS

Toy	Benefit
All of the toys listed on p. 205	Benefits as described on p. 205
Tricycle	Develops coordination and strength and prepares toddlers for learning how to ride a bicycle
Paints, washable markers, easel, modeling clay	Stimulate creativity and develop hand-eye coordination
Simple jigsaw puzzles	Teach toddlers about shapes and spatial relationships and develop fine motor coordination
Puppets, dolls with clothes, small "people," action figures, dress-up clothes	Stimulate pretend play
Building blocks, snap-together blocks, sewing cards	Develop hand-eye coordination and fine motor skills
Cars, trucks, and trains	Develop hand-eye coordination and stimulate pretend play
Board games involving color coordination, not reading	Foster cooperation, following rules, listening

Getting Ready for Preschool

The benefits of preschool for children age 3 and older are indisputable. In the company of trained teachers and other children, they learn to talk better, to listen, to wait their turn, to share.

If your child enjoys being around other children, he's probably ready to try preschool. Many options exist for toddlers, ranging from all-day child care to 2-hour nursery schools. Your choice will be governed by such things as your child's age, whether he's toilet trained, whether you work, and how many days and hours per day you want him to be in school. What toddlers need most from school is a nurturing setting where they can spend most of their time playing, exploring, and making friends. The program should focus on social and emotional development, not on academics. When the time comes, children have an easier time learning how to read and write if they've first learned to trust others, enjoy their company, and feel good about themselves, which is what preschool is about.

Preparing Your Child for Preschool

Some children are so excited by the sight of a room full of toys and children that they rush off without looking back at Mom or Dad. But most are clingy and wary at first. So prepare your child for preschool beforehand. Here are some things to do.

■ *Spend some time apart.* Get your child used to separating from you by leaving him with a baby-sitter or a friend or relative from time to time before he starts school.

■ *Talk about school.* Tell your toddler that he will be starting school soon, and describe what it will be like. Show him picture books about young children in school. Be upbeat.

■ *Take him to see his school* and, if possible, his classroom before the first day to familiarize him with the surroundings. Spend some time there visiting.

■ *Promise your child that you'll stay with him at first.* Any school worth considering will let you do this.

■ *Assure him that you (or a trusted caregiver) will pick him up.* Make sure to be on time.

Keeping Your Child Healthy

The regular checkups that were so much a part of your life when your child was an infant become less frequent during the toddler years. You are the front line for health care for your 1- or 2-year-old, so watch for symptoms such as rashes, fever, fatigue, and diarrhea, which may signal the need for a call or visit to the doctor's office. For general guidelines on how to handle such symptoms see Chapter 10, What to Expect When Your Child Is Sick.

Now that your child has a mouthful of teeth, you'll need to pay closer attention to his dental health. Schedule his first trip to the dentist by the end of his first year (see p. 139). Starting at age 3, your child will need to see a dentist every 6 to 12 months.

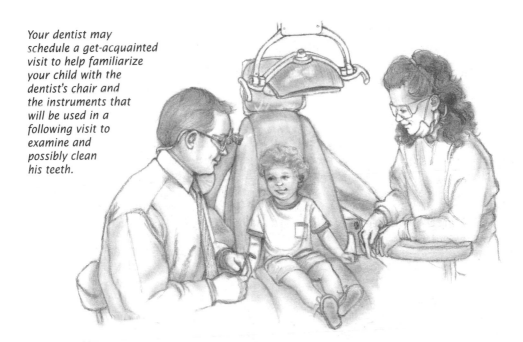

Your dentist may schedule a get-acquainted visit to help familiarize your child with the dentist's chair and the instruments that will be used in a following visit to examine and possibly clean his teeth.

Checkups

Your toddler will need a medical checkup at 15 months, 18 months, and 2 years. The health care practitioner will follow the usual routine, measuring your child's weight and height and plotting them on the growth charts. Head circumference is measured and plotted until a child is 2 years old, the period when its growth is most rapid.

In addition to doing a general physical exam of eyes, ears, chest, legs, feet, genitals, and other body parts, the doctor will pay close attention to your child's teeth. She'll count how many have come in, note their position, and determine whether they have cavities. The doctor will also examine your child's skin for signs of moles that may be changing, for skin rashes, and for infections. She will check for excessive bruises or other injuries that could be signs of a health problem.

During these visits be sure to tell the doctor if you have any concerns about your child's development. Tell your doctor if you notice any of the following problems:

▌ Your 15-month-old says no words.

▌ Your 18-month-old doesn't hold a spoon.

▌ Your 2-year-old doesn't talk in two-word sentences.

▌ Your toddler at any age shows little or no interest in other children.

▌ Your 2-year-old is losing already mastered language or motor skills.

No concern is too trivial (see **Developmental Problems,** Part 5). Parents are more likely than doctors to spot signs of developmental problems in a child. So your observations are crucial for helping the doctor determine whether to refer your child to a specialist for developmental assessment and therapy.

For information on immunizations at this age, see Childhood Immunization Schedule, page 110.

QUESTIONS PARENTS ASK
Exercise

Q: Does my child need to exercise?

A: Toddlers need to run, climb, crawl, ride tricycles or other riding toys, throw balls, and, in general, burn off energy. Because toddlers are naturally active, your child will get enough exercise if you give him space to run around and play. Make sure he has the chance to be physically active every day. Let him run around in the backyard or in a room in your home. Or take him to a local park or an indoor play space. Your child might enjoy taking a gymnastics class or swimming class intended for toddlers and a parent or caregiver. But he doesn't need special classes to get the exercise he needs.

Going to the Dentist

Your child has probably already visited the dentist at least once. Dentists recommend a first visit within 6 months of the appearance of your baby's first tooth or by 1 year at the latest. Beginning at age 3, your child should visit the dentist once every 6 months. Unless your doctor has detected a problem, the purpose of these early dental visits is mainly to get your child comfortable with the routine of going to the dentist every 6 months to 1 year. The dentist will examine your child's teeth and will check to be sure that there are no problems, such as baby bottle tooth decay (see *Cavities*, Part 5), and will provide you with information on how to care for your child's teeth.

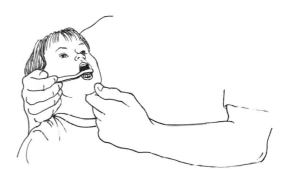

To brush your child's teeth, stand behind her, tilt her head up with one hand, and, with your free hand, hold a soft-bristle toothbrush at a 45-degree angle against the gums of her front teeth and move the brush back and forth gently, in short, tooth-wide strokes.

The dentist may ask whether your water supply is fluoridated and, if so, whether you use tap water for drinking and cooking. If the dentist thinks that your child needs extra fluoride, he may recommend fluoride supplements, which come in liquid or chewable form and are taken daily. See *Cavities*, Part 5, for more on fluoride.

Note: Children with heart conditions, including congenital heart disease, previous endocarditis, acute rheumatic fever, mitral valve prolapse, and conditions requiring any prosthetic material (artificial valves or shunts) in the heart are at risk for bacterial infection during dental procedures such as teeth cleaning, scaling, or periodontal surgery. Mention any of these conditions to your child's dentist, who will provide a dose of antibiotics (amoxicillin) about 1 hour before the procedure and again 6 hours later. Children with other conditions, such as sickle-cell disease, immune deficiencies, and rheumatic fever, may also need antibiotics before and after a dental visit for protection against infection.

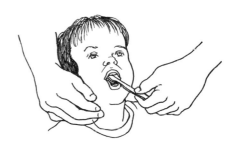

After brushing the outer and inner surfaces of the front and back teeth, brush the chewing surfaces.

Brushing Your Child's Teeth

You can begin to use fluoridated toothpaste to brush your child's teeth when he is around age 2. Until this age, it is best to use just water to avoid excess fluoride consumption (see *Cavities*, Part 5). Use a small amount of toothpaste, no larger than a pea. Several toothpaste brands are now made to taste good to children. If your child doesn't like toothpaste, you can continue brushing with just water. The mechanical action of the brush is more important than toothpaste.

If your child wants to brush his teeth by himself, let him, but make sure that you have a turn, too. A toddler's idea of brushing his teeth is usually to chew on the brush. Make sure to clean all areas of his teeth: the front, back, sides, and chewing surfaces.

Keeping Your Child Safe

Turn your back for a few seconds, and your child may be running across the parking lot, or teetering over the side of the deck, or rummaging in the medicine chest. The toddler years are probably the most demanding in terms of child safety. If you have baby-proofed your home (see p. 141), you have a big leg up. But your child's growing need for independence presents new safety issues at home and on the road. Here are some problems you may face and how to handle them.

Driveway Hazards About 100 young children from age 1 to 4 are killed each year after being hit by an automobile, often when the vehicle is backing out of the driveway. To reduce the risk when you go out, make sure that someone responsible keeps your child away from the car as you are backing out. Before getting into your car, walk behind it to check for children. Be especially careful when driving a minivan or sport utility vehicle, which ride high and make seeing a child behind them more difficult.

Traveling by Plane Don't be tempted to cut costs by having your toddler sit on your lap rather than buying him a seat. Children this age are at higher risk of injury during a crash or even a turbulent flight if they're not strapped into a car seat that you bring with you and secure with the airplane seat belt. Your child needs to sit in a car seat on an airplane until he weighs 40 pounds.

Backyard Swing Sets Install swing sets at least 6 feet from fences or walls. Cushion the ground beneath them with at least 10 inches of sand or 12 inches of wood chips or with rubber mats. Check regularly to make sure the swing set is securely anchored, and remove splinters or protruding nails or other hardware that could cause injury. Avoid sets with monkey bars.

Pets Dog and cat bites are a leading cause of toddler injuries. Young children are most vulnerable because they don't know how to behave safely with a pet. Never leave your child alone with a dog or cat—even one that appears gentle and good-natured. For more information, see *Bites, Animal and Human,* Part 5. Resist the temptation to get a pet iguana or another lizard, a turtle, or a rodent, such as a hamster or gerbil, because they often carry salmonella—a bacterium that is a common cause of illness. If your child touches any of these animals, make sure he washes his hands with soap and water immediately afterward.

Sunburn Before your child plays outdoors, apply a UVA/UVB (broad-spectrum) sunscreen with a sun protection factor (SPF) of at least 15 to prevent sunburn. Reapply the sunscreen if your child swims or otherwise wears or wipes it off. Give him a hat and sunglasses, too. Getting your child into the routine early will help make sun protection a lifelong habit.

SAFETY ALERT

Poisoning

Toddlers know no bounds and are at considerable risk for getting into poisonous substances. In fact, 50 percent of all poisonings in the United States involve children under the age of 5. To do your best to prevent your child from being poisoned, carry out the four *R*s of poison prevention.

Recognition: Survey the house to identify any poisonous plants, caustic cleaners, or other harmful household products. For help in identifying such plants or products and for other suggestions about poison-proofing your home, contact your local poison control center.

Removal: Throw away toxic household products. Use safe substitutes instead of corrosive cleaners or strong pesticides. Lock up hazardous substances and medications in cabinets that are shoulder height or higher. Make sure that all your medicines have child-resistant caps.

Readiness: Keep your local poison control center's telephone number near your phone; put it on speed-dial if you can. To locate your local poison control center, look in your phone book, or contact the American Association of Poison Control Centers (see Appendix: Parent Resources).

Response: Know what to do in case of poisoning. See Chapter 11, Preparing for and Handling Emergencies, page 415.

Tick-Borne Illnesses Check your child from head to toe for ticks each evening after he's been playing outdoors if you live in an area that ticks inhabit. Dressing your child in long pants, long sleeves, and socks and shoes is also helpful. For more information on tick-borne illnesses, see *Lyme Disease,* Part 5.

Child Abuse

Each year, millions of children are maltreated or neglected by their parents or care-givers. The problem crosses all economic and social barriers. Young children are especially vulnerable because of their size and relative helplessness. It is important to recognize the signs of child abuse in order to protect your child and other children in your community. Child abuse means any of the following:

▎ Physical harm, such as punching, burning, or in some other way inflicting injury; spanking (see p. 202) is not considered child abuse unless it is hard enough to cause injury

▎ Physical neglect, such as refusal or delay getting medical treatment, withholding food, or inadequately supervising a child

▎ Emotional neglect, such as might result if the parents beat each other or use drugs around the child

▌ Mental injury, including behavior ranging from belittling the child to inflicting bizarre punishments, such as locking him in a closet

▌ Sexual abuse, including fondling a child's genitals, exhibitionism, intercourse, rape, or any other sexual contact with a child

Signs of abuse aren't always as obvious as bruises. Other symptoms include abnormal behavior, such as aggression or social withdrawal, as well as low self-esteem, compulsivity, hyperactivity, and excessive tantrums. Under federal law, every state must have a system for preventing and responding to child abuse incidents. Most states have a child protection agency that investigates child abuse reports and helps families in which abuse has occurred or in which a child appears at risk. Anyone can report child abuse incidents to the state, but people who work with children are legally obligated to do so. They include teachers and others who work in schools, doctors, nurses, psychologists, social workers, and other health care providers.

A Parent's Life

When your child makes the transition from infancy to toddlerhood, your role as a parent changes. Now, instead of simply nurturing and meeting your baby's every need, you must begin coping with and nurturing your child's new, more independent self. That means making many new decisions about how much to give in to the many things your child wants (eating candy, watching TV, avoiding bedtime, etc.). Here are some ways to meet the new challenges and cope with the stresses of the toddler years.

Coping with Stress

Just when you are finally getting the hang of parenting, the playing field changes and you've got to relearn how to be a parent. Many of the old rules don't work anymore. It's one thing to have an infant who cries and fusses at times but who is basically under your control. It's another thing to have a toddler who cries and fusses, disagrees with you, and generally challenges you at every turn. How do you cope? Maintaining a sense of humor and remaining flexible will help. If one approach doesn't work, try something else. Rigid notions of how things should be have no place in parenting a toddler.

Saying No Without Guilt

Saying no isn't easy. Parents often feel guilty denying a child what he wants. No one wants to be a killjoy. But you owe it to yourself and your child to learn to say no when the circumstances demand it. Your child may cry, but, deep down, he'll feel more secure when you set consistent limits than when you don't. Setting limits is a parent's job. If your child cries and misbehaves, try to take it in stride by remembering that it is normal for a toddler to behave this way and it's normal for a parent to say no.

Coping with Your Anger

Inevitably, you will feel angry with your child on occasion. Children constantly test their limits and, in the process, may push you to your snapping point. Here are some strategies for controlling your anger at those explosive moments:

- Recognize when you're angry. You may even notice physical signs, such as an increased heartbeat or shortness of breath.

- Put your child in a safe place, and remove yourself from the situation that's angering you, for example, by going into another room to be alone for several minutes.

- Release your anger by punching a pillow, taking deep breaths, or talking to a friend. Once you have calmed down, look closely at the cause of your child's behavior and think about whether you're expecting too much from your child or from yourself.

- Realize that your child is not trying to hurt you when he acts up, but he may be begging for attention or imitating other people.

- Once you and your child are calm, discuss what made you angry with your child, reassuring him that although you are angry about the particular behavior, you still love him.

- *Do not* hit or shake your child.

- *Do not* call your child names or use other hurtful language.

Limiting TV and Videos

Years ago, no one thought that toddlers understood much of what they saw on TV. The assumption was that they were merely entertained by the music, the talking, and the movable feast of colorful images. But research has disproved this assumption, finding that even 1-year-olds remember what they see and relate it to real life. Some of this learning is positive, as when a toddler points to the letter E on a sign after having seen it on an educational program. But some of what children learn from TV is negative.

Many disturbing images appear on television, often during the commercials (advertisements for movies, for example) that appear during the most harmless shows. Even educational television and videos can inhibit your child's creativity. TV is a

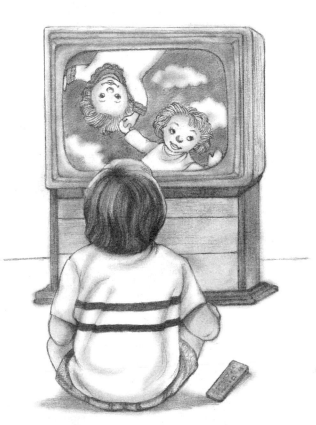

It may be tempting to use television programming or videos to keep your child occupied. Keep in mind that too much television can impair a young child's brain growth and development. Children thrive best on positive interaction with adults and other children.

passive activity that teaches your child to be a spectator. The more time a toddler spends sitting in front of a TV, even while watching educational television, the less time he's spending interacting with parents or caregivers and actively doing things that stimulate learning and development. Research has shown that watching a lot of television before preschool is associated with behavior problems and delays in reading readiness when children enter school. For this reason, the American Academy of Pediatrics urges parents to avoid television altogether for children under 2 years old and limit TV time to no more than 1 or 2 hours a day of high-quality educational shows and videos for children 2 years old or older.

If you start early, you can prevent your child from getting into the habit of watching show after show, video after video. Pay attention to what he is watching. You may find viewing a program with your child helpful. This gives you the opportunity to use it as a focus for discussion. You can point out, for example, how the activities on TV may differ from those in real life.

To help parents determine which television shows are appropriate for their children, the TV industry has a system for rating programs based on such things as violence and sexually suggestive content. The ratings appear next to many TV shows listed in the local newspaper.

In addition, newly manufactured televisions with V-Chips installed allow parents to block certain programs based on their ratings. Televisions with V-Chips present parents with an on-screen guide with which they can choose, for instance, to block programs containing sex, violence, or vulgar language. Many stores carry V-Chip set boxes, which can be attached to older sets. For more information on V-Chips and television ratings, see Appendix: Parent Resources, Parenting. Keep in mind that although the ratings system and V-Chip technology may be helpful, they are general and can never replace good parental judgment as to what is appropriate for your child to watch.

Tuning Out Violence

Toddlers shouldn't watch violent TV shows, movies, or videos. That includes cartoons that have a lot of hitting, punching, and other displays of physical force or abusive language. Young children are especially vulnerable to the negative effects of violent shows, because they have trouble telling the difference between fantasy and reality. Some children respond to violent programming by becoming more aggressive toward others or less sensitive to the pain and suffering of others. They may also become fearful. All these things can interfere with a child's ability to make friends and interact socially with other people.

Your Preschool Child

6

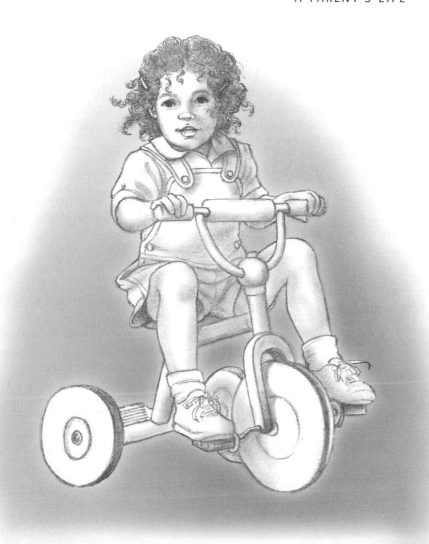

Preschool children have a lot to say, and most of it takes the form of questions. Their curiosity is endless, extending to everything that they see, hear, and experience. So be prepared with short and simple answers. You are your child's guide to the world around her.

Because children grow and change so quickly during their preschool years, the developmental part of this chapter is separated into two sections: Your 3-Year-Old and Your 4-Year-Old. The sections on health care, basic care, and parenting address the needs of both 3- and 4-year-olds.

Your 3-Year-Old

Three-year-olds can do many things for themselves, like getting in and out of a car seat, undressing, washing hands, and maybe even using the potty. They may proudly state their name and age. And their speech is usually clear enough for most people to understand. A child who is often more agreeable and cooperative and less likely to have tantrums is your reward for surviving the toddler years. This isn't to say that your child obeys your every command. Instead of throwing tantrums, your child is likely to throw words at you in the form of arguments. If you say, "Dinner first, then ice cream," she's likely to challenge you verbally: "No, ice cream first!" Life with a 3-year-old sometimes feels like being on the debating team.

Growing and Moving

By now, most of your child's growth is in the legs and torso—she's growing longer and leaner. That little potbelly of the last 2 years is beginning to disappear as your child grows taller and her abdominal muscles become stronger.

SO BIG!

At 3 years, the average boy is
- 36¾ to 38¾ inches tall.
- 29¼ to 34 pounds.

At 3 years, the average girl is
- 36¼ to 38½ inches tall.
- 28¼ to 33¼ pounds.

For more information, see Appendix: Growth Charts.

On the Move: Gross Motor Skills

Children at this age are more agile. They walk and run more fluidly than they did a year ago. Your child can probably climb stairs using alternating feet—one foot on one step, the other foot on the next—rather than putting first one foot and then the other on each step. But your child may still descend the stairs one foot at a time, because going down is more difficult than going up. From your child's viewpoint, riding a tricycle may be the most important physical achievement!

Handling New Tasks: Fine Motor Skills

Your child is also learning to coordinate the fine muscles of her hands, which results in many new skills. Many 3-year-olds can snip paper with safety scissors and may have enough control over a pencil to copy simple shapes. Try

▬ DEVELOPMENTAL MILESTONES

Age	Most Children	Some Children
3 years	Jump with both feet at the same time	Play simple board games
	Balance briefly on one foot	Brush their teeth without help
	Throw a ball overhand	Dress themselves without help
	Ride a tricycle	Explain the use of common objects
	Say their name, age, and gender and name a friend	
	Engage in imaginative play	
	Stack eight blocks	
	Use adjectives often	
	Use action verbs	

As you review this list of milestones, remember that children who are within the normal range will have some areas in which they excel and others in which they are slower. Not achieving a particular milestone at the designated time is not always a matter of concern. If you and your child's doctor are concerned about your child's overall development or any of your child's developmental skills, such as language, hearing, vision, or motor skills, seek the help of the appropriate specialist. For more information, see *Developmental Problems,* Part 5.

drawing a simple cross on paper, for example, and see if your child can do it, too. She may even be able to write some letters of the alphabet, although she probably can't yet hold a pencil in the proper writing position. Most children still clench their pencils in a fist or grip them with a thumb on one side and fingers on the other.

Your child's improved dexterity and hand-eye coordination may now give rise to a broader range of artistic expression. Instead of merely stacking blocks, she may now attempt to construct houses and other structures with blocks or snap-together toys. With some help, a child can flatten clay or dough and shape it with cookie cutters. She can glue pieces of paper and paint a picture with a brush or finger paints.

Communicating

At age 3, your child now understands most of what you say, and you should understand most of what she says. Children at this age routinely use sentences composed of four or five words, often with connectors like "because," indicating that they understand cause and effect. Children now refer to themselves as "I," and use other pronouns, although they may get "him" and "her" confused. Plurals and numbers are also part of their language. Your child may eagerly tell anyone who asks that she's 3 years old (often holding up three fingers), and she may be able to count three or more objects.

Grammatical errors and mispronunciations are common. Many children have trouble with certain consonant sounds, like *l, r, s,* and *th.* For example, it's normal for

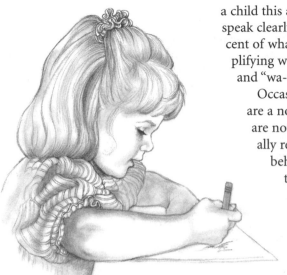

a child this age to say "dis" instead of "this." But most children speak clearly enough for a stranger to understand about 75 percent of what they say. At this stage, children gradually stop simplifying words with babyish talk like "noo-noos" for "noodles" and "wa-wa" for water.

Occasional problems, some of which sound like stuttering, are a normal part of language development at this age and are not a reason to be concerned. Occasional stuttering usually resolves itself. However, if you notice any unusual behavior, such as your child contorting her face while she tries to speak, discuss it with your child's doctor or a speech-language pathologist. Parents are usually the first to know if their child has a speech or language problem. So trust your instincts, and seek help if you think your child may need it.

At age 3, scribbling gives way to more precise strokes of the crayon. Your preschooler may be able to copy shapes, draw letters, or draw a simple stick figure.

Learning Language

Surprisingly, some of the common grammatical mistakes children make provide evidence that they are learning grammatical rules. For example, 3-year-olds understand that adding *s* to the end of a word makes it plural and that adding *ed* to the end of a verb converts it to the past tense. But they often overgeneralize by saying things like "mouses" instead of "mice" and "goed" instead of "went." The nearly universal tendency for children to make these errors shows that children learn language by rules rather than simple imitation. If they were just imitating the adults around them, they would say "mice" and "went."

QUESTIONS PARENTS ASK
Suddenly Silent

Q: My son talks a lot at home, but when he's with other adults—even people he knows fairly well, like baby-sitters and his friends' parents—he hardly says a word. Sometimes he won't answer when someone asks him a question. Is something wrong?

A: Even a 3-year-old who's typically talkative and outgoing around the house can be shy around people outside his immediate family. Sometimes children this age respond with gestures rather than words. For example, if asked his age, a child may put up three fingers rather than say "three." You needn't worry as long as your child talks well with some people and tries to communicate with words or gestures. But tell your child's doctor if he shows signs that he doesn't hear or understand when spoken to—for example, if he usually looks confused or doesn't respond at all.

Learning

At around age 3, many children start showing an interest in letters and numbers. They may recognize some letters of the alphabet. They can also count to 3 and possibly higher. These intellectual feats are something to be proud of. You can help your child develop them further by talking about letters and numbers during play and everyday observations. But don't push. Otherwise, you risk taking the fun out of your child's natural curiosity about letters, numbers, and other things and—worse— risk making her feel that she's not doing well.

Children this age are eager to learn. If your child wants to know something, she won't hesitate to ask. She'll ask about something else, and something else after that. Sometimes it will seem that every other word out of your child's mouth is "Why?" Be patient and receptive to her questions; it helps her soak up new information.

Playing and Learning

Despite the seemingly endless questions, most of your child's learning still revolves around play. Many children at this age understand spatial relationships (how shapes fit together and how objects are oriented to one another) well enough to do beginner puzzles. And the more puzzles they do, the better their grasp of spatial relations. Your child may now be able to identify colors; that means she's ready to play games involving color recognition. Playing these games is good practice in cooperating, listening, and following rules—social skills that children need to learn before starting school. But don't expect too much. Children this age like to play by their own rules, and they have a hard time losing, so you may find it best to downplay rigid rules, as well as winning and losing. The idea is for your child to have fun and learn something in the process—not to cause tears.

Imaginative Play

At age 3, a child's pretend play involves more storytelling than before, a sign of her growing ability to think in terms of symbols, cause and effect, and timing. The stories usually mirror

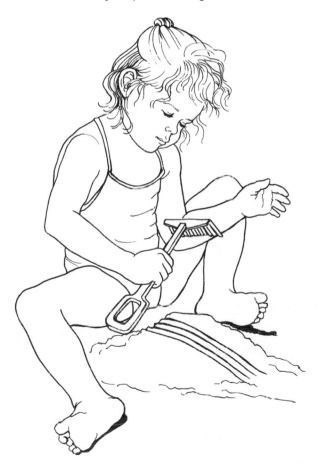

The simple act of playing with sand toys is a learning experience for preschoolers. Through such play, your child's understanding of cause and effect and how objects fit or work together is enhanced.

either familiar rituals or situations from books, tapes, or CDs. With toys as props, a child may invent a story of a daddy duck teaching a baby duck how to swim or a kitten being scared and going to its mommy for protection. A child sometimes plays a part in the stories she invents. For example, she may get on her tricycle and say that she's driving to the supermarket to buy a long list of food. It helps her rehearse real events and relationships with family members and friends in the safe environment of make-believe.

Although 3-year-olds seem to know that this sort of play is make-believe, they cannot always tell fantasy from reality. At Halloween she may not know that the strange creatures at the door or the party are really other children dressed as ghosts or skeletons. Even cartoon characters on TV or in computer games can seem real. Such confusion may extend to the way a preschooler sees her parents. She may believe, for example, that Daddy can actually stop the rain or that Mommy controls when the sun goes down. No amount of logical explanation from you will convince her otherwise.

TOUCHPOINT

"I'm Scared"

Is your child suddenly scared of barking dogs? Fire alarms? Does she scream when she sees a spider? Is she afraid of the shadows on her bedroom walls at night? It's normal for 3-year-olds to become fearful of things that previously didn't faze them. This doesn't mean they're regressing. To the contrary, fear is a sign of their growing awareness of the world around them—a dog's growl may remind a child of an angry dog she once saw. But it is also a way for children to come to terms with the stormy world within. Preschoolers have aggressive feelings toward other children and sometimes toward their parents. Kids may act on these feelings by hitting or yelling, but they're scared of these feelings all the same. Because they're incapable of saying that their wild feelings frighten them, they project their fears onto bugs, shadows, loud noises, and other wild things.

You can help by talking to your child about her feelings and acknowledging that her feelings are real, even if the things she is afraid of pose no true threat. Not that a heart-to-heart talk can wipe away fears, but knowing that you're listening can comfort your child. You can also show your child safe and socially acceptable ways to handle anger. When you're angry, try not to lose control. It is better to talk calmly but firmly, and if you do fly off the handle, say you're sorry. In other words, let your child see that it's natural to get angry and that it's possible to get over it. And during this fearful period, be especially selective about the TV programs and videos that your child watches, screening out those with sinister characters and violence.

Source: Touchpoints Project (see p. 81).

Social and Emotional Development

More than before, children this age crave the company of other children. Their time together is much friendlier than it used to be. Although much of their play is still side-by-side (so-called parallel play), they're beginning to play cooperatively. Some children can share their toys with other children at least some of the time, and they're often willing to take turns. If one child hops on a friend's tricycle, the friend is less likely to throw a tantrum than he was 6 months or a year ago.

Three-year-olds often unconsciously act out their feelings with their playmates. They'll hug each other one minute and tease each other the next. They'll test to see how far they can push a playmate with teasing or anger or other emotions and still have that child as a friend. At different times, a child may regard a particular friend as a baby to be protected, as a parent figure to be worshiped, or as a rival to be fought.

In addition to acting out their feelings, 3-year-olds often can describe them. Your child probably tells you if she's sad, scared, or tired and notices other people's moods, too. She might point to a drawing in a book of a person who's frowning and say, "He looks grumpy." You can help your child with this important social skill of recognizing the feelings and emotions on another person's face by pointing out people who look sad, angry, happy, or surprised in books and magazines and on television.

When your child is scared or angry, she can better control her emotions than she could have even a few months ago. She might hug her special blanket for comfort when she's upset, rather than automatically crying—at least some of the time.

Recognizing Limits

As their self-awareness grows, children reach another important social and emotional benchmark: They begin to accept that they can't do everything by themselves. Whereas they used to scream in frustration if they had trouble with a task, now they

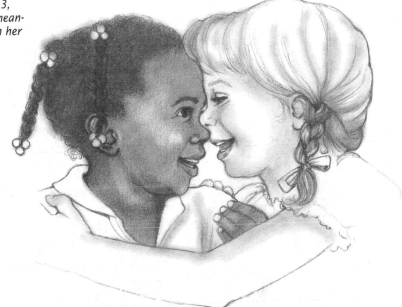

You'll find that at age 3, your child will enjoy meaningful friendships with her playmates.

sometimes ask for help. They'll watch what a parent or someone else does and then try to imitate it. This new sense of perspective helps children cooperate more with playmates. Cooperation is a social skill that will help them in play groups, preschool, and, of course, well beyond.

Becoming More Independent

As children gravitate more toward other children, they eventually separate from their parents more easily. In general, morning good-byes at preschool may be less tearful than they used to be, because children have worked through the anxiety they once felt when apart from their parents. Still, the process is one step forward and one step back as your child experiments with her growing independence. Don't be surprised if she separates easily from you one day but clings and cries the next.

As in the past, your child will test the limits of your authority. But the difference is that now she's doing it more skillfully, with words. If you say, "You need your rain boots today," she may reply, "No, I don't." Sometimes she seems to be looking for an argument, like when she asks for a cookie before dinner and, anticipating that you'll say no, quickly adds, "Only one." If you agree to one, she may well say, "No, two." Don't let yourself get drawn into these arguments. The way to avoid them is to present the child with concrete choices. If she wants a snack, offer her a couple of healthy alternatives to choose from, such as apple slices or whole-wheat toast. To avoid clothing battles, set out a couple of choices and allow her plenty of time to decide.

A FATHER'S STORY
Snow Boots on the Beach

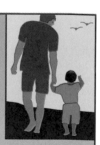

The day we left for vacation at the beach, Rachel insisted on wearing her snow boots. I said no, but she kept pleading. Finally, my wife gave in just to get her to stop arguing with us.

I was still opposed. I thought it was our responsibility to teach Rachel right from wrong, and wearing snow boots in July is definitely wrong. I imagined people staring at us and thinking we were nuts.

Just as I expected, people stared at us when Rachel wore her boots on the boardwalk. But most of them smiled at us in a friendly sort of way. They were probably the ones who knew what life was like with a 3-year-old.

Rachel couldn't have been happier. For most of the week, she seemed cheerful and undemanding. I came to realize that letting her wear snow boots on the beach was good for two reasons. Rachel got what she wanted—which gave her a sense of control. The rest of us got a peaceful family vacation. I learned to choose when to take a stand and I decided that making a battleground over what she wears on her feet is not usually worth it. Unless she wants to go barefoot in the snow!

Play Dates

When planning play dates, two's company and three's a crowd. Children this age can easily get overwhelmed when more than two children are together at once. Take your child's lead on this question. If she plays happily with two other children, feel free to invite two. If she retreats to her room or gets cranky, next time limit her to one friend, or none, if she doesn't seem to want company on a particular day.

Rituals and Transitions

A child's need for rituals grows stronger at this age. A bedtime ritual in which the bath is always followed by the bedtime story, which is always followed by a song, which is always followed by lights out and a kiss, gives a child a sense of security in knowing what comes next.

A child at this age also needs time for transitions. Don't be surprised if your child balks when you try to get her to put down her toys to put on her jacket for a car trip. Three-year-olds have difficulty making the transition from one activity to the next. Give her a warning ("In five minutes, we're going out") and then another warning so that she can gear up for the next event.

Your 4-Year-Old

A 4-year-old is proud to be 4. This is the first birthday that a child can really antici-pate, and many children talk about their fourth birthday for weeks or months before it comes. Of course, their ever-growing awareness extends well beyond the calendar. Many show an interest in recognizing and writing the letters of the alphabet and take great pride in reading their names and in counting objects.

Four-year-olds show maturity in other ways, too. Most can use the toilet and dress themselves with little or no help and can put away their toys or clothes—with coaxing. But their "grown-up" behavior one minute is at odds with their silliness the next. Kids this age love singing goofy songs and talking nonsense—and nothing prompts more uncontrollable laughter than bathroom humor. Don't worry: This, too, shall pass.

Growing and Moving

For about 2 years, your child's posture has been maturing. At this stage, children tend to stand more like an adult, with their feet approximately as far apart as their shoul-ders. They can walk downstairs using alternating feet, and their balance is good enough for skipping, hopping, walk-ing on a curved line without tripping, and possibly even walking along a low balance beam.

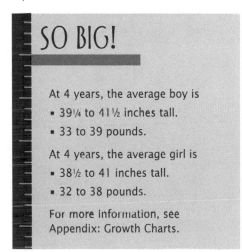

SO BIG!

At 4 years, the average boy is
- 39¼ to 41½ inches tall.
- 33 to 39 pounds.

At 4 years, the average girl is
- 38½ to 41 inches tall.
- 32 to 38 pounds.

For more information, see Appendix: Growth Charts.

DEVELOPMENTAL MILESTONES

Age	Most Children	Some Children
4 years	Draw a person with four parts (i.e., head, body, and legs)	Balance on each foot for 4 to 5 seconds
	Brush their teeth	Name two opposites
	Dress themselves	Draw a person with six parts (i.e., head, body, arms, legs)
	Give their first and last names	Form letters or write their first or last name—or even both
	Tell about their daily activities and experiences	
	Hop on one foot	
	Ride a bicycle with training wheels	
	Play board or card games	
	Count three blocks	
	Copy a circle and a cross	
	Name four colors correctly	

As you review this list of milestones, remember that children who are within the normal range will have some areas in which they excel and others in which they are slower. Not achieving a particular milestone at the designated time is not always a matter of concern. If you and your child's doctor are concerned about your child's overall development or any of your child's developmental skills, such as language, hearing, vision, or motor skills, seek the help of the appropriate specialist. For more information, see *Developmental Problems*, Part 5.

On the Move: Gross Motor Skills

Children's growing physical strength and agility at this age open new opportunities for them. Sometimes it may seem that your child never stops moving. Many communities have sports teams and classes beginning around this age. Don't push, but if your child seems interested in sports or dance classes, such as soccer, gymnastics, swimming, skiing, skating, or ballet, now may be a good time to start.

Now is the time to begin playing catch with your child, but don't expect her to keep her eye on the ball just yet. Many 4-year-olds tend to close their eyes when the ball is coming toward them. That's why they miss many of the balls you throw. It takes years for most children to learn how to catch and throw well. But practice definitely helps develop dexterity, coordination, and confidence.

Handling New Tasks: Fine Motor Skills

The development of children's fine motor skills is especially apparent in the artwork that they turn out. A year ago, your child may have been able only to make tiny, random snips in a piece of paper (using safety scissors). Now she may have enough control to cut in a straight line. Her drawing is changing, too. She has gone beyond those circular scribbles and sketchy crosses of a year ago to carefully copying a circle and a cross and possibly even drawing a person with a head, a body, and arms or legs. She may even be able to write her name.

As for day-to-day activities, your child's fine motor skills are now progressing to the point where she may be able to dress herself, buttoning shirts, zipping pants, and fastening straps. She may still have trouble snapping her jeans, and tying shoes will be too difficult for another year or two.

Communicating

Remember the days when you had to coax your child to talk? By this time, your child may need no encouragement. In fact, she may never seem to stop talking until she falls asleep. Nothing will get in her way—least of all your conversations with another adult. If anything, seeing you talk to someone else is like an invitation to interrupt in order to recapture your attention. Remind your child not to interrupt, but don't expect her to have the self-control to do as you say just yet. Here are two ways to help her control herself. One is to suggest that she say, "Excuse me," when she has something to say. The other is to structure family conversations so that everyone gets a turn to talk, including your child. Help her feel that others are listening to and valuing what she has to say.

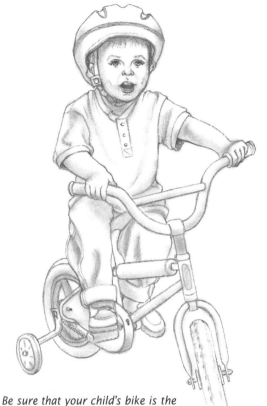

Be sure that your child's bike is the right size for him (the balls of both of his feet should touch the ground while he's holding the handlebars) and that he never rides near the street. Whether riding a bicycle or tricycle, your child should always wear a helmet that fits.

Four-year-olds know around 1,500 words, and many use them in complex sentences to tell stories about what happened during the day and to describe things they've seen or heard. Unlike what they grasped a year ago, most children now have a firm understanding of words that relate one idea to another, like "if," "when," and "why." They use these words to ask endless questions about how things work and why people act the way they do.

Children's language use and understanding, as well as their speech, still have limitations at this stage. For example, though your child may understand concepts like big and little, and same and different, she probably can't yet grasp time concepts like yesterday and next week. She may describe in rich detail something that happened at preschool, but be unable to tell you whether it happened yesterday or a week ago.

Normal Mistakes

Mild stuttering (dysfluency) is still normal at this age as your child's eagerness to speak seems to create a traffic jam of words. Mispronunciations are less common than a year ago, but they're still part of a 4-year-old's speech. The sounds children mispronounce most often are *f, l, r, s, v, sh,* and *th.* So, "very" might come out like "berry" and "the" like "duh." And your child is still probably making many of the same grammatical errors that she was making a year ago, like "mouses" for mice and "brang" for brought. Treat these errors as you have all along, by using the correct words rather than by telling your child that she said something wrong. For example, if your child says, "I brang my snack outside," you might say, "I see you've brought your snack outside." As long as they hear language spoken correctly, children usually learn to correct their own grammar by about age 6.

Early Reading and Writing Skills

Your preschooler's communication skills may also include some reading and writing. Many 4-year-olds can recognize all the capital letters of the alphabet (recognition of lowercase letters comes later), especially if they've spent a lot of time being read to and looking at books by themselves. Listening to and responding to stories in books are important activities for your child's written and spoken language development.

QUESTIONS PARENTS ASK
Pretend Reading

Q: Our 4-year-old has memorized many books that he's familiar with, and he "reads" them out loud without missing a word. Is he teaching himself how to read?

A: This is considered a significant early step toward learning to read. At its most basic level, your child is learning that the words on the page are separate from the pictures. But he's also noticing that the pictures help tell the story. Some children seem to be reading a book when what they're really doing is reading the pictures and making up their own story around them. Other children have truly memorized the book's words after hearing them over and over again. Eventually, your child will look at the print, begin to recognize the capital letters, and later on notice that specific groups of letters correspond to the words he's memorized. He'll also recognize simple words that appear frequently, like "a," "I," and "the." In the meantime, he's exercising his memory and power of concentration.

Learning

Four-year-olds learn by asking, and they've got a lot of big questions on their minds, like these: Why is the sky blue? How was the world made? What keeps the moon up in the sky? Who is God? Why do we die? If you're expecting another baby, your child will probably want to know how babies are made and how they come out.

Answer these questions honestly. Instead of fairy-tale explanations, like "An invisible giant holds the moon up," give simple but realistic explanations: "The moon spins around the earth like a ball on a string." Avoid elaborate physics or biology lessons, which will only cause your child to lose interest and change the subject. For guidance, you might show her books for preschoolers about subjects like the solar system and the human body.

Despite her preoccupation with fantasy, your child understands the difference between fantasy and reality much of the time. Though she may still believe in Santa Claus, this year when the monsters come trick-or-treating at Halloween, chances are that she'll know that they're just kids dressed up. In addition, she can better distinguish between fantasy and reality in the light of day than at nighttime, when a chair in her room may look like a monster. When it comes to TV or videos, you'll need to carefully select programs and games and sit with your child through some of them to interpret them for her (see p. 214).

Logical Thinking

Your child's thinking is also becoming more logical. Many children this age can count to about 15 and figure out which number is smaller (or larger) when asked to compare the value of two numbers under 10. But their logic goes only so far. For example, they may assume that a nickel is worth more than a dime because it's bigger.

In one classic experiment, children watch as an adult shows them two vases that hold the same amount—one tall and thin, the other short and fat. Then an adult fills the tall vase with water and pours the water into the short vase. Preschoolers asked which vase has more water usually say the tall, thin one. They believe that this is so, even when told that no water spilled or was left over when poured from that vase into the other one. What the children can't yet grasp is that the amount of water doesn't change just because it's transferred to another container.

Museums and Plays

Going to children's museums and concerts and short plays for children can be a wonderful way to spend a day with your preschooler. Just don't get too ambitious. The idea is to spark your child's interest in the world around her. Many local libraries have activities and live performances created with the preschool child in mind.

Most preschoolers have neither the attention span nor the temperament to sit quietly for long stretches and "behave." You're best off starting with exhibits and performances geared to young children. Many parents find that they can take their preschoolers to a museum but can't stay for more than about an hour. And don't expect to linger at a picture or an exhibit for more than a moment—your child will likely race from one to the next. When your child starts to fidget and whine, it's time either to leave or to go to the cafeteria.

When deciding which cultural attractions to go to, take your cue from your child. If she's interested in art, take her to an art museum. If she likes animals, go to an aquarium or a zoo. If she enjoys learning about dinosaurs (a popular subject with preschoolers), a natural history or science museum with dinosaur fossils and bones is a good choice.

School Readiness

Every public school district and every private school has its own date by which a child must be 5 years old in order to start kindergarten. But many parents whose children are old enough still wonder if their children are ready.

Wide variations exist in the normal rate of development of children between the ages of 4 and 5. And within these normal limits, no hard and fast rules exist for determining which children can handle the social and academic demands of kindergarten. To a large extent, the answer depends on the school, the child, and the family involved.

If you're concerned about your child's readiness, discuss her development with your doctor and the educators at the school your child will attend and ask whether a formal preschool evaluation is in order. Public schools usually have psychologists or other specialists to do the evaluation. Or your child's doctor can refer you to a doctor who is a specialist in child development. Even if your child's development lags in a few areas, she may be able to start school if she has therapy ahead of time and her school offers the kind of special education that she needs. All public school systems are required by federal law to provide special education services for children age 3 and older who are found to have academic learning delays. The schools should develop an individual education plan describing each child's needs and the services that will address them.

If you are considering holding your child back at kindergarten age, weigh the advantages and disadvantages. A child slightly older than her peers may handle the academic and social challenges better than a younger child. On the other hand, she may not feel challenged enough. Also, she may feel physically large and out of place among her younger classmates. And several years later, your child may enter puberty sooner than other children in the class—a situation that may result in social and behavioral difficulties for a child.

Preparing Your Child for School

The best way to stimulate interest in reading, writing, and arithmetic is not to drill your child with flash cards, but to make learning part of her everyday life and, especially, part of things that interest her. Doing this makes learning meaningful and fun. Here are some ideas:

▮ Keep your home well stocked with markers, pens, pencils, and paper. Many studies show that the preschoolers with the highest levels of written language development are those who have the easiest access to writing tools.

▮ Cut out magazine pictures of babies, animals, cars, and toys, and help your child create her own scrapbook of familiar objects. She'll "read" it over and over again.

▮ Encourage your child to help you make a grocery list. Ask her if she wants to make her own list or scribble some "words" on yours.

▮ Take dictation. Have your child make up a story (or make up a story with her). Write down what she says word for word to give her practice organizing her thoughts for writing.

▮ Point out words that your child often sees at home and in the neighborhood, like stop signs, sports logos, and your street sign. Being aware of the words around her will help her learn to read.

SCHOOL READINESS

Areas of Readiness	What to Look For	What to Do If Your Child Lags
Social	Child enjoys preschool; she doesn't cry excessively or show other signs of distress. For children not in preschool: Child separates easily from you, plays well with other children.	Work with your child's preschool teacher on easing her anxiety. Ask your doctor if your child's difficulties are within normal limits and, if not, how to ease your child's anxiety about separation and help her play cooperatively.
	Child follows instructions.	Practice having your child follow a set of instructions you give her at home.
	Child can concentrate on a task for several minutes and sit still for several minutes.	Ask your doctor whether your child's behavior is within the normal range. Also, ask whether your child should be evaluated by a psychologist or another specialist at your elementary school or by a neuro-developmental specialist to help identify the cause of your child's difficulty.
Developmental	Child can speak clearly.	Ask your doctor about speech therapy to improve your child's pronunciation.
	Child can hold a pencil in position for writing and can copy a circle or draw pictures.	If your child is not drawing at all, a neurological assessment might be in order to determine why. Or ask about occupational therapy to improve your child's fine motor skills.
	Child can count to 3 and knows some colors.	If your child is not counting, ask your doctor for an assessment that would help explain whether the cause is a developmental delay (such as a language or perception problem).

▌ Give your child many opportunities to see her name, whether on labels or by writing it out (in all capital letters) yourself and hanging it in her room. A child's name is often the first word she learns to read and write.

▌ Visit the library with your child, and be sure she has access to plenty of age-appropriate books.

▌ Look at picture books together. They'll encourage you and your child to talk about what's going on in the story, thereby sharpening her ability to understand what she sees and hears. Ask her progressively harder questions about what the illustrations show, starting with questions like, "What color is the house?" and building to, "Who lives there?" and "Why is he going out?"

▌ Count. Seize the opportunity to practice counting whenever your child asks, "How many?" Make it a game to see how high your child can go.

▌ Talk about different sizes, shapes, and weights. When your child helps you cook, show her that a tablespoon is bigger than a teaspoon. And as you look at road signs, posters, and even the moon, talk about their various shapes.

Social and Emotional Development

Children this age love to make friends. Many 4-year-olds declare that they have a "best friend," although this person may change from one week to the next. Chances are, your child will want to look and behave like her closest friends, asking to wear the same clothes, eat the same breakfast cereals, and get the same toys. Boys may prefer playing with boys, and girls with girls. Your child may choose toys and activities based on gender, rejecting those that seem to be intended for the opposite gender. Four-year-olds are moving out into the world as never before.

Cooperating with Other Children

The play of 4-year-olds is truly cooperative. They can play board games, build with blocks together, play ball games, play house, or act out elaborate fantasies involving action figures, stuffed animals, costumes, and other props. They share their toys much more easily than they used to, because they've learned from experience that their toys will be returned. They've also learned that sharing is a handy way to get other children to play with them and to get to play with other children's interesting toys.

Play doesn't always go smoothly, however. Sometimes 4-year-olds still squabble. But they do so with less pushing and shoving and more with words, like "I hate you" or "You're not my friend anymore." Don't be alarmed if you hear your child saying things like this, or worse. Children can get very angry, and venting anger is natural. Expressing themselves with words is not only safer than using fists, but also more appropriate for their age.

Gender Differences

Are girls really partial to dolls and boys to trucks and trains? As a parent, you may want to encourage your child to be open to all kinds of play by giving your daughters trains and trucks and making sure your son has at least one doll. It is common for girls to play with trains and for many boys to play house. But despite your efforts, you may find that your child often prefers toys that are traditional for her gender. Research shows, for example, that boys as young as 1 year old show less interest in dolls than do girls, regardless of their parents' attitudes, suggesting that the preference for gender-specific toys may be at least partly inborn.

This preference grows stronger during the preschool years because of a developmental shift that occurs at around age 3 to 4. By now, children know not only whether they are boys or girls but that they will remain males or females. They also continually pick up cues about what it means to be male or female. They may observe, for example, that Daddy fixes broken things around the house and Mommy does the cooking, that girls and women sometimes wear dresses but boys and men don't. While watching TV, children see girls playing with dolls and boys with toy cars and action figures. They absorb these and other gender stereotypes from books and videos, teachers, playmates, and relatives. As part of their ongoing search for who they are, preschoolers want to fit the mold. They tend to gravitate toward playmates of the same sex, as well as toys and clothing that they associate with their gender.

What about a child who breaks the mold—a boy who plays dress-up at nursery school or a girl who'd rather be with boys? You needn't try to change your child's behavior. A 4-year-old boy might want to try on a colorful feminine hat or jewelry because it looks like fun, and a girl can dislike playing with dolls (and other girls who play mostly with dolls) and still be perfectly normal. The only cause for concern comes when a child shows no interest in same-sex play or playmates: A boy wants to dress like a girl most of the time; a girl shuns other girls and does not imitate her mother or other women. Such extreme behavior can sometimes reflect psychological problems with the child or the family as a whole; discuss this behavior with a doctor.

QUESTIONS PARENTS ASK
Body Exploration

Q: Our neighbor called to say that our 4-year-old son and her daughter pulled down their pants in front of each other. Should we say anything to our son or punish him?

A: Preschoolers have a strong sense of curiosity and a natural interest in their (and other children's) genitals, so they may want to sneak a peak. This is normal and innocent. They know that genitals define gender, and this is an age when children identify with their own gender and become fascinated with the differences between girls and boys. Don't reprimand your son, who may be traumatized if a parent reacts with anger and harsh punishment, but tell him that he shouldn't pull his pants down in public—that's something he should only do at home—and that he certainly should not let anyone touch his private parts. Remind your child to tell you if someone touches his private parts.

Though some sexual behavior (such as masturbation, talking about genitalia, or even examining another child's genitals) is normal for preschoolers, other sexually related behavior is not. Excessive exhibitionism or modesty, persistent attempts to see or touch others' (children's, parents') genitals, or assuming a coital position with another child is a cause for concern, possibly signaling that the child has been sexually abused. Or it might indicate that the child is observing sexual behavior that he shouldn't be viewing, either in real life or on television, on videos, on the computer, or in magazines. It's up to you to monitor what he is seeing. Ask your child's doctor for guidance if you have concerns about his behavior.

Fantasy Play, Imaginary Friends

The pretend play that children have been engaging in since toddlerhood reaches new heights by around age 4. Many children enjoy playing with action figures or dolls or replicas of movie characters. Creating, or reenacting, scenes with these figures is one way that children express their emotions. Don't be concerned if you see your child using one action figure to clobber another, shouting words like, "I'll kill you." This sort of play is a safe outlet for a child's aggression.

Some 4-year-olds also have imaginary friends or imaginary siblings. They might even blame these imaginary pals for things that they themselves have done wrong. Using a pretend friend as a scapegoat gives a child an escape when she knows she's done something wrong and she feels ashamed, but she doesn't know how to cope with her feelings. It's normal for children to do this occasionally. However, it is a concern if a child blames an imaginary friend for her bad behavior continuously, or if such a friend replaces real friends. If either of these things happen, consult your child's doctor.

TOUCHPOINT

Tantrums Again?

Remember the tantrums of the toddler years? They often resurface in 4-year-olds in the form of angry words and defiant behavior. Tell your child that it's time to leave her friend's house, and she may shout, "No!" and run off. Deny her a much-desired piece of candy, and she may say things like, "I hate you" and "Shut up."

Chances are that your child wasn't so rebellious last year. What's changed is your child's growing awareness of her identity. She is aware of her gender, her skin color, perhaps whether she has been adopted. She knows the labels, but she's not sure what they mean. And this uncertainty may make her feel insecure at times. Challenge what she does, and she may think you're challenging who she is.

Being rude and rebellious is your child's way of testing the limits of her independence, and your love. The worst thing you can do is explode with anger. Take a deep breath, be patient, and show understanding. Say that if she's mad at you, you'll talk with her about her feelings when she calms down. This is also the time to tell her that rude language ("shut up," for example) is unacceptable. If her behavior escalates to a tantrum, ignore it if possible (see p. 188 for more on coping with tantrums). This may also be the appropriate time for a time-out (see p. 203).

You can prevent much defiant behavior by avoiding small battles. Clothing is a good example. If it's important to your child to wear a beloved jumper that's missing buttons—and she needn't look her best—let her have her way.

Source: Touchpoints Project (see p. 81).

A FATHER'S STORY
Daddy, Will You Marry Me?

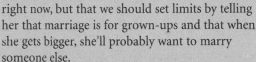

My daughter has been saying that she wants to marry me. She says that she and I will live in our house, and Mommy will live in the house next door. When Julia first started talking about this, my wife and I thought it was cute. But when she continued the fantasy, we got a little nervous. It just didn't seem normal. After all, she's the kid and we're the couple. Doesn't she understand that?

I started wondering if maybe I was fueling her feelings by being too affectionate with her. I felt uneasy even giving her a hug when I returned from work. I stopped knowing how to behave with my own daughter!

My wife talked with the pediatrician about what was going on. The doctor said that 4-year-olds commonly want to marry or flirt with the parent of the opposite sex. She explained that we shouldn't make Julia stop right now, but that we should set limits by telling her that marriage is for grown-ups and that when she gets bigger, she'll probably want to marry someone else.

We tried what the doctor suggested. At first, Julia said, "I'll marry Daddy when I'm a grown-up." But a few days later she announced that she planned to marry someone else—a boy from her school. I felt relieved. But, I have to admit, I began to wonder how I'm going to feel in 10 or 20 years when she says the same thing.

Caring for Your Preschool Child

Now that your child is willing and able to participate in much of her own care, your job will gradually become less hands-on and more supervisory. You can provide nutritious foods, remind her to use the bathroom, and help her select clothes. The days of feeding, dressing, and diapering are gone.

Instead of dressing and feeding her yourself, your job now will be to find ways to motivate your child to do what she needs to do. Just because a child is capable of getting dressed doesn't mean that she'll always do it. Many parents are driven to anger upon entering their child's room expecting to see her dressed for the day, only to find her lolling on the floor in her pajamas. Children this age delight in dawdling—while they eat, dress, or play. And it takes more than nagging to get them to finish a meal or dressed and out the door on time. Eating habits, discipline, and good hygiene habits are among some important concerns during this time. The following pages provide some advice and suggestions on caring for and protecting your 3- or 4-year-old child.

Eating

Mealtime with a preschooler can be messy and tense, or it can be more relaxed, enjoyable, but still messy, depending on how you approach it. Feeding a preschooler is less labor-intensive than feeding a younger child. Your child can use a spoon and fork now, and less food is likely to land on the floor and clothing than when she was a toddler. You no longer have to cut most foods into tiny pieces to prevent choking. But chewy meats still have to be cut into small, easy-to-swallow pieces of no larger than ½ inch.

Feeding Picky Eaters

Like toddlers, preschoolers can be picky, unpredictable eaters. Your child may insist on nothing but yogurt for breakfast every day for several weeks, then suddenly declare, "I don't like yogurt." She may refuse to eat anything green (or another color), or she may want cereal for dinner and a cheese sandwich for breakfast. Many children won't eat two foods they normally like if the foods are touching each other or mixed together on the plate. Such quirks can be frustrating to parents, but they're not worth fighting over. There's no harm in your child's eating breakfast food for dinner or separating her carrots from her chicken soup, as long as the foods she eats are nutritious.

To make sure that your child eats well, eat healthy food yourself. Lots of whole grains, fruits, and vegetables are good for the entire family. Also, control the food you bring into the house, avoiding junk foods, such as high-fat chips, cakes, and cookies, and cereals in which the first or second item on the list of ingredients is a form of sugar, such as sucrose, fructose, glucose, or corn syrup.

Offer 3- and 4-year-olds three meals and two or three snacks a day. Don't be concerned if your child eats only one substantial meal on a given day—she may not be particularly hungry that day. Rely on finger foods, such as cooked carrots or whole-wheat bread and finger-size pieces of fish or chicken, more often than foods that must be eaten with a fork or spoon. Introduce new foods regularly. The more often you offer new foods, the greater the variety of foods your child will eat. Don't stop offering a food just because your child has rejected it several times. Keep on trying!

Also, make it a household policy that no one eats in front of the TV. Though many parents find that turning on the TV during mealtime is a convenient way to get their children to sit still and eat, the drawbacks outweigh the benefits. Research shows a relationship between TV watching and obesity in children (see *Overweight,* Part 5).

QUESTIONS PARENTS ASK
Cholesterol and Triglycerides

Q: My father had high cholesterol and then had a heart attack at age 50. When I had my own cholesterol tested recently, it was high. Should I be concerned about my 4-year-old son?

A: All parents can help their children, after age 2 years, develop heart-healthy eating habits by limiting their children's fat intake (particularly the saturated fat in meat and dairy products) to no more than 30 percent (but no less than 20 percent) of total calories a day. A child like yours whose family members have high cholesterol levels or early heart disease should have a blood test to check his cholesterol levels. Certain children will also need to have a triglyceride screening. About 3 to 5 percent of children in the United States have a tendency toward high cholesterol that runs in their family, and about 1 in 100 kids has very high levels that might require medication after age 10. According to the American Academy of Pediatrics, a test of blood cholesterol (blood lipids) should be performed for any child

■ whose parent or grandparent was diagnosed with coronary artery disease (atherosclerosis) at age 55 or younger.

■ whose parent or grandparent had a heart attack, angina, stroke, or sudden cardiac death at age 55 or younger.

■ whose parent has total blood cholesterol of 240 milligrams per deciliter (mg/dl) or higher.

■ whose family health history is unknown.

Other children who may need to be screened if their physician recommends it are those who have risk factors, such as obesity and a diet high in saturated fat. Overweight adolescents who also smoke may be screened. Obese children and those with high cholesterol, diabetes, or a family history of high triglycerides should also be screened for triglyceride levels.

A basic blood cholesterol screening is usually done first. No special fasting or diet is required. If the total blood cholesterol count is more than 200 mg/dl, then a more in-depth "lipid profile" will be used to test for the different kinds of cholesterol. This test requires a 12-hour fast—usually overnight.

The results will distinguish between "good cholesterol" and "bad cholesterol." One way to remember the difference is this:

L for "lousy" is the LDL, or low-density lipoprotein.

H for "happy" is the HDL, or high-density lipoprotein.

The results of cholesterol screening and recommended treatments are as follows:

■ *Acceptable (LDL cholesterol below 110 mg/dl):* Provide education on healthy eating and repeat the test in 5 years.

■ *Borderline (LDL cholesterol 110 to 129 mg/dl):* Place the child on a "Step 1" diet. This is a basic, healthy diet of no more than 30 percent of total calories from fat. Saturated fats found in meat and dairy should be limited, but healthy fats such as those found in natural peanut butter and foods prepared with olive oil and canola oil are acceptable. The child should be monitored by a health professional and tested again after 3 months.

■ *High (LDL cholesterol 130 or higher):* Put the child on a more stringent "Step 2" diet of no more than 30 percent of calories from fat, less than 7 percent of which may come from saturated fat, each day. Since it is difficult to drop saturated fat intake to below 7 percent without risking various kinds of malnutrition, this diet requires careful planning and should only be undertaken under the close supervision of a health professional, such as a dietician.

Cholesterol-controlling medication is not recommended for children age 10 or younger, except in unusually severe cases after consultation with an expert in pediatric cholesterol problems.

Your child's doctor may also recommend screening for triglycerides. This can be done as part of the lipid profile that also includes the cholesterol screening. A normal triglyceride level in children is below 100 mg/dl. The problem with high triglycerides is that they can lower the level of the good HDL cholesterol in the blood. High triglycerides are common in children who consume too much of their daily calories as simple sugars, such as juice, sodas, sugary cereals, candy, and baked goods. If your child's levels are above 100, encourage your child to exercise more and reduce sugar consumption.

One Meal for All

Don't fall into the trap of becoming a short-order cook for your preschooler. Prepare one meal for the family each night, but make sure that at least some parts of it appeal to a child's taste for plain foods. If you are grilling chicken, for example, hold the barbecue sauce on some pieces if your child doesn't like it. If your child refuses to eat it, don't let her talk you into making something else for her. Don't offer dessert unless she has eaten a healthy portion of the regular meal.

Using the Food Pyramid

A healthy diet can reduce the risk of obesity and other conditions, including heart disease and cancer. As a result, the U.S. Department of Agriculture designed the food guide pyramid to help people plan healthy meals—that is, those high in grains, vegetables, and fruits; and low in fat, cholesterol, sugar, and salt.

The pyramid is divided into six sections, each representing a different food group. The point is to serve foods in the large sections in the pyramid's bottom half more often than those in the small sections at the top. The bread, cereal, rice, and pasta group should constitute the largest share of the diet, with six servings a day for chil-

▬ HEART-HEALTHY, RIGHT-FAT DIET

Instead of . . .	Choose . . .
Whole milk	Skim milk or 1 percent milk
Ice cream	Fat-free ice cream or frozen yogurt
Butter/shortening	Olive oil, canola oil, nonfat spreads
Hot dogs	Low-fat hot dogs
Potato chips, corn chips	Pretzels, nonfat chips, plain popcorn
Chocolate	Cocoa-containing foods (fudge pops, right-fat brownies)
Sugary foods	Low-sugar foods, whole fruit
Cream cheese	Fat-free cream cheese, almond butter

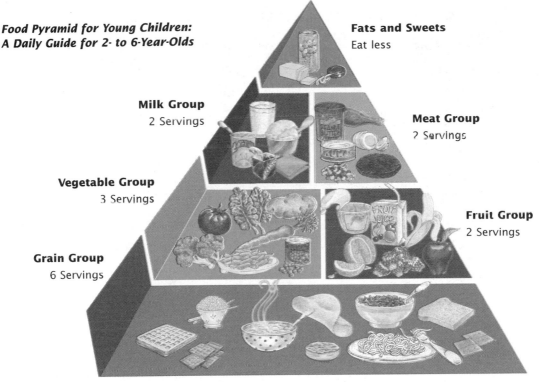

Food Pyramid for Young Children:
A Daily Guide for 2- to 6-Year-Olds

Fats and Sweets
Eat less

Milk Group
2 Servings

Meat Group
2 Servings

Vegetable Group
3 Servings

Fruit Group
2 Servings

Grain Group
6 Servings

Source: U.S. Department of Agriculture

dren ages 2 to 6, followed by vegetables (three servings), and fruits (two servings). Dairy products (milk, yogurt, and cheese) and meat should be relatively minor players, with just two servings a day. In fact, meat is optional; other proteins, including dry beans, eggs, and nuts, can do just as well. Serve the foods at the pyramid's peak only sparingly, if at all. They are fats (which include butter, oil, and high-fat foods, such as potato chips) and sweets.

Snack Time

You can't fault a youngster for wanting snack foods that taste good and are fun to eat. It's unrealistic to expect your child to be satisfied only with fruit and carrot sticks between meals. But snacks needn't be limited to cookies or chips. You can stock up on snack foods that are high in both nutritional value and kid appeal; see the chart on page 238 for suggestions.

Tooth Care

At this age, your child needs to see a dentist for a regular checkup every 6 months. The dentist will clean your child's teeth, monitor their emergence, and discuss fluoride treatments.

▬ CHOOSING HEALTHY SNACKS

Offer More Often	Offer Less Often
Cereal, unsweetened	Candy
Crackers	Cheese-filled crackers (store-bought)
Carrot, cucumber, and celery sticks	Chips
Dried fruit	Fruit rolls
Fresh fruit (grapes, apples, bananas)	Cheese-coated popcorn
Low-fat cookies: vanilla wafers, fig cookies, animal crackers, or graham crackers	High-fat cookies (chocolate, iced, or cream-filled)
Frozen or regular yogurt, low-fat	Ice cream
Pretzels	Frozen fruit pops
Rice cakes	Soda
Plain popcorn	Peanut butter

Your job as a parent is to help keep your child's teeth clean and to limit sugary, sticky snacks. Children usually need help brushing their teeth until at least age 6. Let her do as good a job as she can, then tell her that it's Mommy's or Daddy's turn. To find out whether your child can brush well enough on her own, let her do it for a day or two before a dental checkup, then ask the dentist how clean your child's teeth look. One way to make sure she is brushing long enough is to have her hum the alphabet song twice while she's brushing.

Toileting

By age 4, most children can use the toilet by themselves during the day, although not necessarily at night (see p. 199). After your child learns to use a potty routinely, she'll need to make the transition to a toilet so that she'll be able to use the bathroom at school. Children usually make the switch without any difficulty or parental coaxing. Put a step stool in the bathroom to make it easy for your child to climb onto the toilet. Some children don't want to sit on the toilet, because the opening is too big, and they're afraid of falling in. To help your child overcome this fear, get a child-sized toilet seat that fits over the regular one. Praise her for her toileting successes.

When Toilet Training Fails

Many preschoolers still wet their pants occasionally, especially if there's been some stress in their lives, like a new school or sibling. But even without stress, many preschoolers wet their pants if they hold in their urine too long. When this happens, it's usually because they were so involved in playing that they didn't go to the bathroom in time. Parents can usually help control this problem by reminding their child to go to the bathroom regularly, especially before leaving the house, as well as after meals and before bedtime. Some children have accidents at preschool because they are timid about telling the teacher they need to go. To help your child, pretend that you are the teacher and have your child practice the words she needs to say.

Many children at this age stay dry during the day but wet the bed at night. It is common and normal for a 3- or 4-year-old to wet the bed at night. If your child continues to wet the bed on a regular basis after this age, tell your child's doctor; he may examine and assess your child for a possible medical problem (see **Bed-Wetting,** Part 5). Most cases of bed-wetting simply mean that your child's urinary control is maturing more slowly than average.

QUESTIONS PARENTS ASK
A Boy Who Sits

Q: Our son still urinates sitting down. Should we insist that he stand up?

A: "Insist" is not an attitude that's likely to get you far, especially with a subject as prone to power struggles as toilet use. Your son doesn't need to meet any deadlines for accomplishing this skill. For now, let him watch his father and, if they're willing, older brothers or male cousins. Preschool boys are so eager to imitate their fathers and other boys that, with time, your son will want to use the toilet the way they do. In addition to motivating your son, you'll need to address a technical issue: Many preschool boys aren't tall enough to urinate in the toilet while standing up, so they'll need to stand on a step stool.

Sleeping

"I'm not tired." "One more story, pleeeze!" "I need a drink of water." "Mommy, can you rub my back?"

Sound familiar? One skill that children master during the preschool years is the art of stalling at bedtime. Experts often refer to reappearances after a child has been put to bed as "curtain calls." Many children have trouble winding down at night. Small children have trouble accepting that they need to go to bed when everyone else in the family is still awake and, presumably, having fun. But don't let the delaying tactics get out of hand. It's one thing to get your child a glass of water or read her one more story, but if she expects a second glass of water and yet another story, you need to start saying no.

Establishing a Routine

Keeping to a regular bedtime ritual of reading a set number of books or creating a sequence of things, such as bathing, putting on pajamas, playing music, talking, or singing to your child, can help her settle down on time and get the rest she needs. If you stick to a set routine with clear time limits, she'll get used to it and come to expect it. What's more important, it will set your child's internal "clock" to be ready to fall asleep at the same time each day.

Helping Your Child to Sleep

Preschoolers need 10 to 11 hours of sleep in a 24-hour period, either at night or combined with an afternoon nap. But if your child balks at going to bed night after night and if it usually takes her a long time (say, longer than half an hour) to fall asleep, you could be expecting her to get more sleep than she needs. Monitor your child's nighttime sleep and daytime nap schedules to see if she is having any of the following problems:

▌ If your child is still napping at age 4, napping for longer than an hour a day, or napping too late in the day (after 4 P.M.), then she may not be able to fall asleep until late at night.

▌ If your child is going to bed early (say, 7 P.M.), she may have trouble falling asleep, wake up in the middle of the night, or wake up early in the morning.

▌ If your child sleeps relatively late in the morning (from 8 A.M. to 10 A.M.), she may not be able to fall asleep until after 10 at night.

Here are some steps you can take to help your child get adequate, regular sleep:

▌ If your child takes a long time to fall asleep after she goes to bed, move her bedtime to the time she actually falls asleep. The more swiftly she falls asleep after the lights are out, the less likely she will resist going to bed.

▌ Next, to get your child to go to bed earlier at night, start waking her earlier in the morning. Children who don't have to get up early for preschool can easily get into

---

A MOTHER'S PERSPECTIVE

Monster Spray

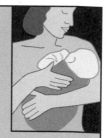

My daughter was resisting going to sleep because she was worried about nightmares. She thought the shadows on her wall from the streetlight outside might become monsters. She'd cry until I came back into her room, then want me to crawl into her bed and sleep with her.

One of the mothers in my parent group had a solution: monster spray. She said to take a plant sprayer, fill it with water, and tell my daughter that it had magic powers to scare the monsters away. I did what she said. I even had my daughter draw a scary picture and then tape it onto the bottle of monster spray for extra effect.

I never even had to use the monster spray. Ever since my daughter started keeping the bottle next to her bed, she hasn't been worried about nightmares. Or if she has, she hasn't needed my help.

the habit of sleeping late. But the later they sleep in the morning, the later they will stay awake at night. Pleasant as it is (especially on the weekends) to have a child who sleeps until 8:30 A.M., you can't have it both ways. Either your child goes to bed early and rises early or she goes to bed late and rises late.

Discipline

Many parents find that the discipline methods they used a year ago are losing their power. Preschoolers are more difficult to distract than toddlers, and other methods, such as time-out, may be wearing thin. During a time-out, for example, your child may refuse to stay in her time-out spot. Or, once the time-out is over, she'll go right back and do the same thing that the time-out was supposed to stop. By around age 4, children can be defiant, so parents need to be more resourceful.

First of all, don't overuse the time-out. The more you use it, the less seriously your child will take it. As in the past, reserve the time-out for the two or three worst kinds of behavior, like hitting or rudeness, and ignore behavior that's simply obnoxious, like whining for attention. Ignoring a behavior is often effective, because it withholds your attention—exactly what your child may be seeking by misbehaving in the first place. Or, you can divert your child's attention by taking out a toy, a puzzle, or some crayons and start using them alongside her. Again, she may be seeking your attention, and when she gets it, she will stop the negative behavior. Most importantly, try not to lose control of your emotions or become angry—patience is your best ally.

A FATHER'S STORY

The Wish List

Our daughter's demands for toys were getting out of hand. Stephanie would leaf through toy catalogs and point to something that she wanted on practically every page. Going shopping with her was a nightmare of "Can you buy me this?" And when we'd say no, she'd throw a tantrum.

I got so sick and tired of this that one day when she asked for something, I said, out of sheer frustration, "Just put it on your list." Instead of whining or crying, she said OK and dropped the subject. The next time she demanded a new toy, my wife and I tried this again. And again it worked.

Eventually, Stephanie stopped asking us to buy her so many toys and started naming the toys that she was going to put on her list. Sometimes she'd even take a pencil and paper and scribble a "list" herself. I think that, for her, having the power to put a toy on her list was sometimes as good as having it. Having the list was good for us, too. When the time was right to buy her something, we used it to find out what kinds of toys she would enjoy.

Immediate Rewards and Consequences

Preschoolers still have short attention spans, but they understand rewards and consequences. So reinforce good behavior with rewards (a hug or a healthy snack or some play time). Make an effort to catch your child doing something good, and praise the behavior. This will boost her self-esteem while reinforcing the good behavior. Tell your child that for every day she behaves well (such as dressing herself without a fuss) she gets a sticker, and once she has accumulated 10 stickers she can pick out a special treat or a toy. Limit your use of this technique to just one or two kinds of problems at a time, and only on a short-term basis—until the behavior has stopped long enough to indicate that the habit has been broken.

GOOD TOYS FOR PRESCHOOLERS

Toy	Benefit
Sports toys: tricycle, bicycle with training wheels, plastic bat and ball, roller skates, ring toss	Provide exercise; give a sense of physical accomplishment.
Puzzles with 20 or more pieces (by about age 3½)	Promote hand-eye coordination and understanding of spatial relationships; encourage child to concentrate and complete a task, a valuable preschool skill.
Simple board games (which involve no reading)	Encourage cooperative play, following rules.
Toy musical instruments	Preschoolers love to listen to music, sing, and dance. Musical activities stimulate brain development in ways that are important for learning math.
Dress-up costumes and clothes	Many preschoolers delight in dressing up for dramatic play, and doing this fuels their imagination.
Action figures, dolls, dollhouses, doctor kits, toy farms, airports, etc.	Promote fantasy play, an integral part of preschool development.
Art supplies: clay, paint, brushes, safety scissors, nontoxic markers, construction paper, paste, beads, and string	Encourage creative expression; help develop fine motor skills.
Building blocks and snap-together plastic pieces	Promote creativity, spatial relationships, and hand-eye coordination.

You can discourage negative behavior with an immediate consequence, particularly one directly connected with the undesirable behavior. Telling your child that she won't be able to attend a birthday party next week is not immediate enough. Taking away the rest of the popcorn she just threw at her brother sends the right message—no popcorn throwing.

Choosing Toys

Many of the birthday presents and other toys you buy may be things that your child requests—the action figure that Andrew has, the bike with the bell that Julia has. Many of your children's desires will be also influenced by television commercials. But some types of toys are worth buying, because they are challenging and interesting to preschoolers and help develop important physical and mental skills. Use the chart on page 242 as a guide.

Keeping Your Child Healthy

Get used to it: Your child is going to scrape her knee, bloody her lip, and catch illnesses that she's never had before. Preschoolers are prone to injuries and infections, because they are growing more active and spending more time with other children. But you can limit the number of accidents and illnesses.

Lower the risk of serious injury by seeing that your child continues to use a car seat, wears a helmet when she's riding a bike or skating, and is never in or near a swimming pool or another body of water without an adult's close supervision.

To keep your child healthy, concentrate your efforts on prevention and early detection of serious problems. Yearly checkups will assure that her immunizations are current and that difficulties with hearing or vision are picked up and treated early, before they impair development and learning.

Checkups

Take your child to the doctor for annual checkups at ages 3 and 4. The annual checkup is a time for the doctor to assess your child's physical health and developmental progress.

The checkup should include a blood pressure screening, a height and weight check, and an examination of

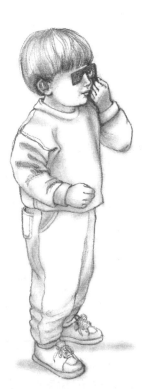

At age 3 or 4, your child should have his first vision test. Your doctor will check your child's visual acuity and examine his eyes for any abnormalities that would interfere with his learning.

the body, including skin, eyes, ears, nose, throat, lymph nodes, lungs, heart, abdomen, genitals, hips, and back. The doctor will assess your child's muscle tone, walking gait, reflexes, growth patterns, and recent patterns of illness. A hearing and vision test will probably be given at age 4.

The annual checkup is also a time to ask your doctor about any concerns you have about your child's physical, developmental, and emotional health. Is your child fully toilet trained or still wetting at night? Tell your doctor. Is she communicating effectively? Can she play in groups and get along with other children? All these things can inform your doctor about the state of your child's health and development. He may ask about sleep patterns, social adjustment, temperament, developmental progress, and family status.

Screening Tests

For immunizations, see Childhood Immunization Schedule, page 110. In addition to regular immunizations, your child's doctor may recommend a blood lead level screening, which is required in many states. Additionally, the following tests may be performed on 3- and 4-year-olds at high risk for particular illnesses:

▌ Blood cholesterol level and triglycerides for children with a parent or grandparent who has early heart disease or high cholesterol (see p. 235)

▌ Tuberculin test (PPD) for children with risk factors for tuberculosis, such as exposure to someone with the disease or living in areas where it is prevalent

▌ Hemoglobin and hematocrit (blood test) for children at increased risk for anemia

Overcoming Fear of the Doctor

Preschoolers have many fears, and one of the most universal is the fear of visiting the doctor. Some children come to associate the doctor with pain and discomfort, such as the gagging sensation caused by the tongue depressor and, of course, shots. Unlike younger children, preschoolers can anticipate doctor visits and ask such questions as, "Am I going to get a shot?" Here are some things that you can do to ease your child's fears:

▌ *Be positive.* Explain that the doctor is there to help your child get healthy if she's sick and stay healthy if she's well.

▌ *Tell your child about an upcoming checkup.* Preschoolers need time to prepare mentally for a checkup by asking you questions and talking about their concerns. But don't give her too much time to worry about it. Tell your 3-year-old the morning of a checkup, and give your 4-year-old a day's notice.

▌ *Be honest.* If your child asks if she's going to get a shot and you know that she will, say yes. If she asks whether it will hurt, say that it may hurt for a few seconds, but that it will help prevent her from getting sick, which hurts a lot more.

▌ *Get a toy doctor's kit.* Playing with the toy stethoscope and blood pressure gauge and other instruments can make the checkup routine less mysterious to a child.

▮ *Discuss your child's fear of shots.* If your child is fearful about an upcoming immunization, talk to your doctor about methods to reduce the pain. A doctor can help make immunization shots less painful by putting pressure on or vibrating the skin near the injection site or by prescribing a painkilling cream for you to apply to your child's arm about 1 hour before the shot.

QUESTIONS PARENTS ASK
Frequent Sickness

Q: My daughter had five colds this past year. Could there be something wrong with her that's making her so prone to getting sick?

A: It's hard to imagine a normal, healthy preschooler being sick *less* often. When children start day care or preschool, they're especially vulnerable to infections because they're exposed to more children—and more germs—than ever before. It's not unusual for a 3- or 4-year-old to have four to eight colds a year. Other infections that are common at this age are strep throat (see *Sore Throat/Strep Throat,* Part 5), Coxsackie virus (see *Hand-Foot-and-Mouth Disease,* Part 5), *impetigo* (see Part 5), and *chicken pox* (see Part 5). Children are less likely to get sick if parents and care providers encourage them to wash their hands regularly, especially before eating.

How Not to Get What She's Got

Your child isn't the only one in the family who's bound to get sick often. Whatever is going around at preschool often goes around at home as well. You can't avoid catching some of these illnesses (after all, your child needs close contact with you when she's sick). But you can reduce your chances of catching what she's got. Here's how:

▮ Wash your hands with soap after blowing your child's nose or touching her tissues. Encourage her to do the same.

▮ Encourage your child to cover her nose and mouth when she coughs or sneezes, preferably with a tissue.

▮ Don't share towels. Damp towels, washcloths, and sponges are breeding grounds for germs. Launder them frequently.

▮ Don't share food, utensils, or glasses. Don't let your child spread germs by reaching into pretzel bags and other food containers that the rest of the family uses. At mealtimes, don't allow everyone to reach into the same food bowl. Put separate portions on each person's plate.

Keeping Your Child Safe

With preschoolers' growing independence come the following safety considerations. For information on water safety, fire safety, and car seats, see Chapter 11, Preparing for and Handling Emergencies.

Car Safety   A child needs to be in a car seat until she weighs at least 40 pounds or her head is higher than the back of the car seat when sitting (see p. 369). Some states require that a child be in a car seat or a booster seat until age 5, even if she weighs more than 40 pounds. As long as a child needs a car seat or a booster seat, she must use it when she takes the school bus or van trips with her preschool or day care. Don't allow your child to sit in a front seat, where she is more likely to be injured in an accident and where passenger-side air bags also may cause injury. The backseat is safest.

In addition, never leave your child alone in a parked car, even to dash quickly into a store. Preschoolers have injured themselves and others by releasing the emergency break or shifting into gear and setting a vehicle in motion. Leaving a child in a parked car in warm temperatures is very dangerous because the temperatures can rise rapidly, causing heatstroke (see p. 412). And don't let your child play near a parked car; it may suddenly start moving, and the driver may not see your child.

Bike Helmets   Once your child starts riding a bicycle with training wheels, she needs a helmet. Helmets protect children from serious head injuries by absorbing and distributing the impact of crashes. Bike helmets reduce the risk of brain injury by 90 percent and other head injuries by 85 percent. Look for a helmet with a sticker indicating that it meets or exceeds safety standards set by the Snell Memorial Foundation or the American National Standards Institute. Make sure that the helmet fits comfortably on your child's head and doesn't slip around.

Strangers   Without going into an elaborate explanation that might alarm your child, simply tell her never to talk to strangers. Also tell her never to go anywhere with someone (even someone she knows) unless you have given her permission. Instruct her not to go anywhere by herself. If an unfamiliar person approaches her when she is not with an adult, even someone who seems friendly, instruct her to yell "No!" and run away and tell a trusted adult immediately. Rehearse these instructions by having someone play the role of the stranger and having your child practice her response.

A Parent's Life

A preschool child's growing independence gives parents a bit of a breather. No longer are you spending every waking moment tending to your young child's needs. In addition, you can do more activities as a family. You can go to museums, puppet shows, movies, and casual restaurants. You may be able to try boating and short hikes. Remember when you were stuck at home, exhausted from caring for an infant around the clock, and your friends promised that life would get better? This is what they meant.

Family Vacations

If you were somewhat travel-shy when your child was younger, you may feel ready to plan your first "real" vacation (that is, other than a trip to visit relatives or friends) now that she doesn't need constant care and a caravan of paraphernalia. But to make the vacation enjoyable for the whole family, keep a few things in mind.

For one thing, just because you think that traveling is fun doesn't mean that your child will agree. Strange surroundings may scare or unsettle her. Sitting in a car or an airplane for hours can make her restless and cranky, setting the entire family on edge. Clearly, this wasn't what you had in mind when you were reading the travel brochures.

Planning a vacation with a preschooler takes more than just reservations. You also need to plan for your child's needs. When traveling by car or plane, try these tips:

▌ *Stock up on small toys.* Crayons and coloring books, stickers and paper, and magnetic drawing toys can keep a preschooler occupied en route.

▌ *Bring snacks.* Preschoolers get hungry every few hours. Bring juice packs, pretzels, raisins, crackers, and other easily packed foods.

▌ *Take breaks.* When traveling by car, stop every 2 hours for your child to use the bathroom and stretch her legs. On a plane, walk your child up and down the aisles when she gets bored.

▌ *Keep a change of clothing within easy reach.* That way, if your child spills juice down her shirt or wets her pants, you'll be prepared.

▌ *Bring drinks or chewable candies if you are traveling by air.* Having your child suck, chew, or swallow can help prevent ear pain caused by changes in air pressure.

▌ *Bring sunscreen, hats, long-sleeved shirts, and insect repellents.* You'll need insect repellents if you're traveling to an area where there is a risk of infections that are transmitted by ticks or mosquitoes (e.g., Lyme disease, encephalitis, malaria, and yellow fever). Choose one that contains no more than 10 percent deet, a chemical potentially harmful to children. Sunscreen is important if you plan to spend time outdoors in summer or winter. The reflected sun off snow or water can burn even if the air is cool.

If your family enjoys boat outings together, make sure that everyone is wearing a personal flotation device (PFD). Be sure to choose one for your child that is appropriate for her weight and height. The PFD should not be loose and should always be worn as instructed with all straps belted. A label on the jacket should say that it has been approved by the U.S. Coast Guard and has been tested by Underwriters Laboratory (UL).

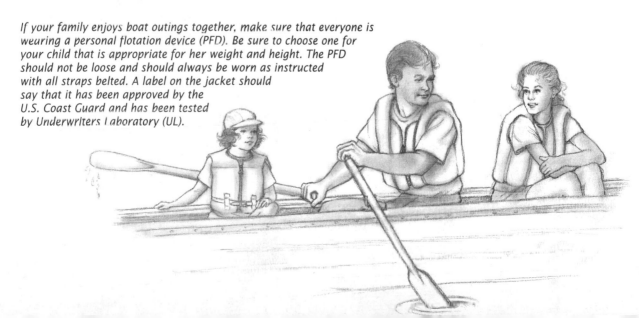

7 Your School-Age Child

SEE HOW THEY GROW

CARING FOR YOUR CHILD

KEEPING YOUR CHILD HEALTHY

SPORTS AND YOUR CHILD

A PARENT'S LIFE

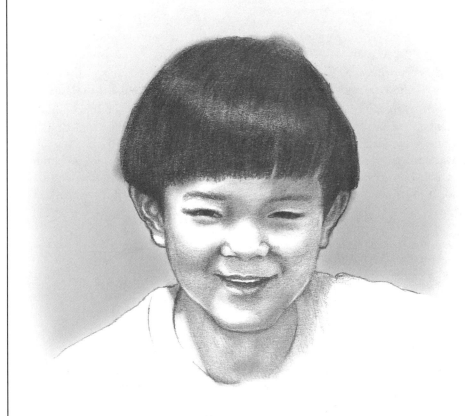

The first day of school is a turning point for both parent and child. Looking ahead over the next several years, you can imagine your child reading, writing, learning math, telling you facts about nature or history, hitting baseballs, trying a musical instrument, making friends, and having sleep-overs. The prospects are thrilling, and you are one proud parent. Already, your child may be a fledgling reader and writer. He probably knows his letters, and he's counting higher and higher. Now he's ready to build on what he knows, learn new skills and facts, and develop new ideas.

From your child's perspective, attending school is both exciting and scary. Entering kindergarten, a child who is fairly self-sufficient and at ease with other children may still be nervous about how he will blend in with a new group with different rules and new ways of doing things. And parents, while enjoying their child's new accomplishments and independence, also find it hard to let go. They know that the first day of school is the beginning of a long and gradual move away from home and toward a world in which other children take center stage while parents play a supporting role. You may tell yourself that the tissues you brought to the bus stop on the first day of school are for your child, but you may find yourself using them.

See How They Grow

It's an exciting time, as you watch your child's baby fat melt away to reveal a taller, stronger, wiser, and more savvy youngster ready to take on the world—at least sometimes. At other times your school-age child will cling to you for reassurance and look to you for guidance. Being there for him when he turns to you, and letting him go when he's ready to take on new challenges, will be a fine balance for both of you.

Developmental Milestones

Starting school is just one reason why a 5-year-old is at a pivotal moment in his life. Another has to do with his development. By this age he will likely have reached the majority of major milestones that doctors use to gauge whether there are any basic developmental problems. Sure, he'll learn to run faster and jump higher. His cognitive abilities will expand as he learns in school and in life. But at this point his basic skills are in place. The foundation for further growth has been laid.

Growing and Moving

Look in any kindergarten class, and you're bound to see striking variations in the children's body types, height, and weight. It's not unusual to see a 3-foot, 8-inch child

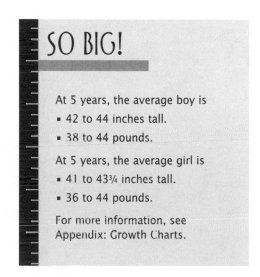

SO BIG!

At 5 years, the average boy is
- 42 to 44 inches tall.
- 38 to 44 pounds.

At 5 years, the average girl is
- 41 to 43¾ inches tall.
- 36 to 44 pounds.

For more information, see Appendix: Growth Charts.

▬ DEVELOPMENTAL MILESTONES

Age	Most Children
5 years	Get dressed without help
	Know their address and telephone number
	Count on fingers or count up to five items
	Copy a triangle or a square
	Draw a person with six parts (i.e., head, body, arms, and legs)
	Recognize most letters of the alphabet
	Print some letters of the alphabet
	Understand and name two opposites
	Use and recognize complex language (e.g., "I didn't play on the slide, but I played in the sandbox")
	Play make-believe and dress up
	Balance on each foot for 6 seconds
	Can skip

As you review this final list of milestones, remember that children who are within the normal range will have some areas in which they excel and others in which they are slower. Not achieving a particular milestone at the designated time is not always a matter of concern. If you and your child's doctor are concerned about your child's overall development or any of your child's developmental skills, such as language, hearing, vision, or motor skills, seek the help of the appropriate specialist. For more information, see *Developmental Problems*, Part 5.

weighing a mere 40 pounds standing next to another who's 4 feet tall and weighing nearly 60 pounds. Both these sizes and weights are normal for 5-year-olds. Dramatic variations in size can be found among children throughout their early school years.

Body types tend to remain stable. A child who enters kindergarten with a tall, lanky frame is likely to start middle school with a tall, lanky frame. And a husky child will probably stay that way. Some shorter children may catch up later, when they go through their preadolescent growth spurt.

Regardless of their body types, sizes, and growth rates, all children undergo certain physical changes during their early school years. For one thing, they become stronger because most of their weight gain goes right to their muscles. You can see more muscle definition in their arms, legs, shoulders, backs, and chests. In addition, their faces mature. Their noses become larger and their faces narrower, making it possible to imagine how your child might look when he's grown up. Skin becomes less luminescent and more adultlike. And many blond children's hair begins to darken.

Toothless Grins

Without a doubt, the most dramatic change is in children's smiles, which can be transformed in an instant with the loss of a tooth. Children usually lose their first tooth at age 5 or 6. The exact age when your child's first tooth falls out will depend on how old he was when his first baby teeth appeared. The earlier your child's first teeth appeared, the earlier he will lose them. Once a child's baby tooth falls out, the permanent tooth usually takes about 2 months to come in fully.

Building Physical Skills

Early school age is also when improvements in children's fine and gross motor skills enable them to become more accomplished in writing and art as well as sports. Now that your child has sufficient strength, stamina, and coordination, he can probably shoot baskets, play soccer, or execute a tricky dance move. On the playground, children this age may also hang upside down on the trapeze and cross the monkey bars hand-over-hand. Swimming, diving, playing a musical instrument, singing in a chorus, and learning tap dancing or ballet are among the many activities within an elementary school child's capabilities.

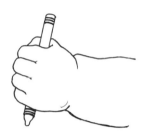

You can expect much more precision in hand movements and drawings from your school-age child.

In art, instead of drawing figures with circles and sticks, children gradually learn to sketch and paint realistic images of people, animals, and objects. The way your child holds his pencil or crayon will also change. The full-fisted grasp of the preschooler gives way to a more conventional position in which he holds the pencil between the index finger, middle finger, and thumb. (See the illustration.)

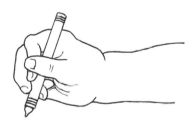

More so than before, children this age display a wide range of talents. One 7-year-old excels at chess, another at swimming. One 8-year-old can multiply three-digit numbers in his head, and another can play the violin. Your child's strengths in particular areas will depend on his innate gifts, his opportunities for training, and his drive to practice.

GIRLS AND EARLY PUBERTY

Girls show the first signs of puberty several years earlier than boys. For decades, medical textbooks stated that it was abnormal for girls to show these signs, which include underarm hair and breast swelling, before age 8. But new research has confirmed what doctors and parents have observed for years: Many girls do start puberty that young. It is not uncommon for some girls to begin the early stages of puberty before age 8. Even so, your child's doctor should be notified in case this early start is indicative of a medical problem. More likely, reasons for early puberty have to do with differences in weight and nutrition—factors known to affect puberty onset. For example, heavier girls with a higher percentage of body fat tend to mature earlier than others. Lean girls, with minimal body fat, mature later. But the age at which puberty begins for girls or boys is mainly hereditary. If a girl's mother or her father's female relatives started puberty earlier, she is more likely to do so.

Chubby or Overweight?

Many parents worry if they have a child who appears to be heavier than other children. The percentage of schoolchildren who weigh too much has increased in recent decades. A child is considered obese if his weight is more than 20 percent of that considered normal for his height. Consult the Appendix: Growth Charts, and ask your doctor if you are concerned about your child's weight.

School-age children do not have "baby fat." Although all children have some fat on their bodies, most truly overweight children have overweight parents, and therefore a genetic basis probably underlies their problem. But other contributing factors exist, such as overeating, especially high-fat snack foods, a habit children often learn from their parents. An equally important cause, however, is thought to be the lack of physical activity. Studies have shown a definite connection between obesity in children and hours spent watching television.

An overweight child should not diet, meaning cut calories or meals, without the direction of a doctor or dietitian. Dieting can interfere with his growth. Instead, give your child two important things to do. First, encourage him to get more exercise—ride his bicycle, play basketball with a friend, take dance classes. Second, he should adopt healthy eating strategies by substituting low-fat foods for high-fat ones (like skim milk instead of whole milk), eating lean meats and fish (skinless chicken or broiled fish instead of hot dogs or cheeseburgers), and choosing healthy snacks, such as fruit or pretzels instead of potato chips and ice cream. Children, in general, should eat more fruits and vegetables and less fatty foods. Above all, keep in mind that your child is watching what you eat. The biggest influence on your child's eating habits is your own! For more information, see *Overweight,* Part 5.

Communicating

"Knock, knock."
"Who's there?"
"Sarah."
"Sarah who?"
"Sarah doctor in the house?"

School-age children love jokes and riddles. This reflects their growing ability to use and understand more complicated language. Hearing and telling jokes is a fun way for children to strengthen these language skills. A 5- or 6-year-old might delight in a simple knock-knock joke, but as he gets older he'll gradually come to understand more subtle jokes and riddles involving puns and other forms of word play.

Learning Grammar

The more your child talks, the better his speech becomes. In fact, the mispronunciations and grammatical errors that used to be common become less frequent throughout the school years. When a schoolchild does make a speech error, he's apt to correct himself. Among the grammatical errors you're most likely to hear are incorrect verb forms, like "Billy hided the toy." Don't correct your child directly; instead, correct using proper grammar yourself ("Billy hid the toy") as a way of teaching him the right way to say something. But if your child continues struggling with such things as noun-verb agreement ("He go home" instead of "He goes home") or speech intelligibility, discuss the problem with a speech-language pathologist, a doctor, or a teacher to see if your child needs further speech evaluation.

Expanding Vocabulary

Your child's ability to express himself is expanding in many directions. Between the ages of 6 and 8, his vocabulary doubles. He can better remember and understand words he hears, and he's exposed to more words as he learns to read. With so many new words at his disposal, a child can tell stories and talk about his feelings and experiences in richer detail than before.

Understanding the Meaning of Language

When children are learning to read and write, they're working to recognize words and associate them with their sounds and meanings. These nuts and bolts are so all-consuming that children may not understand much of what they read at first. But by about age 9, a great leap occurs. As the processes of reading and writing become more or less second nature, children's minds are free to concentrate on the content of what they read. They can now write much longer, more detailed passages.

For all their monumental strides in communication, elementary school children may occasionally stumble over the finer points of language and grammar. For example, before age 10, most children can't grasp the figurative meanings of words. A child may understand that a tiger is a wild cat, but he may not understand that the word could also refer to a powerful and assertive person.

LEARNING A SECOND LANGUAGE

Children have an easier time learning a new language and are most likely to speak it like a native if they learn it during the elementary school years—or even better, during their preschool years, while living in a bilingual home. Fortunately, more elementary schools offer foreign language instruction either during the regular school day or after school. Foreign language camps are available in some communities.

The best way for children (and adults) to learn a new language is to spend time with people who always speak that language. The ideal situation would be to live in a foreign country for several months. But, because this isn't possible for most people, the recommended option is to try to simulate the experience of living abroad by finding a foreign language course that uses a method of teaching called immersion. Lessons are conducted exclusively in the new language, and games and songs are used to help children learn.

Learning

In some ways, a first-grader's way of thinking doesn't seem different from a preschooler's. Children in both age groups enjoy pretend play, are in awe of superheroes, and talk about magical happenings, such as the tooth fairy's leaving money under the pillow or Santa's bringing toys down the chimney. But a closer look reveals significant changes in the working of a schoolchild's mind. He's beginning to think more logically, like an adult. Most of what a preschooler knows is based on his observations and experiences. But more and more of an older child's knowledge comes from his ability to reason.

Thinking Logically

A classic experiment underscores the shift toward logical thinking that occurs during the early school years: When 4-year-olds are shown two containers, one tall and one short, and then see water poured from one container into the other, most assume that the tall one contains more water because it looks bigger. But by age 6, most children know that the amount of water held must be the same because none of it spilled when it was being transferred. They can't be fooled into believing that the quantity of water has changed just because the size or shape of its container has changed.

Usually by the time a child is 8, she'll begin reading books on her own.

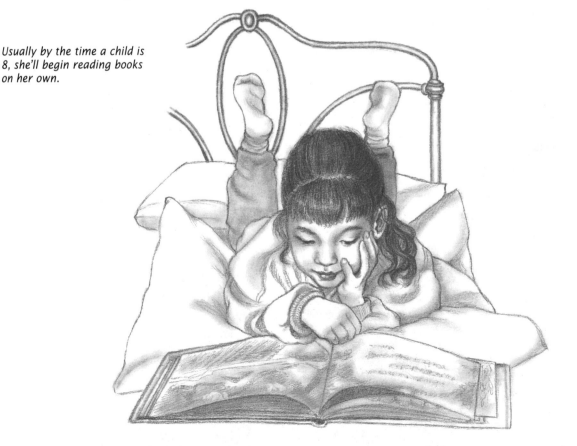

In addition to thinking more logically, your child's memory is expanding and his attention span is growing, because his brain is operating more efficiently and at a higher level than it used to. A younger child's brain keeps creating new connections without regard to the usefulness of the information they hold. A schoolchild's brain, in contrast, has the capacity to order and categorize information and perform step-by-step operations, which is important in higher-level thinking. For example, school-age children perfect their understanding of cause and effect: "It's been raining for 3 days, so our basement is wet." They can absorb information and make inferences or draw conclusions in a way that younger children cannot.

With this maturity of brain functioning, your child is ready to sit in a classroom and learn. During the first 2 years of elementary school, a child learns the fundamental skills related to the tasks of reading, writing, and arithmetic. By third or fourth grade, these skills become tools for further learning. A child reads, not to sound out words, but to absorb knowledge about history, geography, nature, and other subjects. He writes, not to practice forming letters, but to describe what he's learned. He's also learning how to learn: how to organize his time for studying and to develop tricks for remembering things.

Successful Students: Born or Made?

How much influence do you and your child's teachers have on academic performance? Will a bright child do well even in a mediocre school? Can a challenging school help a child of average intelligence excel? These are the questions parents ask as their schools evaluate their children and they in turn evaluate their schools.

How well your child does in school depends to a large extent on his intelligence, which is shaped by the interplay of his genes and his life experiences. Intelligence takes many forms: verbal, logical, spatial, social, musical, visual, and others. Like adults, children have strengths and weaknesses. Your child's intelligence in these and other areas is influenced by the full gamut of life experiences, from the amount of time he spends reading to the amount of love he gets from you. A high IQ (intelligence quotient) isn't the only ingredient for academic success or success in life. Children also need both motivation and understanding from their parents and their teachers. They tend to do best in school if their parents value high academic achievement and their teachers set high standards. Your child's achievements also depend on his learning environment. If he sees his parents reading, he will also read. If members of the family often discuss ideas, he will learn thinking skills.

Encouraging Your Child to Learn

Motivating a child to strive for excellence takes more than leaning on him to do his homework. It requires that you and your child's teacher help him believe that he's up to the tasks expected of him. Children who lack confidence tend to underachieve because they are afraid of failure. Teachers can help by giving schoolwork that is hard enough to be challenging but easy enough for the child to feel successful when doing it. Parents can help by providing a little extra encouragement. Tell your child, "I

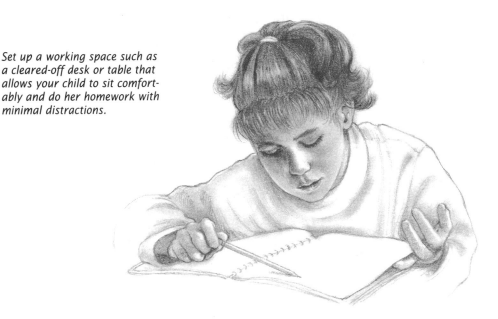

Set up a working space such as a cleared-off desk or table that allows your child to sit comfortably and do her homework with minimal distractions.

know you can do it," especially after he's struggled with an assignment or gotten something wrong. Knowing that you believe in him will help him believe in himself. Letting him know failing is OK—that he can learn something from it and try again another time—will give him confidence to try new things. The most important thing is that he does his best.

To encourage your child to try a new task, try saying something like, "That looks pretty easy." If your child thinks a task is easy, he'll be apt to believe he can do it, whereas if he thinks it's hard, he may assume that trying is useless. If it ends up being too difficult, say, "It wasn't as easy as it looked," and help your child find a similar task at a level he can accomplish.

Computers and Learning

Computers keep pushing the boundaries of learning. Software is available to help children write their own homework reports and books and make their own movies. Some computer programs can make every subject imaginable come alive with moving images, sounds, and commentary. On the Internet, children can find help with their homework, locate "key pals" around the world to correspond with, and plug into electronic field trips such as geological expeditions to the thermal ponds of Yellowstone National Park and the cliffs of Iceland. Many parents feel that a computer is the best technological product that they can get for their children.

But there are downsides. Computers pose some dangers in terms of mature content and access to strangers. As with TV, Internet sites bombard children with commercials. Here are some strategies for helping your child use the home computer as a learning tool while minimizing the problems.

■ Locate the computer in the family room or another well-traveled area of the house. This makes it easier to monitor your child's travels on the Internet.

■ Before buying software, preview it through a store demonstration or on a friend's computer. Make sure it's appropriate for your child.

■ Limit your child's computer time to about an hour a day. However marvelous it is, the computer is not a substitute for books, homework, or playing outside, and virtual pals are not substitutes for time with real friends.

■ Explain to your child that the Internet can be dangerous if used inappropriately.

■ Make sure your child knows that people on-line are not always who they say they are and that he should *never* give out personal information without your permission.

■ Sit at the computer together. Spend some time using the software and surfing the Web while talking with your child about it.

To shield your children from inappropriate material on the Net, you can purchase software programs that prevent your child from accessing a predetermined list of inappropriate sites. These programs vary in their effectiveness and methods. Some offer warnings about pages that contain bad language or images; others warn about a site's ability to disclose a name, an address, or a phone number. To obtain this software, ask for "blocking" software from your software dealer. Because the Internet is constantly changing and growing, you will need to update this software periodically. You can also ask your Internet provider to block adult sites.

Be sure to show an interest in hearing about your child's latest browsing discoveries—that way you'll have a better idea of what your child is doing on-line. Visit your child unannounced while he's surfing, and monitor the sites he visits. In addition, you can use the following methods to make sure that he is not visiting Web sites that you consider inappropriate. For older children and adolescents, set the rules for what types of sites are off-limits beforehand. Keep in mind that it is your responsibility as a parent to monitor your children's activities through adolescence. Here are some steps you can take to stay on top of your child's Internet use:

■ Open your computer's Net browser, and look at the "bookmarks" or "favorites" list to see what sites your child has visited and added to the list.

■ To discover which sites your child has visited most recently, click the down arrow next to the location box where the Internet address is usually typed. The last eight to ten sites visited are listed there, and you can click on them to go right to those sites. Or, if your child is currently on-line, you can click the "Back" and "Forward" buttons to see the pages he has most recently viewed.

▌ To examine your Internet browser's history files, which show sites recently visited, search the hard drive for files or folders with names that contain the word "history."

▌ To find images your child may have downloaded, search for files containing .gif, .jpg, .sit, .tip, or .zip.

▌ Review your computer's e-mail files for saved incoming messages.

Assessing Your Child's Learning

At the beginning of each school year, teachers often tell parents about the curriculum and what the children in class are expected to learn. (If the teachers have no occasion to convey this information, such as holding a meet-the-teacher night, call your child's teacher to find out.) The children in a class aren't expected to learn at the same pace; nor are they expected to learn all subjects equally well. Just because your child isn't in the top reading group doesn't mean he's doing poorly. If he is fortunate enough to be a top reader, he may still find multiplication and division difficult.

You'll get a sense of how well your child is doing in school by seeing his report card, having conferences with his teacher, looking at the work papers he brings home from school, and looking over his homework. Is he easily frustrated by assignments? Does he get many problems wrong? If your child's teacher says that he's lagging in some or all areas, the first thing to do is give him extra support. More time with him on his homework and additional attention from the teacher in school might be enough to make a difficult subject come into focus. Parent-teacher communication is crucial here. Find out when your child's teacher is available, and talk with the teacher on a regular basis by phone, in person, or by e-mail (many schools have teachers on-line). Or write a note if you have a concern. A single parent-teacher conference is not enough to keep the lines of communication open, so you'll have to take the initiative to find out how your child is doing and to ask the teacher about any concerns you may have.

If Your Child Is Having Learning Problems

If your child is underachieving, you need to find out why. Closely examine his behavior. Does he seem bored or unmotivated? Does the teacher say that he frequently misbehaves in school? Is he restless in school, and does he have a hard time sitting still? Is he having trouble keeping up with homework? If the answer to at least one of these questions is yes, or if he's underachieving in several subjects, arrange for him to be evaluated as soon as possible for learning problems. It is also possible that early speech and language problems may underlie learning difficulties. By law, public schools must provide free evaluation and treatment for children suspected to have learning disabilities, as well as behavioral and emotional problems that can interfere with learning. Schools are also required to develop an individualized education program (IEP) to provide appropriate educational services for children with disabilities (see *Learning Disorders,* Part 5).

Once the evaluation is complete, your child's school should schedule a meeting with you and your child to discuss the findings and the options for therapy. Because this meeting may be confusing, it sometimes helps to bring along someone you trust and who can interpret the information given. The person could be a knowledgeable friend, a psychologist, or, if possible, your child's doctor. If you disagree with the findings, don't sign the report. You have the right to appeal the school's treatment recommendations as part of the IEP process.

Learning disorders are sometimes accompanied by problems paying attention. An estimated 1.5 to 9 percent of all schoolchildren and at least 20 percent of children with learning disabilities have an *attention deficit disorder* (ADD) (see Part 5), which is an inability to concentrate for as long as is normal for their age. Some of these children have attention deficit/hyperactivity disorder, or ADHD, which means that they are hyperactive, as well as inattentive. Attention disorders are usually diagnosed in the first year or two of elementary school, when a child should have enough self-control to sit still and pay attention for several minutes at a time.

Social and Emotional Development

Socially and emotionally, these are relatively easy years. Children can usually control their disappointment and frustration without going to pieces. They feel some pressure from their classmates to conform—to play certain sports, for example, to wear certain clothes, to get a certain hairstyle, or to collect sports cards. Children this age are often eager to please—not only one another, but also adults.

As children enter their school years, they become more aware of other people's thoughts and feelings. Unlike a preschooler, a school-age child can often anticipate what a classmate or one of his parents is about to do in a particular situation. He may show that he understands another child's viewpoint during fantasy play, which is popular with young elementary school children. Whether they dress up or simply use makeshift props, children often act out scenes from real life by playing house or school. This reveals their understanding of the adult world by imitation.

A 5-year-old has a budding sense of morality: telling right from wrong, honesty from dishonesty. If a playmate cheats during a game, a child this age may show outrage (although this outrage may apply only to other people's behavior, not to his own). But young elementary school children's moral thinking goes only so far. They may know right from wrong, but may not understand whether the "wrong" was done by accident or on purpose.

Throughout elementary school, children crave one another's company. Happiness is a good friend. At some point, however—and this varies from child to child and from school to school—children become aware that some classmates are more popular than others. And they focus on what it takes to be popular. Your child may

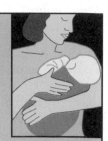

A MOTHER'S PERSPECTIVE
The Truth about Santa

When Jenny was 8, I thought she couldn't possibly still believe in Santa Claus. But at Christmastime she kept talking about Santa coming, so I certainly wasn't going to spill the beans.

Christmas morning, Jenny looked as thrilled as ever to enter the living room and see the presents. Christmas day went along much as it had since she was about 2.

On New Year's Day, Jenny and I were working on a puzzle together when she said, out of the blue, "I know there's no Santa Claus."

I was dumbstruck.

Then she said, "I would've told you earlier, but I didn't want to spoil your Christmas."

become more aware of how he looks and become concerned about wearing or doing something that will embarrass him or that other kids might make fun of. Much of this focus may be on having the right hairstyle, clothing, or decorative toy hanging from a backpack. Suddenly, your child may stand in front of the mirror and primp before going out.

Don't be alarmed by what may seem like too much emphasis on superficial things, like looks and possessions, although now may be the time to point out that material things are not as important as personal values and character. Understand that your child is learning how to get along with his peers and how to function within a social network—valuable skills for later in life. Some children are, by nature, more socially adept than others, but all must learn by trial and error how to fit in. You can help your child deal with difficult social situations. Role playing is often helpful. Have him practice what he will say or do in a difficult situation.

Boy-Girl Friendships

As their gender identity increases, boys naturally gravitate toward boys and girls toward girls. Many elementary school children have nothing to do with classmates of the opposite sex, who may suddenly become "yucky," and some are blatantly hostile toward them. But most children manage to be friendly with both boys and girls at least some of the time.

Recent research suggests that being able to get along with both sexes may be a sign of leadership. On the other hand, an inability for a boy to make friends with other boys or a girl with other girls is a cause for concern. It may indicate that a child is having difficulty with social adjustment—a problem that can lead to social isolation or loneliness.

Some children develop crushes on members of the opposite sex in their age group. This interest can develop as early as kindergarten, depending on the child and the school, but it becomes more common in the upper grades. Some children show their feelings by flirting, while others keep their feelings to themselves. Both kinds of behavior are normal, as is the affection behind them. The flirtatious behavior doesn't indicate that a child is likely to become sexually active anytime soon. On the other hand, children this age are quite curious about their own and other children's sexual anatomy. At some point, some exploration of genitals is likely (see What Your Child Needs to Know About Sex, p. 280).

QUESTIONS PARENTS ASK
How Do I Protect My Child from Bullies?

Your child may not tell you if he's being bullied or bad-mouthed by other children at school, but there are signs: Your child suddenly resists going to school; he regularly asks for extra lunch money or school supplies; or, in extreme cases, he comes home scratched and bruised. Bullies can be boys or girls. When girls bully another child, it is more likely to take the form of verbal taunts or rejection from a peer group, rather than physical threats. Girls can bully boys, and vice versa.

You can do several things to help make a bully stop bothering your child, but be fore-warned: The two pieces of advice that many parents give to their children—either to fight back or to ignore the bully—don't work. Instead, teach your child how to show some self-confidence and not to give the bully the satisfaction of seeing him suffer. Pediatricians, schools, and education groups are taking the problem of bullying more seriously than ever. These experts have the following recommendations for parents:

■ *Urge your child not to cry in front of a bully.* Crying makes bullies tease and taunt their victims even more.

■ *Teach your child how to show self-confidence.* Suggest that he look the bully in the eye and say something like, "Stop it. I don't like what you're doing," then walk away with head held high and shoulders square.

■ *Role-play with your child.* Help him practice being assertive, like standing up straight and looking the bully in the eye. Recommend things he can say to throw the bully off guard. For instance, if the bully calls your child stupid, your child can respond with something like, "That's not true. I'm smart; I get good grades."

■ *Advise your child to travel in groups.* Children are less likely to be bullied if they're with friends.

■ *Talk to other parents.* If your child is being bullied, chances are that other children at school are being bullied, too. Their parents may have suggestions.

■ *Tell the bully's parents.* If all else fails, this technique may be effective. Because many bullies learn intimidation from their own parents, some parents may be defensive. Others, with the interest of their own child's reputation at heart, are likely to intervene.

▌*Meet with the teacher and principal.* To be most effective, the meeting should involve several parents whose children are also being bullied. Don't act emotional, lest you be dismissed as overly protective. Calmly say something like, "Our kids are scared to go to school because they're being bullied. What can we do about the problem?" Suggest the school incorporate an antiviolence and respect program into the curriculum.

Caring for Your Child

With each passing year, your child will assume more responsibility. When your child first starts school, he is able to dress himself and remember to bring home items he brought to school. By age 10, your child may be ready to stay home alone for short periods, make his bed, prepare some meals for himself, take his own medicine, and organize his time well enough to do his homework without your having to sit down and do it with him. Caring for your school-age child involves helping him make the leap in responsibility with countless how-to's, ranging from how to floss his teeth to how to use the stove safely. It also involves coaching your child on the proper ways to behave in various social situations, from having friends over, to dinner out with friends and their parents. As academic and social pressures increase, caring for your child also means being there on his side, an emotional port in the storms of life.

Eating Well

Your child eats some healthy foods—a bowl of yogurt here, a glass of orange juice there—but is his overall diet good enough? If he's like most schoolchildren, the answer is no. Only 1 percent of U.S. children ages 2 to 11 meet all the national recommendations on nutrition. Fewer than 30 percent consume the recommended amount of fruit, grains, meat, and dairy, and just 36 percent eat enough vegetables.

Buried in the bad news are signs of hope. Elementary school children are fairly knowledgeable about nutrition. In one survey, half of 6- to 9-year-olds could name all of the food groups (milk/dairy, meats, vegetables, fruits, and grains), and 65 percent knew that what they eat can affect their health.

So, how can you encourage your child to apply what he knows about good nutrition, say, to choose milk over soda, carrots over candy, grapes over chips? Here are four parent-tested ways to get your child to eat better:

▌*Appeal to his mind.* Explain why particular foods are good for him. Be matter-of-fact, not preachy. Say, "Drinking milk every day is important, because it's got a lot of calcium, and you need calcium to build strong bones right now." Or: "If you eat more fruits and vegetables, you might get fewer colds, because fruits and vegetables have vitamins and minerals that help your body fight germs."

▌*Appeal to his stomach.* The it's-good-for-you argument goes only so far. If your child doesn't respond, tell him that a particular food or dish (that's good for him) is delicious. Serve and eat it yourself. Make an effort to prepare and present foods that look appealing and taste good.

▌ *Give him choices.* If your child doesn't like milk, let him choose other high-calcium foods and drinks (see below). Take your child to the market, and let him pick out some healthy foods that he'd like to eat.

▌ *Limit his choices.* Don't bring junk foods into the house. Don't buy foods with saturated or hydrogenated fats or sugars as the first or second ingredient. You do the shopping. You can control what's available to eat—at least at home.

▌ *Make healthy snack foods easy to eat.* Your child is more likely to help himself to cantaloupe instead of cookies if it's been cut up and put in a plastic container in the refrigerator than if it's whole.

▌ *Set a good example.* Children often find what they see on their parent's plates attractive. So if you are eating vegetables, whole grains, fish, and lean meats, chances are that your child will surprise you and gradually follow suit.

Vitamin supplements are generally not necessary for children in this age group. Instead, help your child get the nutrients he needs from the food he eats. The chart on page 264 lists the nutritional needs of children ages 5 to 10 and some examples of good food sources. Use it to assess your child's eating habits and identify areas for improvement.

Don't be fooled by bread and muffin labels with the words "whole-wheat" or "whole-grain" on the label. Many of these products contain only minimal amounts of whole-wheat flour. Instead, look on the list of ingredients. Whole-wheat flour should be the only flour listed, or at least the first ingredient listed. Otherwise, it's not whole-wheat bread.

Calcium Crisis

Most children don't get enough calcium. The lack of calcium is especially critical for girls, because starting at around age 8 they enter a period of 3 or so years when they create more bone than they will at any other time in their lives. Later in life, when female hormone levels drop, women begin losing calcium from their bones at a rapid pace, which leads to the weakened bone condition known as osteoporosis. Children need calcium to build strong, thick bones that will last them a lifetime.

Calcium supplements are not necessary for most school-age children. Calcium is readily available in everyday foods. Milk and yogurt are among the best sources of calcium, but they're not the only ones. Here are some other sources that many children like. The foods at the top of the following list are higher in calcium than those at the bottom:

▌ Calcium-fortified orange juice (some have as much calcium as milk)

▌ Calcium-fortified soy milk

▬ *YOUR CHILD'S DIETARY NEEDS*

Food Groups	Daily Servings	Good Sources	Serving Size for Age 4–6	Serving Size for Age 7–10
Fruit	2–3, including one high in vitamin C	Apples, oranges, bananas, peaches	½–1 small	1 medium
		Fruit juice[1]	½ cup	½ cup
		Canned or cooked fruit (applesauce)	4–6 Tbs.	¼ – ½ cup
		Fruits high in vitamin C: oranges, grapefruit, kiwis, mangoes, strawberries	½ –1 small	1 medium
Vegetables	3 or more, including at least one high in vitamin A (spinach and other green, leafy vegetables; squash; sweet potatoes; broccoli)	Cooked vegetables	3–4 Tbs.	¼ –½ cup
		Salad	½ cup	1 cup
		Raw vegetables	Few pieces	Several pieces
Grains	6	Whole-grain bread	½ slice	1 slice
		Cooked rice, pasta, cereal	⅓ cup	½ cup
		Whole-grain crackers	3–4	4–5
		Bagel or English muffin	½	½
Dairy[2]	2–3	Low-fat or nonfat milk or yogurt	½ – ¾ cup	¾ –1 cup
		Soy milk fortified with calcium and vitamin D	½ – ¾ cup	¾ –1 cup
		Cheese	1 ounce	1 ounce
Protein	2–3	Cooked lean meat, fish, chicken	1–2 ounces	2–3 ounces
		Tofu	4–6 ounces	6 ounces
		Eggs	1	1–2
		Cooked peas or beans	4 Tbs.	5 Tbs.
Fats, oils, and sweets	Small amounts	Oils, butter, sweets	Total from all foods eaten (including those listed above) should be no more than 30 percent of total daily calories.	

1. Fruit juice is high in sugar and low in nutrition. Look for products that are 100 percent juice, and limit consumption to no more than 8 ounces per day.
2. See discussion on calcium, p. 263.

- Cheese: cheddar, Edam, Monterey Jack, mozzarella, Parmesan, provolone, ricotta, Romano, Swiss, cottage
- Sardines
- Ice cream, ice milk, and nuts and vegetables such as almonds, greens (collard, mustard), spinach, and broccoli. While these foods contain calcium, they are not a practical source, since the amount of calcium in each is either minimal or, in the case of vegetables, not easily absorbed (the fiber interferes with the body's ability to absorb the calcium).

Preventing Eating Disorders

In movies, on TV, and in school, children quickly get the message that thin is beautiful. It doesn't take long for them to take a critical look at their own figures and wonder if they're thin enough. A preoccupation with thinness can begin in early elementary school, and it may lead to eating disorders, such as anorexia nervosa and bulimia nervosa. Ninety percent of eating disorders occur in girls.

True eating disorders in children are rare. Most children go through periods of food struggles with their parents. Refusing to eat, hiding food, or throwing food away (or feeding it to the dog under the table) are common—if occasional—acts, as is sneaking sugary or high-fat snacks now and then. A true eating disorder is one in which the child develops an enduring pattern of behavior associated with serious health problems and emotional disturbance. The types of eating disorders include the following:

- *Anorexia nervosa:* extreme fear of weight gain, which causes a failure to maintain adequate weight
- *Bulimia nervosa:* frequent binge eating followed by vomiting or excessive exercising in order to eliminate the calories consumed
- *Binge eating disorder:* frequent, severe episodes of binge eating, followed by excess weight gain

The treatment of eating disorders is complex, involving psychotherapy, nutritional counseling, and medical intervention when necessary. If you suspect that your child has an eating disorder or if you notice unusual eating patterns or abnormal weight gain or loss (see Appendix: Growth Charts), consult your child's doctor.

Because most eating disorders appear in adolescence or later, the best thing you can do now is to lay a healthy groundwork for good eating habits and attitudes. You can't prevent your child from thinking that a lean figure is attractive, but you can help prevent this thinking from taking an extreme and unhealthy turn.

To help your child establish healthy eating habits and a good sense of how much to eat at one sitting, don't insist that your child finish everything on the plate. Instead, use this rule of thumb: Stop eating when you begin to feel full. Your child can learn to rely on the feeling of fullness as the signal to stop eating—a useful skill to use throughout life.

Getting Enough Sleep

Bedtime usually undergoes some upheaval during the school years. The first major shift often comes when children enter kindergarten. Many children who had become night owls because they could sleep late in the morning must go to bed earlier now that they need to wake up early for school. Five-year-olds still need about 10 to 11 hours of sleep a night. Shifting your child's bedtime earlier shouldn't be difficult once school starts. He'll be so exhausted from the early morning wake-up, the excitement of attending a new school, and possibly the need to adjust to a longer school day that he should be ready for bed by around 8 to 9 P.M., even if he was previously accustomed to staying up later.

By about age 7, another shift often occurs. Children's sleep needs can decrease to as little as $9\frac{1}{2}$ hours a night, so they may not feel tired enough to fall asleep at their usual bedtime. By age 10, many need only 9 to 10 hours of sleep. (See p. 108 for an age-by-age sleep chart.)

You can't expect to have the same degree of control over your child's bedtime when he's 7 that you had when he was 5. But don't give up control entirely. If you do, your child may stay up so late that he won't get enough sleep. Lack of sleep won't just make your child cranky. It could make concentrating difficult for him, leading to underachievement in school. It may also interfere with his growth. During deep sleep, which occurs in the first third of the night, the body releases human growth hormone, which regulates growth. You'll do yourself, and your child, a favor if you get him on a regular schedule that allows for enough sleep so that he wakes up by himself in time to get ready for school.

Discipline

Your 7-year-old's bedroom is a minefield of toys and dirty clothes. How can you make him clean up his mess? During an argument, your 8-year-old yells a curse word at you. What should you do? It's 8:45 P.M., and your 10-year-old still hasn't finished his homework. How can you get him to do his homework on time, next time?

Schoolchildren are expected to be polite, to follow rules, and, as they get older, to assume more responsibility for themselves, like doing their homework and performing chores around the house. Of course, all children misbehave occasionally. But failure to behave appropriately most of the time will no longer be forgiven by teachers and other adults. It is taken as a sign of rudeness and a lack of self-control.

In some ways, children are easier to discipline as they get older because you can reason with them. Tell your child that it's rude to say "I hate that" when offered a food that he doesn't like, and suggest polite alternatives.

The Parent Traps

In a desperate attempt to get their children to listen to them, parents often fall into one of several traps: They shout. They nag. They may even hit their children. These responses tend to make a child's behavior worse. When you shout, your child will probably shout back, and you'll both get angrier. When you nag, your child is likely to ignore you. When you hit, not only do you increase the chance that your child will keep misbehaving, but you are modeling a behavior that you do not want to see in your child.

Spanking school-age children is associated with a later increase in antisocial behavior such as bullying, lying, and cheating. The more children are spanked, the more anger they report as adults, the more likely they are to spank their own children, and the more likely they are to approve of hitting a spouse. Spanking is also associated with higher rates of physical aggression, more substance abuse, and an increased risk of crime and violence when older children and adolescents are spanked. Instead, maintain a positive, loving emotional environment while setting consistent rules and limits.

How do you enforce those rules and limits?

- *Listen to your child.* Not only will you show him that you respect him (which will make him more inclined to do as you say), you'll pick up clues as to why your child misbehaves in certain ways.

- *Stay calm.* Children are more likely to listen when you look them in the eye and speak in a normal tone of voice.

- *Set a good example.* If you routinely say "please" and "thank you" and treat others with respect, your child will, too.

- *Make it clear that you mean business.* Provide incentives for your child to behave properly, and tell him the consequences if he doesn't (such as no play dates the following day). When you set consequences, enforce them.

- *Remove privileges.* Let your child know that if he does not adhere to the rules and limits you set, then he will lose something he wants—his favorite TV show, video game, or a sleep-over with a friend, for example. Then follow through every time. Make the consequence in proportion to the offense, or you'll have trouble following through.

- *Catch him being good.* Point out and reward good behavior, especially when your child does something good without your having to ask him to do it.

THREE WAYS TO DISCIPLINE YOUR CHILD

Strategy 1: Talking

Explain to your child why a particular behavior is good or bad.

Used For . . .

- Teaching manners. Tell your child what to say and do in different situations. For example, you might teach him to say "please" and "thank you," to put his napkin in his lap, and not to get a snack for himself without offering one to his playmate.

■ Explaining how to avoid danger. For example, you might tell him to look both ways before crossing the street, to ride his bike on the right side of the street, and not to talk to strangers.

■ Explaining the social consequences of a particular behavior, such as why it makes you or others angry. This approach works especially well with 9- or 10-year-olds, who are sensitive to other people's opinions.

Strategy 2: Withholding or delaying privileges
Warn your child that he won't be able to do something that he enjoys (such as watching TV or having a play date) unless he does what he's supposed to do. For older children, grounding is an effective technique if used in a limited way. Do not issue punishment impulsively. Always warn the child first.

Used For . . .

■ Encouraging your child to do homework on time, clean his room, do other chores, or meet other responsibilities.

Strategy 3: Rewards
Put a sticker on the calendar for every day that your child behaves well (does homework on time, straightens his room, etc.). Once he's accumulated a certain number of stickers, he gets a reward, such as a new toy.

Used For . . .

■ Preventing one or two common behavior problems (repeatedly putting off homework, forgetting to put away toys, dawdling before school, missing the bus). When used sparingly as directed, this strategy can help jump-start a routine of good behavior. But when overused, it can backfire, weakening a child's motivation to behave well.

Teaching Your Child About Money

When you get cash from the ATM, does your child think the money is free? Should your child save or spend the birthday money from his grandparents? How much allowance should he get, and should he be expected to do chores to earn it? The school-age years are when children gradually develop a grasp of the abstract concept we call money. That is why these years are the perfect time to help your child develop some money management skills.

   The biggest questions for parents often revolve around allowances. Allowances are not simply a handout. They are an opportunity to help your child discover how quickly those dollars and cents can slip through their fingers if they don't plan carefully. Some parents choose to tie the payment of an allowance to chores. If you choose this route, make sure the required chores are well within your child's abilities, and then use a chart to record whether he performed them. Otherwise, the pay-for-chores system loses its meaning.

Other parents prefer to separate the chores from the allowance based on the idea that helping out at home is simply part of being in a family. In this case, the allowance is mainly a tool for teaching a child money management skills.

Whichever route you choose, once you begin paying an allowance, try to step back and wait to see whether your child's inclination is to save or spend. Some children are natural squirrels. Others will require some encouragement to save.

Setting Saving Goals

Next, help your child create specific saving goals. Younger children can save for less expensive items that may require only 2 to 3 weeks' worth of saving, such as a special baseball cap, hair ornament, or movie. Older children can set larger goals. Allowing your child to spend some money each week on a small item while saving the rest for longer-term goals will help teach money management skills.

Determining the Allowance

Set the amount of money based on your family's financial level and your own values regarding how much money a child should have. You, as a parent, are the best judge of the correct amount.

Birthday Money

Birthday and other gifts are a different issue because they come in larger amounts. Your child can combine the gift money with the allowance savings and save it for the long-term goals. But first consider allowing your child to spend some of the gift money immediately, because, after all, it is his birthday!

Opening a Bank Account

Once your child has accumulated some money of his own, you can open a savings account in his name and encourage him to make deposits. Some banks require a minimum deposit in order to open an account without incurring service charges. If so, you can have your child accumulate money in a piggy bank at home until he has enough. Once he has a bank account, explaining how a bank works and how interest accrues will be challenging but worthwhile.

Keeping Your Child Healthy

The older children get, the less often they get sick. They're more resistant to infections now that their immune systems have been strengthened by years of exposure to viruses and bacteria, although they still get minor illnesses occasionally. But other problems can emerge at this time. It's no accident that many children start wearing glasses in first or second grade—this is when nearsightedness (see **Vision Problems,** Part 5) tends to be diagnosed. As your child becomes more active in sports, he may experience his first sprained ankle or strained finger. In fact, injuries are the main health threat to a school-age child and are the leading cause of death in this age group. Emotionally, increasing academic demands and complexity of peer relationships can contribute to problems like depression.

Your child will see the doctor less often than in the past. The average school-age child sees the doctor at most only two to three times a year. As in the past, annual checkups are important for diagnosing problems early, but being aware of warning signs and reporting them to your child's doctor is equally important. Where sports injuries are concerned, the key is prevention with safety equipment, good sportsmanship, and appropriate warm-up and conditioning time.

Checkups

Your child's annual checkup should includes a physical exam, blood pressure screening, vision and hearing screening, height and weight measurements, and a check of the spine for straightness. The doctor will use your child's height and weight to assess whether he's growing and gaining weight at a normal rate. To do this, she will look at a chart that tells what percentile your child's weight falls into in relation to his height. If the doctor is concerned that your child's weight in relation to his height puts him at risk for obesity, the doctor will advise you and your child on increasing exercise and reducing the fat in your child's diet (see *Overweight,* Part 5).

If your child's weight in relation to height is too low, the doctor will determine whether your child is ill. The doctor may question whether your child is eating enough, and may refer your child to a nutritionist for counseling. An older child whose weight remains low might be at risk of an eating disorder (see p. 265).

Social and Emotional Concerns

In addition to evaluating your child's physical health, the doctor will probably try to assess his emotional and psychological well-being. She may do so by asking him things like whether he is happy in school, likes his teacher, and has friends. If you have concerns along these lines, mention them to the doctor privately ahead of time, so as not to embarrass your child. If your child seems to be struggling socially, emotionally, or academically, discuss the possibility of a referral to an appropriate therapist. For information on behavioral problems, see *Anxiety Disorders* (Part 5), *Behavioral Problems* (Part 5), and *Depression* (Part 5).

Finally, at some point, you can ask your child's doctor how to handle sex education. She'll probably ask how much you have already discussed with your child, and she might recommend some books to help you through these landmark parent-child talks. For help with these topics, you can ask your doctor to talk directly with your child about the physical changes to expect during puberty. But most of this information will need to come from you.

Screening Tests

See the Childhood Immunization Schedule on page 110 for the full description of immunizations your child will need before starting kindergarten. In addition, the following screening tests may be required:

▌ Hearing

▌ Vision

▌ Tuberculosis (PPD): Recommended only for children who live in areas with a high prevalence of tuberculosis or who may have been exposed to the disease, although some doctors include this as a routine test for all children.

▌ Lead screening: Some states require this test before entrance to kindergarten.

Annual blood lead screening is not necessary after age 6, because the school-age child's brain is no longer as susceptible to damage. School-age children do not tend to put their hands and other objects (that might contain lead dust) in their mouths as frequently as do younger children. Children with autism or other pervasive developmental delays, however, still do and may require continued lead screening (see *Pervasive Developmental Disorder,* Part 5). Anyone, including adults, can get acute **lead poisoning** (see Part 5) from exposure to large amounts of lead by such things as removing lead paint with a heat gun or living near a lead manufacturing smelter without proper environmental controls.

Promoting Mental Health

Your child's doctor is one of the most reliable sources of information about your child's mental well-being. Tell your doctor if you notice anything unusual about your child's behavior. For example, some disobedient or willful behavior should not be taken at face value but may instead be a symptom of an underlying behavioral disorder or mental health problem. *Depression* (see Part 5), for example, may result in low school performance or a withdrawal from family social life. Phobias or *anxiety disorders* (see Part 5) can cause a child to resist attending school or participating in other activities that make him anxious. Obsessive-compulsive disorder (see *Anxiety Disorders,* Part 5) can cause a child to engage in seemingly senseless repetitive behavior. In situations like these, the usual discipline methods are not only inappropriate but may be harmful—your child cannot control this behavior, so punishing him or expecting him to respond to the usual rewards or incentives is counterproductive. Instead, discuss any behavior that concerns you with your child's doctor, who may refer you to counseling for your child.

Seek help from your child's doctor and a mental health professional (child psychologist or psychiatrist) if you notice any of the following signs:

▌ Changes in your child's behavior, such as sleep problems, sudden mood changes, constant complaints of pain or illness with no apparent cause, inability to socialize with peers, sudden interest in adult sexual activity, use of drugs or alcohol, excess self-stimulation

▌ Behavior that seems unusually immature for your child's age

▌ Aggressive behavior, such as fighting or bullying others, cruelty to animals

▌ Panic attacks or anxiety reactions

▌ Compulsive behavior, such as repetitive hand-washing or excessive repetition of ritual behavior

▌ Unusual unresponsiveness to parental suggestions, guidance, or other interactions

▌ High-risk behavior that threatens the child's safety, including fire-setting and fascination with fire

▌ Antisocial behavior, violations of the law, stealing, destruction of property

▌ Suicidal thoughts, talk, or attempts

Your Child's Teeth

Your child should continue to have a dental checkup twice a year, or as directed by the dentist. During the checkups, your child's teeth will be cleaned and the dentist will examine their overall health. He'll look for cavities and make sure that your child is losing his baby teeth at a normal rate and in the normal order (see *Cavities,* Part 5). If not, problems could occur, such as a missing permanent tooth.

The dentist will also look at the position of your child's permanent and baby teeth. If they're crooked or too crowded, the dentist may refer you to an orthodontist for a consultation to see if orthodontic help is needed once all permanent teeth are in.

Once your child has his 6-year molars (which, true to their name, appear around age 6), the dentist will probably recommend that dental sealants be applied to their chewing surfaces to prevent cavities. These surfaces are where 84 percent of cavities occur. Sealants are clear, tasteless, odorless plastic coatings that are painted on the teeth and then dry to form a hard coating. See *Cavities,* Part 5, for more information.

Sports and Your Child

At this age, children have many opportunities to participate in organized sports. No sooner do they start school than they bring home notices for soccer leagues, baseball leagues, gymnastics classes, and football. Playing a sport is an excellent way for a child to get exercise, gain self-confidence, make friends, hone social skills, like cooperation and sportsmanship, and constructively channel pent-up energy. But risks exist, both physical and emotional. Children—and parents—can easily get swept up in sports fever.

The result may be that a child signs up for too many teams and classes, then gets burned out in a few years. A recent survey found that 75 percent of children who participated in sports in elementary school stopped playing altogether by age 15. The most common reasons that children gave were that they weren't having fun or learning anything.

In terms of physical risks, the International Sports Medicine Congress (ISMC) reported that although children playing organized sports are no more likely to experience traumatic injuries (broken bones, sprains, lacerations) than those who do not, they are more likely to experience overuse injuries caused by repetitive training workouts. Because of this, the ISMC recommends that children avoid specializing in particular sports until at least age 10. Before this, children should be encouraged to participate in a broad range of activities that will enhance motor development.

Here are some guidelines for parents who want their children to have positive, long-lasting participation in sports.

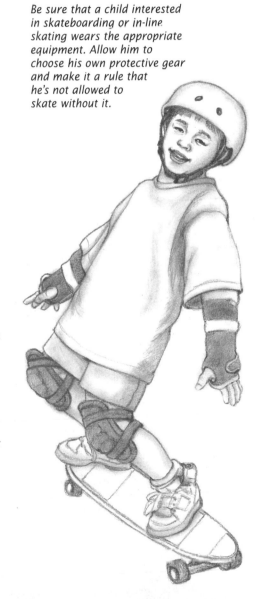

Be sure that a child interested in skateboarding or in-line skating wears the appropriate equipment. Allow him to choose his own protective gear and make it a rule that he's not allowed to skate without it.

- **Don't push.** Let your child choose which sports he wants to learn and play, even if they're not your first choices. If your child shows no interest in trying any sports, offer gentle encouragement or suggest noncompetitive activities like bicycling, skating, or dancing. Many children lose interest in playing sports during middle to late elementary school, especially if they feel that they're not good. But lack of exercise in school-age children is associated with an increased risk of obesity and cardiovascular disease years later. If your child doesn't like competitive sports, encourage recreational activities instead, like swimming, biking, dancing, boating, and hiking.

- **Shop around.** Not all sports classes and leagues are created equal. Find out (either through observation or by talking to other parents) whether a particular one emphasizes competition over fun. A hard-driving coach who benches children who don't play well may win a lot of games, but in the end she does more harm than good. Coaches and teachers should be supportive of all children, regardless of their abilities, giving them instruction and playing time.

- **Make safety a priority.** Some questions to ask: Is safety equipment available during games and practice sessions? Are children pressured to play even after they've been injured? In contact sports like football, is an effort made to combine children of similar sizes? Injuries often occur when a large child collides with a small one.

- **Don't specialize.** Children under 10 are best off with broad-based training in basic sports skills like swimming, catching, throwing, running, skating, and kicking. They can also get this training by playing games like soccer, baseball, hockey, and touch football. Intensive training in just one sport is too demanding, both physically and emotionally, for young children.

▌ *Participate.* Parents must actively participate in the process of coaching and training their children in sports.

SAFETY ALERT

Coach Training

The parent volunteers who serve as coaches often have little or no training. But it is important for volunteer coaches to get training in sports safety for children. The American Red Cross and the U.S. Olympic Committee have collaborated to create a nationwide system of coach training sessions. Contact your local American Red Cross office for information on coach training in your area. The National Youth Sports Safety Foundation also has information on coaching youth sports. See Appendix: Parent Resources, Safety.

Playing It Safe

In recent years, youth sports organizations have attempted to reduce the incidence and the severity of injuries by instituting safety regulations and requiring that children use safety gear such as helmets, mouth guards, athletic cups, and protective eyewear during games and practice sessions. Elementary school children are less likely to wear protective equipment than high schoolers, and girls are less likely to wear equipment than boys, probably because parents and coaches assume that smaller children are not at risk of serious injury. But serious injuries can occur at any age and among either girls or boys.

Parents and coaches need to insist that children wear protective equipment in order to participate in sports. Eye protection, for example, should be worn for sports involving close body contact or the use of a ball or stick. Helmets specifically designed for a particular sport will protect against brain and head injuries. Bicycle helmets, for example, reduce the risk of head injury by 85 percent and the risk of brain injury by almost 90 percent. Helmets are recommended for the following sports:

▌ Baseball	▌ Hockey	▌ Skiing
▌ Bicycling	▌ Lacrosse	▌ Snowmobiling
▌ Boxing	▌ In-line skating	▌ Softball
▌ Horseback riding	▌ Skateboarding	▌ Wrestling
▌ Football		

SPORT-BY-SPORT SAFETY

All sports: Keep water and sports drinks always available for when children are thirsty during games and practice sessions. Children become overheated more quickly than adults and risk dehydration or heat exhaustion. Have children wear the appropriate protective equipment during games and practice sessions.

Sport	Precautions
Baseball	Children under age 8 should not pitch, because of the risk of injury to their elbows. Older children shouldn't pitch more than 300 pitches or three innings a week, to prevent overuse injuries to the elbows and shoulders. All children should wear helmets with face guards while batting or catching and wear soft spike shoes. Soft-core balls are safest.
Basketball	Children should wear mouth guards, and those who need corrective lenses should wear sports safety glasses. Cut fingernails short, and don't allow children to wear dangling jewelry or rings. Make sure that the playing surface is free of debris and that areas such as nearby walls or posts are padded. Check that footwear is designed for playing basketball.
Field hockey	Field hockey is a contact, collision sport that requires the use of shin guards, mouth guards, and eye protection. Shin guards should cover the shoe and the leg to prevent foot injuries.
Football	Properly outfitted with well-fitting equipment, children age 10 and up can safely play tackle football. Players should wear spiked footwear. Make sure that helmets fit properly, have face masks, and are reconditioned and recertified each year. Other gear, such as shoulder, hip, and knee pads, should fit properly. Have children always wear mouth guards, and match players according to size.
Gymnastics	Don't allow gymnasts to practice without a qualified spotter who is there to reduce injuries from slips and falls. Make sure that equipment is properly maintained, secured, and set up, with sufficient mats placed appropriately. Clothing should allow for freedom of movement but not be so large as to hinder a safe performance. Make sure that coaches are certified and trained in safety precautions.
Ice hockey	Players must have the following safety gear: helmet with face shield, mouth guard, shin pads, shoulder pads, gloves, elbow pads, padded shorts to protect hips, and a protective cup for boys. Choose skates that fit properly; skates that are too large can cause injury. Wipe skate blades clean after use. During play, prohibit checking from behind.
Skateboarding and in-line skating	Wear helmets and knee, elbow, and wrist guards. Skate and skateboard away from traffic in areas designated for the sport.
Soccer	Soccer is a contact, collision sport that requires the use of shin guards, mouth guards, and eye protection. Soccer goals must be well padded and properly secured. Heading the ball (hitting the ball with the head) may cause concussion, brain damage, and possible memory and intellectual impairment. Choose a number 4 soccer ball. Make sure that shoes have molded cleats or ribbed soles. Children should avoid shooting on goals until they complete warm-up and stretching exercises.

Anabolic Steroids and Dietary Supplements

As children grow older and more competitive in sports, they may hear about others who are trying to enhance their athletic performance by using anabolic steroids or over-the-counter dietary supplements, such as creatine monohydrate, which are meant to mimic the effects of steroids. People in the United States are spending more than $100 million a year on black-market anabolic steroids, and even some preadolescent children are taking them.

Anabolic steroids are male hormones sometimes prescribed by doctors to treat specific diseases. But they are not appropriate for use by athletes without a doctor's prescription. Nonmedical use of these drugs is both illegal and dangerous. Numerous short-term and long-term health side effects result from the use of these drugs. According to the National Clearinghouse for Alcohol and Drug Information, major side effects include the following:

▌ Liver tumors

▌ Yellowing of the skin and eyes (jaundice)

▌ Fluid retention

▌ High blood pressure

▌ Severe acne

▌ Trembling

▌ Weakness of tendons, which may result in tearing or rupture

▌ Stunted growth in adolescence

▌ Mood swings, irritability, impaired judgment, aggressiveness (known as "roid rage")

In males only, there are additional side effects:

▌ Testicular shrinkage

▌ Reduced sperm count

▌ Baldness

▌ Development of breasts

In females only, anabolic steroids have other side effects:

▌ Facial hair

▌ Irregular menstrual cycle

▌ Enlargement of the clitoris

▌ Deepened voice

People who take anabolic steroids often develop drug dependence and experience withdrawal symptoms once they discontinue use of the drugs. Adolescents who use these drugs are also more likely to abuse other substances as well. Discuss the dangers of anabolic steroids with your child before he may be tempted to use them.

Even more popular than steroids is creatine monohydrate, an over-the-counter dietary supplement used by athletes hoping to enhance performance. Taken in high doses, creatine can damage the kidneys and cause dehydration and cramping. Because there have been no long-term studies of creatine use in young people, this dietary supplement represents an unknown, untested substance that is not appropriate for use by children or adolescents.

A Parent's Life

There's no question that your life gets easier once your child reaches school age. Your child is more interested in playing with other children than with you now and can take care of many aspects of his own physical needs, like feeding, dressing, and washing. If you work outside the home, you may no longer need full-time child care. If you stay home or work part-time, you may now have longer stretches of time to devote to other activities. And when your child starts sleeping over at friends' homes, you've hit the jackpot: a Saturday night out without having to find a baby-sitter.

This isn't to say that you'll have a lot of free time. Many parents find that they're busier than ever once their child starts school, because they're helping with homework and music lessons; transporting children to friends' houses, after-school programs, and sports activities; and attending parent-teacher organization meetings. Also, during these years, many parents decide to reenter the workforce after having taken time to be home with small children. In scheduling family activities, don't forget to leave unscheduled time. It's during the moments when you've got nothing to do except sit on the couch that you can keep in touch both with what your child is doing and with who he is.

You and Your Child's School

Parent volunteers are the lifeblood of a good school. Increasingly, financially strapped schools rely on parents to provide services that they don't have money to pay for, like monitoring games during recess, teaching after-school enrichment courses, and typing manuscripts that children have written in class. Your involvement can help your child feel good about school and do well academically. It also can be fun and rewarding to get to know your child's teachers and his classmates' parents.

You can become involved in many ways, even if you're pressed for time. If you've got a demanding full-time job, you're probably too busy to volunteer to lead regular committees. But you can take part of a morning to read to your child's class, or you can help plan one of the class parties, go on a field trip, or sell tickets to a fundraising event. Get involved with your school's parent-teacher organization. What's important is that you be a part of your child's education.

If you can't visit your child's classroom, stay in regular contact with the teacher. Scheduled parent-teacher conferences are not enough. You must call the teacher or write her a note if you've got concerns. Contact the teacher if you suspect any academic problems—for example, if your child is consistently struggling with certain homework assignments or if his homework is too easy for him. Bring up social issues, too. Is your child getting along well with the other children? Don't bother your child's teacher with every spat he has with a classmate, but if your child is upset or afraid to attend school, or if he seems not to be making friends, discuss it with the teacher. The teacher should be able to help identify the problem and suggest solutions.

QUESTIONS PARENTS ASK
Getting Information from Your Child

Q: Every day, I ask my 8-year-old daughter how school went, and her response is usually just "Fine." How can I find out more from her?

A: By the time you ask your child what happened in school, it's ancient history to her. She may have forgotten. Or it could be that so much happened that she doesn't know where to begin. One way to tease out more revealing answers is to ask more targeted questions: What did you do in art class today? Did you play dodgeball at recess? What did you have at lunch? Did you do any math today? If your child's answer is one syllable or nonexistent, try another topic. The most important thing you can do is to learn to walk the fine line between showing an interest and respecting her privacy. If you do, she'll open up when she's ready.

Home Alone

You've got to pick up your younger child at a party, but your 9-year-old has just started playing a game. He doesn't want to go with you any more than you want to have him along complaining. Can you leave him home alone? Most experts agree that the average 10-year-old is mature enough to stay home alone for short periods (about a half hour), but leaving children younger than 10 is controversial. In many states, leaving children under age 10 home alone for several hours on a steady basis is illegal. Find out what your state laws require. Leaving children under age 10 at home occasionally for 20 minutes or so is a gray area. Ask yourself these questions: What if a fire broke out? Would your child know what to do? What if someone you didn't know came to the door?

Of course, you can never be completely sure that you're doing the right thing the first time you shut the door to your home with your child inside. But there are several ways to tell if your child is ready for a dry run. First of all, he says that he wants to stay home alone. Second, he's demonstrated that he's mature enough to think before he acts. A child who habitually opens the door whenever the doorbell rings without first asking who's there is too impulsive to stay home alone. Third, he's capable of following two-step or three-step instructions without forgetting anything. Tell your child how to reach you or whom to call in an emergency, and be sure you feel confident that he will act on your instructions.

Before Leaving Your Child

Before leaving your child for the first time, lay down some ground rules.

■ Don't let him use the stove, oven, microwave, or other heat-producing appliances, such as space heaters, blow-dryers, or bread machines. These appliances probably won't cause a fire or injury, but don't take any chances.

■ Keep the door locked, and tell your child not to open it except for a family member.

■ Teach him to call 911 in an emergency and to exit the house as fast as possible in the event of a fire (see Fire Safety, p. 371).

■ Role-play with your child. Imagine a fire starts. Imagine a stranger shows up. Imagine his sister cuts herself badly with a pair of scissors.

■ Don't let strangers know that your child is alone, and instruct your child not to tell anyone who calls that you are out. If a caller asks for you, have your child say that you're too busy to answer the phone.

■ When you go out for the first time, don't go far and don't go for long. Leave a phone number where you can be reached, or if you can't be reached by phone, give him the number of a trusted neighbor. Let the neighbor know that you'll be out briefly.

■ Tell your child exactly when you'll be back, and don't be late.

■ Once you and your child feel comfortable with his being home alone for short periods, it's tempting to go to the next step and let him watch his younger brother or sister. Don't. No matter how good a job he does taking care of himself, a child under age 12 is not ready to baby-sit.

■ Don't make leaving your child alone a regular routine: after school while you work, for example. Instead, sign him up for a supervised after-school program, or hire a sitter or "companion."

The Big Talks: Sex and Substance Abuse

Many parents choose to discuss these topics by the time a child is about 9 years old, before he goes through puberty, hears a lot of misinformation from classmates, and feels significant peer pressure to smoke, drink, try drugs, or have sex. But many parents feel ill at ease bringing up these subjects with their children. They're difficult subjects to talk about. Parents may fear that the information will make their still-innocent children lose their innocence too soon, or that it will somehow make them want to experiment with sex, cigarettes, alcohol, or drugs. Parents may also feel uncomfortable about their own personal experiences. Can you comfortably instruct a child not to do something that you yourself have done?

The answer is yes. Children need this information to be well prepared for the changes they will face in the years ahead. They also need to know the limits of acceptable behavior—you can decide what is acceptable for your child's age and maturity level. Children will hear about sex, drugs, tobacco, and alcohol from various sources: teachers, classmates, movies, TV. Many schools routinely present programs on these topics to children. Find out if yours does. But even if your child's school is running such programs, you should be his main source of information. Talk to your child about what the school is teaching. This will help to reinforce the message.

What Your Child Needs to Know About Sex

Chances are that you won't have to sit your child down to have a big talk about sex. Instead, discussions about sexual development will grow out of questions that your child asks, like, "How do you make babies?" or "What's sex?"

These questions may catch you off guard because you weren't expecting them and you haven't planned out what to say. Many parents become flustered by questions about reproduction and sex, because they assume that they must answer them with a description of intercourse. But they needn't—at least not right away. All that's required is a direct answer to the child's question. For young school-age children, answer their questions briefly without elaboration. Long explanations will probably overwhelm them, and information will get lost in the shuffle. Many good books that address these subjects are available for parents to read with a child. Ask your child's doctor for suggestions on books and other resources.

You can try answering the question "Where do babies come from?" with a discussion of sperm and eggs: Men produce sperm, and women have eggs inside them. When sperm fertilize an egg, a baby grows. This scientific explanation may satisfy a 5- or 6-year-old. But at some point down the road the child is bound to ask a follow-up question, like, "How does the sperm get to the egg?" Then answer *that* question in simple and direct terms, such as, "The man puts his penis inside the woman's vagina, and the sperm swim out into the woman, where an egg may be waiting to be fertilized—this is called sexual intercourse and it happens when a man and a woman love each other."

Your child probably won't ask you all the important questions about sexuality and puberty, so be prepared to initiate some conversations. One way to start is to ask your child how much he knows about subjects pertaining to sex and reproduction. The average age at which children begin to experience sexual attraction is age 10—so knowing much of the following information by that time is good for them. Attraction, however, is only the first stage, distinct from the emotional feelings, sexual desire, and then sexual behavior that emerge in teenage years. It is then that your talks about sex should shift to discussions on the social and emotional aspects of sex and about your values. For now, here are some of the things your child will need to know about.

Puberty Explain that puberty is a hormonal process by which boys' and girls' bodies gradually change and develop (including breast growth, pubic hair, menstruation, and wet dreams), with the result being the maturity of a young woman's and a young man's body to jointly create a baby.

Human Reproduction Intercourse should be discussed in the context of something good and loving between a man and a woman. Describe how babies are created and the ways that they can be delivered. Name the parts of the male and female bodies that are involved in reproduction and how they function. Use the proper names for sex organs, to avoid leaving the impression that there's anything dirty or shameful about them.

Masturbation Discuss masturbation as a normal part of sexuality for both boys and girls.

Sexually Transmitted Diseases, Including AIDS Explain that various diseases can be transmitted through sexual contact, and describe how to prevent them. For more information on *HIV/AIDS Infection,* see Part 5.

Birth Control Describe the purpose of birth control in family planning, name the various forms of contraception, and describe generally how they protect against pregnancy. Explain which forms of birth control (condoms) protect against sexually transmitted diseases.

Homosexuality Your child should know about different sexual orientations. You can't explain why some people are gay, because the answer is unknown. But you can explain that same-sex relationships are built on love, as are heterosexual relationships. And be sure to say that criticizing or making fun of anyone because of sexual orientation is wrong.

Preventing Smoking, and Drug, Alcohol, and Inhalant Abuse

As with so many aspects of parenting, to influence your child's behavior, you must set a good example. So if you don't want your child to smoke, drink excessively, or use illegal drugs, don't do these things yourself. But you need to do more than avoid this behavior.

By the fifth grade, some children have already begun experimenting with tobacco, alcohol, and inhalants—which include any chemical-based substance, such as cleaning solvents, markers, or glue, that children breath into their lungs to get high. This form of substance abuse has become increasingly common and has the reputation for being a gateway to alcohol and drug use.

Other children this age are dead-set against substance abuse (for now, at least). An effective way to begin discussing substance abuse with your child is to ask him what he knows. Then follow up with questions about what he thinks about smoking, drinking, inhaling, and taking drugs. Give your child clear statements about what *you* think about these activities. Make sure that he understands your values and expectations.

Tailor the content of your talk to your child's responses. For example, if, like many elementary school children, your child confuses illegal drugs with medical drugs, set him straight. Or, if your child thinks that all drinking is bad, including the occasional glass of wine that you have with dinner, explain the difference between social drinking and drinking to excess. He may think that sniffing glue or correction fluid isn't harmful, because these products are found at home or in school. Be sure he understands that these products are poisonous if not used the way they are intended.

Avoid being preachy, or your child will tune you out. But be consistent, and make it clear that you disapprove of excessive drinking or any tobacco or illegal drug use. Enlist teachers, scout leaders, and clergy to help set a "drug-free" tone for your community.

During your discussions, keep two goals in mind. One is to give your child information about tobacco, alcohol, and drugs and the harm that they can do to him. But the other goal is more important: to stimulate your child's thinking about these substances—why and how people use them and the consequences. In the end, the child who has thought these things through is in the best position to make the right choice when he's alone with a friend who says, "Come on, just try it."

QUESTIONS PARENTS ASK
A Parent's Past

Q: What do I say if my child asks me if I used drugs as a kid? Should I lie and say that I didn't, or should I tell the truth?

A: If your child asks point-blank if you ever smoked marijuana or used some other drug, tell the truth. But don't volunteer more than you have to. Make your answer brief, and back it up with a message that your child can use. You might try saying something like this: "Yes, I smoked marijuana, but that was a long time ago. I was confused and didn't know what I was getting into. If I'd known then what I know now, I wouldn't have done it." Make it clear that you strongly disapprove of drug and tobacco use now.

Learn the Warning Signs of Drug Abuse

Parents can take several steps to help prevent their children from becoming involved in drug use or to catch it early when it begins. Remember that because alcohol is the most widely available recreational drug, it is also the most commonly abused drug.

Start Young Discuss the dangers of drug and alcohol use with your child starting at about age 8, or even younger if your child has questions. Drug abuse both harms a child's health and can also prevent a child from achieving success in areas important to him, such as sports, school, and social life.

Look for the Signs It's not easy, but you can watch for certain signs. Some drugs make a child's eyes red or bloodshot. You child may start dressing or acting differently and become withdrawn. Don't jump to conclusions, however, because some of these changes may occur whether or not a child is using drugs.

Look for the Physical Evidence Some parents actually find drugs or drug paraphernalia in the child's room or clothing pockets: solvent-soaked clothes or handkerchiefs, pipes, forceps, roach clips, spoons, cigarette rolling papers, alcohol burners, syringes, unidentified pills. Other, less obvious signs include the use of air freshener and mouthwash to disguise smells from drug use. Any of the following products found in your child's possession may be a tip-off to inhalant abuse: solvent-soaked clothes or handkerchiefs, aerosol sprays, cans of spray paint, butane lighters, and leather-cleaning sprays.

Disappearance of Money or Valuables The disappearance of cash or other valuables from your home or your child's room can indicate that your child is taking these things to buy drugs or alcohol.

Behavior Changes Behavioral changes include the following:

▌ Acting more secretive, irritable, withdrawn, or hostile

▌ Acting depressed, apathetic, or unmotivated

▌ Leaving old friends behind and spending a lot of time with a new group of friends

▌ Being reluctant to talk about the new friends or to bring them home to meet you

▌ Acting more forgetful, less able to think fast

▌ Showing less interest in school performance

▌ No interest in sports or school/community activities

▌ Disheveled appearance, poor personal hygiene

If you notice these or other changes, talk with your child to find out if drug use may be the cause. Ask your child if he has friends who use drugs. Ask if he understands the dangers of drugs. Ask to get to know his friends. Offer to drive him and his friends to activities. If you suspect drug use, let your child know clearly that you cannot allow it, because it is illegal and dangerous to his health.

Understand when you talk to your child about drug use that he may be under strong peer pressure to use drugs or alcohol. Seek professional help from a counselor or therapist trained in substance abuse counseling.

SIX SYMPTOMS OF SUBSTANCE ABUSE

▌ Red eyes, glazed appearance

▌ Slowed speech

▌ Wandering attention

▌ Rash around the nose and/or mouth (inhalant abuse)

▌ Excessive sniffling or clearing of throat

▌ Chronic coughing

PART THREE
GETTING HELP

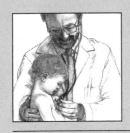

CHAPTER 8

YOUR CHILD'S DOCTOR AND HEALTH PLAN

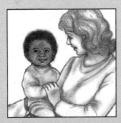

CHAPTER 9

LEAVING YOUR CHILD IN THE CARE OF OTHERS

8

Your Child's Doctor and Health Plan

CHOOSING A HEALTH PLAN
CHOOSING YOUR CHILD'S DOCTOR
WORKING WITH YOUR CHILD'S DOCTOR
ADOPTION HEALTH CONCERNS

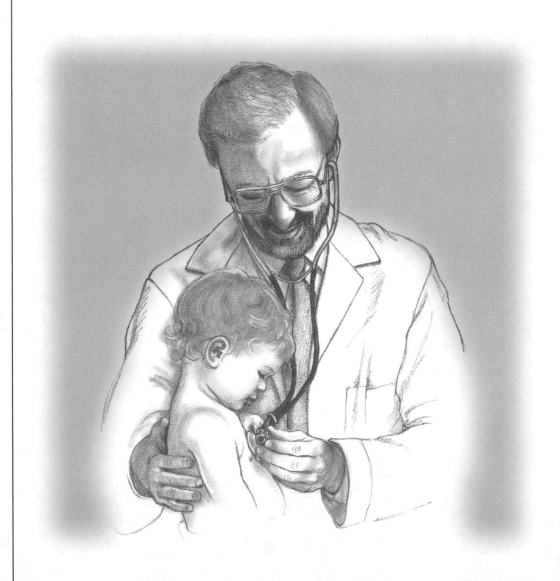

f, like many people, you see a doctor only occasionally for an examination or a test, things will change once you have a child. In your child's first year of life alone, you will visit your child's doctor or other health professional at least six times for regular checkups, and more if your child has any of the common fevers, flus, rashes, or infections that occur in infants and young children.

Think of your relationship with your doctor as a partnership. Both of you will play a role in keeping your child healthy. As a result, choosing your child's doctor carefully is important, and to do that, you must also decide what health plan your child and your family will subscribe to. A good relationship with your child's doctor will grow over the years into a partnership of trust.

Choosing a Health Plan

In today's changing health care environment, deciding which health plan to join can be as important as choosing the right doctor for your child—and more confusing. Because many health plans restrict your choice of doctors, choosing your health plan may determine which doctors you can use. There are many important things to consider in comparing health plans, once a child is in the picture.

If you don't have health insurance, or you have it for only yourself, explore your options to find a plan that will include your child. Or, if finances are very tight, you can find a health plan that covers only your child—state and local agencies or your local hospital will assist you in finding health coverage for an uninsured child. See Appendix: Parent Resources, Medical/Financial Assistance.

QUESTIONS PARENTS ASK
Maternity Benefits

Q: We are planning to have our first child. Will my health insurance from work cover my pregnancy and childbirth costs?

A: Right away, call your health plan and ask whether pregnancy and childbirth are fully covered, including regular prenatal visits, hospital expenses, and any necessary newborn medical care. Most plans cover maternity, but some cover more expenses than others. Once you are pregnant, you'll be in the doctor's office frequently. That means you're better off having a plan that fully covers these office visits or requires only a small co-payment (your out-of-pocket payment). If you are not yet pregnant and your maternity coverage is not as comprehensive as that of another available plan, now is a good time to change plans. Start early. Many employers allow you to switch plans only at a certain time of year. If you miss that open enrollment period, you may be stuck with your current plan.

Consider both prenatal care and at-the-hospital childbirth expenses. Make sure your plan has no restrictions on your choice of anesthesia during childbirth. And, before your baby's birth, obtain health coverage for your newborn, either through a family plan or an individual plan for your child.

Types of Health Plans

Choosing a health plan for your family may be one of the more complicated things you do in your life. Don't just throw up your hands and choose the plan your friends or co-workers have. Ask their opinions about their plans, but make sure to examine the available plans closely to see which one best meets your needs. For example, if you are planning more children, full prenatal and maternity coverage will be important. If you have a child with a particular medical condition, make sure the plan you choose offers you the options you want—such as easy access to a wide choice of specialists. *Choosing a plan that is well known and widely respected in your area is a good start.*

Health care coverage has changed dramatically in recent years. Traditionally, a health insurance company allowed you to choose your own doctors and specialists and covered all your in-hospital costs and a percentage (usually 80 percent) of your outpatient medical costs, and you paid the rest. To keep the premiums down, these plans sometimes carry a deductible figure, such as $500 per year, that the patient must pay out of pocket before the insurer pays the medical bills. This kind of plan, known as an indemnity plan, still exists but is now uncommon and usually quite expensive.

Now, many health insurance plans practice what is known as managed care, which means that, in an effort to control consumer and employer costs, the health plan contracts with a specific group of doctors and sets policies regarding your health care coverage. These policies may require that you use certain doctors and hospitals and may restrict the types of drugs, the number of expensive tests, or the length of a hospital stay that the plan will pay for. Managed care plans often emphasize preventative care (e.g., well-child checkups and immunizations) as a means of controlling costs as well as promoting good health.

Some plans require larger co-payments (the amount you pay when you visit the doctor). Some cover the cost of prescription drugs and medical equipment, and some don't. Some allow you to use a doctor outside the plan (often at a higher fee), and others require you to use only the doctors and specialists in the plan. Plans vary widely in the types of coverage they offer and in the quality of their doctors and services.

The first thing to understand about a health plan is what type of plan you are considering. Examine the individual plan, and compare its benefits to your needs and lifestyle. Make sure your plan fully covers regular doctors' visits, immunizations, urgent care visits, and emergency coverage for your child.

Questions to Ask About a Managed Care Health Plan

Don't be afraid to ask questions when considering a managed care health plan. Go to your employer's health benefits department, or call the health plan's customer service or member services department. If you can't easily get answers to these questions, try another plan. There are many good questions to ask, some of which concern the quality and availability of doctors:

■ *Is your child's doctor or another preferred doctor on the plan?* If not, why not? Find out how the plan chooses its doctors.

■ *How many doctors on the list have practices open to new patients?* Some plans have a long list of doctors, but many of their practices are closed to new patients.

■ *How does the health plan make sure its doctors are competent?* Many health plans admit any doctor who wants to be part of their network. Others are more choosy. Some even track their doctors' outcomes and patient satisfaction record. Look for a plan with high standards.

■ *How are the doctors compensated?* Many managed care plans give doctors financial incentives to keep costs down. But if those incentives interfere with getting the tests, procedures, or care your child needs, the health plan may not be a good choice.

■ *Who decides which procedures, tests, or specialists your child needs?* Look for a plan that leaves most of the medical decisions in the hands of the doctor and yourself, not an administrator.

■ *Do you need to get permission from your child's primary care physician to see a specialist?* More plans are now offering "open access" to specialists within the plan's network.

■ *Is a second opinion covered?* Some plans cover the cost of a second opinion. Some will cover a second opinion only if you stay in the network.

Some questions about a health plan address the quality of the plan itself:

■ *What kind of accreditation has the health plan received?* Ask if the plan has been reviewed by any of the following accreditation organizations: the National Committee for Quality Assurance, the American Accreditation Healthcare Commission, or the Joint Commission on Accreditation of Healthcare Organizations. Find out the accreditation status of the plan. See Appendix: Parent Resources, Medical/Financial Assistance, for ways to contact these organizations.

■ *How many complaints were filed against the plan or the physicians in the plan in the last year, and how many were upheld?* Ask the health plan or your state insurance department or state medical licensing board for this information.

■ *How do consumers rate this health plan?* Check with your employer, state insurance department, state Medicaid agency, or regional Medicare offices. Also check your local library or computer on-line services. Some plans voluntarily publish their own surveys and performance information.

■ *What is the procedure for filing an appeal?* If your child has been denied coverage for a particular service, or if you feel your child's health care has been inadequate in any way, learn how to file an appeal with your health plan.

You should also ask questions about specific benefits and services of the health plan:

▌ *What benefits are covered, and what are the limits of the coverage?* Review the list of what is covered, including office visits, hospital stays, home care, prescriptions, medical equipment, mental health, and maternity. Are there limits to the amount the plan will pay or limits to the number of visits or procedures allowed? Make your decision based on your family's needs.

▌ *Can you go to the doctor or hospital you want?* If there is a specific health care provider (doctor, hospital, laboratory) you prefer, find out if you can use the provider while covered under this plan.

▌ *Can you go out of the plan for specialized care?* If the plan offers you the option of seeing doctors or using out-of-plan hospitals, find out how much extra you will have to pay.

What Services Does Your Child Need?

The best time to review a health plan is before you enroll. If you are already in a plan, most employers offer a chance to switch insurance at a certain time each year, or if you are purchasing health insurance independently, many trade groups and business organizations offer group plans you can purchase. Either way, collect information from all the plans your employer or organization offers, and compare them.

Health care is expensive. Office visits, prescriptions, tests, and hospitalizations add up rapidly, especially if your plan's coverage is incomplete in some areas. So choose the plan that offers the most complete coverage for your family's particular needs. Here are some other steps you can take:

▌ Read the contracts and the description of services carefully.

▌ Write down the services that are most important to you and your family: Maternity coverage? Prescriptions? Preventive care? Mental health coverage? Physical or occupational therapies? Learn how much is covered.

▌ Talk with your employer's human resources department or with the health plan's member services department if you have questions.

▌ Talk with people you know who are members of the plan.

▌ Call the member service phone line, and ask questions about the plan in order to determine the level of customer service.

▌ Check the list of doctors and other providers that the health plan issues to see if your doctor or one you want is on the list. Is there a wide choice of doctors in your area?

▌ Find out whether the plan contracts with a hospital with top-notch pediatric services.

▌ Insist on answers. Many health plans provide glossy brochures and information that promote the plan but do not give specifics on coverage. Ask to see lists of doctors in the plan and specific coverage details.

The chart below describes the most important services a health plan for children can offer. No plan will offer all these services, so decide which are the most important for your family.

When choosing a plan, consider your family's needs and read the description of coverage carefully. The following sections describe some of the most important services that families with children will need.

Preventative and Primary Care Services

Your child will need regular checkups for immunizations, developmental progress, blood tests, and vision and hearing screening, as well as diagnostic exams and tests when she is sick. Most plans cover doctor's visits when the child is sick, but some do not cover the regular checkups and immunizations that will make up most of your child's visits—particularly in the first year. Make choosing a plan that covers well-child checkups and immunizations a top priority.

Hospitalizations

Find out where your child would be hospitalized for illness if she needed it. Are you satisfied with the facility? Is it reasonably convenient to your home? Does it have a well-staffed pediatric unit? Or is pediatric care only a minor sideline? Is your child's doctor on staff there? If not, your doctor will not be able to attend to your child if she is hospitalized. Discuss with your doctor which local hospitals are most appropriate for pediatric care and where he has admitting privileges. Many doctors can admit patients to more than one hospital.

Emergency Care

In the past, you could jump in the car and head for the nearest emergency room whenever the need arose. Not anymore. Many plans now require you to use the

WHAT TO LOOK FOR IN A FAMILY HEALTH PLAN

Preventative and Primary Care	Medical Services	Special Care
Routine checkups and exams	Consultations with pediatric specialists	Mental health counseling or hospitalization
Doctors' visits for sick children		
Dental checkups	Hospital services in a children's hospital	Coordination of care for a disabled or chronically ill child
Health education		
Immunizations	Diagnostic evaluations and tests by pediatric specialists	Equipment and supplies
Laboratory and X-ray services		Physical, speech, or occupational therapy
Pregnancy and childbirth costs		
Prescription drugs	Emergency and ambulance services	Long-term treatment of a chronically ill child at home or in a treatment facility
Speech, hearing, and vision tests		

emergency room in the plan and to get authorization before you go. Find out the plan's policy for emergencies. Some of the questions you should ask include these:

▌ Must you call first before going to the emergency room?

▌ What if the situation is life-threatening?

▌ What hospital should you go to?

▌ What is the co-payment required?

▌ Is the hospital reasonably convenient to your home?

▌ If you are in another area, can you use a different emergency room?

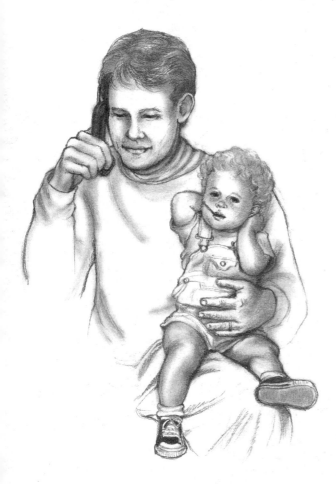

Unless the situation is life-threatening, some health plans require you to call and get authorization before going to the emergency room.

Pregnancy and Childbirth Coverage

Whether you are waiting for your first child or are planning your next, comprehensive maternity coverage should be a top priority. Not only does early prenatal health care improve your chances of having a healthy baby, but a plan that covers all your in-the-hospital expenses can be immensely helpful to new parents who are already faced with the other substantial costs associated with having a baby, from baby clothes and equipment to child care or reduced work hours. Some plans offer complete coverage of all maternity costs. Others will expect you to pay all or part of various expenses, ranging from prenatal checkups to in-hospital pediatric exams—or even, in some cases, elective anesthesia during childbirth.

Care for Chronic Conditions or Special-Needs Children

If your child has chronic medical conditions or special needs, check to make sure that the plan covers any medical needs your child may have. If your child has been previously treated for chronic conditions such as asthma, diabetes, or epilepsy, or a disease such as cystic fibrosis or muscular dystrophy, the plan may not cover the condition. Federal laws now restrict the length of time your child can be excluded for a preexisting condition (see Preexisting Conditions, p. 294), but even a few months without coverage for some illnesses can mean a severe financial burden.

Find out whether the plan covers the cost of specialized equipment such as wheelchairs or other assisting devices and technology. Also, home health care services are important for a chronically ill child.

Find out what provision the plan makes if your child is diagnosed with a developmental delay or impairment. Will your child be covered for a variety of therapies, such as speech, physical, or occupational therapy, and related testing? Will the plan cover family counseling, including assistance to help you cope with the demands of caring for a special-needs child? Comprehensive plans will offer all of these.

Health plans vary. Many are reluctant to pay for items not considered part of traditional medical care, and they frequently do not provide home care. But talk with your doctor and your health plan's member services department about these expenses to try to get some of these expenses covered. It is imperative that you act as an advocate for your child. Frequently, getting coverage is a matter of asking often and loudly for services and coverage that you otherwise may not get.

Despite your efforts, expenses that are not covered will occur. Networking with groups that offer advice and support for families with special-needs children is critically important. Your child's doctor or nurse may be able to give you the names of local parent support groups that you can enlist for help. The names of organizations that can refer you to local support groups are also listed in the resources appendix of this book. Support groups help in several ways: For instance, they can write letters to help convince local insurance companies to cover certain costs. They can also give you information about local volunteer groups that may provide home care and other services at little or no cost.

Supplemental Security Income   The Supplemental Security Income (SSI) program is a federal program that supplies cash assistance and health insurance for children with disabilities. Many children who would qualify for these benefits are not getting them, because their parents have not applied, according to SSI. For information on contacting SSI, see Appendix: Parent Resources, Medical/Financial Assistance.

Early Intervention   If you have an infant or child up to 3 years old with medical or developmental needs, contact the early intervention services in your area. The early intervention program provides services for infants and toddlers to identify and treat a problem or delay as early as possible. Early intervention services are available for all children at risk of developmental problems without regard to income level or insurance status. Services can range from prescribing glasses for a 2-year-old, to providing speech therapy for a child with a speech delay or physical therapy for an infant with cerebral palsy. Early intervention services are often paid for through the local public school system or the local department of public health. These services are mandated by the federal government through legislation such as the Individuals with Disabilities Education Act.

Each state determines which agency will handle early intervention services. Your child's doctor can tell you how to contact the program in your area. You can also call the National Information Center for Children and Youth with Disabilities, which is listed in the Appendix: Parent Resources, Disabilities/Special Needs.

When you contact the local early intervention program, explain that you think your child may need services and that you would like to arrange for an evaluation and assessment. If your child is evaluated and found eligible for early intervention services, there usually will be no cost to you, although a few states have a sliding scale based on the parents' income.

Preexisting Conditions

If your child has an ongoing medical problem (preexisting condition), you may worry that if you or your spouse change jobs, you will not be able to insure your child's health. But federal law now offers some security for people in this position. The law says that insurers may impose only one 12-month waiting period for any preexisting condition treated or diagnosed in the previous 6 months. Your prior health insurance coverage will be credited toward the preexisting condition waiting period as long as you have maintained continuous coverage (including coverage for your child) without a break of more than 62 days.

For example, if you had health coverage for a year and you switch jobs and join another plan, the new health plan must insure you and your child with no waiting period. The plan cannot impose another waiting period. But if you or your child have never been covered by an employer's group plan and you take a job that offers such coverage, you may have to wait 12 months before medical care for your child's preexisting condition is covered.

Another federal law, known as COBRA (Consolidated Omnibus Budget Reconciliation Act of 1985), requires employers to offer the same insurance coverage for 18 months (at your expense) after you leave your job. In other words, as long as you can pay, your previous employer cannot drop you from the plan for 18 months. COBRA also covers divorced spouses and dependent children under 21 years old.

What Is Not Covered?

Coverage varies widely from one plan to the next but many carry similar restrictions. Expenses not covered often include the following:

▍ Eyeglasses (although insurers sometimes cover routine eye exams)

▍ Hearing aids

▍ Elective cosmetic surgery

▍ Dental expenses (although some plans will cover some preventative dental or other services)

Some plans will cover complications arising during pregnancy but not normal pregnancy. Many plans limit mental health coverage to only a certain number of outpatient visits or hospital days.

Health plans will generally not pay duplicate benefits, so if your child happens to be covered under your plan and under your spouse's plan, your benefits will not exceed 100 percent of the cost of the expense. Which insurance plan covers your family's health care needs depends on which plan is designated as primary and which as secondary. This is something the insurance companies will determine.

Because many plans cover only the cost of visits to doctors in their plan, some new parents discover that the exams by the pediatrician at the hospital shortly after their baby's birth are not covered. Check with your plan and your hospital in advance to arrange for a doctor who participates in your plan to visit your newborn at the hospital. If you go to the hospital designated by your health plan, you will be able to arrange for a doctor from your health plan to examine your child.

Self-Insured Plans

Self-insured plans are health insurance plans that employers create and fund for their employees. These plans are usually created so that the employer can offer health insurance while saving costs. Although some self-insured plans are administered by an insurance company, others are administered by the employer. Some state and federal laws that apply to most health plans may not apply to self-insured plans. If your employer's self-insured plan is not regulated by the state, you may need to consult an attorney who specializes in health law if problems arise.

The Uninsured Child

If your child has no health insurance, you are not alone. Millions of children in the United States are uninsured. Most of these children are not living at poverty level. The U.S. Census reports that most uninsured children are the children of working parents who cannot find affordable health insurance.

The federal government, which covers the cost of health care for children of families who meet the Medicaid program's income guidelines, has somewhat relaxed the income standards for Medicaid coverage. The result is that more children are now covered by Medicaid, and many more would receive this coverage if their parents were aware of the program and applied for coverage. If your child has no medical insurance, ask about the income requirements for Medicaid in your state.

But many working people who cannot afford to buy health insurance do not meet these income guidelines, and these are the people who need alternative programs. Don't assume that you must do without health care coverage altogether because buying a family health insurance plan is too expensive. Various programs, many of them based at the state level, provide full or partial health care coverage for children, families, and pregnant women on a sliding scale according to your income. Some states have laws requiring hospitals, health plans, and health care centers to provide free health care to uninsured or underinsured people.

Also, if you have health insurance for yourself but your employer doesn't offer—or you can't afford—a plan that includes your children, some health insurance companies offer low-cost health plans just for kids. Children are less expensive to insure because they don't usually get serious illnesses that require expensive procedures, tests, and hospitalizations.

Here are some ways you can find out what is available to you and your children:

▌ Call your state's department of public health.

▌ Go to your local hospital's patient finance department, and ask for information.

▌ Inquire with your employer's health benefits department.

▌ Call area health plans, and ask about low cost insurance plans for kids.

▌ See Appendix: Parent Resources, Medical/Financial Assistance, for organizations to contact for help finding health coverage for your uninsured child.

Choosing Your Child's Doctor

One of the first things you must do as a new parent is choose a doctor for your child. It's a good idea to choose your child's doctor before your baby is born so that he will be available for questions and checkups in the first few days of your baby's life. During your baby's first year, you will be visiting and calling this doctor frequently, so choose a doctor you have confidence in and feel comfortable with. The practice of medicine is said to be partly art and partly science. In pediatrics, probably more than any other specialty, the "art" of medicine lies in the doctor's ability to communicate and develop trust with the parent and child. Visit and interview one or more doctors in person. If you choose well, this doctor will be caring for your child from the first diaper rash all the way through adolescent acne.

If you choose your child's doctor while you are still pregnant, this doctor may be available to perform your baby's first exam while you are still at the hospital. And, once you are home with your baby, you will know whom to call for any problems and where to go for your baby's first checkup.

Pediatrician or Family Practice Physician?

When you ask friends or family members for recommendations, you may find that some parents take their children to a pediatrician and others to a family physician. These doctors have trained in different specialties, but their training overlaps in the area of child health.

Family Practice Physician

A family physician is a doctor educated and trained in the medical specialty known as family practice. This doctor is trained to provide continuing and comprehensive care for the whole family, and often serves as a primary care physician for children as well as adults. A family physician may be a good choice for your family if you like the idea of the entire family seeing the same doctor. Choose a family physician who is board-certified by the American Board of Family Practice (see Appendix: Parent

Resources, You and Your Child's Doctor), which conducts exams and grants certificates to family physicians who meet its qualifications and pass the examination.

Pediatrician

A pediatrician is a doctor trained in caring for children from infancy through adolescence. Pediatricians are trained to manage your child's total health care, including growth and development, illness, nutrition, immunizations, injuries, and physical fitness. A pediatrician, who is trained in child development, can also work with you on issues such as behavior, emotional or family problems, and learning or other school-related problems. Choose a physician certified by the American Board of Pediatrics. You can look for this certificate, which will probably be on display in the doctor's office.

Other Health Care Practitioners

In most pediatric practices, many phone calls and routine visits will be handled not by doctors, but by trained health professionals, including nurse practitioners, pediatric nurse practitioners, and physician's assistants.

- *Nurse practitioners* have completed nursing school and then received additional graduate school or certified nurse practitioner program training. Nurse practitioners who have national certification may use the title N.P.

- *Pediatric nurse practitioners* are nurse practitioners with a specialty in pediatrics. Both nurse practitioners and pediatric nurse practitioners are qualified to take health histories, give physical exams, handle common illnesses and developmental difficulties, and provide health information under a physician's direction.

- *Physician's assistants* (PAs) are health professionals trained to work under a doctor's supervision. PAs are trained in a 1-year course of study to take patient histories, perform physical exams, and treat minor health problems under the physician's direction.

Shopping for a Doctor

Whether you have just had your first baby or are about to, or you have recently moved and need a new doctor, find a doctor while your child is well so that you will know where to go in case of illness or injury or for checkups or immunizations. Here are some steps you can take:

- *Get recommendations.* Ask friends, family, and neighbors to recommend doctors. Ask your doctor to recommend someone. Ask at the local hospital or a children's hospital for the names of pediatricians or family physicians in your area. Get a list of doctors from your health plan.

- *Check the location.* Finding a doctor who is conveniently located in your area is important, given that you will need to make frequent visits, particularly during your baby's first year.

▮ *Interview the doctor.* Schedule a 15- to 20-minute interview with two or three recommended doctors.

▮ *Check the doctor's credentials.* Look for diplomas at the office, or call the office and ask where the doctor attended medical school and completed residency and whether the doctor is board-certified. Check these credentials by sending a request with the doctor's name and a self-addressed stamped envelope to the American Medical Association Physician Data Services, 515 North State Street, Chicago, IL 60610. Call your state medical board and ask if the doctor has ever had any malpractice judgments against him or ever been disciplined for wrongdoing (license suspended or revoked). Many states sponsor Internet sites that provide information about physicians practicing in the state.

Schedule an Interview

By meeting with more than one physician, you can compare and contrast the doctors' styles, philosophies, and methods. Schedule an appointment, and make it clear that you are coming to interview the doctor as a possible choice. Plan on about 15 to 20 minutes with the doctor, but allow extra time to talk with staff and look around the office and waiting areas. While you are there, find out some things about the doctor and how he practices. How long has the doctor been in practice? Is the doctor always at one office, or does he have more than one location? What hospitals is the doctor affiliated with, and would you feel comfortable taking your child to these hospitals? Does the doctor work with other physicians as partners? How accessible will your doctor be by telephone or for an emergency office visit?

A physician should have admitting privileges at a children's hospital or a general hospital with a respected pediatric service. If the hospital where the doctor has admitting privileges is affiliated with a medical school, the physician may be more likely to know highly qualified specialists and have access to the latest diagnostic techniques, treatments, and research findings.

While you are waiting to meet with the doctor, look around. Is the office area clean? Is the staff friendly and responsive to your questions, or do you have trouble getting anyone's attention? Is there a children's play area with age-appropriate toys? Is there a separate waiting area for healthy and sick children? What is the atmosphere in the waiting room? Crying babies and restless, irritable children are not unusual in a pediatric office. But if even the adults seem restless and annoyed, it's not a good sign. Ask someone waiting in the office how long they usually have to wait to see the doctor.

Here are some other questions to ask the staff:

▮ Are the well-child checkups performed by the doctor, or by the nurse practitioners or physician's assistants? The more exams done by the doctor, the better.

▮ What are the office hours?

▮ How difficult is it to get an appointment? How far in advance do you need to make an appointment?

- If it's a group practice, can you request that the same doctor see your child during most visits?

- How long is the average time in the waiting room?

- How are billing and payment handled? Is payment due at the time of the visit?

- Does this doctor accept your insurance?

- How are insurance claims from your plan handled?

- How is emergency care handled?

- If your child is sick at night or on weekends, whom do you call?

- Will your child usually see the doctor, nurse practitioner, or physician's assistant for minor illnesses?

- Does the doctor have daily call-in hours for everyday medical questions?

- Who provides coverage when the doctor is away?

What Kind of Doctor Do You Want?

When you talk to the doctor, look for certain characteristics. Above all, your doctor should be a good listener. New parents have many questions and uncertainties. You don't want a doctor who makes you feel as if you must apologize for asking questions. Think in advance about what kind of doctor you want. Are you looking for a young, energetic doctor with all the latest equipment? Are you looking for a kind, nurturing doctor who will spend lots of time talking with you and your child? Do you prefer an older doctor with years of practical experience?

Try to get a feel for whether the doctor likes children. If you have your child with you, does the doctor turn to the child and try to talk or interact with her in a kind and caring way?

As a way of drawing your doctor out, ask if he has a philosophy of care. There is no correct answer to this question, but the doctor's response will help you get a feel for how the doctor sees his role in your child's life. Ask a variety of questions, and get a feel for whether you would like to work with this doctor. Your relationship with your doctor should be a partnership, and part of the doctor's role is to help you to be a good observer of your child's health. You, as the parent, are in the best position to watch for troubling signs of illness; the doctor can show you what to look for.

Ask the doctor about when he is likely to refer your child to a specialist. Think about your preference on this matter. While some parents prefer to see an allergist if their child has allergies and a dermatologist if the child has a rash, other parents prefer the convenience of having one doctor handle most conditions.

Here are other questions to ask the doctor:

- What is your pediatric background? Where have you practiced, and for how long?

- Do you have a specialty area or an area of pediatric interest?

▌ What hospital are you affiliated with? (If at all possible, look for someone affiliated with a children's hospital or a teaching hospital affiliated with a medical school.)

▌ If my child enters that hospital, will you be there attending to her?

▌ Who examines newborns at the hospital? (Group practices often rotate doctors.)

▌ What is your opinion on breast-feeding, child nutrition, discipline (and other parenting topics)?

▌ If my child is sick, can I expect to see you, or will another doctor or a nurse practitioner be likely to see my child?

▌ If I have a minor question, when is the best time to call? Will I talk with you or a nurse? How long will I wait if I want to talk to you directly?

▌ Is there anything you need to know about my family or my child? (If the doctor shows interest and asks questions, that's a good sign.)

▌ How often do you or the other doctors take "on-call" duty for the practice? (Commonly 1 to 2 days a week.)

▌ If my child is ill, can we be seen in the office that day? (The answer should be yes.)

Working with Your Child's Doctor

Now that you have chosen your child's doctor, you can expect to see him frequently. The American Academy of Pediatrics recommends checkups at ages 1, 2, 4, 6, 9, 12, 15, 18, and 24 months, and then every year after that. The age-by-age chapters in this book describe in detail what will happen at each of these visits, but the following are some general guidelines on developing a partnership of trust with your child's doctor.

The Doctor's Visit

A parent is not a passive onlooker in a child's checkup. The more you prepare and participate, the more likely you are to get the kind of health care you want for your child. Your goal should be to develop a strong partnership with your child's doctor. The regular checkups with your child's doctor are a good way to build that relationship. Here are some steps to help you do so:

▌ Go to the doctor's office knowing as much as possible about your family's health history (allergies? vision problems? epilepsy?) and your child's health history. Bring a health record for an older child.

▌ Bring any records you can obtain from your child's previous well-child visits, immunizations, and hospitalizations.

▌ Purchase a notebook that you use exclusively to write down information about your child's health. Keep a folder for your child's papers and records.

WHAT DOES THE DOCTOR DO?

Your child's doctor must not only monitor and treat your child's health but also advise and counsel parents in the many issues of parenting, including nutrition, development, learning, and behavior. Here are some things your child's doctor does:

- Conducts newborn exam and subsequent physical exams.

- Gives advice on feeding and early infant care.

- Tracks your baby's growth and development; administers immunizations.

- Diagnoses and treats minor illnesses or injuries.

- Diagnoses and treats emergencies and serious illnesses.

- Provides advice and information by telephone.

- Refers more complicated cases to specialists.

- Informs you about how to keep your child healthy and safe.

- Answers all your questions.

- Watches for family problems that might interfere with your child's health.

- Before the doctor's visit, write down your questions or concerns.

- Write down any symptoms your child has.

- If your child is old enough to talk, let her answer some of the doctor's questions. You can fill in with more information after she answers.

- Help the doctor detect problems. Think in advance about any unusual symptoms or behavior you have noticed or any child care problems you are having.

- Inform the doctor of any possible problems in following a prescribed treatment— your child won't take a particular medicine, for example.

The First Visit

You will probably be asked to fill out a health history for your child and your family. Your child's doctor will want to know about any diseases and conditions that run in your family in order to watch your child for signs and symptoms. The doctor also needs to be aware of any complications that occurred during pregnancy and childbirth.

Your doctor will ask you about any problems or questions you might have. When describing symptoms or problems, tell the doctor the whole truth. Neglecting to mention certain details, such as the fact that you suspect a medicine is not working, will hinder the treatment. Your child's doctor will also perform a physical exam (see Your Baby's First Checkup, p. 85).

Keep Your Child's Doctor Informed

If you have any problems at home that are interfering with your ability to be a good parent, talk to the doctor about it. Is an older sibling causing problems and distracting your attention from the baby? Are you going through a separation or divorce? Tell your child's doctor. Studies show that family stress can increase a child's risk of developing certain medical problems, such as asthma and ulcers. Your child's doctor may make suggestions on how to deal with your parenting problem or may refer you to someone who can.

Find Out When to Call and When to Visit

The first visit is also a good time to discuss procedures with your child's doctor. What should you do if your child is sick? What symptoms might warrant a call to the doctor? During this discussion, the doctor will help you learn to identify symptoms of illness and distinguish less serious symptoms from those that warrant a call or a visit to the doctor.

Don't Push for Drugs

If the doctor says that a particular drug or treatment is not appropriate, there is probably a reason. For example, parents often ask for antibiotics (which treat bacterial infections) when the child has a virus. But antibiotics will not cure a virus, which must run its course before your child will recover.

Do Push for Help

On the other hand, if you feel your child has a problem that needs attention from a specialist, advocate for your child. In today's cost-cutting environment, primary care doctors often are under pressure to treat by themselves the problems that might formerly have been referred to more expensive specialists or therapists. Don't sit still for this. If you think your child should see a specialist, speak up, and keep speaking up. Many plans require you to get permission from your child's primary care physician to see these specialists.

Ask Lots of Questions

If you don't understand or don't agree with something the doctor says, speak up. You may avert a misunderstanding. Keep asking questions until you get a clear answer. If you have any complaints, ranging from something in the doctor's manner to the attitude of the office staff, say so. It's up to you to get your child the best health care you can. But also understand that even physicians can have a bad day. Don't give up on the doctor's advice too easily.

Keep Your Eye on the Bottom Line

Read your health plan and know your coverage. For example, if you do not have prescription coverage, tell the doctor. Your child's doctor may be able to prescribe a generic version of the same drug or a less expensive drug that does the same thing. If you anticipate having trouble paying your bills, many doctors are willing to arrange an installment plan that lets you pay smaller amounts over a longer period, or they may even reduce your fee if you pay with cash up front.

Helping Your Child Feel Comfortable

Doctor visits can be unsettling or frightening to children at all ages. Infants are often upset by being undressed, placed on a scale to be weighed, and stretched to be measured. Older babies are frightened of being handled by people they don't know, and children of any age are upset by the pain of immunization shots.

One method of comforting your child is to stick close during the visit. Many doctors do at least part of the exam while you hold your baby in your arms or on your lap. When the child must be on the examining table without you, stand nearby and talk to her in a comforting voice. You can comfort a somewhat older child in advance by telling her about the upcoming doctor's visit and explaining what will happen. Try to dispel her fears by telling her that you will be with her the whole time and that nothing bad will happen. But don't give her too much warning—you don't want her fretting unnecessarily for a week in advance. You can also prepare your young child by playing doctor with her, using a set of toy doctor's instruments.

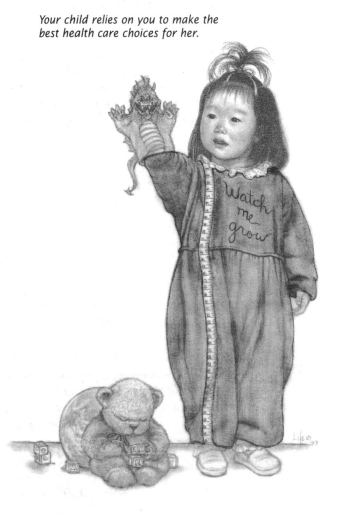

Your child relies on you to make the best health care choices for her.

During the visit, be respectful of your child. Let her do some of the talking once she is old enough. Then you can fill in the details if necessary. When talking about your child to the doctor, remember that she is present and hears what you are saying. Explain, or have the doctor explain, some of what is going on. Probably the most effective way of helping your child feel calm about visiting the doctor is to remain calm yourself. Your positive attitude toward health care is something you can give your child that will last a lifetime.

Complementary and Alternative Medicine

Complementary and alternative medicine (CAM) describes techniques outside of so-called conventional Western medicine that are used to treat illnesses or health conditions or to maintain health. Claims that these therapies are successful are sometimes based on historical tradition, rather than on objective evidence obtained through rigorous scientific testing. That is why you won't hear about most of these treatments and health care practices from your doctor. They are not yet widely taught in medical schools; nor are they ordinarily used in hospitals or reimbursed by medical insurance companies.

As a parent you will no doubt read about or hear about a number of these treatments. The reality is that some alternative therapies may be useful and others may be downright harmful. It is therefore imperative that you discuss any plans to use CAM with your doctor. Ask your doctor about alternative treatments used for your child's specific health problem. The doctor should provide you with the appropriate information, and you may find that he will recommend an alternative therapy and refer you to an appropriate specialist.

Some alternative therapies have attained credibility as complementary to mainstream medicine. For example, physical therapy (see **Back Pain,** Part 5) is useful as a complementary measure for children recovering from musculoskeletal injury or for those with a chronic illness like *cerebral palsy* (see Part 5). Biofeedback, in which a child learns to control the pain with imaging techniques, is of known value in the treatment of childhood migraine *headaches* (see Part 5). Guided imagery may help prepare children for surgery, painful procedures, or anxiety-producing situations. Acupuncture, a practice originating in China that involves puncturing the body with needles at specific points with the purpose of curing illness or relieving pain, has been used successfully to treat postoperative pain in children, but needs further study on its effectiveness for other conditions.

Other types of CAM are promoted without scientific basis and should be viewed by parents with appropriate skepticism. For example, the practice of burning mercury indoors to promote good health will contaminate the house while exposing your family to mercury poisoning, with serious neurotoxic and other consequences. Acupressure alone—which involves massage with the fingers applied to areas of the body used in acupuncture, has been shown to be unhelpful in relieving children's postsurgical nausea or vomiting. Chiropractic spinal manipulation (a method that bases its effectiveness on the correction of partially dislocated vertebrae) has not been found to alter the course or severity of childhood asthma.

Herbal remedies have become increasingly popular. Again, never give one of these remedies to your child without discussing it first with your child's doctor—the consequences can be serious. Some herbs, such as aconite, artemesia, pennyroyal, comfrey, and sassafras, can be quite harmful to children (and adults) and should be avoided. Others, such as Chinese patent medicines, can be contaminated with arsenic or lead. Still others contain chemicals such as caffeine, natural coumarins (anticlotting agents), or phenylbutazone (an anti-inflammatory drug that can cause bone marrow failure), all of which can be harmful to children.

Many herbs and so-called dietary supplements may be safe for adults but potentially harmful to children for many reasons. Because of their smaller size, children often receive a larger dose of the chemical components of the supplement. Infants especially have a different physiology than do older children and adults, including a less efficient system for detoxifying chemicals in the liver and kidneys. As a result, infants may be more vulnerable to unusual side effects. Their growing, developing bodies are sensitive to chemicals that might perturb cellular growth and differentiation, making them more vulnerable to herbs affecting cell growth and metabolism. Parents should weigh carefully, in consultation with their child's doctor, the potential benefit of such herbs versus their risk of inducing serious illnesses in children.

Herbs such as echinacea, feverfew, and chamomile may have value for treating childhood conditions. (More than 25 percent of our commercial drugs were originally derived from herbs and plants.) Nevertheless, these herbs still need more extensive testing.

Faith, a positive mental attitude, meditation, and prayer have always played a major role in healing. Good nutrition, relaxation techniques, and restful sleep, all of which might be considered complementary measures, are especially important for good health. Activities such as art, play, creative writing, reading, music, and exercise promote the physical and emotional well-being of children.

The importance of being informed about any particular CAM therapy before making choices about its potential usefulness for your children cannot be emphasized enough. Do not allow interest in CAM for your child delay or interfere with good medical management provided by your child's doctor.

If you are planning to consult a CAM practitioner, contact the professional organization that credentials the competency of the practitioner (e.g., schooling, licensure, certification, and malpractice experience). For addresses of some of these professional organizations, turn to Appendix: Parent Resources, Alternative Medicine.

Adoption Health Concerns

Adopting a child is an exciting and a stressful process. For many families, the long journey of applying and waiting for an adoptive child seems to end when the agency calls to say that a specific baby or child is available. But this moment actually begins a new process for parents—the process of gathering as much information as possible about the child, her background, and her health status. Health information, in particular, is crucial to making an informed decision about adopting the child who is available to you.

Getting the Health Information You Need

Most states now have laws that require adoption agencies to gather and disclose health information on children placed for adoption. These laws were created during the past decade, when several important court decisions found in favor of adoptive parents who sued adoption agencies for "wrongful adoption"—failure to disclose, or misrepresentation of, the health status or background of an adopted child when the child was placed.

State policies vary on how much information adoption agencies and state social service agencies are required to disclose. Some states' policies require release of all "non-identifying information" to parents, that is, all information that does not specifically identify the birth parents. The reason for this approach is that it serves no one to withhold information. Adoption agencies, in the past, have been found guilty of withholding certain information that might interfere with the child's being accepted by an adoptive family (such as information that the child's birth mother was hospitalized for schizophrenia). But withholding this kind of information leads to a situation in which parents unknowingly adopt a child with problems far more severe than they may be able to handle financially and emotionally.

If this kind of information is presented clearly and completely, parents can make an informed decision about their adoption choices. Some parents willingly adopt children with special needs, and these adoptions are often quite successful because the parents know in advance what to expect and can mobilize a network of professional, medical, financial, and personal support to help their family along the way.

Obtaining the child's medical record is crucial, of course, but information about a child's life experience—abuse or neglect, for example—is equally important for parents to understand fully what kind of commitment they will be asked to make when adopting a particular child. Adoptive families should receive the following information—ask for it if you are considering adopting a particular child and haven't received it. This information is worth digging for.

■ What is known about the birth mother's pregnancy, childbirth, and the events immediately after? Was the birth difficult or easy? Did the birth mother drink alcohol, take drugs, or smoke during pregnancy? How much? Did the infant show any signs of this substance use at birth?

■ What is the child's complete medical history from birth to present? Was the infant full term or premature? If she was premature, by how many weeks? Were there any pregnancy or childbirth complications? What childhood illnesses or special conditions, such as asthma, have been diagnosed? Look carefully at the doctor's comments on the child's medical record, especially if the doctor suggested certain tests be done. Were they? Ask for the results.

■ What genetic or health information is available about the birth parents? Did the parents have any identifiable genetic diseases or other conditions that may have a genetic component? (A wide range of diseases, from schizophrenia to asthma, tend to run in families, although they are not specifically "genetic" diseases and may or may not affect the child you are seeking to adopt.)

▌ If the child was in foster care, how and why did she come into foster care?

▌ With whom has the child lived? Include everyone from birth to present.

▌ Why was the child moved from one placement to another? Find out the reasons for each move.

▌ What attachments has the child formed? How did the child relate to her birth family or foster family? Can she bond with others? Does she visit with siblings?

▌ What adjustment problems has the child had? How did her behavior change when she was moved to another home?

▌ What are the child's positive characteristics? What are her likes and dislikes?

▌ How does the child react to stress?

Whether you are adopting a child through a domestic agency, an international agency, or a private arrangement, finding out all you can about the child's medical, personal, and family history will give you valuable information toward making your adoption decision. For more information on adoption, see Appendix: Parent Resources, Adoption.

9

Leaving Your Child in the Care of Others

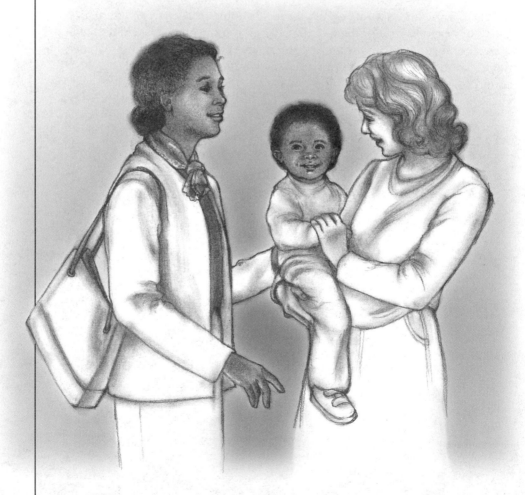

D uring the months preceding your baby's arrival, before life revolves around the whimpers and smiles of the tiny new being in your care, thoughts of finding good child care may be low on your list of concerns. But after a few weeks of nonstop parenting, even the most organized planners may be surprised to discover how much time and effort it takes to find high-quality, reliable child care when they need to return to work—or even to go out for a few hours! This chapter is a guide to finding high-quality child care and to reducing the anxiety most parents feel when making these choices.

Child Care and Your Child

If you're like most parents, you may worry about whether placing your child in a child care center or in the care of a nanny or another child care provider will be good for him. You may wonder whether a paid caregiver will hold or feed your baby the right way. And you may think about the big picture: Will your baby be safe and happy? Will being away from your child change your relationship with him or weaken the strong bond that you've forged?

Many parents feel twinges of guilt when planning to leave their child in the care of others. But life's realities require most parents to find help caring for their children at least some of the time. In the United States, about 11 million children live with a single parent who is working. Child care is necessary for these families, as well as those families in which both parents work outside the home. Even families in which one parent stays home full-time may need to hire child care help at least occasionally.

Returning to Work

If you choose to return to work, take comfort that you are not alone. The U.S. Census Bureau reports that a little over 10 million children under 5 years old—more youngsters than ever—take part in some form of alternative child care arrangement.

Although there is strength in numbers, these statistics don't address the basic question: Will placing a child in the care of others be detrimental to him? Child development experts have been trying to answer this question for years, and there is no shortage of opinions.

The latest research indicates that as long as everything is going well at home, *high-quality* child care is not detrimental to a child's well-being. For instance, an ongoing government-funded study of more than 1,300 children found that as long as a parent has already established a loving bond with the child, quality child care won't interfere with parental bonding during a child's first year, an issue that has long been under dispute. The same study, conducted by the National Institute of Child Health and Human Development, also found that high-quality group child care, to some extent, boosts the social and cognitive (thinking and learning) development of infants and toddlers. The results did indicate, however, that the quality of interaction between parent and child in the home has a greater impact on a child's overall self-esteem and well-being than what's going on at child care.

Once you do start looking, keep these basic rules in mind:

▌ Seek out high-quality child care with providers who are responsive to your child's needs.

▌ Choose a form of child care that is a good match for your child and your family.

▌ When you are home, spend time holding, playing, and talking with your child.

Even high-quality child care is no substitute for quality time with a parent. Parents and children need time together truly to know and understand each other and to feel connected.

Limiting Work Time

In an ideal world, children would spend more time with their loving, enthusiastic parents than with a child care provider. But the realities of work and finances often separate parents from their children for more time than they like. That's why a mix of work and child care may be best for both parents and children. The goal is to find a balance.

Many parents know this instinctively. That's why so many parents limit their work schedules or find ways to cut back once they have children. If both parents work, the answer may lie in flexibility. Fortunately, corporate America is beginning to respond to the need for parents to spend more time with their children. Some companies, for instance, offer part-time schedules or a compressed 40-hour work week that allows parents to work, perhaps, four 10-hour shifts, instead of five 8-hour shifts. Others offer job-sharing options, in which two workers work part-time, "sharing" one full-time job. Thanks to computer technology, you may even be permitted to telecommute from home—cutting out that hour or two of commuting gives you several more hours with your child each week.

If you are considering whether and how much to continue working after the birth of a child, explore the following possibilities:

▌ Part-time work for one or both parents

▌ Job-sharing with someone at work

▌ An extended leave of absence from your job

▌ Working at home, at least some of the time, to gain flexibility and reduce commuting time

▌ Starting your own business so that you can set your own hours

▌ Working a different shift from your spouse so that one parent is always home

Staying at Home with Your Child

Parents who choose to stay home with their children need not fear that their children are deprived of the kind of activities and social interaction that child care centers and preschools provide. A parent who chooses to stay home can provide the same stimulating activities, healthy environment, and nutritious meals and snacks available at quality child care centers, plus an extra dose of loving devotion that only a parent can deliver. Parents at home with children can organize play dates, join play groups, and plan their own creative activities for their children. Many books have suggestions for playing creatively with children at all ages. Even a trip to the playground or park provides stimulating activity and social interaction for a small child. Parents at home with their children can review this chapter for ideas and advice about creating a healthy, safe environment for their own child and can turn, when necessary, to the section on finding the occasional baby-sitter that every parent needs once in a while.

Choosing the Right Child Care for Your Child

Different types of child care arrangements work best for different types of children and families. For example, a toddler who tends to become overwhelmed and disorganized in a room full of noisy, active children might do better with an in-home nanny or a family child care provider with fewer children. Parents who work in a home office may like the idea of hiring a child care person to come into their home while they work or may prefer the solitude gained by taking the child to a center. Considering both your child's needs and your own will make for the best child care choice.

Some new parents have a relative nearby who is available to provide child care. Other parents who work part-time may create a child-swapping arrangement in which they share child care responsibilities with a close friend who also works part-time but on a different schedule. If these options aren't available to you, you have three choices when it comes to child care: at-home care, child care centers, or family child care (a caregiver who takes children into her home and cares for them "family-style").

PLANNING AHEAD

A Time Line for Getting the Care You Need

If you are planning to return to work within a few weeks or months after giving birth, give yourself enough time to find child care:

■ *Centers:* Start searching during your pregnancy, as soon as you know that you will need the care. Many centers have long waiting lists. If you plan to work part-time, you may need to reserve far in advance the weekdays that you will need.

▌*Family child care:* Don't start searching aggressively more than 2 or 3 months before you need care, because most family child care providers cannot guarantee a space too far in advance. However, it's never too soon to get a list of licensed providers in your area, and you can start interviewing them to find out which ones you like. Visit those in your area, and talk with the providers in advance about your concerns.

▌*At-home care:* Start searching during your pregnancy, as soon as you know you will need the care. Whether you are going through an agency or are advertising in a local newspaper, finding a nanny you feel you can trust usually takes time.

Identifying Your Needs

Everyone's needs are different when it comes to child care. Before you start your active search, consider which of the three options best suits your individual situation. Do you have irregular working hours? An at-home caregiver can provide this kind of flexibility. Does your child crave the company of other children his age? A child care center with groups organized according to age may be a good choice for you. Consider the factors discussed in the following sections.

Cost Unlike some countries, where child care costs are mostly government-subsidized, paying for child care in the United States is expensive. In 1993, American families with one child paid an average of 8 percent of their family income in child care costs. Rates vary greatly depending on where you live, with the highest rates tending to be in or near the larger cities.

Environment Consider what setting you want your child to be in during his hours without you. Do you want him at home? Although child development experts say continuity of care by the same caregivers is more important than the setting, many parents of young infants feel strongly about the sense of security that being at home provides. If a home atmosphere is important to you and at-home care is too expensive, you might consider family child care.

Your Schedule Check out a center's schedule. Are they open during the hours you work, and do they stay open long enough for you to get there when your day is done? Are they closed at certain times of the year for vacation? Do they allow you to choose your own days? For someone who works nights or weekends, in-home care is sometimes the only option.

Program Size Family child care centers are usually run by one person, and the groups of children are therefore smaller than in child care centers, although some centers offer smaller groups within the larger center. In a center, however, because of the long day, your child may have more than one adult caring for him daily. If your child is sensitive to new adults, a family child care center or in-home child care may be a better choice.

Child Care Provider Checklist

Complete this checklist for each provider you are considering. Use it to sort out the pros and cons of each provider. First, complete these general items:

▮ Provider's name, address, and phone number

▮ Provider's fees

▮ Hours available

▮ Is the provider licensed?

▮ For how many children?

▮ What is the ratio of caregivers to children?

▮ Is the provider trained in child care or early childhood development?

▮ Is the location convenient?

▮ Is transportation provided?

▮ Are parents always welcome to visit?

▮ What fees are imposed if you are late in picking up your child?

▮ What is the policy if your child has a fever or another illness?

Next, record your observations about the caregiver:

▮ Does the caregiver seem to enjoy and understand children your child's age?

▮ Does the caregiver interact closely with and show affection toward your child?

▮ Does the caregiver set and maintain reasonable limits for children?

▮ Are you comfortable with the caregiver's philosophy on discipline?

▮ Do you feel comfortable talking with the caregiver?

Next, address these issues of health and safety:

▮ The center or home is clean.

▮ Caregivers wash their hands and keep diaper areas sanitized.

▮ The center or home is childproofed for safety.

▮ Procedures for emergency evacuation are posted.

▮ The provider is trained to perform CPR and other first aid procedures.

▮ Smoke detectors are present and in the proper place.

▮ The room is spacious and well ventilated.

▮ Children have room to play freely outdoors.

▮ There are barriers to outsiders' having access to the children without permission.

▮ The center is secure, and there are procedures in place for releasing children only to authorized adults.

▮ The center or home does not have lead-based paint, asbestos, molds, or other indoor toxic hazards.

For infants and toddlers, you need to assess these aspects of the child care facility:

▌ The babies' play space is comfortable for floor play.

▌ Clean and comfortable changing areas and sleeping spaces are separate from cooking and eating areas.

▌ There are a wide variety of interesting and safe toys to play with and spaces to crawl in.

If you have a preschooler, evaluate these conditions:

▌ The children and caregivers seem interested, busy, and relaxed.

▌ Toys and materials are organized so that children can get them themselves.

▌ A wide variety of materials, such as blocks, puzzles, toys, and games, is available.

▌ There is a daily schedule with time for active and quiet play.

▌ There are "theme weeks" and an organized curriculum in place.

At-Home Care

This child care provider can be one of several types. She may be a nanny who comes to your home each day to care for your child. Or she may be a live-in nanny or an au pair who watches your children for a set number of hours each week. She could be an older woman who has raised her own children or a young person studying early childhood education in college. At-home care is a popular option for parents of

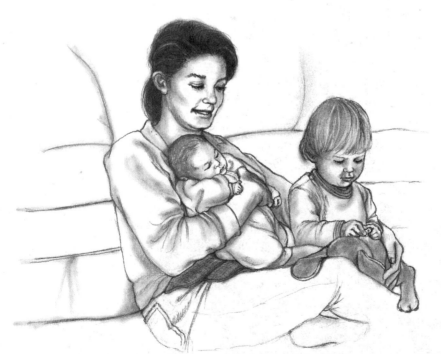

If you hire a nanny, your young children are surrounded by the comforts of home and may receive more individualized care than they would in an out-of-home setting with other children.

young children because of the one-on-one attention the children receive in their own home. A relatively expensive option for one child, it can be cost-effective for families with multiple children.

Nanny, Au Pair, and Baby-Sitter

The differences between a nanny, an au pair, and a baby-sitter are described below:

▌ *Baby-sitter:* When you think of your typical baby-sitter, you probably think of your teenage neighbor or niece. Baby-sitters, who are of all ages, are generally hired occasionally by parents who want to get away for a few hours.

▌ *Nanny:* Nannies are professional caregivers who earn their living caring for children in the child's home on a regular basis, usually full-time.

▌ *Au pair:* An au pair is a young person from another country who comes to the United States to experience the American lifestyle. An au pair will care for the children in a family for a set number of hours in exchange for room and board and a weekly stipend.

QUESTIONS PARENTS ASK

What Are the Pros and Cons of At-Home Child Care?

Advantages of at-home child care:

▌ Comfort and consistency in familiar surroundings

▌ Individualized care from the same person

▌ Child exposed to fewer illnesses from other children

▌ Consistent coverage for working parents even when child is ill

Disadvantages of at-home child care:

▌ Child care provider may have no training in the basics of child care or in early childhood development

▌ Less structure, equipment, and resources than center care provides

▌ Child care person isolated and unsupervised

▌ Difficult for parent to assess the quality of care being provided

▌ Less opportunity for child to socialize

▌ Often the most expensive option

▌ Potential for child care to be disrupted suddenly if provider becomes ill or quits suddenly and no backup is available

Finding Quality At-Home Child Care

Hiring at-home child care offers some special benefits. If parents work long hours or have unusual schedules, this option allows flexibility. Parents don't have to rush a baby or small child through a trying morning routine to get out the door on the way to the child care center. If a child is sick, the parents can still go to work.

It may seem ideal. But keep in mind, as you search for the perfect person, that a nanny is like any other employee. She is human. She has a life outside her job, and your child may or may not be her first priority. Remember that this is an employer/employee relationship and it is your responsibility to set standards and expectations for your nanny to meet right from the start.

This person, a total stranger in the beginning, will spend a significant amount of time alone with your child with no oversight. That is why choosing an at-home child care person carefully is extremely important. Here are some important things to consider before you hire an at-home nanny.

To start, you'll need to gather names of prospective nannies:

▌ Ask friends and colleagues for recommendations.

▌ Check and post notices at area colleges, religious organizations, the local YMCA, bookstores, supermarkets, or community bulletin boards.

▌ Advertise in local papers, especially community newspapers.

▌ Contact a reputable nanny agency. Using an agency to find a provider can reduce the time and energy it takes to find one, because it presents you with a list of pre-screened, qualified candidates. This process, however, is expensive, so find out what you are paying for. For instance, some agencies offer training and ongoing support to their nannies and some don't. Some will offer you a replacement if you are not happy with your nanny, and some will make you pay again and start from square one. To locate agencies in your area, check the yellow pages or call the International Nanny Association. See Appendix: Parent Resources, Child Care.

▌ Contact an au pair agency. Au pairs go through a screening process that checks their references, police records, and health records, and provides a psychological profile. Several organizations in the United States are authorized by the U.S. Information Agency to bring au pairs into the country. For more information on training and screening of au pairs, contact the U.S. Information Agency. See Appendix: Parent Resources, Parenting.

Defining Your Expectations

Before you search for candidates, have a clear picture of your needs and your expectations of the nanny's duties. Ask yourself these questions:

▌ Do you want your caregiver to live in or live out? (Sometimes live-in care is less expensive.)

▌ What days and what hours will she be required to work?

- Will you provide transportation, or will she need to drive and have her own car?

- What household responsibilities, such as laundry, cleaning, or cooking, will she have (if any) in addition to caring for your child?

- Do you have an age preference?

- How long will you need her? Six months? A year? Indefinitely?

- Will you expect her to care for your child when your child is sick?

- If she lives in your home: Can she smoke or drink there? Can she entertain friends? Will you give her a curfew?

Determining Salary and Benefits

A nanny's performance will be influenced by how much you pay her. If you treat her like a professional—pay her well, offer her certain benefits—she will be happier with her job and take her responsibilities more seriously. When you are calculating a salary, keep in mind that this employee is watching precious cargo. When you hire a nanny, you are legally responsible for filing local, state, and federal withholding taxes and paying employer's Social Security contributions. Health benefits are not required, but some employers provide them as an incentive. The following questions will help you establish a fair salary and benefits package:

- *What can you afford to pay per hour of care?* Rates vary depending on where you live. For the going rate in your community, contact the International Nanny Association (see Appendix: Parent Resources, Child Care).

- *What can you afford to pay in benefits?* Giving the nanny perks, like a paid vacation, holidays, and/or health insurance reinforces the idea that she is a professional.

- *What will you pay in overtime?* This is particularly important when you are considering live-in help, who often work more hours than live-out help.

Interviewing a Prospective At-Home Caregiver

Most parents find it convenient to interview first over the phone to screen out clearly inappropriate choices. During the phone conversation, ask about the person's experience and background. Find out where she lives, if she has a car, and if she is available during the hours you need her. Then describe the salary, benefits, and basic house rules and policies regarding the use of your car and television, friends and visitors, and safety considerations in your home.

Use the phone interviews to develop a list of two or three good candidates. Next, set up a face-to-face interview. When you interview the candidates, first hand them a written job description that reviews all the duties and responsibilities (see box on the next page). This way the candidates won't misunderstand your expectations. If possible, have both parents on hand for the interview. Ask the candidate to bring references. Watch her interact with your child while she is there.

Here is an example that you may want to use as a guideline for a written job description. Parents who have used at-home care will tell you that you can never be too specific.

Sample Job Description

At-home care is needed between the hours of 8:30 A.M. and 6:00 P.M., Monday through Friday, for 6-month-old James and 3-year-old Madeline. The provider must have previous experience caring for young children, particularly infants, and must have a car. The parent will pay $_ per hour (or per week) and will pay an additional $_ per each half hour of overtime worked. Benefits will include (list any perks, such as paid vacation time or health insurance benefits).

For this fee, the provider's duties include watching the children carefully and protecting them at all times; taking James for a walk in the stroller each day (weather permitting); picking up Madeline from nursery school promptly at 11:30 A.M. on Tuesdays and Thursdays; preparing lunch and snacks as directed; planning creative and fun activities for Madeline each day and allowing her time for free play; engaging, talking to, and playing with James; washing, drying, and folding laundry once a week; and keeping the house reasonably tidy (i.e., picking up toys, cleaning up spilled food, washing the dishes used, and keeping the rugs vacuumed).

Pay attention to whether the caregiver arrives on time and whether her appearance is neat and clean. (You want someone punctual and concerned about hygiene.) Next, ask questions. Here's what you'll need to find out and observe:

▎ *Qualifications:* What are her qualifications, including previous experience, formal training, and language abilities?

▎ *References:* Ask for the names of previous employers, and call them to ask about her reliability and other qualifications. Make sure that references are recent, and ask about any gaps in her career.

▎ *Availability:* Is she available when you need her and for as long as you think you will need her? Are there outside interests such as schooling that will interfere with her availability? Has she family members who depend upon her?

■ *Child care philosophy:* What are her attitudes toward such things as discipline, nutrition, and toilet training, and do her attitudes match yours?

■ *Planning activities:* Ask the prospective nanny what she plans to do with your child to find out whether she knows how to plan activities and take the time to understand your child's abilities and interests.

■ *Health considerations:* Is there anything about the prospective caregiver's health that may interfere with her job? Try not to hire a smoker, because secondhand smoke is linked to various medical problems.

■ *How does she interact with your child?* Observe whether she tries to interact with your child during the visit even though your child may not warm up to her right away.

Nanny on Board

Once you have chosen the best candidate, try to arrange at least one paid trial day so you can really observe how the caregiver handles your child, and go through the child's routine with the caregiver. Do it on one of your days off, and plan to be there for part of the day and leave for a few hours. Pay close attention to how the caregiver treats your child. Is she someone you and your child can feel comfortable with?

Once you have hired your child care provider, drop in on her unannounced on a regular basis to make sure things are running smoothly. If your baby is crying when you arrive, don't be dismayed—babies cry. Your nanny should be trying to calm him. But if your baby is crying every time you stop in or if the television is always on, your child may not be getting the kind of care he deserves. You and your nanny should not view these visits as spying—most working people have supervisors who observe their work. Let her know that you will be dropping in from time to time. If you have trouble getting home from work in the middle of the day, ask a trusted relative, friend, or neighbor to make an occasional visit.

Child Care Centers

Over the years, as the number of mothers returning to work has grown, so has the number of child care centers throughout the country. Many parents choose center-based care because they want their child to interact with children of the same age or because they prefer to have their child in a setting where there is oversight of the child care providers. All child care centers are required to be licensed by the state, and they must meet minimum health, safety, and staffing requirements. Although a few are open during the evening, most child care centers are set up to accommodate the nine-to-five worker and are open roughly from 7:30 A.M. to 6 P.M., throughout the year. Some centers also provide before- and after-school care for the school-age children of working parents.

QUESTIONS PARENTS ASK
What Are the Pros and Cons of a Child Care Center?

Advantages of child care centers:

▌ In most states, licensing requirements ensure that basic health and safety standards are met.

▌ Oversight and the presence of other staff members ensure more accountability that your child will receive proper care.

▌ The program is usually geared directly to your child's age group and developmental level.

▌ Workers may be better trained and relatively better paid than caregivers in less formal settings.

▌ Other children provide an opportunity for daily social interaction.

Disadvantages of child care centers:

▌ Staff turnover may be high, requiring your child to adapt to new caregivers frequently.

▌ Expensive, particularly if you are sending more than one child.

▌ Children in a group setting are likely to be exposed to more illness.

▌ Less individualized attention, particularly if the child-to-staff ratios are high.

▌ Hours may be less flexible than other child care settings.

▌ Children usually cannot attend if they are ill.

Finding a Quality Child Care Center

To a new parent who is unfamiliar with them, the words "child care center" may conjure up images of a cold, institution-like atmosphere. But the truth is that a walk through a good child care center should leave you feeling happy, if not excited, about the opportunities your baby or young child will have. At a quality center, you can be assured that your children won't be deposited in front of the television for hours. Each day has a schedule of creative play activities planned that provide learning opportunities for children, including playing with water, blocks, or sand; making orange juice; planting flowers; or music and dancing. Child care centers usually include a "circle time" group experience in reading or singing or other activities. Child care researchers report that good child care centers help children develop social skills.

Gathering information for selecting a day care center is easy, because plenty of public information on centers is available, more than there is for the other two child care options. The following are the best sources of information to locate child care centers in your area:

▌ Your child's doctor

▌ Other parents in your neighborhood or workplace

▌ The local library

▌ Your church or synagogue

▌ The local board of health or welfare board

▌ Your employer (check to see if your place of employment has a child care facility on-site)

▌ The local YMCA

▌ Local child care resource and referral agencies

▌ The National Association for the Education of Young Children (NAEYC), a professional organization of early childhood educators, which provides names of accredited child care centers and preschools (see Appendix: Parent Resources, Child Care)

What You Should Find Out About a Prospective Child Care Center

As you investigate prospective child care centers, do so with a skeptical eye. Although excellent centers exist, they are not in the majority. One survey of 400 child care centers found that only one in seven provides a level of quality that promotes healthy development. That study, conducted in four states by four universities, also found that one out of every eight centers has safety problems. Infant and toddler programs fared worse than preschool programs. To ensure that a center you are considering is of high quality, the first step is to question the program director about the following.

Is the Center Licensed?

When you tour the facility, ask to see the center's state license, which should be displayed prominently. Check to be certain it is current. You can also check with your state child care licensing agency, which may be able to give you a list of licensed child care centers in your area. A state license is a must.

Is the Center Accredited?

The standards for child care vary so much among states that the NAEYC has set up the National Academy of Early Childhood Programs (NAECP) to administer an accreditation system for all child care centers, preschools, kindergartens, and school-age programs. To become nationally accredited, a program must meet standards well above those required by many states. NAECP accreditation is additional assurance that a center's administrators are concerned about quality. Because accreditation is voluntary and relatively new, however, you needn't discount a prospective center only because it isn't accredited. For a list of accredited centers, contact the NAEYC. See Appendix: Parent Resources, Child Care.

What Is the Teacher-Child Ratio?

The number of children for whom each teacher or caregiver is responsible profoundly affects the quality of care. A better teacher-to-child ratio provides several benefits:

▌ More individual attention for each child

▌ Safety—the teacher can watch each child more carefully

▌ Less anxiety or distress—the teacher can respond to the child's needs more quickly

▌ Developmental progress—the teacher can adapt care and activities to each child's stage of development

The chart here gives American Public Health Association/American Academy of Pediatrics (APHA/AAP) recommendations by age for group size and child-to-staff ratio. For example, children age 24 months and younger should be in groups of no more than six with at least one staff member for every three children (a ratio of 3 to 1).

▬RECOMMENDED GROUP SIZE AND CHILD-TO-STAFF RATIO FOR CHILD CARE CENTERS

Age	Maximum Group Size	Child-to-Staff Ratio
0–24 months	6	3 to 1
25–30 months	8	4 to 1
31–35 months	10	5 to 1
3 years	14	7 to 1
4–6 years	16	8 to 1

What Is the Cost?

The general rule is that you get what you pay for. Although there isn't a big difference in price, child care research suggests that good-quality services cost more than lower-quality services. That's because hiring teachers with early childhood training; providing low ratios of children to adults; buying insurance; and providing a safe environment, appropriate equipment, and nutritious food all cost money. Also, keep in mind that infant care is more costly than care for older children. Some centers offer lower rates for families of limited income.

What Are the Qualifications of the Staff?

Although most states do not require teaching credentials for licensing, look for some evidence of training and expertise in early child life or child development. Directors and some teachers at many quality centers have degrees in early childhood education and should have several years' experience in the field. Staff training has a significant impact on child care quality. Ask if the center provides for ongoing, in-house teacher training. Also, at least one staff person trained in CPR and first aid should be on duty at all times.

How Long Has Each of the Teachers Been on Staff?

Be wary of a center with a high turnover rate. This raises questions about the quality of the program and creates a less stable atmosphere for your child.

How Are Meals and Snacks Handled?

Nutritious food should be offered frequently over the course of the day. The American Academy of Pediatrics recommends at least one meal and two snacks or two meals and one snack for children in child care for up to 8 hours a day. Children in child care for more than 8 hours a day should have at least two meals and two snacks. Although some centers provide lunch, often parents must provide a boxed lunch and snacks. A center that offers milk for lunch and snack times is a plus, because milk must be stored cold. Research shows that more than 8 ounces of juice a day for small children is unhealthy. Alert the staff to any food allergies or special diets your child may have. Ask to see a few sample meal and snack selections.

How Are Illnesses Handled?

The program should have a clear policy regarding sick children that lets you know when you must keep your child home, under what conditions the provider will call you to pick your child up, and when your child can return to the center. That policy should closely resemble the guidelines on page 335.

Sick children should have a safe place separate from other children, where they can await their parent or caregiver. If your child has a chronic illness and requires medication or special care, you should describe these needs to the staff early in the process and find out how the center can accommodate them.

Must Children Be Immunized?

Centers can take many precautions to prevent the spread of disease. One of them is to be sure that all the children are immunized at the appropriate ages (see Childhood Immunization Schedule, p. 110). Providers should also be fully immunized.

How Are Emergencies Handled?

Centers should have clear policies for handling medical emergencies and evacuations in the case of disasters, such as fires or chemical emergencies. Upon your child's enrollment in a center, you should be asked to fill out a form that provides the center with a list of emergency contacts. You will also be asked to fill out a consent form that permits the staff to administer first aid or transport the child to receive emergency care if needed.

What Is the Center's Policy on Dropping Off and Picking Up a Child?

The center should keep a closely monitored log for signing children in and out and a file of the names, addresses, and telephone numbers of any person authorized by you, the custodial parent, to pick up your child. The center should not allow anyone other than those on the list to pick up your child unless you give prior written

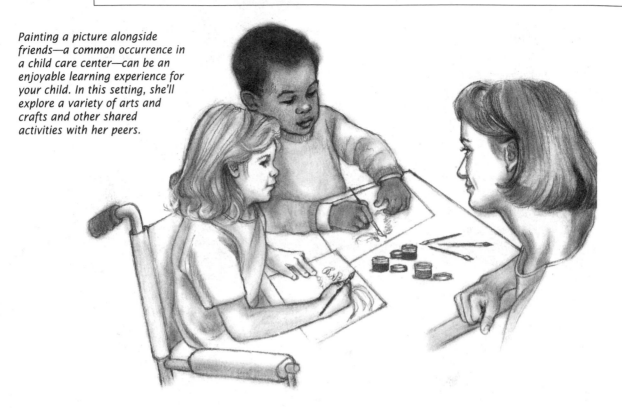

Painting a picture alongside friends—a common occurrence in a child care center—can be an enjoyable learning experience for your child. In this setting, she'll explore a variety of arts and crafts and other shared activities with her peers.

consent. Telephone authorization should never be allowed, because a person can easily pretend to be a parent over the phone.

What to Look for When You Visit

A series of visits to the child care center is one of the best ways to evaluate whether you want to send your child there. Schedule a tour with the director, and then return for one or more unscheduled visits. The center should not have a problem with your dropping in unannounced, but should require that you identify yourself at the front office before wandering around. Good centers welcome and even encourage such visits. As you walk through, here are some questions to ask yourself.

How Do the Caregivers Interact with the Children?

Pay attention to how the adults interact with the children. Consider visiting during a time of day when the children are most difficult, such as just before nap time or early when parents are dropping the children off. This way, you can observe how the providers handle disputes, behavior problems, or children upset at having just been separated from a parent. Look for the following types of interaction for different age levels.

Infants and Toddlers Close interaction with a caregiver responsive to your baby's needs is the key to a baby's development. Infants and toddlers should be held, cuddled, and talked to often. Providers should make eye contact with babies and respond to their smiles and emerging skills and interests. Make sure that when feeding the infants, caregivers don't prop the bottle but hold the baby close. Toddlers should be fed family style in groups, around a child-size table, which allows them to talk to other children. The caregiver then has the opportunity to demonstrate good table manners.

Preschool Children Caregivers should be working with children on a variety of games, arts and crafts projects, and other forms of play for the children and should partake in those activities. Pay attention to how children are disciplined. Providers should be encouraging your child's independence while setting consistent limits. Spanking or any form of physical punishment should not be used.

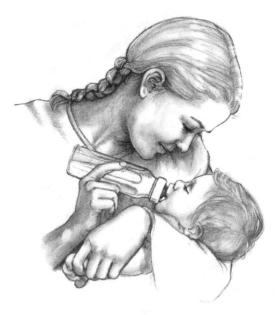

Look for a provider who cradles and interacts closely with your baby during feedings.

School-Age Children Providers should organize sports and games, but also provide time for independent and free play. Quiet time should be available for homework and reading. Look for a caregiver who offers a strong sense of guidance and support for the child while providing individual and group learning opportunities.

How Do Caregivers Interact with Parents?

It's important to establish a good relationship with your caregiver. For the lines of communication to remain open and honest, you'll want to feel comfortable sharing your feelings and concerns with this person. Take note of her attitude toward you. Does she welcome all of the many questions you may have, and is she comfortable answering them? Is she defensive or short with you? Does she place a priority on communicating with parents? Do you like her?

What Happens in a Typical Day?

Look for programs that provide a mix of activities but also quiet time. Some group activities should be planned, along with time for free and individual play, snacks, and lunch. Outdoor play, including stroller walks for young infants, is also important and should be provided each day, weather permitting. When evaluating the program's activities, remember that each age group has particular needs.

Infants Infants should have a wide range of places to sit and lie. If you have a non-mobile infant, be sure that he is able to play freely, yet is protected from other children. Some centers have a raised, gated platform reserved for pre-crawlers. Others may use a playpen. If that's the case, be sure that toys are available for him to play with and that he will be spending only brief periods of time in it. If you see a playpen on your tour, ask why it's there and how much time your baby will spend in it. Cribs should be used for napping only.

For infants of all ages, toys and other safe items should be available to look at, reach for, and explore. The baby should be routinely engaged in verbal exchanges linked to daily events and experiences. Providers should name objects and sing rhymes to the baby and should be responsive to the baby's expression.

Toddlers Opportunities allowing toddlers to explore, make choices, and carry out their own ideas should be provided. The children should be able to move at their own pace, away from and back to the security of a loving caregiver. Look for a program that has plenty of age-appropriate toys, climbing structures, and large blocks of time for free play.

Preschoolers Academic instruction shouldn't be emphasized, but learning should be achieved through the context of play and experiences. For instance, reading readiness, writing, math, science, and social studies skills can be naturally integrated through such activities as playing with toys, painting, drawing, storytelling, dancing, cooking, and field trips.

School-Age Children School-age children need a wide range of supervised activities that offer a change of pace from the school day. These can include team sports, cooking, dramatics, art, music, crafts, games, free time, and time to read, relax, or do homework. Children should be encouraged to explore new interests and develop peer relationships.

Is the Facility Clean?

When touring the facility, be sure that these basic guidelines set by the U.S. Centers for Disease Control and Prevention are met:

▮ Providers routinely wash the children's hands and their own hands, particularly after using the toilet or having changed diapers, after handling pets or a pet object, before and after eating, and after playing on the playground. Sinks should be close at hand for both diaper-changing areas and bathrooms.

▮ The diaper-changing areas are equipped with disposable coverings that are removed from beneath the child after each use. The underlying surface should be disinfected with a mild bleach and water solution after each use.

▮ Toys that infants and toddlers put in their mouths should be washed and disinfected with a mild bleach solution and rinsed between uses by individual children.

- Surfaces that children have the most close contact with, such as floors, bathrooms, or play tables, should be routinely cleaned and disinfected.

- Areas where blood or other body fluids have spilled are immediately cleaned and disinfected.

- Wounds, including cuts, scrapes, and bites that break the skin, are cleaned and disinfected with peroxide. (For information about the risk of transmission of blood-borne illnesses through biting, see *Bites, Animal and Human,* Part 5.)

- Small, flushable toilets or modified toilet seats are recommended over potty chairs, which are difficult to keep clean. If the provider uses potty chairs for toilet teaching, they should be kept clean and only in a bathroom area, out of the reach of children.

- Safe food preparation and handling techniques should be followed, and eating utensils should be washed and disinfected.

Is the Facility Safe and Secure?

Look to see if the following guidelines from the U.S. Centers for Disease Control and Prevention have been met:

- The building and grounds should be well lighted and free of hazards. The rooms should be comfortably warm in cold weather and ventilated with fresh air.

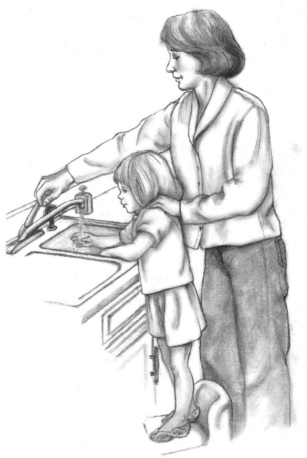

Hand washing should be as routine as diaper changing at child care centers.

- Furnishings, equipment, and materials used in a child care facility should be safe for children. Child-sized furniture and equipment adapted for children's use helps prevent falls and other injuries. No items should have sharp or unprotected corners, protruding nails or bolts, rusty or loose parts, or small parts that can be swallowed.

- Toys and play equipment should be in good repair.

- Floors, walls, and ceilings should be smooth and in good repair with no peeling paint or worn wooden surfaces that might cause splinters. Floors should be free from bare concrete, cracks, dampness, drafts, splinters, and sliding carpets.

- Stairways, steps, and walkways should be kept in good repair and well lighted. Stairways should have securely mounted handrails on both sides. Gates should be mounted at the top and bottom of stairs in infant or toddler areas.

- Indoor and outdoor surfaces should be cushioned with materials such as carpet or wood chips in areas with climbers, slides, or swings.

- Playground areas should be enclosed with a fence or natural barriers. They should be clean and safe, with no debris, dilapidated structures, or broken or worn equipment. The ground under play equipment should be a soft surface such as sand, wood chips, or resilient matting.

- Electrical outlets within the reach of children should be covered with child-resistant covers. Electrical cords should be out of children's reach.

- Toxic materials should be stored in a locked cabinet.

- An inspection certificate should be posted showing that there are no lead or asbestos hazards.

- Smoke detectors should be installed on the ceiling, or 6 to 12 inches below the ceiling, every 40 feet on each floor. Fire extinguishers with instructions for their use should be installed in accordance with local fire marshal recommendations.

- All staff members should know what to do in the case of a medical emergency. Emergency phone numbers should be posted by every telephone.

- A written plan for evacuation in the event of a fire should be posted in a visible area.

Does Enough Space Exist for a Variety of Activities and Equipment?

The NAEYC recommends that there be at least 35 square feet of usable playroom floor space indoors per child and 75 square feet of play space outdoors for each child. There should be enough space for afternoon naps. Each child should have an individual bed, mattress, or mat to sleep on, and adults should have enough room to walk between sleeping children. A place, such as a cubby, should be kept for each child's personal belongings, including a change of clothes.

QUESTIONS PARENTS ASK
Is a New Center a Better Center?

Q: Should I look for a new facility with lots of up-to-date toys and new equipment?

A: Many excellent child care programs are housed in old buildings and use old equipment, recycled objects, and teacher-made materials. Parents must look beyond initial impressions. More important than new toys is the quality and stability of the staff. Although toys and equipment should be clean, safe, age-appropriate, and plentiful, new and expensive toys and facilities do not guarantee a good experience for your child.

Family Child Care

The "family" in family child care is what appeals to most parents who choose this arrangement. Unlike most child care centers that are housed in less cozy, classroom-style settings, these group programs are situated in the home of the provider—often a mother raising her own children.

Like siblings in a household, the children you find in family child care are usually of different ages, which appeals to many parents. Another plus is the group size. Generally, although not always, the group is smaller in home-based care than in center-based care.

In most states, family child care providers must be licensed by or registered with the state; must meet minimum health, safety, and staffing requirements; and must adhere to state limits on the number of children of different ages they may have on hand at one time. Although state-imposed limits vary depending on where you live, you can usually expect to find from four to six children in a high-quality arrangement. In homes with a larger group, someone is usually there to assist the provider. Be careful, though: Many family child care sites remain unlicensed, which may mean inadequate safety and health policies.

QUESTIONS PARENTS ASK
What Are the Pros and Cons of Family Child Care?

Advantages of family child care:

▮ The arrangement provides a homelike environment.

▮ Children can socialize with children of varying age groups.

▮ Family child care may have more flexible hours than a child care center.

▮ It may be less expensive than other options.

Disadvantages of family child care:

▮ Quality depends on the individual providing the care.

▮ The arrangement may not provide enough age-mates for a child—particularly 3- and 4-year-old children, who like to play with other children their own age.

▮ Child care plans may be disrupted if the caregiver or her child is sick.

▮ Children usually cannot attend if they are ill.

Finding Quality Family Child Care

Family child care, run in a private home, is the most popular type of out-of-home child care for infants and toddlers in the United States, in part because of the homelike atmosphere it provides and the small group sizes. It may also be less expensive and offer more flexible hours than child care centers. Because these small home-based businesses are run independently, they vary considerably in quality. The level of accountability is not as high as it is at child care centers, which are much more heavily regulated.

Excellent family child care homes are available, but other child care homes, often unlicensed, have substandard conditions. The following are the best sources when you are initially gathering information:

▌ State and local child care resource and referral agencies

▌ Friends and neighbors

▌ Local colleges with early child care programs

▌ Your local elementary school

▌ Your local library

▌ Your church, synagogue, or other community organization

▌ Your local paper

To find a local resource, contact the National Association of Child Care Resource and Referral Agencies, Child Care Aware, or the National Association for Family Child Care. See Appendix: Parent Resources, Child Care, for more information.

Screening Prospective Family Child Care Providers

The following are questions to ask the caregiver over the phone in your initial conversation. Remember to be considerate of the situation that family child care providers are in. Just because they are home doesn't mean that they can talk to you. Most of the time they are busy caring for children. Call to make arrangements to talk during a time, perhaps in the evening, when the caregiver can answer your questions.

Licensing Is the provider licensed by the state or local health department to provide child care in her home?

Cost Find out the hourly or daily fee as well as whether you must pay for days your child does not attend, such as sick days, snow days, or vacation days. Also ask if the provider will provide a tax identification number and a receipt for your payment, which you will need if you deduct child care costs for income tax purposes.

Qualifications Many family child care providers with no formal training run excellent programs based on their own experiences and perhaps some self-education. But some education in early childhood education or development is certainly a plus. If you find a provider who is accredited by the National Association of Family Child Care, put her on your short list. To become accredited, providers must receive 45 hours of documented training in such areas as child development, health, and safety. Then, a national commission decides whether to accredit them based on all the information, which also includes parent surveys.

Children's Ages Find out the ages of the other children in the program. For children over age 2, having other children in their age group is a plus.

Backup Care If the provider becomes ill, an emergency arises, or she plans to take vacations, she should have a qualified substitute to care for your child. Find out how many days she had to close unexpectedly in the last year. What does she do if she cares for her own child and the child becomes sick?

Smoking Secondhand smoke has been associated with many medical problems and is known to cause allergies, asthma, and respiratory infections. If somebody in the house smokes, look elsewhere.

Provider-to-Child Ratio Check to see that a prospective provider is at least meeting state requirements for the maximum number of children she has in her care. States limit the number of children according to the ages in the group. For instance, a provider can take in fewer infants than she can preschoolers.

Illnesses As with child care centers, a family child care program should have a clear policy regarding sick children that lets you know when you must keep your child at home. The home should have a safe and separate area where sick children can await a parent.

Meals Be sure that meals and snacks are nutritious, appropriate to your child's age, and based on a planned, written menu. The American Academy of Pediatrics recommends at least one meal and two snacks, or two meals and one snack, for children in child care for up to 8 hours a day. Children in child care for more than 8 hours a day should have at least two meals and two snacks.

Other Adults or Children Who Live in the Home Ask about others living in the house, as well as others who come and go regularly.

References References take on great importance in this type of child care setting, for which you have little to go on outside your observations. Call the references, and ask pointed questions about their experiences with the provider.

What to Look for When You Visit

Be sure to visit the home while the children are there so that you can observe the structure of the day and how the caregiver responds to the children. Ask the provider if you can bring your child along to observe the caregiver's interaction with your child and to observe how your child interacts with the others. Stay for at least a couple of hours to get a feel for what a regular day is like. Look for the following things:

▌ *A warm, nurturing personality:* Make sure the caregiver is someone with whom you feel comfortable leaving your child. She should be warm, at ease with her situation, and energetic. She should convey a sense of self-esteem and a love for children and her job.

▌ *Discipline philosophy:* Look for someone who uses positive guidance instead of punishment. She should set clearly defined rules and limits that are followed consistently. One way to determine this is to observe the children. Is there a minimum of fighting? If not, the provider may not have consistently set her rules.

▌ *Parent-friendly attitude:* She should make you feel welcome in her home and encourage your input. You want to feel as though she is your partner and that you can work out problems that may arise.

▌ *Daily routine:* Look for the same mix of activities and free play that you would look for in center-based care (see p. 324). A broad array of well-maintained, age-appropriate toys should be available.

▌ *Sufficient space:* The facility should have a spacious, inviting, and comfortable place for the children to play in that allows the caregiver to maintain visual contact with all children. The kitchen should be adjacent to the play area so that she can keep her eye on the children when she is preparing snacks or lunch. The facility should also have a place to eat and nap and a designated "quiet area," where children can read or be alone.

▌ *A safe, secure, and clean home:* When touring the home, look to see if the same basic health and safety standards required of center-based child care facilities are met (see pp. 326–328).

Finding Quality Child Care for a Child with Disabilities

Nowadays more options exist for children with disabilities than ever before. That is in part thanks to federal legislation such as the Americans with Disabilities Act, which requires that reasonable accommodation be given to people with disabilities, and the amendments to the Education for All Handicapped Children Act, which require states to develop special education programs for all children, including preschool children.

As a result of these developments, more and more child care programs for children with disabilities are opening their doors. In addition, some states are requiring child care centers to accept applications from children with special needs.

What Kind of Child Care Is Right?

The American Public Health Association and the American Academy of Pediatrics are encouraging the complete integration of children with disabilities and children without disabilities in the least restrictive environment. They have created guidelines to enable child care providers to adapt their facilities accordingly. Sending a child with a disability to child care can be beneficial to the child because of the social contact, physical exercise, and various experiences of a group program. Every child has individual needs, and the appropriate child care setting will vary with each child.

If you are considering child care, your best referral source is your child's doctor. Also check with your state education office or local health department. Once you have choices, evaluate the child care arrangement according to the guidelines provided earlier in this chapter. Be sure that the following guidelines are also met:

■ The staff is specially trained and has a written plan for the care of special needs children developed in consultation with a multidisciplinary team of professionals experienced in the care and education of special needs children.

■ The program should have at least one physician consultant who is active in the development of policies and procedures affecting the disabled children in the group.

■ The facility has a written emergency medical plan for each child with special needs. Make sure you have a copy of this plan.

■ Children without disabilities should be prepared to have children with special needs participate in the program through an education program that uses age-appropriate books, puppets, brochures, guest speakers, and parents of children with special needs.

■ Disabled children should be encouraged to be as independent as their abilities allow, within the bounds of safety. They should be restricted only in the activities that might be dangerous for them or that have been prohibited by doctor's orders.

■ The program should offer special equipment and activities for disabled children.

■ The program should be willing to accept instruction from the child's doctor or therapists.

A Parent's Responsibilities in Regard to Child Care by Others

Relief may be your first emotion once you have made your decision about child care and firmed up your arrangements. Now is the time to prepare your child for the transition.

Preparing Your Child for Child Care

Leaving your child with a new caregiver for the first time is often a difficult moment for parent and child. Your child may cry uncontrollably, reach out for you, and make leaving difficult. Many parents share their children's anxieties at this time and find it difficult to turn their back and walk away. Here are some ways to make the transition easier:

■ *Visit in advance:* Take your child to visit the center before the first day, introduce him to his new caregivers and the children, and encourage him to play. Spend some time there on one or more days to allow your child to become comfortable and familiar with the people and the place. If you are hiring an at-home caregiver, you can go through a similar preparation by having the nanny spend time with your child on one or more occasions while you are present.

▌ *When the day comes:* No matter how much preparation you do, your child is likely to protest when you leave. You can make the transition gradually by staying longer the first day and shortening the time you stay a little bit each day. The transition will become easier over time; most children settle down shortly after their parents leave.

▌ *Bring teddy:* Bring your child's favorite blanket, doll, or stuffed animal.

▌ *Leave swiftly:* After waiting for as long as you feel necessary to console your child, leave swiftly without allowing your child to detain you again and again.

▌ *Once you have left:* Do not reappear unless you plan to take your child with you. In most cases, once the parent is out of sight, children adapt to the situation fairly quickly.

Child Abuse in Child Care

The stories you may have heard in the media about child abuse in child care are enough to make any parent uneasy about leaving a child with anyone else. But the truth is that although abuse does sometimes occur, it is rare. Parents can follow some commonsense precautions to ensure that their child is in good hands.

▌ Thoroughly examine the program before you enroll your child.

▌ Make unannounced visits to check on your nanny or the child care program. If you can't visit, ask a friend or neighbor to drop by for you. If the provider discourages such visits, look for a new caregiver.

▌ If you notice that the provider does not respond to the children's requests for help or daily needs or looks past them when talking to them, find a new situation.

▌ If the caregiver seems unhappy or overwhelmed with the work and responsibilities of caring for children, seek another situation.

▌ Inquire at the state licensing office about whether any complaints have ever been filed against the center or the staff.

How to Detect Abuse

Pay attention to the following signs:

▌ An injury that has no reasonable explanation, or repeated injuries that appear accidental

▌ Hand-shaped bruises or burns or marks in the shape of a cord, a belt, or another object

▌ Pain, itching, bleeding, fluid, or rawness in the genital areas

▌ Sudden bed-wetting, nightmares, or fear of going to bed for no discernible reason

▌ Acting out inappropriate sexual activity

▌ Rebellious behavior that is out of character

▌ A sudden change in your child's attitude toward child care (most often, this is due to a developmental change, but look for explanations regardless)

If any of these signs are present, don't assume the worst. But if you think your child may have been abused, immediately take your child to the doctor for a complete examination. If any injuries or signs of abuse are found, the doctor will report it. You can also contact your local child protection agency for more information.

What to Do If Your Child Becomes Sick

If you send your child to a family child care home or a child care center, you occasionally will get that dreaded phone call from your child care provider asking you to pick up your child because he is sick. Or you will get up one morning ready to dash off to an important meeting only to discover your child has a fever and a cough.

Symptoms that Require a Child to Be Kept or Sent Home from a Child Care Setting

Your family child care or child care center should have a policy that clearly states what symptoms require a child's removal from the home or center. (For more information on these symptoms, turn to Part 5.) That policy should closely resemble the following guidelines set forth by the Centers for Disease Control and Prevention:

▌ Fever, accompanied by sore throat, rash, vomiting, diarrhea, earache, body rash, irritability, or confusion

▌ In a child care situation, fever is defined as
100°F or higher, taken under the arm
101°F or higher, taken orally
102°F or higher, taken rectally
101°F or higher, taken rectally, for infants age 4 months or younger

▌ Diarrhea (i.e., runny, watery, or bloody stools)

▌ Vomiting two or more times in a 24-hour period

▌ Sore throat with fever and swollen glands

▌ Severe coughing: child gets red or blue in the face or makes a high-pitched whooping sound after coughing.

▌ Eye discharge (i.e., thick mucus or pus draining from the eye or pinkeye)

▌ Yellow skin or eyes (see *Jaundice,* Part 5)

▌ Child is crying continuously or requires more attention than the provider can give without jeopardizing the health and safety of the other children

There may be other symptoms, not on this list, that compel you to keep your child home, some of which are a judgment call, such as a headache or an earache with no fever. A cold is not a condition that requires staying home, but if the symptoms are bad enough, you may decide that keeping him home is what's best for your child.

The American Academy of Pediatrics suggests keeping your child home in the following circumstances:

▌ He is too sick to participate comfortably in regular activities.

▌ Caring for him would interfere with the caregiver's or teacher's ability to care for other children.

▌ He has a contagious illness.

Guide to Selecting the Occasional Baby-Sitter

Having a baby doesn't mean you have to give up parties, movies, or your weekly tennis match. In fact, taking a break from parenthood just to pamper yourself for a few hours is highly recommended for recharging your domestic batteries. So even if you don't need regular child care, you may want to hire a baby-sitter on occasion. Hiring someone who is mature, experienced, and trustworthy is important.

Starting Your Search

The following are the best sources of prospective baby-sitters:

▌ Family, friends, and neighbors

▌ A baby-sitting service at a local college placement service

▌ Notices at local high schools, churches, or civic organizations

What You Need to Consider

Even if you're going out for just a few hours, be sure you're leaving your child in the hands of someone responsible enough to comfortably handle anything, from a tantrum-throwing toddler to an emergency. The following sections present some points to consider in your search for a sitter.

Age Consider your personal age preference. When you ask around your neighborhood, a teenager will probably be recommended by neighbors. Teenagers who love children make excellent baby-sitters, but they will need guidance from you concerning the care of your child. You will also need to check out the teenager's history with other families by calling references. When calling references, be particularly curious about the baby-sitter's level of responsibility. Does the sitter show up on time? Does the sitter listen carefully to the parent's instructions and carry them out? The oldest teenager isn't always better, since levels of maturity vary at any given age. Still, keep age 12 or 13 as your lowest limit when choosing a sitter to watch your children when you are out.

Background and Experience   The more experienced the sitter, the better. Be willing to teach a promising candidate basic skills, such as diapering and feeding. Hire a baby-sitter who is trained in first aid, CPR, and choking rescue procedures or is willing to be trained. Local hospitals and organizations such as the Red Cross offer baby-sitting classes and certification.

Personality   Ask the prospective sitter over for tea or a meal with your family. Try to get to know the person a bit. Look for someone who appears to love children and is mature, experienced, and capable. You want a person who listens to you and takes the responsibility seriously. The sitter should show enthusiasm and appear more interested in playing with and entertaining your child than watching television. The following are some questions to ask a prospective baby-sitter in an interview.

For Baby-Sitters for Children of All Ages

▌ How long have you been a baby-sitter?

▌ What do you like about baby-sitting?

▌ What do you think are the most important duties of a baby-sitter?

If Your Child Is an Infant

▌ Have you ever cared for a baby this young?

▌ Do you know the basics of baby care, such as feeding and diapering?

▌ How will you play with him?

▌ If you go for a walk, what precautions will you take?

▌ What will you do if he won't sleep on his back or side?

▌ What if he starts to cry or won't stop crying?

▌ What if he refuses to eat?

If Your Child Is a Toddler or Preschooler

▌ Have you ever cared for a child this age?

▌ What will you do when I go out? What kinds of games will you play?

▌ What precautions will you take if you go outside?

▌ What will you do if he doesn't obey you?

Finally, describe in detail the baby-sitter's duties and responsibilities, discuss an imagined emergency situation, and ask how the sitter might handle it. When you find a baby-sitter you are happy with, discuss the hours and fees for service. Also, write down the sitter's name, address, telephone number, and driver's license number if your sitter has one.

Topics for Review with a New Baby-Sitter

Have your new baby-sitter come to your home a day or so before you plan to have the sitter stay with your child in order to meet your child and spend a little time with him. If that's not possible, ask the baby-sitter to arrive at least a half hour before you depart.

During this time, make sure that you let the sitter know exactly where you will be and how you can be reached. Write down the telephone number and address of where you will be. Also, make a list of emergency telephone numbers, including a friend or relative, the child's doctor, the police department, the fire department, an ambulance service, and the poison control center, and clearly post it. If you have hired a teenager, try to be sure your sitter has access to a reliable adult, such as a trusted neighbor or the sitter's parents if they live nearby.

Take the Sitter on a Tour

Next, take the sitter on a tour of the house, pointing out any first aid equipment, fire extinguishers, and all doors and possible exits. If the sitter will be driving your child, review car safety precautions (see Car Seat Safety, p. 369).

Give the Sitter the House Rules

Give specific instructions, such as these:

- Lock all doors. Show how to lock them and how to get out in case of emergency.
- Keep the children away from dangerous objects (such as knives in the kitchen, tools in the basement) or chemicals, and watch children carefully to prevent household accidents.
- Do not have visitors or friends over unless approved by the parents in advance.
- Do not leave the children alone in the house or outdoors at any time.
- Check the children regularly after they are sleeping.
- If the telephone rings, ask the caller to leave a message by saying, "I'm sorry, she can't come to the phone right now." Do not inform the caller that the parents are not home.
- Do not open the door to anyone unless the parents have given prior permission.
- If the children are in a public place, watch them closely and do not permit them to wander. Avoid sending children to public restrooms alone.

Show the Sitter What to Do

Finally, review issues specific to your child. Review the child's routine, his food preferences, or any allergies he might have. Let the baby-sitter know what your child likes to do. Pull out a favorite game, or leave out favorite books. Make sure the sitter is clear about bedtime and any ritual that makes your child feel comfortable settling in. Here is a list of specific issues to review:

If Your Child Is an Infant

▌ How to heat a bottle and hold your baby during feedings

▌ The location of bottles and baby food

▌ The location of diapers and how to dispose of used diapers

▌ The safe use of baby equipment, such as the changing table

▌ Use of the pacifier

▌ The proper way to put a baby to sleep: on his back

▌ Why soft items like a pillow or stuffed animals should not go in the crib

▌ How to use the baby monitor

If Your Child Is Between 1 and 3 Years Old

▌ Potty-training routine or routine for changing diapers

▌ What foods to avoid, such as whole grapes, raw carrots, or hot dogs, and why

▌ Use of safety gates and other childproofing items

▌ Appropriate television viewing and videos

▌ Routines for putting on pajamas, washing up, and before-bed activities, such as reading a story

If Your Child is 3 Years of Age or Older

▌ Snacks or meals

▌ Favorite toys or games

▌ Off-limits areas of the house

▌ Bedtime routine

▌ Location of night-light or other light that might be left on for the child

Again, and most important, be sure to leave a list of phone numbers, including a number for where you can be reached, that of a nearby adult, your child's doctor's number, and emergency numbers such as fire, police, and poison control.

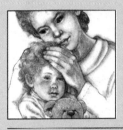

CHAPTER 10

WHAT TO EXPECT
WHEN YOUR CHILD IS SICK

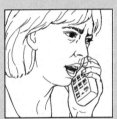

CHAPTER 11

PREPARING FOR
AND HANDLING EMERGENCIES

10 What to Expect When Your Child Is Sick

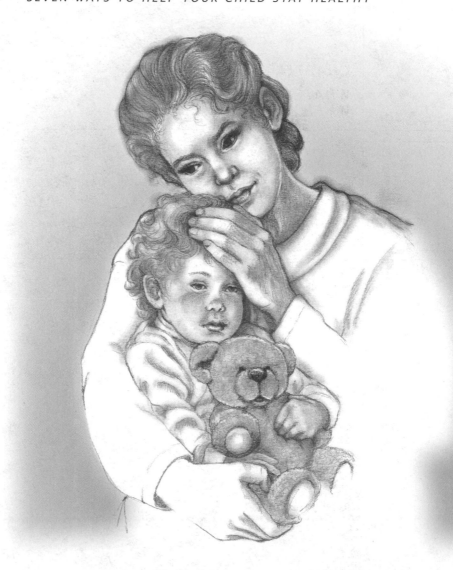

"Mommy, my tummy hurts." "Daddy, I don't feel good." When heard at 6:30 A.M. on a Monday, those words can send a household into a tailspin. First, there's the flood of anxiety that washes over parents with sick children. Second, a child's illness—with its potential trips to the doctor's office, the time taken away from other responsibilities, and the exhaustion of sleepless nights of caring for a sick child—nearly always disrupts the family's routine.

Without doubt, a child's illness is a stressful event for most families. In this chapter, we show you the steps you can take to relieve some of that stress and make the right decisions for both you and your child.

Is My Child Sick?

From the first moment you took your new baby into your arms, you became not only her parent and guardian, but also her at-home doctor. Indeed, staying alert to signs of illness and caring for your child when she's not feeling well is primarily your responsibility—at least for mild illnesses. You'll learn that when you hear that plaintive cry, she just might have a fever and that her loss of appetite and drop in energy just might mean she's catching a cold. You'll soon figure out what you need to do to help her feel more comfortable and return to health.

In this quest, you're not alone. Your principal source of support is, of course, your child's doctor and staff, including nurse practitioners, nurses, and physician's assistants. Their knowledge and expertise are available with just a phone call.

WHEN TO CALL THE DOCTOR
Symptoms Requiring Medical Attention

If you're like most new parents, your first instinct may be to run to the doctor's office at the first sign that your child is ill. However, a simple cold or mild case of diarrhea may not require medical treatment. If you're unsure whether to take your child to the doctor, call the doctor's office first. Your doctor's staff can help you decide whether your baby needs an examination. But the American Academy of Pediatrics recommends calling the doctor *immediately* if you notice any of the following symptoms:

- A fever in a baby younger than 6 months

- Fever and vomiting at the same time

- Vomiting, with or without diarrhea, lasting more than 24 hours

- Diarrhea in an infant less than 1 month old

- Bloody diarrhea or diarrhea that lasts several days

- A rash accompanied by a fever

- Any cold or cough that doesn't improve or that grows worse after 7 days

▌ Ear pain, ear drainage, or both

▌ Cuts that could require stitches

▌ Bleeding that can't be stopped

▌ An inability to move an arm or a leg

▌ Sharp, unremitting pain in the abdomen

▌ Poisoning

▌ Burns

▌ Convulsions

▌ Difficulty breathing

▌ Head injuries with loss of consciousness

▌ Gray or ashen skin color

▌ Blood in the urine

▌ Lack of energy or inability to move

For more advice on when common illnesses require a doctor's attention, look up the name of the illness in Part 5, Guide to Common Childhood Illness, Injury, and Conditions. For what to do in emergencies, see page 377.

Tracking Down the Symptoms

An infant can never tell you if she's sick (at least not in words), and even a 5-year-old can't always identify her discomfort as an illness. That leaves you to interpret the symptoms and make decisions about what to do next. Is her stuffy nose a reason to keep her home from day care (and you home from work)? Is your baby's fever high enough to warrant a call to the doctor?

Far more than any single symptom, like a fever or cough or stomachache, your child's behavior provides the most information about her health. Before you assume the worst after hearing "Daddy, I don't feel good" in the morning, ask yourself how she behaved the night before. Did she eat a good dinner, play with her usual gusto, and sleep well? If so, then she may be OK, especially if she's not running a fever or having bouts of diarrhea or vomiting. But if she refused food, became cranky or lethargic before bed, had trouble sleeping, and still doesn't seem like herself this morning, she might well be coming down with a cold, an intestinal flu, or another illness.

Also watch for symptoms that start suddenly. Is she lethargic? Not eating her usual hearty breakfast? In the end, it's best to follow your instincts—as long as you put your child's needs first. If she's a toddler who usually stays at home with you, you can easily watch to see if any other symptoms develop. But if you have to decide whether or not to keep her home from day care or school—and stay home from work to be with her—the question about illness becomes more urgent.

Resist the temptation to pack your child off to day care or school despite some early warning signs. Keeping her home for a day when she's feeling run-down might prevent her from contracting a more serious infection if you put her in the company of kids with colds and other viruses. For more specific guidelines on when to keep your child home from day care or school, see page 335.

How Long Is It "Catching"?

One of the most common questions asked by parents and teachers is, Exactly how long are common illnesses contagious? The good news is, usually not long. The bad news is that illnesses are often contagious even before symptoms appear. That means your child can "catch" a cold from a playmate who appears and feels perfectly well.

▬ HOW LONG IS IT CATCHING?

Illness	Infectious Period
Chicken pox	Begins 24 to 48 hours before the rash appears; lasts until all lesions are crusted over, usually about 7 to 10 days
Colds	Usually from 7 to 10 days after symptoms appear, but can last as long as 3 weeks
Conjunctivitis	Bacterial infections: until 24 hours after antibiotics are started. Viral infections: for 5 days
Head lice	Until treatment begins
Strep throat	24 hours after antibiotic treatment begins
Stomach flu	As long as the child has diarrhea or a fever

Balancing Work and Sick-Child Care

Balancing work responsibilities with the needs of a sick child is never easy. Although the percentage of working mothers has risen in the past five decades or so—up from 12 percent to 58 percent for those with toddlers and up from 27 to 76 percent for those with school-age children—child care options remain extremely limited for ill children.

If you're a working mother, the burden probably still falls most heavily on you. A recent Gallup poll revealed that 80 percent of workdays missed by mothers occur because of their children's illnesses, not their own. A 1989 study conducted by the U.S. Bureau of Labor Statistics showed that mothers with children 6 years of age or younger had the highest absentee rates of all employees. Fathers, too, are taking time off to care for sick children and are often losing pay and productivity. The financial hardship of this trend is tremendous: More than 28 percent of working mothers have no paid sick time—every day they take off means a day of lost wages. Sadly, the challenges facing poor women are even greater, with only 20 percent of poor women having jobs that offer paid sick leave.

Fortunately, innovative programs that offer either in-home care provided by a trained aide or care in a sick-child center are springing up. Most are funded and managed by large corporations or consortiums of smaller companies. In some cases, employers foot the whole bill for the service; in others, the employee pays a percentage.

Many employers require that parents take their own sick days to care for their sick children or lose a day's pay. If you fall under that umbrella, pay extra attention to finding someone you trust—a sibling, a neighbor, a relative—to pinch-hit when you can't take time off from work.

A working parent can take several steps to help avoid a crisis on those days when a child is unexpectedly too sick to attend day care or school. Most involve advance planning.

▌ Talk with your supervisor about your company's policy for taking time off to be with a sick child. Find out which is most appropriate: taking a sick day, a vacation day, or a personal leave day.

▌ Arrange for a friend or family member who is home while you work to look after your sick child.

▌ Call around to find parent-in-a-pinch agencies that will supply baby-sitters on a moment's notice. You may need to register in advance. These agencies can be expensive, but if missing work will jeopardize your job, it may be worthwhile for a day or two.

▌ If you have the type of job that makes taking time off extremely difficult, consider hiring a child care provider to come to your home, either during the day or as a live-in, instead of enrolling your child in a day care center. The advantage is that the regular in-home caregiver will show up even when your child is sick.

Five Common Symptoms

The vast majority of common childhood illnesses are accompanied by one or more of the following symptoms.

1 Fever

A fever usually is a sign that your child's body is responding appropriately to an attack from viruses or bacteria by stimulating its disease-fighting immune system. Because an infant under 6 months of age has an immature immune system unable to fight even mild infections, even a low fever (over 100.2°F rectal) may require immediate attention. (See *Fever*, Part 5.)

WHEN TO CALL THE DOCTOR
Fever

Call the doctor immediately in the following situations:

▌ A fever over 100.2°F (rectal) occurs in a baby under 6 months, or 102°F in other children.

▌ Your child cries inconsolably with fever.

▌ You have trouble waking your child.

▌ Your child cries when you touch or move her, or she has a stiff neck or purple spots on her, which may indicate a serious brain infection called meningitis.

▌ The fever in a child over 6 months lasts longer than 2 or 3 days.

2 Constant Crying

Babies, particularly those younger than 3 months, frequently cry for long periods. Although constant crying during early infancy may be attributable to *colic* (see Part 5), it also may indicate that your baby is ill. Until you sort out the problem, it's best to stay home with your baby rather than leaving her with a sitter or bringing her to day care, but that's a decision you and your baby's doctor can make together. For ways to respond to an infant's crying, see Coping with Crying, page 106.

3 Cough

A cough is a reflex action of the body to remove any irritating substance— such as a foreign object, mucus from an infection, or airborne irritants like cigarette smoke—that enters the respiratory tract. Like a fever, coughing is a symptom rather than an illness itself. Keep in mind that a cough is only as serious as its underlying cause, of which several exist. Most coughs are caused by viral infections, such as those that cause the common cold (see *Colds/Flu,* Part 5), *croup* (see Part 5), and *bronchiolitis* (see Part 5). For more information, see *Cough,* Part 5.

4 Diarrhea

The frequent passage of abnormally loose or liquid stools is one of the most common reasons parents call the doctor. In fact, the only conditions to occur more frequently than diarrhea during childhood are respiratory tract infections, like colds. In infants, diarrhea is usually caused by a virus, although any time a baby eats a new food, loose stools can occur as a sign that her digestive system is adapting to previously unknown substances. Diarrhea episodes may last just a day or up to a week or two. As long as your child continues to drink plenty of liquids, diarrhea is not a cause for alarm. Note, however, that newborns and infants can dehydrate within a matter of hours, which makes it even more important to maintain and monitor their fluid intake. For more information about diarrhea and how to treat it, see *Diarrhea,* Part 5.

5 Vomiting

Vomiting—the violent expulsion of the stomach contents through the mouth—occurs when the body needs to rid itself of a substance that it cannot tolerate. As a rule, a viral infection triggers vomiting. Most cases of vomiting only once or twice need no treatment other than replacing lost fluids. For more information about vomiting and how to treat it, see *Vomiting,* Part 5.

Working with Your Child's Doctor

Gradually, most parents learn to recognize when their children are sick enough to need a doctor's attention. You know when your child is sick. Generally speaking, call your child's doctor whenever you feel that your baby looks or acts differently from normal—especially if she has a fever or other symptoms—or any time you're unsure how to handle her symptoms. (See When to Call the Doctor, pp. 343 and 347.)

Making the Most of Your Call to the Doctor

When your child is sick and you need to call the doctor for advice, get organized *before* making the call. Make a list of questions you want the doctor to answer and information you want him to know about your baby. Be sure to have a pen and paper handy to write down the doctor's or nurse's instructions and advice. Put your baby in a safe place, and give her something to occupy her while you are on the phone, so you can concentrate on asking your questions and hearing what the doctor says. Be prepared to answer the following basic questions your doctor or health care staff probably will ask when you call:

■ *Is your child running a fever?* Take your baby's temperature before you call the doctor, and write down the result, the method (oral, axillary, rectal, ear), and the time you took it.

■ *How long has your child been sick?* Consider when you first noticed your baby's symptoms and whether they've changed since then.

■ *How is your child behaving?* Help the doctor gauge your baby's condition by describing how she is acting. Is your child just a little fussy or highly irritable, a little less active than usual, or extremely listless or sleepy? Have you noticed changes in your child's eating habits, urination, or bowel movements?

At the Doctor's Office

A trip to the doctor's office when your child is ill will probably be difficult for both of you. Your child's illness might cause her to be cranky and uncooperative, and you might be more anxious than usual. Faced with these distractions, you might forget to tell your doctor an important symptom or fail to remember exactly what he tells you about your child's condition. That's why it's important to write down symptoms, questions, and concerns before the appointment and to write down the diagnosis and any instructions your doctor gives you afterward.

Your doctor will be able to diagnose most—but not all—common childhood illnesses by asking about your child's symptoms while examining her. In most cases, a complete physical exam won't be necessary, and the doctor will concentrate on tracking down whatever symptoms brought your child to the office. He may check her ears, eyes, and throat and listen to her lungs and abdomen as a way to find the cause of her illness.

Sometimes, however, your doctor may want to run laboratory tests, such as urine and blood tests, X rays, or even more extensive tests to confirm or rule out a suspected diagnosis. Not surprisingly, you and your doctor may not always agree about the need for various tests. Doctors often favor doing further tests to rule out uncommon—but potentially very serious—problems, while parents worry more about the negative effects of the tests on their children, including pain, discomfort, and fear.

No simple answer exists. Every time your child is ill, you and your doctor must work together to decide the appropriate course of action. That's why it's important that you find a doctor you can trust. If further tests aren't necessary, you and your child should be on your way within an hour or so. Before you leave the doctor's office, make sure you know the answers to the following questions:

▌ What's making my child sick?

▌ What further symptoms should I expect, and what is the course of the illness?

▌ What treatment is required, and when will it take effect?

▌ How do I care for my child while she's sick with this illness?

▌ Should I schedule a follow-up visit?

▌ If the condition is contagious, when is it safe for her to be around other children?

When Your Child's Doctor Prescribes Medicine

Although most common ailments that children get are caused by viruses, which do not usually require medication, your child sometimes may need a prescription to treat an illness. Administering the correct medicine, in the right dose, and when and for as long as the doctor prescribes is extremely important. Before you leave the doctor's office, make sure you have answers to the following questions. If you forget to ask them of the doctor, or you don't understand something about the prescription, ask the pharmacist.

▌ What is the exact dose of the medicine? What is the recommended way to measure a dose? How precise must I be about the dose?

▌ How often do I give my child the medicine? What happens if I miss a dose? What happens if I give two doses too close together?

▌ How can I tell if the medicine is working? How long does it take before it starts to work?

▌ How long should I wait before calling the doctor if the medicine doesn't seem to be working?

▌ What side effects can this drug cause? What side effects should I report to the doctor?

▌ Does my child take this medicine with food? If not, how long before or after meals should she take it?

▌ How many days should my child take this medicine?

▌ If my child feels better, can she stop taking the medicine, or does she need to finish the prescription?

▌ If my child vomits after taking the dose, should I give her another dose immediately?

▌ Will the medicine interact with any other medicine my child is taking, either prescription or over-the-counter?

▌ Should I refrigerate the medicine? If so, should I warm it up before giving it to my child?

▌ How long can I keep unused portions of the medicine for future use?

What to Do at Home

The illness might last just a day or two, or it might last as long as several weeks, but your child will require special attention during her illness. The motto here remains "Be prepared." Before your child becomes ill, make sure that the medicine cabinet is well stocked. Today, while she's healthy, learn the recommended way to take your child's temperature and to give medicine.

Supplies to Have on Hand

A well-stocked medicine chest can mean the difference between an emergency trip to the pharmacy or doctor's office with a sick child in tow and quick relief for a minor illness or injury. Organize your medicine cabinet for easy adult access, and make sure to throw out unused or outdated prescriptions or over-the-counter medications. Ask your doctor before giving your child any medication, and keep medicines in child-proof cabinets at shoulder height or higher.

Medicines

Keep these items handy to cope with almost any minor problem:.

▌ *Acetaminophen or ibuprofen* (infant or child formula) to relieve fever and mild pain. Acetaminophen and ibuprofen both act as pain relievers (analgesics) and fever reducers (antipyretics). Doctors no longer recommend aspirin for children, because aspirin is associated with the development of Reye syndrome, a rare but serious illness that often can affect the brain and the liver. Acetaminophen and ibuprofen are the generic names of the medications found in many brand-name pain relievers. Both acetaminophen and ibuprofen come in child-strength formulas. Use only medications made for children, to prevent excess dosing. Make sure you follow the dosing instructions with care. Use the liquid form of acetaminophen for children who do not yet have their first molars. After molars come in, you may switch to the chewable tablets. For fever or pain lasting longer than 24 hours, always consult your doctor.

▮ *Antibiotic ointments* to help prevent cuts and scrapes from becoming infected.

▮ *Antihistamines* as recommended by the doctor to relieve itching, hives, insect bites, and allergic reactions. Before giving your child an antihistamine (especially for the first time), consult your doctor.

▮ *Hydrocortisone cream* to relieve rashes and other skin irritations. Hydrocortisone cream, a mild steroid medication, is now available without prescription. However, before using a steroid cream for rashes, even minor ones, consult your doctor. Steroids may paradoxically worsen the condition. Never use hydrocortisone on chicken pox, burns, open wounds, or infections.

▮ *Ipecac* to induce vomiting in poison emergencies. Use ipecac only under the advice of a doctor or poison control center personnel. Some substances can be more harmful coming up than going down, so inducing vomiting after your child swallows a toxic substance (see p. 417) is not always appropriate.

Other Supplies

Keep the following supplies handy:

▮ *Adhesive bandages* to cover cuts and scrapes after they've been cleaned

▮ *Antibacterial soap* or antiseptic solution to cleanse dirty wounds

▮ *Calibrated spoon* or medicine dropper to measure medicine doses accurately

▮ *Cotton balls* to apply lotions and antiseptic solutions

▮ *Cotton swabs* to clean the nostrils and the external ear (never insert the swab into the ear canal, as it can injure the eardrum)

▮ *Gauze bandages* to cover cuts or deeper wounds

▮ *Ice pack* to reduce swelling after a bump or another injury

▮ *Irrigating eyewash* to cleanse the eye of irritants

▮ *Petroleum jelly* to lubricate rectal thermometers and to treat **diaper rash** (see Part 5)

▮ *Saline nose drops* to clear stuffed-up noses

▮ *Sunscreen,* with a sun protection factor (SPF) of 15 or higher, to protect against damaging sun rays

▮ *Thermometer* to measure fever (see information below)

▮ *Tweezers* to remove splinters partially embedded in the skin (always sterilize first)

▮ *Vaporizer* or humidifier to help loosen cough and minimize throat and nasal irritation that's exacerbated by dryness in the air

Taking Your Child's Temperature

Today, various options exist for taking your child's temperature. The five main types of available thermometers are: mercury (glass), digital, infrared tympanic (ear), pacifier, and instant underarm (axillary). (Fever strips that are placed on the child's forehead do not provide an accurate reading and are not recommended.) There are also several methods for taking your child's temperature: rectal, oral, tympanic (ear), and axillary (under the arm). The rectal method is the standard that doctors use. If you use a different method, you may need to adjust the reading according to the directions here to make it comparable to the rectal standard. The chart will help you choose a thermometer for your child and show you how to use it correctly.

▬ TYPES OF THERMOMETERS: PROS AND CONS

Type	Pros	Cons
Mercury	Very accurate Quiet	Numbers can be hard to read Fragile Takes 2 to 3 minutes
Digital	Easy to read Accurate Beeps when ready	Needs batteries Takes at least 1 minute Beep may wake a sleeping child
Pacifier	Safe Will not wake a sleeping infant	Needs batteries 3 minutes recommended for accuracy
Tympanic (ear)	Quick (3 to 5 seconds) Eliminates contamination risk associated with oral and rectal methods	Needs careful placement in ear canal for accurate reading Not accurate in infants Needs batteries Expensive
Instant underarm (axillary)	Quick (2 to 3 seconds) Eliminates contamination risk associated with oral and rectal methods	Child may squirm Expensive

Taking a Rectal Temperature

Use a mercury (glass) or digital thermometer, and follow these simple directions:

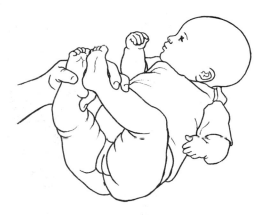

1. If you're using a mercury thermometer, shake it briskly a few times (over a bed or another soft surface to avoid breakage if the thermometer drops) to make certain that the top of the column is below 98.6°F.

2. Lubricate the thermometer bulb with petroleum jelly.

3. Lay your baby on her back, and remove her diaper. Have an older child lie on her side.

4. If you're using a digital thermometer, turn on the switch.

5. Lifting her legs with one hand, gently insert the thermometer into her rectum about 1 inch.

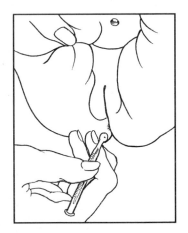

6. Hold it in place for 3 to 5 minutes for a glass thermometer or until the digital thermometer beeps; then remove and read.

7. Clean the thermometer thoroughly after each use.

If you prefer laying your baby across your lap, hold her in place by pressing the palm of one hand against her lower back. With your other hand insert the lubricated thermometer about 1 inch.

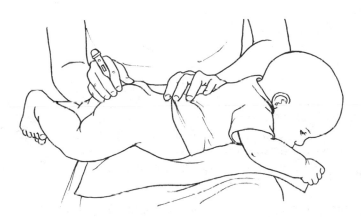

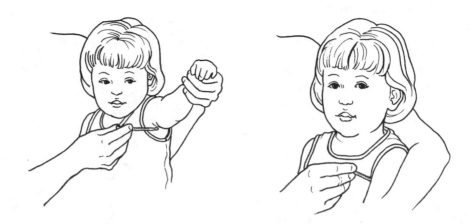

Taking an Axillary (Underarm) Temperature

Use either a mercury or digital thermometer, and follow these steps:

1. Turn on the switch if you're using a digital axillary thermometer. If you're using a mercury thermometer, shake it until the column is below 98.6°F.

2. Place the thermometer in your child's armpit, and hold her arm tightly against her chest.

3. Wait either 4 to 5 minutes for a glass thermometer or until the digital thermometer beeps. If you're using an instant underarm thermometer, the reading will appear in 2 to 3 seconds.

4. Add 1°F (if you want to compare the axillary reading to the rectal method). *Note*: The instant underarm thermometer adds the degree for you.

Taking a Tympanic (Ear) Temperature

When using a tympanic thermometer, be sure to seal your child's ear canal completely. If your child has been lying on her side, especially with her ear against a warm surface, wait 5 minutes before taking her temperature to prevent trapped heat from raising the temperature reading. Make sure your child has been indoors for at least 15 minutes in cooler climates. Cold outdoor air can make the reading inaccurate.

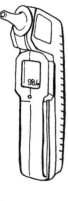

1. If you are right-handed, hold the thermometer in your right hand and take the temperature from your child's right ear. If you are left-handed, use your left hand and place the thermometer in your child's left ear.

2. Gently insert the end of the thermometer into the ear with the lens angled slightly forward.

3. Using your free hand, gently pull the outer ear back (if the child is over 1 year of age, pull back and up). This will straighten the ear canal, allowing it to become fully sealed.

4. Once the thermometer is positioned snugly, press the start button.

5. Read your child's temperature after 3 or 4 seconds.

6. If you have children under 3 months old, children under 3 years old with health concerns, or if you're learning to use the tympanic thermometer, take your child's temperature three times and use the highest reading.

7. Change or clean the lens filter after each use.

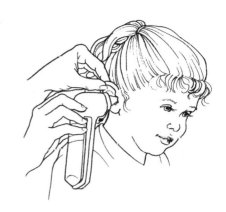

Taking an Oral Temperature

Allow 30 minutes after your child eats or drinks before taking your child's temperature to avoid altering the reading.

Pacifier Thermometer The pacifier thermometer is a safe and accurate way to take the temperature of an infant or a small child. The thermometer is intended for taking temperatures only, and should not be substituted as a regular pacifier.

1. Press the power button located in the front of the pacifier.

2. Position the pacifier bulb in your child's mouth.

3. Read your child's temperature after 3 minutes. To make a comparison between an oral reading and a rectal reading, add 0.5°F to the temperature displayed on the pacifier thermometer.

4. Clean the pacifier bulb thoroughly after each use.

Digital or Mercury Thermometer Once your child is about 5 or 6 years old (or old enough to follow instructions), you can take an oral temperature using either a mercury or digital thermometer.

1. Ask your child to open her mouth and to lift her tongue.

2. Turn on the switch if it's a digital thermometer. If you're using a mercury thermometer, shake the column down to below 98.6°F.

3. Place the thermometer under your child's tongue toward the back of the mouth, and ask her to close her mouth—very gently, if you're using a mercury

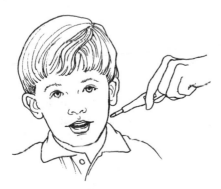

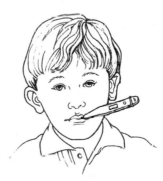

thermometer. Warn her not to bite down, but rather to hold the thermometer in place by placing her tongue behind her lower front teeth.

4. Leave the thermometer in place for about 1 to 2 minutes (or according to manufacturer's instructions). Never leave your child alone with a thermometer in her mouth. Remove and read.

5. Add 1°F to compare to rectal temperature.

Giving Your Child Medicine

When the doctor prescribes medication, he will also tell you about how much, when, and in what manner to give the medication. Be sure to follow these directions with care. If you do not understand something about your child's medical problem or the medication prescribed, ask the doctor to explain further.

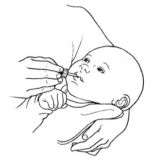

Most medicines for babies and children come in sweet-tasting liquid forms. You'll need to measure the dose of liquid drugs with a specially marked measuring dropper, syringe, or spoon tube you can buy at any pharmacy. Older children often like taking medicine and may learn to take it themselves with your supervision. If your child hates taking liquid medicine, ask your doctor if you can mix it with a bit of juice. Generally speaking, children can start taking pills at about 6 years old, but the age varies considerably. Keep a careful watch on your young child until she gets the hang of swallowing pills on her own. If your older child finds taking pills difficult, your doctor may tell you to crush them into some jam or other food—but be sure to ask.

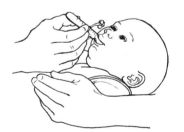

Liquid Medications for Infants and Toddlers

Follow these steps to give your toddler or infant liquid medicines:

1. Hold your baby in the crook of your arm. Gently open her mouth by pulling down on her chin. If your baby is particularly squirmy, and no one else is available to help you, you may find it easier to place your baby on a safe surface, such as a changing table or in the middle of a bed.

2. Use a calibrated spoon, dropper, or syringe—not a regular spoon—to measure and administer the medicine.

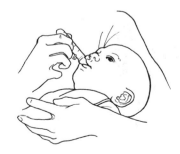

3. Place the calibrated spoon on your child's lower lip, lift the spoon, and let the medicine run into her mouth. If you're using a dropper or syringe, place it in the corner of her mouth and release the medicine.

Here are some further tips to help you give your baby medicine:

▌ If your baby struggles, have someone else hold her while you administer the medication. You can wrap her arms and legs in a blanket to lessen her squirming.

▌ If your baby spits out the medicine, try pouring the medicine further back in her mouth, then gently hold her mouth closed until she swallows. You can also try giving the medicine in several smaller doses using a medicine dropper.

▌ If your child vomits less than 20 minutes after taking the medication, check with your doctor immediately. Your baby may not have gotten enough medication into her system and may need another dose.

Making Fluids Taste Better

Infants are more likely than older children to become dehydrated when ill. To combat dehydration, your doctor may recommend using an over-the-counter oral rehydration drink specifically designed to replace electrolytes and fluid. But if your child seems to dislike the taste and refuses to drink the solution, you can try flavoring it using these specific, tested guidelines.

For an 8-ounce serving of the drink, you can add one of these:

▌ ½ teaspoon of sweetened gelatin dessert mix or a sweetened powdered drink mix

▌ 2 ounces of apple juice or, for children over 12 months, orange juice

Do not use other juices or flavoring products, because there is no research on whether they might disrupt the balance of electrolytes in the solution.

Eyedrops

Follow these steps to give your baby eyedrops:

1. Hold your baby still or, if possible, have someone hold your baby still for you.

2. Very gently pull her lower eyelid down, and let the drops fall between her eye and lower lid.

3. Tilt her head slightly so that any excess eyedrops run down her cheek and not into her other eye.

4. For a squirming toddler, it's easier to have someone else hold her hands down from her face while you apply the medicine.

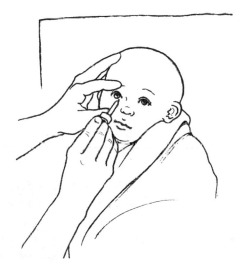

Nose Drops

Here's how to give your baby nose drops:

1. Hold your baby still or, if possible, have someone hold your baby still for you.

2. Tilt her head back slightly, and drop the proper amount into each nostril—2 or 3 drops at a time.

Ear Drops

Follow this procedure to give your baby ear drops:

1. Lay your baby on her side with the affected ear up.

2. Hold her steady while you drop the right amount of medication into the ear, and wait until the drops have run down into the canal.

3. Gently push several times at the tragus, the small bump of cartilage just in front of the ear, to help move the drops down the ear canal.

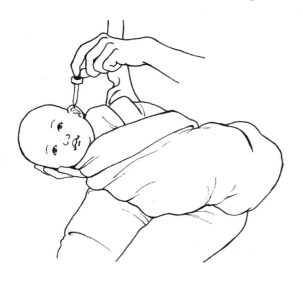

Keeping Your Child Comfortable and Content

As anyone who's helped care for a sick child can tell you, administering medicine and taking the child's temperature are just a small part of the job. You will also spend time comforting your child and helping her feel comfortable. The best way to help your child is to simply be there as much as possible. If you have to go to work and leave your child in someone else's care, make sure you call and talk to your toddler or older child a few times during the day. Other ways you can help include the following.

Providing Quiet Time for Rest

How much rest your child needs depends on how sick she is and with what. Children can assess their own need for rest pretty well, but set some limits so that your child doesn't overexert herself. To decide on how much activity to allow, take your cues from your child's behavior, her symptoms, and your doctor's advice.

Helping Ease Your Child's Symptoms

Your doctor can give you advice on how to help ease your child's symptoms. The doctor may, for example, recommend giving acetaminophen or ibuprofen to reduce a fever or saline drops or medication to help clear congested breathing passages.

Getting Your Child to Eat or Drink

If your child's appetite is low, it's fine to let her eat only small amounts every few hours. However, it is extremely important that both infants and older children drink liquids regularly, especially if they experience diarrhea, vomiting, or high fever, all of which can lead to *dehydration* (see Part 5). Let your child take small sips of fluid, suck on lightly flavored ice pops, or—if she's a baby or toddler—sip drinks from a teaspoon rather than a bottle so that she will take the fluids in small increments. Drinking too much too fast may prompt a child with an upset tummy to vomit. On the other hand, if your child is hungry and hasn't vomited in 12 hours, and your doctor hasn't advised against it, let her enjoy her favorite foods, but reintroduce solid foods gradually.

When Your Child Needs Hospital Care

Your goal, and the goal of your child's health care team, is to keep your child as healthy as possible so that hospital stays are unnecessary. But in some instances, hospital stays are necessary. Dehydration, for example, is one common cause of hospital stays in infants. If your child is scheduled for a hospital visit, there are steps you can take to prepare and make the visit as calm and helpful as possible.

Three Reasons to Go to the Hospital

Despite their best efforts, most parents will make one or more trips to the hospital during their children's lives—usually for one of the following reasons.

1 Emergencies
The number one reason children go to the hospital is to receive treatment for an acute injury or illness, such as a very high fever, respiratory distress, a broken bone, or a burn. When deciding whether to go to the emergency department, err on the side of caution: If you think your baby needs immediate attention, notify your child's doctor and take her in. Before an emergency arises, call your doctor's office or health plan to find out which hospital emergency room to use. You may not be covered if you show up at a hospital not included in your health plan.

2 Diagnostic Tests
If your child becomes ill, your doctor may want to rule out certain problems before making a diagnosis. Certain diagnostic tests and procedures are often—but

not always—performed in a hospital setting. These include complicated X rays, EEGs, CT scans, MRI scans, and cardiac catheterizations, to name a few. (See the Glossary at the back of this book for a description of these procedures.) Some procedures require a hospital stay, while others are performed on an outpatient basis.

3 Surgery

Surgery is another reason your child may need to stay at the hospital. For many minor surgeries, your child may spend only a day at the hospital, arriving early that morning, having surgery, and staying for several hours of observation before you take her home with postoperative care instructions.

Preparing Your Child for the Hospital

Preparation is the key to making sure your child has the easiest possible time at the hospital. If the hospital visit is planned in advance, you can do several things to make hospitalization less traumatic for you and your child.

Educate Yourself

Learn as much as possible about the reason for your child's hospitalization and what will happen at the hospital. Ask your doctor or nurse, or even hospital staff members, to explain in detail what your child faces, so that you aren't surprised or confused when your child needs you to be strong and reassuring. Your doctor may be able to refer you to parent support groups or to families who have had similar experiences, so that you can find out what to expect.

QUESTIONS PARENTS ASK

Informed Consent

Q: I'm not sure I understand what informed consent really means. If I sign a consent form, does that mean the doctors can do anything they want to my child?

A: Before your child undergoes certain diagnostic procedures, surgeries, or treatments, you'll be asked to give your informed consent. In most circumstances—other than dire emergencies, when you or a close relative cannot be reached—a physician and nurse must explain all relevant details and implications of the treatment course proposed by the health care team. When giving written consent, you are acknowledging that you received an explanation of the procedure, understand its risks and benefits, and agree to the proposed care. If the doctor decides that your child needs another type of test or treatment procedure, he will again request your consent and explain all the risks and benefits beforehand.

Be Honest

As always, honesty is the best policy: If your child is facing a painful procedure, don't try to hide it. Prepare her for the surgery or need for hospitalization a few days in advance. That is not to say you should unduly alarm your child or make her anxious. Instead, say that when she wakes up from surgery (for instance), she will hurt for a while, but then she'll gradually feel better over time.

Make sure your child knows that you'll be there as much as possible, and that you and other family members will make the time go more quickly by playing games with her or reading stories to her. Many hospitals provide handouts and booklets written for your child's age group that will explain a particular procedure or familiarize your child with the hospital milieu.

Visit the Hospital Before Your Child Is Admitted

Many hospitals have orientation tours for children of all age groups. If your child's does not, phone the pediatric unit and ask if a nurse might have time briefly to show you and your child around. The more familiar your child becomes with her new, temporary surroundings before being admitted, the less anxious and upset she'll be when she's admitted.

Tell the Hospital Staff About Your Child

Write down any information you think might aid the nursing staff in caring for your child, including her sleeping and eating habits and any fears you know she harbors. Describe your child's bedtime ritual. Does she usually get a story before bed? Does she sleep with a favorite blanket or toy? Pack her pajamas, toothbrush, and other home items she may need. Also, let the staff know if your child has any special foods she likes or any food allergies. Although you shouldn't expect your child's every whim to be indulged, most nurses will try to take special needs into consideration.

Coping with the Hospital Experience

No matter how well you prepare your child for her hospital visit, the event is likely to be quite upsetting both to you and to your child. Knowing some of the issues your child might face may help you better understand her behavior as a patient and help you find ways to minimize her physical and emotional distress.

Separation Awareness

More than any other single aspect of the hospital experience, your child's separation from you is probably the most frightening and upsetting to you both. In general, the younger she is, the more acutely she'll feel the emotional impact of losing your reassuring presence. You'll probably feel anxious and distressed every time you have to leave her as well, and that's perfectly normal and natural, too.

The best solution is to stay by your child's side as much as you can. Hospitals now actively encourage parents to stay overnight to be with their child. Often, a bed is provided for parents in the child's room. Infants appear to tolerate even the most invasive procedures well if they have a constant, loving parent or caregiver nearby. As a toddler, your child may feel as if the hospitalization is a punishment for some minor indiscretion she committed; others may think that you have abandoned them forever. It is especially important for parents to stay with a toddler. Take shifts at the hospital if possible. Although these issues tend to diminish as the child gets older, being away from home and apart from parents remain upsetting situations even to adolescents. Talk to your doctor and the hospital staff about staying with your child and participating in her care as much as possible.

Tiredness

Hospitals are not the place to get a good night's sleep. Nursing or physician's orders may require temperature taking, blood pressure, and pulse checks at odd times in the night. A crying child in another bed may keep your child awake. The bed and room are new and strange. All this may make your child tired, irritable, and not her normal self. And you may find yourself tired and irritable for the same reasons!

Fear

Needless to say, the strange sights and sounds of the hospital unnerve us all, perhaps our children most of all. First and foremost, your child will be scared of the pain or discomfort involved in the hospital treatment—even if it involves just a needle stick or an X ray. Being away from home and in a strange place is just plain scary, too. The following suggestions may help you calm your child's fears and anxieties about being in the hospital.

▌ *Let your child express herself.* Often, the only time children feel free to release their emotions is in front of a parent. When you come to visit, then, you may be confronted with a child who immediately begins to cry, scream, or act out in an aggressive manner. As upsetting as this may be to you, comfort her as best you can. Try not to punish or scold her—it is far better that these powerful emotions, which stem from fear and loneliness, are released.

▌ *Promote trust in the environment and staff.* The way you behave toward, and talk about, the hospital and staff will influence your child's attitude about her experience. The more positive you are, the more secure your child is apt to feel. If you are uncomfortable or uncertain about the quality of care or the personality of health care personnel, talk to your doctor immediately, but don't discuss these concerns in front of your child.

▌ *Take advantage of available resources.* Talk to the hospital social worker, child life specialist, or nurses in the ward about how to give your child's day some social and physical structure. Nurses can foster friendships between youngsters who are well enough to play games together or sit together to watch cartoons on television. Social workers, staff psychologists, and other professionals are also available to help you and your child cope with what happens in the hospital and at home during the recovery process.

Your Child's Surgery

Whether your child is having ear tubes inserted or a hernia repaired, anesthesia will probably be part of the experience. Although feeling concerned about your child is normal, remember that anesthesia is now a safe and standard part of most pediatric surgical procedures.

Anesthesia is the use of medications by an anesthesiologist (a specially trained doctor) to eliminate pain and awareness during a medical procedure. If your child is scheduled for surgery, ask your doctor about the plans for using anesthesia at the same time that you discuss the planned surgery. Three main kinds of anesthesia exist.

▌ *General anesthesia* is by far the most common choice for surgical procedures in children. General anesthesia uses drugs that both relieve pain (analgesia) and produce unconsciousness (anesthesia).

▌ *Regional anesthesia* is much less commonly used for young children. With regional anesthesia the patient remains awake and aware during the procedure while pain and sensation are eliminated in the region of the body affected by the procedure. Regional anesthesia may be used, for example, to relieve sensation from the waist down during hernia repair in an infant.

▌ *Conscious sedation* involves giving medication to calm the child during a procedure, such as placing stitches or giving a test such as an EEG (see the Glossary at the end of this book).

As with any medical procedure, anesthesia poses some risks, ranging from minor side effects to life-threatening conditions. But the science of anesthesia has improved considerably in recent years. New and better anesthetic medications with fewer side effects and new equipment with many built-in safeguards and fail-safe devices have reduced the risks of anesthesia to a point where serious side effects are now rare.

On the day of the surgery, tell the hospital staff and the anesthesiologist if your child has a fever, a cold, a cough, a runny nose, any kind of respiratory infection, or the flu. If so, the procedure may be rescheduled for another day.

Once your child is cleared for surgery, the anesthesiologist will determine the choice of anesthetic drugs and their dosages based on many factors, including the child's age, weight, health status, and the type of procedure being performed. Anesthesia is administered continuously during the procedure through intravenous (IV) lines and an inhalation mask, so that there is no chance that your child will wake up during the operation.

What to Bring

When your child is scheduled for surgery, you will need to make sure the hospital or clinic has certain health information about your child. Frequently, a preoperative (preop) appointment is scheduled, and you can bring this information at that time. If not, make sure the hospital or clinic has the following information before your child arrives for surgery:

▎ Your child's medical history, including immunizations and allergies (ask your doctor's office for it just as if you were enrolling your child in camp or school)

▎ Information about previous surgeries or tests, including surgical records and test results

▎ X rays

▎ Blood test results

▎ Insurance information

▎ A written list of medications your child is taking, including prescription, over-the-counter, or any natural or herbal remedies

▎ A copy of court papers designating your legal guardianship (if necessary)

▎ A written list of questions that you or your child has

Also ask your doctor to fax or send your child's most recent medical evaluation and physical exam results ahead of time.

On the Day of Surgery

Eating and Drinking   Check with your hospital or clinic for guidelines for eating and drinking on the day of the surgery. Children's Hospital Boston has the following suggested guidelines for the day of surgery:

For newborns and infants up to age 6 months:

▎ Do not give your baby anything to eat or drink during the 3 hours before surgery.

▎ Your infant should finish eating solid foods (including cereal mixed with formula) 8 hours before surgery.

▎ Your infant should finish the last bottle of formula 6 hours before surgery.

▎ If your infant is breast-feeding, she should finish her last feeding 3 hours before surgery.

▎ Your infant may have breast milk or clear liquids, including infant electrolyte solution, apple juice, or sugar water, up to 3 hours before surgery.

For children age 6 months and older:

▌ Don't give your child anything to eat or drink during the 3 hours before surgery.

▌ Your child should finish eating everything except clear liquids 8 hours before surgery.

▌ Your child may have breast milk or clear liquids, including clear juice drinks, water, and electrolyte solutions, up to 3 hours before surgery.

The Anesthesia Process

Once your child is ready for surgery, the following procedures will be used to administer general anesthesia:

▌ Older infants and children may receive an oral sedative before entering the operating room. Once in the operating room, the anesthesiologist places a clear plastic mask over the child's nose and mouth to begin the administration of anesthesia. Some hospitals even have scents to give the child's anesthetic a pleasant aroma. Your child may be given a choice of strawberry, banana, or other appealing scents.

▌ The anesthesiologist will decide, in collaboration with the family, if a parent or guardian may accompany the child into the operating room to calm and reassure the child. Once the child is unconscious, the parent will be escorted to the waiting area until the surgery is completed.

▌ During the procedure, the anesthesiologist administers a combination of anesthetic drugs at the appropriate dose, using a combination of an IV line and a mask. The anesthesiologist or a designated health professional trained in anesthesia stays with the patient throughout the entire procedure.

▌ Your child will remain unconscious for the entire procedure. Once the surgical procedure is completed, the anesthesia will be discontinued in the operating room and your child will be taken to the recovery room, where you may rejoin her.

▌ Postoperative pain relief will be coordinated by the anesthesiologist.

Seven Ways to Help Your Child Stay Healthy

Keeping your child healthy at all times is an impossible task: As long as children attend school, play with friends, and use public transportation, colds and ear infections, sore throats, and stomachaches will be an inevitable part of childhood. Nevertheless, you can take the following steps to keep your child as healthy as possible.

Your main goal should be to reduce your child's exposure to infection, which the first six steps address. The last step discusses the significant harm of secondhand tobacco smoke on children.

1. If your child goes to day care, check out the center's infection control procedures:

   • Is food handled safely? Is food refrigerated when necessary?

   • Is the diaper-changing area far away from the kitchen?

   • Are toys, cribs, and other surfaces disinfected on a daily basis (and the diaper area after every diaper change)?

   • Do child care workers wash their hands after changing diapers, wiping runny noses, or playing with a sick child?

   • Are beds or cots placed at least 3 feet apart so that children don't cough or sneeze on each other during nap time?

   • If your center falls short on any of these safety tips, talk to the manager about instituting changes, or switch to another center.

2. Instruct your child to wash her hands thoroughly before and after meals, after playing outside or playing with animals, and after using the toilet.

3. Teach your child to use a tissue to catch a sneeze or cough or to clean up a runny nose, then throw the tissue away and thoroughly wash her hands before touching anything else. *Remember:* If all parents and children followed this advice, your child might be exposed to fewer infections in the first place!

4. Discourage your child from sharing drinking glasses or eating utensils with her friends to avoid picking up or passing on an infection.

5. To prevent the spread of head lice, don't allow your child to wear a hat or cap or use a comb, brush, or hair ornament that belongs to another child.

6. Don't send your child to school sick. Take the advice of your child's day care teachers; if they say your child appears ill and should go home, bring her home and evaluate her there.

7. Don't allow anyone to smoke around your child. The increased risk of cancer from cigarette smoke, even so-called secondhand smoke—is well known. What is not as well publicized is the link between secondhand cigarette smoke and the child's increased risk of asthma, allergies, and respiratory tract infections of all kinds.

Preparing for and Handling Emergencies

11

"When my baby had a terrible attack of croup in the middle of the night, she couldn't catch her breath. We took her to the emergency department at 3 A.M."

"The time my daughter fell from the jungle gym and got a cut over her eye, it looked bad because there was so much blood. But the doctor said it wasn't as serious as it looked."

"I never knew what panic was until I realized my son had just swallowed a bunch of my iron supplements. I knew they were dangerous. I usually kept them far from his reach, but I made a mistake. I was glad I had the poison control center's number handy. They saved his life."

Most parents have an emergency story to tell, and often more than one. Hundreds of kinds of emergencies involve young children. According to the National Safety Council, about one-third of the 100 million emergency department visitors each year are children and teenagers—a statistic that probably doesn't surprise most parents, who know how unaware of danger children can be. In the United States, injuries are the leading health problem in children over 1 year old; they cause more deaths in children than all diseases combined and are the leading cause of disability.

This chapter provides tips on preparing for emergencies, keeping your first aid kits up-to-date, recognizing emergencies, and knowing what to do when emergencies occur. Although most accidents are relatively minor, make sure you know how to identify an emergency and distinguish which medical problems can be dealt with at home and which require medical attention. Be sure also to learn the simple first aid techniques that can save your child's life. When accidents happen—and they will happen, no matter how careful you are—knowing what to do can prevent a tragedy.

Top Eight Unintentional Causes of Fatal Injury in Children

0 to 1 Year Old	1 to 4 Years Old	5 to 9 Years Old
1. Suffocation	1. Fire/burns	1. Motor vehicle occupant injury
2. Motor vehicle occupant injury	2. Drowning	2. Pedestrian injury
3. Fire/burns	3. Pedestrian injury	3. Fire/burns
4. Choking	4. Motor vehicle occupant injury	4. Drowning
5. Drowning	5. Choking	5. Bicycle injury
6. Poisoning	6. Suffocation	6. Unintentional firearm injury
7. Pedestrian injury	7. Falls	7. Suffocation
8. Falls	8. Poisoning	8. Falls

Source: National Center for Health Statistics.

BEFORE ACCIDENTS HAPPEN

The first line of defense against accidents and emergencies is prevention: Making your child's surroundings safe is a top priority (see the safety sections in the age-by-age chapters in this book) in order to prevent accidents, both major and minor. Also, taking courses in cardiopulmonary resuscitation (CPR) for children is an important step for all parents.

As your child grows and changes, the safety precautions you will need to take will change with him. The 2-month-old infant who cannot crawl or walk requires different safety precautions from the older, crawling baby or the preschooler starting to play sports. The age-by-age chapters in this book contain a full description of steps you can take to protect your child from accidents at each age level. But here are some safety precautions that apply to children of all ages.

Car Seat Safety

All children under 40 pounds should be securely strapped into a car seat appropriately positioned for their age group. Parents of infants under 20 pounds often use an infant car seat. For information on choosing an infant car seat, see page 24. For the most up-to-date information on car seat safety regulations, contact the National Highway Traffic Safety Administration (see Appendix: Parent Resources, Safety).

The American Academy of Pediatrics recommends that all parents take a minute to check their children's car seats for safety. Here's what to look for:*

1 *Does your car have a passenger-side air bag?*

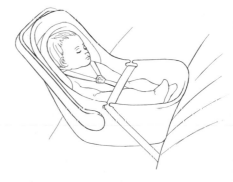

- An infant should never be placed in the front seat of a vehicle that has a passenger-side air bag.

- The safest place for all children to ride is the rear seat.

- If an older child must ride in the front seat of a vehicle that has a passenger-side air bag, place the vehicle seat as far back as possible and buckle the child properly.

---

* Used with permission of the American Academy of Pediatrics, from the All Kids Safe brochure produced by the alliance of Allstate and the American Academy of Pediatrics, 2000.

Car Seat Safety

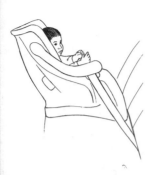

2 *Is your child facing the right way for both weight and age?*

- If you use a seat made only for infants, always face it backward.

- Infants should ride facing the back of the car until they have reached at least 1 year of age and weigh 20 pounds.

- A child over 20 pounds and at least 1 year of age faces forward.

3 *Has your child grown too tall for the convertible or forward-facing seat and is your child at least 40 pounds? Use a booster seat.*

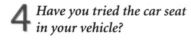

- Use a belt-positioning booster seat to help protect your child until he is big enough to use a seat belt properly.

- A belt-positioning booster seat is used with a lap and shoulder belt.

- Shield boosters, used only with lap belts, are not safe for children over 40 pounds. Children under 40 pounds should use a convertible or forward-facing seat. Shield boosters should only be used without the shield with a lap/shoulder belt.

4 *Have you tried the car seat in your vehicle?*

- Not all car seats fit in all vehicles.

- When the car seat is installed, be sure it does not move side-to-side or toward the front of the car.

- Be sure to read the section on car seats in the owner's manual for your car.

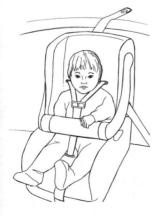

5 *Is the auto seat belt in the right place and pulled tight?*

- Route the seat belt through the correct path (check your instructions to make sure), kneel in the seat to press it down, and pull the belt tight.

- A convertible seat faces backward for an infant and forward for a toddler. It has two different belt paths, one for each direction.

- Check the owner's manual for your car to see if you need to use a locking clip or tethers to help keep the safety seat secure.

6 *Is the harness snug; does it stay on your child's shoulders?*

- The shoulder straps of the car seat go in the lowest slots for infants riding backward and the highest slots for children facing forward.
- The chest clip should be placed at armpit level to keep harness straps on the shoulders.
- Harnesses should fit snugly against your child's body. Check the instructions on how to adjust the straps.

7 *Do you have the instructions for the car seat?*

- Follow them, and keep them with the car seat. You will need them as your child gets bigger.
- Be sure to send in the registration card that comes with the car seat. It will be important if your car seat is recalled.

8 *Has your child's seat been recalled?*

- Call the Auto Safety Hotline at the National Highway Traffic Safety Administration (see Appendix: Parent Resources, Safety) for a list of recalled seats that need repair.
- Be sure to make any necessary repairs to your car seat.

Fire Safety

Making your home safe from fire is an important step in protecting your child from injury. Right from the start, you can take steps such as dressing your child in appropriate, fire-resistant sleepwear.

Sleepwear Safety

You can help protect your child from burns in case of fire by choosing sleepwear that is less likely to catch fire. The Consumer Product Safety Commission recommends that children wear pajamas that are either flame resistant or snug-fitting or both.

Flame-resistant sleepwear has long been considered the safest choice. But new research indicates that cotton pajamas that fit snugly against the skin also protect against burns because they block the flow of oxygen—which fuels a burning fire—next to the skin.

▌ Choose sleepwear that is flame resistant and snug fitting—but not tight and uncomfortable.

▌ Don't allow children to sleep in loose-fitting sweat pants or sweat shirts, bathrobes, or large, oversized T-shirts.

▌ Choose sleepwear with cuffs at wrists and ankles, which block the flow of oxygen and help keep out fire and smoke.

▌ Follow washing instructions for flame-resistant garments.

Making a Fire Safety Plan

Beginning around age 4, tell your child what to do if there's a fire at home. Explain how to get out of the house as fast as possible without stopping to look for family members. Explain what to do if he can't get out: Have him drop to the ground and roll himself in a blanket or rug to shield himself against fire and smoke inhalation until firefighters arrive.

In the United States, more than 1,000 youngsters age 9 and under die in home fires annually. The best way to avoid such a tragedy is to teach your child what to do should a fire start in your home. Warn your child of household dangers, keeping the message simple: "The stove is hot—don't touch." "Matches are only for adults." As your child matures, he can absorb more information. The following paragraphs tell what youngsters need to know and when.

Ages 3 to 5

Teach your child what a smoke detector sounds like and what it means. Tell him not to hide in a closet or under the bed if a detector goes off, but instead to stay near a window and wait for someone to rescue him. Once outside, stress that he should not return to the house for anything, even a pet or a toy. Show him how to crawl under the smoke: Because smoke rises, the air near the floor will be clearer. Teach him your address and phone number, and show him how to dial the emergency number, such as 911—write it on the phone in case he needs to call for help.

Ages 5 and Older

Warn your child that if he smells smoke (at night in his room, for example), he should not open the door until he checks for smoke around the frame. If he sees any, he should go to a window. If he can't see smoke, he should lightly touch the door-knob with his fingertips or feel between the door and the jamb. If the door is cool, he can cautiously open it. If it's warm, he should leave it closed, go to a window, and wait to be rescued.

FAMILY ESCAPE PLAN

Working together with every member of the household, follow these steps.

First, make a plan:

▮ Using a felt marker, draw a floor plan of your house on a large piece of paper or poster board.

▮ Have your children help you identify two escape routes from each room. Mark each exit with a large X. Include windows, doors, and any outdoor features, such as a porch roof or large tree, that may help you and your family get out of the house.

▮ Pick a safe spot well away from the house or building, such as a mailbox, tree, or telephone pole, where family members can meet once they escape from the home. Mark this spot on the plan. Go outside and show your child this spot.

▮ Post the plan on the refrigerator or a centrally located bulletin board.

▮ Make sure everyone knows what to do.

Practice this plan twice a year:

▮ Set off a smoke detector so that your child knows what it sounds like. Explain what it means: Adults and children over age 5 should leave the house immediately, using the designated exits. Younger children should stand by a window and wait for a parent or firefighter to rescue them.

▮ Walk through the house with your family, and point out the exits marked on your floor plan.

▮ Prepare children for the unexpected. Pretend an exit is blocked by smoke, and ask each older child how he would get out.

▮ Everyone should exit from his or her room and meet at the designated safety spot. Children under age 5 should stand by a designated window and wait for rescue. Reiterate that each family member should wait at his or her spot until everyone arrives.

Water Safety

From the kitchen wash bucket to the backyard pool, containers of water present a danger to children. Drowning is among the leading causes of deaths in children of all ages. Water can be dangerous in any location, even in small amounts. Buckets, toilets, and bathtubs are particularly hazardous to infants under 1 year old. Swimming pools, spas, and hot tubs present the greatest risk to children between 1 and 4 years old. Children 5 to 14 years old most frequently drown in open water sites (lakes, rivers, oceans) and swimming pools. Here are some tips for preventing water emergencies:

▌ Never leave your child unsupervised in or near any body of water, even for seconds. This includes everything from toilets, buckets, bathtubs, and wading pools to swimming pools, lakes, and streams.

▌ Empty all containers, such as bowls, buckets, and small tubs, immediately after use, and store them out of your child's reach.

▌ Completely surround swimming pools with fencing at least 5 feet high, with self-latching and self-closing gates. If your neighbor has a pool, be sure that gates and fences are secure.

▌ Furnish your pool area with rescue equipment, emergency numbers, and a telephone. When using a neighbor's pool or a public pool, make sure that rescue equipment and a telephone are available.

▌ Always have your child wear a U.S. Coast Guard–approved personal flotation device when on a boat or near natural bodies of water. Be sure the device fits properly and is fastened correctly. Follow the directions provided on the flotation device.

▌ Learn CPR (see p. 379).

▌ Provide swimming lessons. The American Academy of Pediatrics recommends that children 4 and older have swimming lessons not only for fun but also to help prevent drowning. However, children under 4 may not be developmentally ready for swimming lessons, and parents should not assume that toddlers and preschoolers are safe from drowning because they've participated in swimming lessons.

Foreign Travel Safety

Whether traveling for pleasure or to visit relatives abroad, foreign travel can pose health risks, especially for children. For one thing, some infections (such as travelers' diarrhea, hepatitis A, hepatitis B [see *Hepatitis,* Part 5], and *tuberculosis* [see Part 5]) are more prevalent overseas than in the United States. And children are naturally curious about such things as animals and ponds, which can harbor bacteria and other germs. So if you're planning to take your child to another country, ask your child's doctor what general precautions to take. Also consult your travel agent and check with the U.S. Centers for Disease Control and Prevention Traveler's Hotline for guidelines pertaining to the specific countries you will be visiting (see Appendix: Parent Resources, Safety).

Routine Immunizations

When children travel to developing countries, their risk of exposure to a childhood illness is greater than it is in the United States. At least 8 weeks before your trip, make sure that your child's immunizations are current, and ask whether he should have other routine shots ahead of schedule, or additional vaccinations against such things as hepatitis A.

Water and Food

In developing countries, water may be contaminated with sewage or fecal matter, which may contain bacteria, parasites, viruses, and other germs that cause illness. Don't drink unsterilized tap water or use ice cubes. You can purify tap water by boiling it for 1 minute and then letting it cool to room temperature, or by treating it with water purification tablets. If purification isn't possible, use bottled water for drinking and brushing teeth. Drinking bottled soft drinks is also safe.

Avoid fresh foods, which may be contaminated or washed in contaminated water. These include salads, unpeeled fruits, and seafood.

Travelers' Diarrhea

Travelers' diarrhea, most often caused by *E. coli* bacteria, is the most common medical condition among travelers. Children are most vulnerable to it, as well as to its main complication—dehydration. Avoiding contaminated water and foods is the best hedge against travelers' diarrhea. Pack a commercial oral rehydration solution, and give it to your child at the first sign of diarrhea to reduce the risk of dehydration and to relieve symptoms.

Encourage your child to wash his hands frequently, and be especially watchful to make sure that he doesn't put sand or dirt in his mouth.

Swimming

In tropical regions, don't swim in freshwater ponds, lakes, or rivers, because of the risk of schistosomiasis, a common travelers' illness caused by a parasite that lives on a freshwater snail. Infestation can lead to serious illnesses, such as liver problems and bladder tumors. Other forms of contamination, such as raw sewage, can be found in salt water, including saltwater lakes and ponds. Check with local officials to be sure that swimming areas are not contaminated by infectious agents. Adequately chlorinated swimming pools are the safest option.

Preparing for Emergencies

Panic is a natural and an unavoidable reaction to an emergency situation: Your child is hurt or ill, and all you can think about is making him better. Clearly, you want to stay by his side instead of running to the pharmacy for first aid supplies, looking up a phone number, or racing through town looking for the nearest hospital. Prepare and equip yourself now, so that when an emergency happens, you'll know what to do and have the necessary supplies and phone numbers available.

Preparing for Emergencies

First Aid Kits

Having the necessary supplies on hand will save time and anxiety—possibly even a life—when accidents happen. See page 350 for a list of items every family medicine chest should include. In addition, create one or two portable first aid kits to carry in your car, your camper, and your vacation luggage.

PORTABLE FIRST AID KIT

▌ *Acetaminophen:* Carry a small bottle of acetaminophen with a dropper or medicine spoon to measure the proper dose if you use liquid.

▌ *Plastic bandages:* Carry several sizes.

▌ *Antibiotic cream or ointment:* Use to treat minor cuts and scrapes.

▌ *Syrup of ipecac:* Use in case of poisoning only after speaking with a poison control center or your child's doctor.

▌ *Tweezers:* Use for removing ticks or splinters.

▌ *Rubbing alcohol:* Use (small container or individual packets) as an antiseptic for removing splinters and ticks.

▌ *Sunscreen:* Use sunscreen with a sun protection factor (SPF) of 15 or higher.

Emergency Telephone Numbers

Although 911 is often the only number you need to know in case of a dire emergency, 911 is not available everywhere. Post the following numbers close to the central telephone in your home (usually in the kitchen) and in your office date book or wallet. If you have automatic dialing on your telephone, enter these emergency numbers:

▌ Children's doctor   ▌ Ambulance

▌ Children's dentist   ▌ Fire

▌ Poison control center   ▌ Police

You can usually find a listing for your local poison control center inside the front cover of the white pages of your telephone directory. You can also contact the American Association of Poison Control Centers; see Appendix: Parent Resources, Poison Control.

Know Where to Go

No one wants to have to ask for, and then remember, directions to the emergency department during a crisis. Find out where to take your child if an accident or acute illness strikes while he's at home, at day care, or in school.

UNDERSTAND YOUR EMERGENCY INSURANCE COVERAGE

When it comes to medical emergencies involving your child, the last thing on your mind will be money. Nevertheless, you may avoid the often prohibitive cost of an emergency department visit if you work out the details with your insurance company *before* an accident or acute illness occurs. Ask your insurance company or health plan these questions about emergency care:

▪ *Do you need authorization before going to the emergency department?* Many health plans require you to call ahead in all but the most life-threatening situations.

▪ *Is there a co-payment for emergency treatment?* Many health plans require a co-payment for every emergency department visit. Find out what it is.

▪ *What if an emergency happens away from home?* Within the United States, some health plans allow the hospital to submit claims directly to the plan, so that you won't have to pay up front. However, if you rush to the hospital with a nonurgent condition, you could end up paying part of the bill later.

▪ *What if you're out of the country when an emergency takes place?* Unless you purchase a special traveler's policy, you'll pay on the spot for any medical care received abroad. Some health plans permit you to file a claim after you return, but you'll need complete records of your treatments and the fees charged.

FIRST STEPS IN CASE OF EMERGENCY

Read this section at least once, and then keep this book handy so that you can quickly review these procedures should an accident or acute illness occur.

Evaluating Your Child's Condition

Knowing what to do first may save your child's life. Here are the first steps to take when a serious accident occurs:

1 *Do not move your child.*
The ONLY exception is if the child is in danger of further injury (e.g., lying in traffic, trapped in a burning building).

2 *Make sure your child is breathing.*
Put your face close to his nose and mouth. Can you feel his breath on your face or see his chest moving? If not, begin mouth-to-mouth resuscitation (see p. 380 for an infant or p. 383 for a child) before you attend to other injuries.

3 *Take your child's pulse.*
If no pulse is present, begin CPR as directed on page 380 for an infant or page 383 for a child.

HOW TO TAKE YOUR CHILD'S PULSE

If your child is under 1 year old, place two fingertips over the pulse point on the inside of his upper arm (see illustration, p. 382). An infant's pulse is most easily felt here.

If your child is older than 1 year, place two fingertips over the pulse point on the neck, in the groove beside the Adam's apple (see illustration, p. 385). Do not use your thumb to feel for a pulse, because it has its own pulse.

The following are the normal childhood pulse rates:

Infants (under 1 year)	80–160 beats per minute
Toddlers (1 to 2 years)	80–130 beats per minute
Children (3 to 10 years)	70–130 beats per minute

4 *Check to see if your child is fully conscious.*
If not, turn your child's head to one side to encourage saliva drainage and prevent choking. Do *not* move the head if you suspect a serious head or spinal injury. Try to determine the cause of his unconsciousness, and call for emergency help.

5 *Check for bleeding or other injuries.*
If bleeding is apparent, determine the nature of the bleeding and treat it as necessary (see Bleeding on p. 392). After your child is breathing on his own and the bleeding is under control, treat any other injuries as outlined later in this chapter.

6 *Look for signs of poisoning.*
If you see stains or burns on your child's mouth or pills or other medications or toxic substances nearby, you should suspect poisoning. Call your poison control center, and see Poisoning on page 415 for more instructions.

7 *Call for help.*
Call 911, or if 911 isn't available in your area, call for an ambulance. Be prepared to tell the 911 operator or the health professional what happened. Describe the injuries, your child's general condition, and the state of your child's vital functions and systems, including:

Airway:	Is he coughing, choking, or wheezing?
Respiration:	Is he breathing quickly or slowly?
Pulse:	Is it rapid or slow?
Circulation:	Is he pale or flushed? Are his lips or fingernails blue? Is he bleeding?
Consciousness:	Is he awake? Is he irritated or inconsolable?

8 *Follow the instructions given by the 911 operator or health professional.*
If you're alone with a child who needs constant first aid attention, you will probably be told to stay put and wait for help. In other cases, you may be told to drive your child to the hospital yourself.

9 *Remain as calm as possible.*
By doing so, you'll help your child stay calm as well. The calmer he is, the less pain and discomfort he is likely to feel.

The ABCs of CPR

CPR (cardiopulmonary resuscitation) is a method of restarting a child's breathing and heartbeat using mouth-to-mouth rescue breathing and chest compressions. The reason a child's heart stops is rarely due to heart disease, but instead is more likely caused by a lack of oxygen to the heart muscle caused by a breathing problem. Breathing problems may be caused by suffocation, near drowning, an injury, an airway obstruction, or a lung disease. Once a child stops breathing, the heart may soon stop beating. Quickly restarting a child's breathing using the rescue breathing techniques in this section may prevent cardiac arrest (when the heart stops beating). Chest compressions are a way of helping oxygen-rich blood move through the rest of the body. If CPR is started quickly and emergency personnel arrive swiftly, the child's chances of survival are increased.

CPR includes three basic skills, known as the ABCs of CPR: airway, breathing, and circulation. These skills are explained in the sections below.

Airway

When a child loses consciousness, the muscles relax and the tongue falls backward into the airway, possibly blocking the passage. Because of this, the first step in reviving an unconscious child is to open the airway. You can usually open the airway by tilting the head back, placing two fingers under the chin, and lifting it up and out (see illustration, p. 380). This causes the tongue and its attachments to lift from the back of the throat.

Breathing

When breathing stops, fresh oxygen cannot circulate to the heart muscle and cardiac arrest may follow quickly. Once the airway is cleared, mouth-to-mouth rescue breathing can deliver oxygen to the lungs and heart to prevent cardiac arrest. If the victim's heart is beating, mouth-to-mouth breathing every 3 seconds will supply sufficient oxygen. If the heartbeat has stopped, you will have to perform breathing and chest compressions. That is why it is important to first determine whether the child is breathing and next determine whether the heart is beating.

Circulation

The third skill of CPR is chest compressions, which help circulate blood and maintain some blood flow to the lungs and other vital organs when the heart has stopped beating. Chest compressions must be accompanied by rescue breathing or by breathing provided with a respirator or other emergency medical equipment.

STEP-BY-STEP CPR FOR INFANTS UNDER 1 YEAR OLD

1 *Determine if your child is unresponsive, and shout for help.*

How: Gently tap or shake your baby's shoulder. Do not begin CPR if your infant is asleep. If help arrives, have that person call 911 or an emergency number.

Reason: Shouting for help will summon a person nearby to call for emergency personnel while allowing you to start CPR.

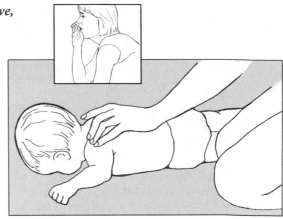

2 *Place your infant on his back on a firm surface.*

How: Turn your infant as a unit, supporting the head and neck. If you suspect a head or neck injury, be especially careful not to bend or turn the neck.

Reason: For CPR to be effective, your baby must be flat on his back on a firm surface.

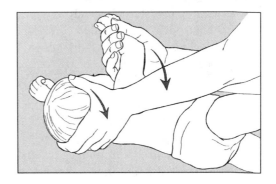

3 *Open the airway (head-tilt/chin-lift).*

How: Lift the chin up and out gently with one hand while pushing down on the forehead with the other to gently tilt the head back. Don't close the mouth. If you suspect a head or spinal injury, open the airway by placing fingers under each side of the jawbone and lifting gently.

Reason: An infant may be unable to breathe because the tongue is blocking the airway.

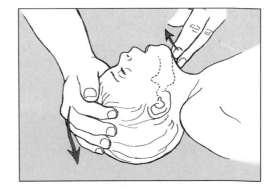

4 *Determine if your infant is breathing.*

How: Turn your head toward your infant's chest with your ear directly over and near the mouth. Listen for the sound of breathing. Feel for breath on your cheek. Watch the chest for movement.

Reason: Hearing and feeling the breath are the best ways to determine whether your baby is breathing. If you see chest movement but don't feel or hear breathing, your infant's airway may be blocked. Do not perform rescue breathing if your baby is breathing.

5 *If your infant is not breathing, give 2 to 5 slow breaths (1½ seconds per breath). Watch for your infant's chest to rise.*

How: Maintain pressure on your infant's forehead to keep the head tilted. With your other hand, lift the chin. Open your mouth wide, and take a deep breath. Cover your baby's mouth and nose with your mouth, making a tight seal. Breathe into your baby's mouth 2 to 5 times, completely filling your lungs with air between breaths. Watch for your infant's chest to rise. If breaths do not cause your infant's chest to rise, the airway is blocked; repeat head-tilt/chin-lift (step 3), and try again. If the chest does not rise with the rescue breath, start the relief-of-obstructed-airway sequence on page 398.

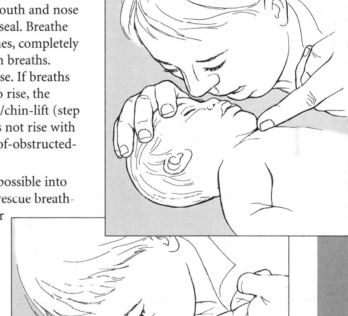

Reason: Getting as much oxygen as possible into your infant is important. If your rescue breathing is effective, you will (1) feel air going in as you blow, (2) feel the air leaving your own lungs, and (3) see your infant's chest rise and fall.

The most common cause of an obstructed airway is that the airway has not been properly opened: Repeat step 3.

6 *Feel for a pulse inside the upper arm.*

How: Place two or three fingers on the inside of your infant's arm, between the elbow and shoulder. Press gently on the inside of the arm with your index and middle fingers. Maintain head tilt with the other hand. Feel for the pulse.

If you can feel a pulse but your infant is not breathing, perform emergency breathing (step 5) at a rate of 20 times per minute.

If no pulse is present, start chest compressions (step 7).

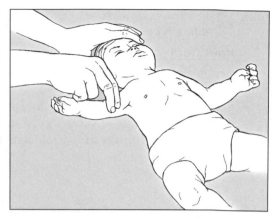

Reason: If the heart is beating effectively, you should feel a strong, rapid pulse within a few seconds. If you do not feel a pulse, begin chest compressions (step 7).

7 *If no pulse is present, begin chest compressions.*

How: Imagine a line across your infant's chest from one nipple to the other. Place two or three fingers on the breastbone about one finger's width below that line. Make sure your fingers are on the breastbone, not below it. Compress the chest downward about 1 to 1½ inches at a rate of 100 times a minute. Compress smoothly and evenly, and release pressure between compressions to allow the chest to return to its normal position. Do not lift your fingers off the chest. Count to maintain a rhythm: "One-two-three-four-five-breathe."

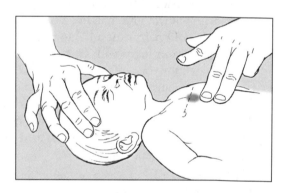

Reason: Proper finger placement will maximize the effectiveness of the compressions and minimize the risk of injury to your infant. Your goal with each compression is to squeeze the heart and increase pressure within the chest so that blood moves to the vital organs.

8 *Give 5 compressions and 1 breath.*

How: After every 5 compressions, deliver 1 rescue breath (step 5). Pause briefly after each 5 compressions to deliver the breath.

Reason: The infant must receive oxygen during chest compressions.

9 *Call 911 or an emergency number at the end of 20 cycles (20 rescue breaths).*

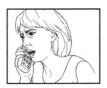

How: Know your emergency numbers. If a second person is available, have him telephone the emergency number while you continue CPR. If you are alone, perform CPR for about 1 minute before calling.

Reason: Notifying emergency personnel at this time allows you to give complete information about your infant's condition.

10 *After the emergency call has been made, resume chest compressions. Check every few minutes for the return of the pulse.*

How: If the pulse returns, check for spontaneous breathing.

If there is no breathing, give 1 rescue breath every 3 seconds (20 breaths per minute), and monitor the pulse.

If breathing resumes, maintain an open airway, and monitor breathing and pulse.

If pulse and breathing resume and are regular and no evidence of trauma exists, turn your infant on his side, continue to monitor breathing and pulse, and await rescue personnel.

Reason: It is important to continue to monitor the baby's breathing and pulse while awaiting the arrival of emergency personnel.

STEP-BY-STEP CPR FOR CHILDREN 1 TO 8 YEARS OLD

1 *Determine if your child is unresponsive, and shout for help.*

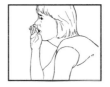

How: Tap or gently shake your child's shoulder. Ask loudly, "Are you OK?" If help arrives, have someone call 911 or an emergency number.

Reason: You should not begin CPR unnecessarily if the child is asleep. Shouting for help will summon people nearby and allow you to begin CPR if necessary.

2 *Position your child on his back on a firm, hard surface.*

How: Turn your child's body as a unit, supporting head, neck, and back. If you suspect a head, neck, or back injury, be especially careful not to bend or turn the neck or back.

Reason: For CPR to be effective, the child must be flat on his back on a firm, hard surface.

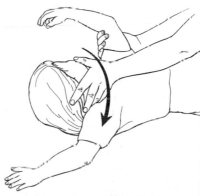

3 *Open the airway* (head-tilt/chin-lift).

How: Kneel beside your child's shoulders. Lift your child's chin up gently with one hand while pushing down on his forehead with the other to gently tilt the head back. Do not close the mouth. If you suspect a head or neck injury, open the airway by placing your fingers under each side of your child's jaw and gently lifting up.

Reason: The airway must be opened to determine whether your child is breathing. Children may be unable to breathe because the tongue is obstructing the airway.

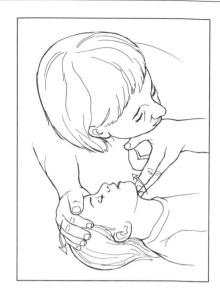

4 *Determine if your child is breathing.*

How: Maintain an open airway. Turn your head toward your child's chest with your ear directly over and close to your child's mouth.

Listen for the sounds of breathing.

Feel for breathing on your cheek.

Look at the chest for movement.

Reason: Hearing and feeling the breath are the best ways to determine whether your child is breathing. If you see chest movement, but you cannot feel or hear air, the airway may still be blocked. Do not perform rescue breathing if your child is breathing effectively. If he is breathing, then the airway is not blocked.

5 *If your child is not breathing, provide rescue breathing. Give 2 to 5 rescue breaths (1½ seconds per breath). Watch for the rise of the chest with each breath.*

How: Pinch your child's nostrils closed with your thumb and forefinger while maintaining pressure on your child's forehead with the same hand. Lift the chin with the other hand. Open your mouth wide, take in a deep breath, and make a tight seal over his mouth. Breathe into your child's mouth 2 to 5 times, completely refilling your lungs between breaths. Watch for his chest to rise. Give each rescue breath for about 1½ seconds, allowing the lungs to deflate

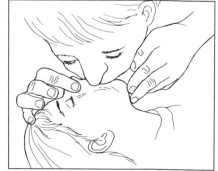

between breaths. If the rescue breaths do not cause your child's chest to rise, the airway is obstructed. Reposition the head, lift the chin, and try again. If unsuccessful, see the clearing-of-obstructed-airway sequence on page 403.

Reason: It is important to get as much oxygen as possible into the child. If your rescue breathing is effective you will (1) feel air going in as you blow, (2) feel the air leaving your own lungs, and (3) see the child's chest rise and fall.

The most common cause of an obstructed airway is that the airway has not been properly opened: Repeat step 3.

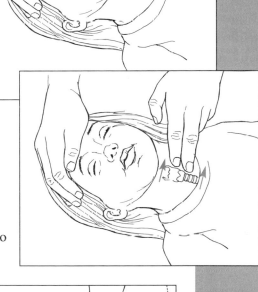

6 *Feel for your child's pulse.*

How: Using the hand at your child's chin, place two or three fingers on his Adam's apple (voice box) just below his chin. Slide the fingers into the groove between the Adam's apple and the neck muscle on the side of the neck near you. Maintain the head tilt with your other hand. Feel for a pulse.

If you feel a pulse and breathing has not resumed, perform rescue breathing (step 5) at a rate of 20 times per minute.

If no pulse is present, start chest compressions (step 7).

Reason: You should not perform chest compressions if a pulse is present.

7 *If no pulse is present, begin the first cycle of chest compressions.*

How: Move the hand that is not maintaining the head tilt to your child's chest. Place the heel of your hand on the lower half of the breastbone (sternum). Do not place your hand over the very bottom of the breastbone. Place your hand two finger-widths above the bottom of the sternum. Compress the chest downward about 1 to 1½ inches at a rate of about 100 times per minute. Compress smoothly and evenly, keeping your fingers off your child's ribs.

Between compressions, release pressure and allow the chest to return to its normal position, but do not lift your hand off the chest. Count to establish a rhythm: "One-two-three-four-five-breathe."

Reason: Proper hand placement is important to maximize effective compressions and minimize the risk of injury to the child. The goal of each compression is to squeeze the heart and increase the pressure within the chest so that blood moves to the vital organs.

8 *Give 5 compressions and 1 breath.*

How: After every 5 compressions deliver 1 rescue breath (step 5).

Reason: The child must receive adequate oxygen.

9 *Call 911 or an emergency number at the end of 20 rescue breaths (approximately 1 minute of CPR).*

How: Know your local emergency number. If a second person is available, have him call local emergency personnel immediately.

Reason: Notifying emergency personnel at this time allows you to give complete information about your child's condition.

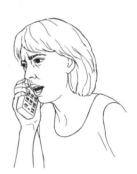

10 *Resume CPR, beginning with chest compressions. Check every few minutes for return of pulse.*

How: If pulse returns, check for spontaneous breathing.

If your child isn't breathing, give 1 rescue breath every 3 seconds (20 breaths per minute), and monitor pulse.

If pulse does *not* return, continue rescue breathing and chest compressions.

If breathing resumes, maintain an open airway and monitor breathing and pulse.

If pulse and breathing resume and are regular and no evidence of trauma exists, turn your child on his side, continue to monitor breathing and pulse, and await emergency personnel.

Reason: It is important to continue to monitor breathing and pulse while awaiting the arrival of emergency personnel. If breathing or pulse stops, resume rescue breathing or chest compressions.

Transporting an Injured Child

In most cases of serious injury, it's best to wait until medical help arrives before moving your child. However, if you need to move your child out of danger or if you are in a remote area or otherwise unable to wait for help, follow these tips:

▪ Give emergency treatment before moving an injured child: Establish breathing (see pp. 384–385), control bleeding (see p. 393), splint fractures (see p. 410), and provide any other lifesaving measures, including CPR (see pp. 379–386).

▪ Carry the stretcher to the injured child, not the child to the stretcher.

▪ If necessary, tie the child to the stretcher so that he won't fall off.

▪ If a commercial stretcher is not available, make one by using a door (be sure splinters and nails are removed) or by using two strong poles with a blanket or other firm material drawn taut between them. If no spinal injury is suspected, a blanket alone can serve as a stretcher, with two sides rolled to provide a grip for carriers.

▪ Bend at the knees, and lift the stretcher gradually, with weight evenly distributed, to avoid injuring your back.

WHEN YOU SUSPECT A HEAD, NECK, OR SPINAL INJURY . . .

▪ Immobilize the child's head between two pillows or rolled-up articles of clothing.

▪ Support the whole length of the child's body as much as possible when you lift him, making sure his head is on the same level as his body. Keep the body lying straight.

Do not . . .

▪ move the injured child unless it is absolutely necessary to save his life.

▪ raise the child's head for any reason.

▪ place pillows or other supports under the head, as this may cause irreparable spinal injury.

▪ let the child's head dangle.

▪ lift the child by the head and heels.

▪ bend the child's spine forward.

See Spinal Injuries, page 419.

When to Go to the Emergency Department

Go to the emergency department immediately if

▪ your child is struggling for breath.

▪ your child has a bone or joint injury, swelling, pain, or deformity.

▪ your child is experiencing serious allergic reactions; is struggling for breath or is wheezing; or has lip and mouth swelling, a spreading rash or hives, and/or diarrhea.

▌ your child is having seizures (convulsions): eyes rolling back, brief loss of consciousness, jerking movements of extremities.

▌ your child has been underwater for more than a few seconds, even if he looks fine.

▌ your child has had a permanent tooth knocked out.

▌ your child has burns to the face, hands, feet, or genitals or any burn larger than the size of his fist.

▌ your child has been exposed to smoke or toxic fumes and has difficulty breathing.

▌ your child has deep or extensive cuts: gaping margins revealing deeper structures; cuts on face, hands, or genitals (see p. 393); uncontrollable bleeding.

▌ your child has had a head injury and a loss of consciousness (even a brief one), confusion, a severe headache, and/or repeated vomiting.

▌ your child is behaving unusually: she is drowsy or confused or is crying inconsolably.

▌ signs of poisoning are present or you know that your child ingested a potentially poisonous substance (call the poison control center).

What to Expect at the Emergency Department

Once you have called your child's doctor, you may find yourself on the way to the emergency department. As you enter the hospital, you may breathe a sigh of relief: Your child is in the hands of professionals.

But then you're asked to wait for what seems like an eternity—even though you suspect that your child broke his wrist when he fell off the backyard swing. The nurse you spoke with at the check-in desk is called a triage nurse. The job of a triage nurse is to sort out the patients who enter the emergency department according to the urgency of their condition. The type of illness or injury, its severity, and the facilities and staff available are the factors the triage nurse uses to rank patients who come into the emergency department. Three basic categories of emergency cases exist:

▌ *Emergent* cases are those in which children are considered at risk for immediate, permanent damage or death. These true emergencies include problems with a child's airway (he's choking, for instance) or with inadequate circulation, asthma attacks, heart problems, signs of internal or severe external bleeding, seizures, loss of consciousness, and severe pain.

▌ *Urgent* cases, such as children with abdominal pain, broken bones, or bad cuts, should be seen within an hour or as soon as possible.

▌ *Routine* cases, including children with ordinary illnesses and injuries, such as scrapes, bruises, fever, and ear infections, are seen as soon as possible.

Helping Your Child Cope

The way an emergency is defined means that your child is probably in some pain and distress. The treatment he must undergo to resolve his medical problems may also be painful, or at least unpleasant. The most crucial ingredient during this stressful time is your attitude and demeanor. If you stay calm, your child has a better chance of handling the situation himself. It's normal to become anxious and upset, but try not to communicate your anxiety to your child. If you are upset, a doctor or nurse may ask you to step outside the procedure room until your emotions are under control. Once you feel strong and settled, follow these tips to reassure and comfort your child:

▌ Stay with your child as much as possible.

▌ Soothe your child with simple explanations.

▌ Ask a nurse for help whenever you need to take a break.

▌ Describe your child's pain honestly, and allow your child to cry.

▌ Stay calm and focused on your child as much as possible. Your fear will frighten him.

▌ Speak up. Don't be afraid to ask questions about procedures or to ask for a second opinion.

If you and your child are in a pediatric hospital, ask whether a child-life specialist works there. These specialists are trained to help children cope with medical settings. They have access to many toys, books, and videos that may distract your child from the problem, or they can help explain to your child what a trip to the emergency department is all about.

COMMON CHILDHOOD EMERGENCIES

Allergic Shock (Anaphylaxis)

Allergic reactions to foods, medicines, insect bites, or stings usually develop rapidly (often within 30 to 60 minutes, sometimes within 30 to 60 seconds!) and can affect your child's entire body. Such reactions can occur in a child who receives his first dose of medication (such as penicillin) or who eats a new food (such as shellfish) for the first time. Anaphylactic shock is the most severe allergic reaction. It usually occurs within seconds or minutes of your child's coming into contact with an allergen—a substance to which your child is allergic. Future exposure to the food or drug usually causes a worse reaction.

Once you know that your child has a particular allergy, it is critical to avoid exposure to the substance that triggers it. But if your child is exposed unexpectedly, this section will tell you how to recognize anaphylactic shock and what to do.

▌Here are some foods that can trigger anaphylactic shock:

Legumes (peanuts, beans, peas)	Eggs
Shellfish (crab, crayfish, shrimp, lobster)	Fish
Nuts (cashews, almonds, pecans, walnuts)	Wheat
Seeds (sesame, sunflower, poppy, cotton)	Milk
Spices (cinnamon, nutmeg, mustard, sage)	Corn
Fruits (apples, bananas, peaches, oranges)	Chocolate
Potatoes	

▌The following medicines can also trigger anaphylactic shock:

Allergy extracts	Insulin
Antibiotics	Local anesthetics
Aspirin	Nonsteroidal anti-inflammatory agents
Corticosteroids	Opiates
Dextran	Protamine
Human gamma globulin	Vaccines (tetanus, measles, mumps)
Heparin	

Signs and Symptoms

▌Flushed skin or bluish gray skin

▌Hives (rash of red, raised, itchy areas of skin)

▌Swelling of any part of the body, especially the face, lips, and tongue

▌Difficult or noisy breathing due to swelling in the throat

▌Tightness in the chest; wheezing

▌A sudden sense of anxiety

▌Itchiness in addition to any of the other symptoms

▌Seizures

▌Confusion, loss of consciousness

▌Shock (dizziness, confusion, rapid pulse)

 Call for emergency help if . . .
your child shows any of the signs of allergic shock.

What to Do

▌Inject your child with epinephrine to control more serious allergic reactions if you know your child is in allergic shock and you have access to an autoinjector. Autoinjectors with a preloaded dose of the drug are prescribed to children at high risk for such reactions.

■ Check your child's airway, breathing, and circulation (see pp. 377–378).

■ Begin CPR, if necessary (see pp. 380 and 383).

■ Call for help, or get someone else to do so. Don't leave your child.

■ Continue CPR until your child is breathing on his own or until help arrives.

■ Give an antihistamine if your child is conscious and you are so instructed by a physician.

Preventing Allergic Reactions

Once you and your doctor identify the substance to which your child has developed a severe allergy, do everything in your power to protect your child from being exposed to the substance. Sometimes an allergist may recommend a series of desensitization injections over time to lessen your child's reactivity to the substance (bee stings, for example). Make sure your child always wears a medical alert necklace or bracelet that identifies the allergy to rescuers and health care workers, in case you're not around when an emergency occurs. For more on determining what triggers your child's allergies and protecting your child from allergic reactions, see *Allergies,* Part 5.

Amputations (Loss of Fingers, Toes, Limbs)

A terrifying, but fairly common, accident involves the loss or crushing of a fingertip or a toe. Get to the emergency department quickly, to increase the chances that the severed or partially severed digit (finger or toe) or limb can be reattached. Bring the severed digit or limb with you, and, if possible, have someone notify the emergency department that you are on the way.

What to Do

■ Control the bleeding (see p. 393).

■ Watch for signs of shock (pallor, dizziness, confusion, and then unconsciousness).

■ Wrap the severed digit or limb in a dry, clean cloth or plastic wrap. Place it in a plastic bag, and pack the bag in cold water or keep it in a cool place.

Do not ...

■ freeze or pack the digit or limb directly in ice, as that can damage blood vessels and other tissue.

If the Limb or Digit Is Partially Severed

Fortunately, if a toe, finger, or limb is only partially severed, the chances of reattachment are high. Reattachment of a fully severed digit or limb is more difficult but can be successful, depending on the size of the severed piece and how quickly your child arrives at the emergency department.

Bleeding

The sight of blood can terrify a child—and you—but most cuts and scrapes children receive are no cause for alarm, even if they bleed profusely. Bleeding is not always obvious, however. A sharp or crushing blow to the abdomen (such as from a fall or from an auto accident) can cause internal bleeding. As you deal with a bleeding emergency, reassure and comfort your child—calming him can slow the flow of blood to the site.

Signs and Symptoms

Symptoms of external bleeding:

▌ Blood pumps or spurts from the wound with each heartbeat (artery cut)

▌ Blood steadily oozes or runs out of the wound (vein cut)

▌ Child shows signs of shock (pallor, dizziness, confusion, or unconsciousness due to loss of blood)

Symptoms of internal bleeding:

▌ Vomit containing specks or streaks of bright red blood or a "coffee ground"–colored material

▌ Child complains of abdominal discomfort after trauma to the abdomen or after a motor vehicle accident

▌ Stools streaked with blood or appearing black, like tar

▌ Child coughs up mucus with specks or streaks of bright red blood

▌ Signs of shock (pallor, dizziness, confusion, or unconsciousness)

 Call for emergency help if . . .

▌ your child is in shock (pallor, dizziness, confusion, or unconsciousness).

▌ bleeding is severe or the wound is gaping.

▌ your child has symptoms of internal bleeding.

What to Do After Calling for Help

▌ Don't leave your child.

▌ Have your child lie still and keep calm.

▌ If head or spinal injury is suspected, do not move your child (see Spinal Injuries, p. 419).

External Bleeding

The first thing to do for external bleeding is to apply pressure. Using gauze or a clean cloth, apply pressure to the wound for at least 2 minutes.

Next, assess the severity of the wound: Hold the cut under cold tap water, or gently pour water from a cup over the wound to make it easier to see. Determine whether an artery or a vein has been cut.

If an artery is cut (see p. 392), place a dressing or clean cloth over the wound immediately, and press with both hands. The pressure must be forceful and continuous, applied with the palms. Steady pressure may cause the child some pain, but is absolutely necessary. If the compress becomes soaked with blood, add a new compress on top of the old one. Do not remove the old compress because you don't want to remove blood clots that have already formed.

If a vein is cut (see p. 392), place thick, sterile compresses or cloths over the wound and apply direct pressure. This type of wound clots more easily than a wound in which an artery was cut, since the blood is oozing steadily, rather than spurting with force. If the compress becomes soaked with blood, add a fresh one on top of the old one. Again, you'll want to be careful not to disturb any forming blood clots.

Finally, lift the bleeding limb or area above the level of the child's heart, without relaxing pressure. Do not do this if the child has extreme pain or evidence of fractures (see p. 409). If the bleeding is from the head, raise the head and shoulders above the heart, unless a spinal or neck injury is suspected.

Do not . . .

▌ move the child if a neck or spinal injury is possible.

▌ release pressure until 10 minutes have passed. If bleeding does not slow down significantly, do not release pressure until you reach the emergency department.

▌ remove bandage dressings.

▌ tie a tight tourniquet or any form of constriction band around a limb.

Deep Cut

Always take your child to the emergency room or doctor's office for immediate medical attention if he gets a deep cut on his hands, face, or genitals; if the cut has gaping edges and is longer than ¼ inch to ½ inch; or if blood is coming from his eye or ear. These areas take special care to be repaired without loss of function and with minimal scarring.

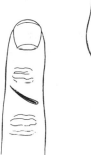
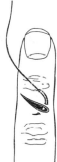
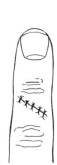

Burns *(side tab)*

Internal Bleeding

▌ Call for emergency help.

▌ Do not give your child anything to eat or drink.

▌ Keep your child lying still; reassure him and keep him as quiet as possible.

▌ Cover him with a blanket or jacket for warmth.

▌ Assess for other injuries. If a head or spinal injury is suspected, do not move your child (see Spinal Injuries, p. 419).

▌ Treat shock (see p. 418).

Burns

Burns are common injuries. More than 27,000 children are hospitalized each year with burn injuries, and another 40,000 are treated in emergency departments, doctor's offices, and clinics. More than half of childhood burns occur in children under 4 years old. In most cases, burns can be treated successfully and leave no permanent damage, but be sure to act quickly if your child is burned.

Burns can be caused by fire, chemicals, heated objects, radiation (from the sun), fluids, or electricity. They can be a minor problem or a major medical emergency. Only small and superficial burns should be treated at home. More severe burns carry the risk of infection, scarring, and shock (see p. 418) and must be treated immediately by emergency personnel.

Signs and Symptoms

▌ Red, raw skin areas

▌ Local swelling

▌ Fluid-filled clear or yellow blisters

▌ A blackened area within a burned area

 Call for emergency help if . . .

▌ the burn is larger than your child's fist.

▌ an extensive burn involves the hands, feet, face, or genitals.

▌ the burn is dirty or appears infected.

▌ second-degree or third-degree burns are present.

Types of Burns

▌ *First-degree burns* are the least serious, because they damage only the top skin layer, causing it to redden and become raw. Although somewhat painful, they usually heal by themselves without needing medical treatment. See page 396 for information on pain relief.

▌ *Second-degree burns* damage both the first layer of skin and the second layer (called the dermis). The area around the burn swells, and fluid-filled blisters develop. Second-degree burns are painful, but usually do not lead to infection or scarring. Nevertheless, be sure to bring your child to the doctor for treatment, especially if the burn is large and/or affects his hands or face.

▌ *Third-degree burns* are the most serious and always require immediate medical attention. They destroy all layers of the skin and may extend into deeper tissues. Patches of skin may appear blackened and charred. Fat, muscles, and even bones may be damaged. Because nerve tissue may be destroyed at the same time, many third-degree burns are often painless until the healing process begins.

What to Do

First, make sure that the cause of the burn has been extinguished or removed. For instance, if your child's clothing is on fire, have him drop to the ground and roll around, or wrap a blanket around him, until the fire is smothered. If a toxic chemical or scalding water spilled on your child's clothing, remove the clothing immediately, or your child's skin will continue to burn. Then, wash the injured skin with cool water.

Next, evaluate the severity of the burn. If it produced anything more serious than a superficial redness of the skin, call your child's doctor immediately for advice. She may advise you to take your child to the office or an emergency department for evaluation and treatment.

Do not . . .

▌ attempt to treat a serious burn at home.

▌ apply any butter or ointments or break open any blisters.

Treating First-Degree Burns

▌ Cool the affected area by placing it under tepid or cool running water for about 10 to 20 minutes, or for as long as your child will tolerate it.

▌ Cover it with a sterile cotton bandage. The area may be tender for several hours, even a few days, but as long as the pain does not worsen and signs of infection don't appear, the wound will heal on its own.

▌ Check with a nurse or doctor for even a mild burn if it is larger than a half-dollar. Sometimes doctors will recommend a tetanus shot for larger, dirty burns or for second- or third-degree burns.

Do not...

▌ apply butter, cream, or petroleum jelly to the burn. These products may slow healing and increase the chance of infection.

▌ apply local anesthetic creams or sprays, as they may also cause allergic reactions or slow healing.

▌ break open any blisters that have formed. This will only increase the risk of infection.

Pain Relief for Mild Burns

First-degree burns, although not severe, can be quite painful. To reduce the pain, keep the affected area raised slightly to decrease blood flow to the area. You can also give acetaminophen or ibuprofen by mouth to diminish the pain.

Treating Second-Degree Burns

Second-degree burns are usually caused by hot liquids, grease, or caustic chemicals, or sometimes by touching a direct flame. Follow these procedures when treating a second-degree burn:

▌ Cool the affected area by placing your child in the bathtub or by using a garden hose or bucket of water to rinse the burned area. Keep the area submerged for 5 to 10 minutes or until the pain subsides.

▌ Cut off any clothing contaminated with hot grease or burning chemicals.

▌ Gently wash off any dirt, chemicals, or other contaminants.

▌ Gently pat the wound dry with a sterile cloth, taking care not to break any blisters.

▌ If an eye is burned, rinse it out gently in the shower, or place your child's face under running tap water. If chemicals are near or in the child's eye, turn the head to keep the injured side down so that water won't wash chemicals into the unaffected eye.

▌ Create a barrier to prevent contamination from dirt or bacteria by loosely covering the burn with gauze or sterile bandages.

▌ Seek medical attention as soon as possible.

Treating Third-Degree Burns

Third-degree burns are usually caused by prolonged exposure to direct flame or electricity. Third-degree burns may be life-threatening. To treat third-degree burns, follow these steps:

▌ Remove your child from harm.

▌ Call for help.

▌ Check for a pulse and breathing. If necessary, start CPR (see p. 379).

▌ Check for and treat shock (see p. 418). Keep your child warm with blankets, and raise his legs above his heart.

▌ Check for and treat bleeding (see p. 392) or other injuries.

▌ Treat burns with cool, wet dressings as described for second-degree burns.

▌ If medical help is delayed, cover your child with a sterile or clean sheet, blanket, or towel to keep him warm and quiet. Do not give any liquids.

SPECIAL SITUATIONS

Follow these recommendations for the following situations:

▌ *Electrocution:* Do not grab a child who has fallen on live electrical wires. Call for help to turn off the power. Use a wooden pole, a rubber sheet, or another nonconductive material to push the child to safety.

▌ *House fire:* Cover your mouth and nose with a wet cloth. Stay close to the ground below the smoke. Move the child to the nearest exit. (See p. 371 for information on fire safety.)

▌ *Clothes on fire:* Use the stop, drop, and roll technique: Cover the child with a blanket or jacket, drop him to the ground, and roll him back and forth until the flames are extinguished. Prevent a child who is on fire from running around.

Choking and Suffocation

Choking and suffocation are two of the top causes of fatal injury in infants and among the most common causes of fatal injury in children. Choking occurs when the airway to the lungs is obstructed by a piece of food, a toy, or any swallowed object. Suffocation is caused by any blockage of the nose, mouth, windpipe, or air passages that restricts breathing.

If your child is choking, see whether he can dislodge the piece of food or other object by coughing before you take any action. If he is breathing and coughing, don't interfere—in this situation, your child's coughing is a more effective way to dislodge an object than anything you can do. If the airway is completely blocked and your child is not breathing, you will need to take action.

Choking and Suffocation: Conscious Infant

Signs and Symptoms

▮ Gasping for breath

▮ Inability to speak

▮ Turning blue

▮ No signs of breathing

▮ Unconsciousness

 Call for emergency help if . . .

▮ your child has any symptom of choking or suffocation.

What to Do

If your child's breathing is completely obstructed, call for an ambulance (or ask someone else to call). Then, follow the steps for clearing the obstructed airway listed here. Be sure to follow the directions specific to your child's age and condition. An infant's body is different from an older child's in many ways. For instance, pay special attention to holding your infant's neck steady as you apply first aid; this is unnecessary in an older child because the neck muscles are more fully developed.

Conscious Infant: Clearing the Obstructed Airway

1 *Determine whether your infant's airway is completely blocked.*

How: Look for breathing difficulty, an ineffective cough or a lack of coughing, a dusky skin color, or an inability to make sounds. If your infant can cough or cry, do not interfere with his attempts to expel the object.

Reason: It is important to determine whether the airway is completely blocked, because if your infant is still breathing and coughing effectively, your attempts to help may actually make things worse.

2 *If your infant is unable to cry or cough effectively, position him correctly.*

How: Supporting your infant's head and neck with one hand, firmly holding the jaw, place your infant facedown on your forearm, keeping his head lower than the rest of his body.

Reason: You must hold your infant's head firmly to avoid injuring him.

3 *Give up to 5 back blows.*

How: With the heel of your free hand, give up to 5 back blows forcefully between your infant's shoulder blades.

Reason: Back blows increase pressure in the airway and may dislodge the object.

4 *Give up to 5 chest thrusts over the lower half of the sternum.*

How: Supporting your infant's head, sandwich him between your hands and arms and turn him on his back, keeping the head lower than the trunk. Using two or three fingers, deliver up to 5 thrusts over the lower half of the breastbone, just below nipple level. Make sure your fingers are not pushing on the very bottom of the breast-bone.

Reason: Chest thrusts can force air upward into the airway from the lungs with enough pressure to expel the object.

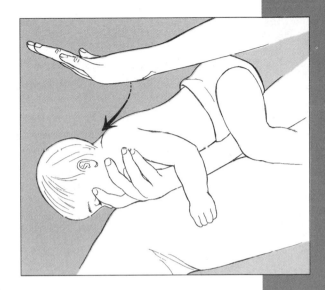

5 *Repeat the sequence of 5 back blows and 5 chest thrusts until the object is expelled or until your infant falls unconscious (see Unconscious Infant, below). Be persistent!*

How: Alternate these maneuvers in rapid sequence: back blows/chest thrusts/back blows/chest thrusts, and so forth.

Reason: It's important to keep going. As your infant becomes more oxygen-deprived, the airway muscles will relax and maneuvers that were previously ineffective may become effective.

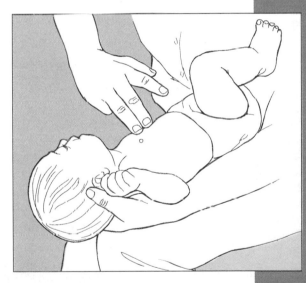

Unconscious Infant: Clearing the Obstructed Airway

1 *Determine if your infant is unconscious. Shout for help. Stay with your infant.*

How: Tap or gently shake your baby's shoulder. Send someone to call for emergency help.

Reason: Shouting will alert bystanders but allow you to stay with your infant.

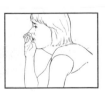

2 *Position your infant on his back.*

How: Turn the baby as a unit, supporting his head and neck.

Reason: This will protect the spine and neck from injury.

3 *Open the airway by performing head-tilt/chin-lift.*

How: Lift the chin up and out gently with one hand while pushing down on the forehead with the other to tilt the head back into a neutral position. Don't close the mouth.

Reason: The airway must be opened for you to determine if your infant can breathe.

4 *Determine if your infant is breathing.*

How: Place an ear over your infant's mouth and watch his chest.

Listen for sounds of breathing.

Feel for breath on your cheek.

Look at the chest for movement.

Reason: You must determine whether your infant is breathing before proceeding.

5 *If your infant is not breathing, give 2 rescue breaths. Look for the rise and fall of the chest with each breath.*

How: With your mouth, make a tight seal over your infant's mouth and nose. Breathe into your infant's mouth and nose twice, completely refilling your lungs with air between breaths. Allow your infant's lungs to deflate between breaths.

Reason: If your infant is found unconscious, you must try to get air into his lungs. If his chest rises when you give rescue breaths, the airway is open. If the chest does not rise, try to reposition the head to open the airway.

6 *If rescue breaths are unsuccessful, try again.*

How: Reposition the head and perform chin lift. Seal the mouth and nose properly, and try again to give rescue breaths.

Reason: Improper head-tilt/chin-lift is the most common reason that airway obstruction is not relieved. Try again to get the position correct.

7 *Deliver up to 5 back blows.*

How: Position your infant by supporting the front of his head and neck with one hand, firmly holding the jaw. Place your infant facedown on your forearm, keeping his head lower than the rest of his body. With the heel of your free hand, give up to 5 back blows forcefully between the shoulder blades.

Reason: Hold the head firmly to avoid injury. The back blows increase pressure in the airway and may dislodge the object.

8 *Turn your infant on his back, and deliver up to 5 chest thrusts over the lower half of the sternum.*

How: Supporting your infant's head, sandwich him between your hands and arms and turn him on his back, keeping the head lower than the trunk. Using two or three fingers, deliver up to 5 thrusts over the lower half of the breastbone, just below nipple level. Make sure your fingers are not pushing on the very bottom of the breastbone.

Reason: Chest thrusts can force air upward into the airway from the lungs with enough pressure to expel an object.

9 *Perform tongue-jaw lift. Check for a foreign object, and carefully remove it if you see it. Avoid pushing the object further into the airway.*

How: Open the mouth with a tongue-jaw lift by putting your thumb in your infant's mouth over the tongue. Lift the tongue and jaw forward with the fingers wrapped around the lower jaw. If you see an object, carefully remove it. Do not perform blind finger sweeps.

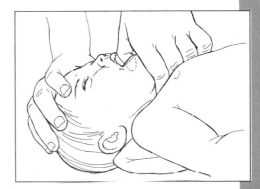

Reason: You may be able to reach a dislodged object if it has not been expelled. Do not perform blind finger sweeps as they may push the object back into or further into the airway.

10 *Open the airway, and try to give rescue breaths. Repeat the sequence until you are successful or until emergency medical help arrives. Be persistent. If you are alone, call for emergency help after 1 minute of rescue attempts.*

How: Seal the mouth and nose with your mouth, and give rescue breaths.

If the airway remains obstructed, alternate the following maneuvers in rapid sequence:

Deliver back blows (step 7).

Deliver chest thrusts (step 8).

Perform tongue-jaw lift, check for foreign body, and remove it if seen (step 9).

Open the airway (step 3).

Attempt and reattempt rescue breathing while maintaining an open airway (step 5).

Reason: Keep trying. As your infant becomes more deprived of oxygen, his muscles will relax and maneuvers that were previously ineffective may now become effective.

11 *When obstruction is removed, check for breathing and pulse.*

How: Open the airway, and check for breathing. If there is no breathing, give 2 rescue breaths. Check for a pulse.

If a pulse is present, provide 20 rescue breaths per minute and continue to monitor the pulse.

If no pulse is present, begin cycles of chest compressions (see CPR, p. 380) and rescue breathing.

If breathing resumes, and your child does not seem to be hurt, place your infant on his side and await the arrival of emergency personnel.

Reason: If your child is breathing, do not perform rescue breathing.

Clearing the Obstructed Airway in a Conscious Child (1 Year and Older): The Heimlich Maneuver

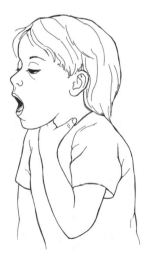

1 *Determine if your child's airway is completely blocked by watching for the sudden onset of signs, including an ineffective cough; increasing breathing difficulty; or blueness of lips, nails, or skin.*

How: The airway is completely blocked if your child cannot speak or cough effectively, or if when asked, "Are you choking?" your child clutches his neck between the thumb and index finger.

If your child can speak or cough effectively, do not interfere with his attempts to expel the object.

Reason: Recognizing the signs of complete airway obstruction and taking action are important. If the child can speak or cough, that means that air is getting past the obstruction and the obstruction is not complete. Interfering with your child's attempts to clear the airway may make things worse.

2 *If a cough is absent or ineffective and your child cannot speak, perform the Heimlich maneuver until the object is expelled or your child becomes unconscious. Be persistent. Don't give up.*

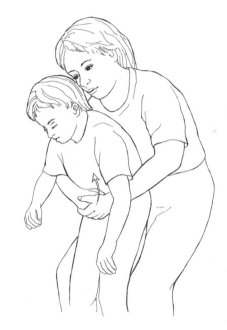

How: The Heimlich maneuver: Stand behind your child, and wrap your arms around his waist. Make a fist and grasp it with your other hand, and place the thumb side of your fist in your child's midline slightly above the navel but below the ribs. Press your fist into your child's abdomen with quick inward and upward thrusts. Give each abdominal thrust decisively to expel the object. Several thrusts may be necessary.

Reason: These thrusts can force air upward from the lungs into the airway with enough pressure to expel the object. Keep trying. As your child becomes more deprived of oxygen, his muscles will relax and maneuvers that were previously ineffective may become effective.

Clearing the Obstructed Airway in an Unconscious Child (1 Year and Older)

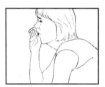

1 *Determine if your child is unconscious. Shout for help.*

How: Tap your child gently, and shake his shoulder to see if he responds.

Reason: Shout for help to alert bystanders to call for emergency help. Stay with your child.

2 *Position your child on his back.*

How: Turn your child on his back, holding the head and body as a unit, by supporting the head and neck.

Reason: This will protect the neck and spine from injury.

3 *Open the airway.*

How: Use the head-tilt/chin-lift maneuver (see p. 384) to position your child's head and open the airway. Place your ear over your child's mouth, and observe his chest.
Listen for sounds of breathing.
Feel for breath on your cheek.
Look at the chest for movement.

Reason: You must determine whether your child is breathing before continuing.

4 *If your child is not breathing, open the airway and try to give rescue breaths.*

How: Use the thumb and forefinger of the hand maintaining pressure on your child's forehead to pinch the nostrils closed. Make a tight seal with your mouth over your child's mouth. Give 2 rescue breaths.

Reason: If your child is unconscious, you must try to get some air into his lungs. If his chest rises, the airway is open. If his chest does not rise, the airway is blocked.

5 *If the first 2 rescue breaths are not successful, reposition the head and try again.*

How: Reposition your child's head and lift his chin. Pinch the nostrils closed. Cover your child's mouth with yours, making a tight seal, and give rescue breaths.

Reason: Improper head-tilt/chin-lift is the most common reason that airway obstruction is not relieved.

6 *If rescue breaths do not restore your child's breathing, perform the Heimlich maneuver up to 5 times.*

How: The Heimlich maneuver: Kneel at your child's hips if he is lying on the floor. Stand at your child's side if he is on a table. If your child is large, you may kneel astride his thighs. Place the heel of one hand on the abdomen midline, slightly above the navel and well below the sternum and ribs. Place the second hand directly on top of the first hand. Press into the abdomen with quick upward thrusts.

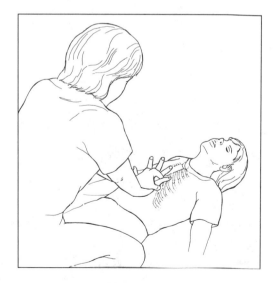

Reason: Heimlich thrusts can force air upward into the airway from the lungs with enough pressure to expel the object.

7 *Perform tongue-jaw lift. Check for a foreign object, and remove it if you see one.*

How: Lift the tongue and jaw forward by putting your thumb in your child's mouth over the tongue and wrapping your fingers around the lower jaw. If you see a foreign object, remove it. Do not perform a blind finger sweep.

Reason: A dislodged foreign body may now be removed by hand if it has not been expelled. Blind finger sweeps may push the object back into or further into the airway.

8 *Open the airway, and try to give rescue breaths. If unsuccessful, reposition the head and try again.*

How: Position your child's head using the head-tilt/chin-lift maneuver. Seal the mouth properly, and try again to give rescue breaths.

If the airway remains obstructed, alternate the following maneuvers in rapid sequence:

Perform Heimlich maneuver (step 6).

Perform tongue-jaw lift, check for foreign body, and remove it if seen (step 7).

Open the airway (step 3).

Attempt and reattempt rescue breathing while maintaining an open airway (step 5).

Repeat this sequence until successful or until emergency help arrives.

Reason: By this time, you must make another attempt to get air into your child's lungs. Keep trying. As your child becomes more deprived of oxygen, his muscles will relax, and maneuvers that were previously ineffective may become effective.

9 *Call for emergency help after 1 minute.*

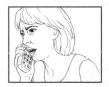

How: If you are alone, call for emergency help after 1 minute of effort.

If there is no breathing, give 2 breaths. Check for a pulse.

If a pulse is present, provide 20 breaths per minute and continue to monitor pulse.

If no pulse is present, begin cycles of compression and breathing (see pp. 385–386).

If breathing resumes and your child does not seem hurt, place your child on his side and await the arrival of emergency personnel.

Reason: It is important to call for emergency help while at the same time continuing your rescue efforts.

Dental Injuries

According to the National Safety Council, more than 2 million teeth are accidentally knocked out each year. More than 90 percent of them can be saved with proper treatment.

 Call for emergency help if . . .

- a permanent tooth is knocked out.
- jaw swelling and pain indicate a possible fracture.
- gum bleeding does not stop despite firm pressure.

What to Do

Time is of the essence. If you save the tooth and bring your child to the dentist within 30 minutes, chances are good that the dentist will be able to reimplant it.

If the tooth is completely knocked out:

- place the tooth in milk, and bring it immediately to the dentist. Do not wash the tooth. Do not touch the root of the tooth. If no milk is available, wrap it gently in a clean tissue or towel and bring it to the dentist.

If the tooth is only partially knocked out:

- push it back in firmly—without washing it—and get your child to the dentist immediately.
- give acetaminophen to help relieve pain.
- apply pressure with a clean cloth to stop the bleeding.

Drowning

Water does not have to be deep to drown a child: Only 2 inches of bathtub water can form a deadly pool for a small child. A bucket of water presents a drowning danger to a toddler who may fall into it head first. Never leave your child unattended near any water.

 Call for emergency help if . . .

- your child is or was unconscious.
- your child is or has been in shock.
- your child has hypothermia (low body temperature).
- your child has difficulty breathing or persistent coughing or wheezing.
- your child was submerged for more than a few seconds (even if he seems fine).

What to Do

1 *Rescue your child from the water.*

- Try to reach your child without jumping into the water yourself.
- If a swimming rescue is necessary, watch your child or the spot where you last saw your child until you reach it. Try to bring a towel, a rope, a life preserver, or another sturdy object for your child to hold onto while being towed to shore. In this situation, there is a strong risk that a panicked child can make you a second victim.
- Do not walk near open ice where your child has fallen through. Instead, extend a hand, leg, pole, or tree branch from firm ice or, preferably, from shore. In this situation too, there is a strong risk that a panicked child can make you a second victim.
- Call for emergency help immediately, or have someone else do so.

2 *Determine if your child is breathing.*

- If your child is not breathing, begin mouth-to-mouth breathing as soon as possible after your child is removed from water. If he does not have a pulse, perform CPR (see p. 380 or p. 383).
- Remove wet clothing. Cover your child with dry clothing or a blanket.
- If necessary, treat him for shock (see p. 418).
- If he still isn't breathing and lacks a pulse, continue mouth-to-mouth breathing and CPR.
- If your child is unconscious but breathing, turn him on his side so that he doesn't inhale more water or some saliva or vomit if he throws up. (Vomiting is common because the stomach often fills with water in drowning.)
- Call for help, but don't leave your child. If you must take him to the hospital yourself, follow the suggestions about transporting an injured child on page 387.
- If necessary, continue rescue breathing until the ambulance arrives or until your child reaches a medical facility.

3 *Do not give up. Don't stop rescue breathing until your child begins to cough and breathe alone.*

Some children have survived long submersions, especially in cold water. For water safety tips, see page 374.

Eye Injuries

Children's eyes are susceptible to three types of injuries—blows, foreign bodies (grit or other particles or objects in the eye), and chemical irritation. Many injuries will not impair vision but will require immediate medical attention. Even a tiny speck of dust can cause irritation and, if it touches the cornea (the transparent outer covering of the eyeball), can scratch the eye if not carefully treated.

Most chemicals, including alcohol and hydrocarbons (e.g., gasoline, lighter fluid), cause only temporary stinging and superficial irritation. However, acids (e.g., car battery acid, rust remover, cement cleaner) and alkalis (e.g., oven cleaner, toilet bowl cleanser, lye) splashed into the eye can severely damage the cornea. When any chemical is accidentally splashed into your child's eye, treat it as an emergency until your doctor or poison control center specialist tells you otherwise.

Signs and Symptoms

▌ Watery, red eye

▌ Reluctance to open eye

▌ Pain, swelling, and irritation

▌ Visible embedded object

 Call for emergency help if . . .

▌ chemicals have come into contact with the eye.

▌ an object is embedded in the eye.

▌ the eyeball is loosened from the socket.

▌ pain persists for more than $1/2$ hour.

▌ your child experiences blurry vision, a loss of vision, or severe eye pain or tenderness, especially after an injury.

▌ the eyelid or eyeball receives a cut.

What to Do

If your child receives a blow to the eye, the eye socket will probably protect the eye itself, but the surrounding area will swell and bruise as tiny blood vessels beneath the skin break. Place a cold compress over the eye until you arrive at the emergency department.

An extremely violent blow to the face, such as in a motor vehicle accident, can cause an eye to be partially torn from its socket. Do not attempt to push the eye into the socket. Cover both eyes loosely with a sterile dressing, and get your child to an emergency department as soon as possible. For more information on what to do about minor eye pain or what the doctor might do, see *Eye Injuries,* Part 5.

Chemical Splashes

▌ Wash the eye immediately and thoroughly with a lukewarm stream of tap water to prevent damage to the cornea. Hold your child's face up under gently running tap water while he is lying down in an empty bathtub or under a shower, or have your child lie down while you continuously pour lukewarm water from a pitcher or a glass into his open eye.

▌ It is very important to try to hold your child's eyelids open during this process, although he will loudly protest. For most chemicals, irrigate (rinse) the eye for at least 20 minutes.

▌ Afterward, watch for persistent pain, swelling, or visual disturbance.

▌ Call the nearest poison control center, and follow their advice. If symptoms persist, they will usually instruct you to seek medical attention.

Foreign Bodies

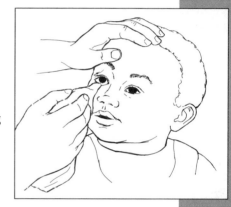

▌ If the particle is in the corner of your child's eye, try to remove it with the corner of a clean cloth or a moistened cotton swab.

▌ If the particle is under the eyelid, try to remove it by opening and closing your child's eye several times while running water over the eye in a gentle, continuous stream. If the object stays on the lid and you can see it, try gently sweeping with a moistened cotton swab to remove it. If you can't see the particle or remove it, call your child's doctor right away.

For information on what the doctor might do for foreign bodies in the eye, see *Eye Injuries,* Part 5.

Fractures (Broken Bones)

A broken bone should always be treated promptly by a doctor for many reasons. The bone has to be set correctly, and your child must be assessed for damage to surrounding organs or tissues. That's why getting medical help as soon as possible is important.

Signs and Symptoms

▌ Snap heard or felt at the time of the injury

▌ Inability to move the limb or joint without intense pain

▌ Swelling, bruising, or both

▌ Deformation of the injured area, possibly caused by a bone's sticking close to or through the skin surface

 Call for emergency help if . . .

▌ your child may have a broken bone.

Fractures

What to Do

If a bone has broken through the skin, or if you can see the broken bone through an open wound, drape gauze or a sterile dressing over the wound. Don't attempt any cleaning, and *don't* touch the wound.

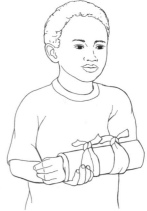

▌ Immobilize the area around the broken bone, and take your child to an emergency department.

▌ Keep blankets over the rest of your child's body to keep him from going into shock until help arrives. Treat shock if necessary (see p. 418).

▌ If you suspect a serious head or spinal injury, do not move your child (see below and p. 419). Immobilize your child's neck by carefully placing weights (e.g., bags of sugar or flour) on either side to keep it from turning.

▌ Call for emergency medical assistance.

▌ If you must transport your child yourself, protect the broken bone by following the directions below.

SPLINTING BODY PARTS

Make a splint with flat objects, such as magazines, boards, or pieces of cardboard. Pad the splint with towels or washcloths. Carefully bind the splints together with strips of cloth, neckties, belts, or similar straps. Tie above and below the break. Make sure that the bindings are snug, but do not cut off circulation.

Head Injuries

The "thud" of a child's head meeting a hard surface can cause your own heart to thud, too, whether it's the sound of a baby falling off the couch or a 5-year-old dropping off the jungle gym. While most head injuries do not result in permanent damage, make sure that a doctor evaluates all but the most minor bumps and bruises. Almost 30 percent of deaths from childhood injuries result from head injuries each year, and about 29,000 children experience permanent disabilities resulting from head injuries.

Signs and Symptoms

▌ Headache   ▌ Irritability

▌ Unconsciousness   ▌ Vomiting

▌ Seizures   ▌ Drowsiness

▌ Dazed state   ▌ A bump or an indentation on the skull

▌ Discharge of blood or straw-colored fluid from nose and ears

▌ Pupils are unequal in size or fail to constrict normally when exposed to light

Call for emergency help if . . .

▌ your child cries for more than 15 minutes after the head injury.

▌ your child has a seizure.

▌ your child is unconscious after the injury.

▌ blood is coming from an ear canal or nose.

▌ your child seems off balance while sitting, crawling, or walking.

▌ your child can't remember getting the injury.

▌ your child has a severe headache.

▌ your child's pupils are not equal in size.

▌ your child has forceful repeated vomiting.

What to Do

Remain calm and stay with your child. Call for help immediately.

If your child loses consciousness, treat him as if he's had a spinal cord injury, and

▌ immobilize his head, neck, and body by padding them with towels, blankets, or jackets, without changing his position.

▌ periodically ask him basic questions (Who am I? Where are we? What day is it?) to assess orientation.

▌ wait for help to arrive.

If your child is conscious and shows no other symptoms,

▌ call your child's doctor.

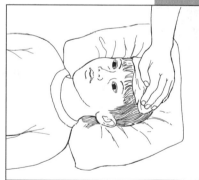

▌ observe him carefully for at least 2 hours after the injury, checking his pupils frequently.

▌ encourage him to lie down and rest.

It's all right for your child to sleep but keep a close eye on him to make sure he doesn't stop breathing and is arousable. If awake, give him only clear liquids and no food until he has gone several hours without vomiting. Don't give your child pain medications unless your doctor tells you to do so. The doctor needs to know your child's reaction to the injury and the effects of medication can confuse the picture.

Do not . . .

▌ move your child if there may be neck or spinal injury, unless he is in a life-threatening situation. (See Emergency Moves, p. 420.)

Heat Exhaustion, Heat Cramps, and Heatstroke

Because children's bodies are less able to disperse heat and cool themselves, children can easily fall prey to heat exhaustion, caused by an excessive loss of fluids in hot, humid weather. A related condition, heat cramps, is less common in children but results in painful, cramped muscles following physical exertion in hot weather. A rarer and more serious condition is heatstroke, which occurs when the body is exposed to extreme heat, causing the body's temperature-regulating mechanisms to break down. Sweat glands fail to work, and the body cannot cool itself in the normal way by producing sweat. Heatstroke can result when a child is left in a closed car in the sun, for example. The body temperature may climb to 104°F or more.

 Call for emergency help if . . .

▮ your child is lethargic or has muscle cramping.

▮ your child is disoriented or confused.

▮ your child's body temperature is 104°F or above.

Signs and Symptoms of Heat Exhaustion

The following symptoms may gradually occur over several hours:

▮ Fatigue

▮ Temperature over 100°F

▮ Pale and clammy skin or red, flushed skin

▮ Dry or sticky mouth

▮ Dizziness

▮ Nausea

▮ Drowsiness

▮ Muscle cramps

What to Do for Heat Exhaustion

As soon as you suspect that your child might be overheated, take him out of the heat and into a cool environment, such as a shady spot or an air-conditioned room or car. You could also try a cool bath. Give him fluids, preferably electrolyte-balanced sports drinks. The beverage should be cool but not ice cold. If he shows no improvement, seek immediate medical attention.

Signs and Symptoms of Heat Cramps

▮ Painful, cramped muscles during or after physical exertion in the heat

▮ Profuse sweating

What to Do for Heat Cramps

Have your child rest in a cool environment. Give fluids, preferably electrolyte drinks. Beverages should be cool but not ice cold. If your child shows no improvement, seek medical attention.

Signs and Symptoms of Heatstroke

▌ Confusion, strange behavior

▌ Body temperature of 104°F or higher

▌ No sweating

▌ Low blood pressure

What to Do for Heatstroke

Heatstroke is a dangerous, potentially life-threatening condition caused by being in an excessively hot environment that impairs the body's ability to cool down. If your child shows signs of heatstroke, follow these steps:

▌ Call for emergency help immediately.

▌ Cool your child's body with ice packs or by submerging his body in cool water.

▌ Do not try to force liquids—your child may not be able to drink cool liquids.

How to Prevent Heat Exhaustion and Heatstroke

Have your child drink a glass or two of water or an electrolyte-balanced sports drink before going outdoors, to keep him hydrated. Avoid serving sugary, carbonated, or caffeinated drinks, such as colas or ice teas, because they often trigger urine production and thus loss of fluids.

Help your child adjust to hot weather gradually. If you're home, have him play outside for just an hour or so if the temperature is unusually hot. If you take him to a warmer climate, it could take 10 to 14 days for him to become fully acclimated. Make sure to limit his outdoor activities during peak heat periods, and monitor him carefully.

You can take other steps to avoid heat exhaustion and heatstroke as well:

▌ Dress your child in loose, lightweight, and light-colored clothing.

▌ Use sunscreen with a sun protection factor (SPF) of at least 15 to prevent sunburn.

▌ In warmer climates, keep outdoor play to a minimum between the hours of 10 A.M. and 3 P.M.

▌ Call for frequent breaks. Interrupt play every 30 minutes, and have your child drink at least 1/2 cup of liquid.

▌ Never ignore complaints about feeling too hot or too tired.

▌ Avoid giving antihistamines while your child is playing hard, because they may contain properties that block the nerves that stimulate sweating.

▌ Keep children cool indoors, too. Don't allow your child to play in poorly ventilated rooms or in any closed space that can heat up.

▌ Do not leave your child in a car unattended or allow him to play in an unattended car; closed cars can overheat rapidly to temperatures as high as 110°F.

Hypothermia and Frostbite

Hypothermia and frostbite are two conditions caused by exposure to cold. Hypothermia results when prolonged exposure to cold causes a child's body temperature to drop below 95°F. Falling overboard from a boat into cold water, even on a warm day, or falling through thin ice into a river or pond are two common situations that may result in hypothermia.

Frostbite is the freezing of body tissue, usually of the hands, fingers, cheeks, ears, nose, and toes. It occurs when certain body parts are exposed to cold temperatures over a long period.

Children are more susceptible to frostbite and hypothermia than adults: They have less body fat to insulate them against the cold, and they tend to lose heat more quickly than adults because their bodies have proportionately more surface area.

 Call for emergency help if . . .

▌ your child's temperature drops below 95°F.

▌ your child seems confused or disoriented or acts strangely.

▌ any symptoms of frostbite appear.

Signs and Symptoms of Hypothermia

▌ Shivering   ▌ Muscle weakness

▌ Numbness   ▌ Drowsiness, incoherence

What to Do for Hypothermia

Call for help immediately. Bring your child to a warm environment. Wrap him with blankets, jackets, or whatever you can find to help him retain body heat.

Do not . . .

▌ expose your child to any direct sources of heat, such as hot water bottles, electric heating pads, chemical heat pads, radiators, or fireplaces.

Signs and Symptoms of Frostbite

❚ Numbness

❚ Blisters

❚ Soft doughy or frozen doughy feeling to the area exposed to the cold

❚ Tingling and burning of the frostbitten area upon rewarming

❚ Aching or throbbing pain upon rewarming

❚ Redness, swelling upon rewarming

❚ Blackness

What to Do for Frostbite

If your child complains of pain, has difficulty moving a finger, a toe, or another body part, or shows other frostbite symptoms, take these steps:

❚ Seek emergency help.

❚ Remove clothing from the affected area, and examine the skin for frostbite.

❚ Slightly elevate the area to decrease pain and swelling.

❚ Place gauze pads between fingers or toes to prevent them from sticking together.

❚ Cover any ruptured blisters with a sterile gauze pad.

❚ Keep your child warm.

Do not . . .

❚ break any blisters that form.

❚ attempt to rewarm the area by using a hot water bottle, warm water, heating pads, fireplace, or other direct heat sources.

❚ rub the area in an attempt to stimulate circulation. This could result in further damage to the skin and underlying tissue.

Poisoning

Many ordinary substances in and around the home are potential poisons. Some are clearly marked: Pesticides, cleaning fluids, rat poisons, and paint thinner are all labeled as hazardous. Others are not so obvious. Consider the possibility of poisoning if your child becomes suddenly ill and acts drowsy or strangely (e.g., irrational, unusually combative, or agitated). If you suspect that your child has ingested poison, call your local poison control center immediately (the number is usually listed inside the front cover of the white pages, or ask your 911 operator to connect you directly).

Signs and Symptoms

❚ Vomiting or diarrhea

❚ Difficulty breathing

Poisoning

▌ Altered consciousness (agitated, drowsy, or sedated)

▌ Burns or redness around the mouth

▌ Breath that smells like chemicals (perhaps paint thinner or gasoline)

▌ An open container of drugs or other toxic substances near your child

 Call the Poison Control Center if . . .

▌ you suspect that your child has ingested any poisonous or toxic substance.

What to Do

The first 1 to 2 hours after a poisoning are the most critical for treatment and recovery. Most poisonings can be handled at home with accurate instructions.

1 *Stay calm,*
and follow these instructions carefully.

• *Mouth:* Sweep any pills or suspected toxic substances out of your child's mouth with your finger. Use a damp cloth to wipe the mouth clean. Inspect the mouth for burns, cuts, or unusual coloring. Do not give your child anything to drink before checking with the poison control center.

• *Eyes:* If a poison has entered your child's eyes, rinse the eyes with a stream of lukewarm water for 10 to 15 minutes. If a powder got into the eyes, flush out any particles (see Eye Injuries, p. 407).

• *Skin:* If poison has spilled on the skin, dilute and rinse the skin thoroughly with lukewarm water (see Burns, p. 394).

• *Inhalation:* Move your child to fresh air. Don't become a second victim! As a rescuer, you can be overcome by toxic fumes after entering an enclosed space. Break a window to ventilate the room before entering. Or, if there's a fire, crawl under the smoke. Watch for signs that your child has breathed a substance into the lungs: coughing, shortness of breath, rapid breathing, skin turning blue, and wheezing. If breathing stops, start rescue breathing (see p. 380 for an infant or p. 383 for a child).

2 *Do not leave your child near the poison.*
Take him with you to the nearest telephone.

3 *Get expert help. Call your local poison control center,*
and provide the following information:

• Child's name, age, and weight

• Your telephone number and location

- The kind of poison you think your child was exposed to
- The ingredients on the label of the pills or medications or other substance
- The exact time (or a good estimate) of when the poisoning happened
- A description of his symptoms, including any vomiting or drowsiness
- If you have an emetic available (a substance, such as ipecac, that induces vomiting)

4 *Follow the instructions the poison control center gives you.*
If the poison control center directs you to the emergency department, get medical attention as quickly as possible—even if your child has vomited and seems fine. Bring the bottle of poison or a sample of whatever your child ingested with you to further aid the medical team in diagnosing and treating the problem.

ACTIVATED CHARCOAL?

Most emergency departments use activated charcoal as an antidote for poisons. The charcoal soaks up the poison, preventing its absorption, and the charcoal-bound poison comes out in the child's blackened stools. Activated charcoal must be given in large amounts (several ounces for most children) and is a black, gritty solution that many toddlers will not easily drink. Thus, charcoal is best reserved for use at the hospital rather than at home. If you have activated charcoal at home, however, and want to give it to your poisoned child, check first with the poison control center.

Using Syrup of Ipecac

Syrup of ipecac, which induces vomiting, should be part of your home first aid kit. It is available in drugstores. Use syrup of ipecac only if poison control center personnel instruct you to do so. Follow these guidelines when using ipecac:

▌ Keep it out of the reach of toddlers.

▌ Do not give to infants under 9 months.

▌ Give 2 teaspoons to children 1 year and younger.

▌ Give 1 tablespoon to children older than 1 year.

▌ Follow the ipecac dose with one or two glasses of water, and spin the child around, which may upset his stomach and cause him to vomit.

Your child probably won't vomit immediately; ipecac can take up to 20 minutes to work. Once begun, vomiting may last 2 to 3 hours. Ipecac can also cause drowsiness.

Do not . . .

▌ give ipecac unless instructed to do so by the poison control center.

▌ induce vomiting with a soap solution, other remedy, or anything except ipecac.

▌ stick your fingers down your child's throat.

In some situations, such as the following, you should *not* induce vomiting:

▌ Your child has ingested any alkaline or acid substance (like drain opener or oven cleaner). That's because anything that burns on the way down will also burn coming back up. Vomiting up these kinds of poisons will only further damage the esophagus and throat.

▌ Your child is unconscious, drowsy, confused, or has had a seizure.

▌ Your child has swallowed a solvent or hydrocarbon (such as turpentine, furniture polish, pine oil cleaner, gasoline).

▌ Your child has swallowed a heart medicine or a medicine that can make him drowsy.

Shock

Shock is a life-threatening condition resulting from sudden decreases in blood pressure, circulation rate, and blood oxygen levels. Vital organs, such as the brain, do not get the oxygen they need to function, and blood pools in other parts of the body, where it isn't needed.

Shock is not an illness by itself but a reaction to another illness or trauma. Shock can be caused by blood loss due to injury, by infections of the blood, by serious injuries, by massive infection, and by many other medical conditions. A child in shock must be treated by medical personnel, who will administer intravenous fluids and medications that raise blood pressure.

Signs and Symptoms

▌ Cool, clammy, pale skin

▌ Weak, rapid pulse

▌ Increased, shallow breathing

▌ Thirst

▌ Dizziness, faintness

▌ Irrational behavior (child may be confused or drowsy)

 Call for emergency help if . . .

▌ your child has any combination of the above symptoms.

What to Do

Whenever a major injury or emergency occurs, watch for symptoms of shock. If your child shows any of the symptoms of shock, take the following steps:

▌ Stay calm; stay with your child.

▌ Call for emergency help.

- Cover your child with a jacket or blanket.
- Check his airway, breathing, and pulse. If necessary, administer CPR (see p. 380 or p. 383).
- Keep your child in the most comfortable position, preferably lying down.
- Do not move your child if you suspect a head or spinal injury.
- If there is no head injury, raise your child's feet above heart level.
- Carefully monitor your child's breathing and pulse until emergency help arrives.

Spinal Injuries

A spinal injury damages the bony spinal column that surrounds and protects the nerves of the spine. These nerves allow us to feel sensation and to move our bodies. Children receive spinal injuries most often as a result of car accidents, bicycle accidents, or sports-related incidents.

Note: Any child found unconscious after a violent injury must be treated as if he has a spinal injury. Do not move the child.

Signs and Symptoms

- Painful movement of arms and legs
- Numbness, tingling, or weak sensation of the arms and legs
- Paralysis of arms and legs
- A deformity or an unnatural angle of the child's head and neck

 Call for emergency help if . . .

- you suspect a neck or spinal injury.
- your child is unconscious.

What to Do

Call for emergency help. Medical personnel need to determine the extent of the damage as soon as possible. In the meantime,

- check for consciousness by calling your child's name.
- check the ABCs—airway, breathing, and circulation—and treat accordingly (see p. 379).
- do not move your child unless he is in a life-threatening situation.
- immobilize the head, neck, and spine by padding them with towels, blankets, or jackets.

Spinal Injuries (cont.)

▌do not change your child's position. If he is conscious, tell him to keep absolutely still.

▌carefully remove your child's shoes, and ask him to wiggle his toes. See if he can feel you as you tickle or gently scratch the bottom of his feet. Ask him to flex his hands and wiggle his fingers. See if he can grasp your hand and squeeze tightly.

▌Let the medical team know what you observed when they arrive.

Do not . . .

▌remove a helmet or hat if your child is wearing one.

▌give your child anything to eat or drink.

EMERGENCY MOVES

The best advice is not to move the injured child. If he is in harm's way (e.g., in the middle of a highway), however, you will need to act fast, even before help arrives. In that case, follow these procedures for moving your child:

▌Stabilize your child's head by placing rolled-up towels, blankets, or other materials on both sides of his head to keep it from moving before you attempt to move him.

▌Firmly grasp your child's sweater or jersey collar with both hands and support his head on your wrists while you pull him out of danger.

▌Another method is to firmly grasp your child's ankles and pull him out of danger. Use this move only on smooth surfaces.

GUIDE TO COMMON CHILDHOOD ILLNESS, INJURY, AND CONDITIONS

Note: A boldface word indicates that the term is also listed alphabetically in this section. For an explanation of the categories in the When to Call the Doctor sections, see How to Use This Book, page xix.

■ *Abdominal Pain/Stomachache*

"My stomach hurts" is one of the most common childhood complaints. But what a child calls a stomachache may not involve the stomach at all. It can signal a problem with the urinary tract, the bowel, the appendix, the lungs, or even the throat. And it's often accompanied by other symptoms, such as a fever or a headache. Whether the cause is the flu or a case of before-school jitters, most bouts of childhood abdominal pain are short-lived and treatable at home.

Signs and Symptoms

- Abdominal pain
- *Fever*
- Poor appetite
- Nausea or *vomiting*
- *Diarrhea*
- Pain with urination or bowel movements
- Fussiness or excessive crying
- Abdominal pain with pain in the back, chest, rectum, or scrotum or down the leg

☎ *When to Call the Doctor*
CALL THE DOCTOR IMMEDIATELY IF

- the pain is severe and lasts more than 1 hour.
- the pain is in the lower right side of the abdomen and is accompanied by fever (signs of *appendicitis*).
- vomiting occurs more than twice.
- blood is in the stool or urine.
- your child recently experienced an abdominal injury or underwent surgery.
- poisoning is a possibility. (Call your local poison control center.)

☎ CALL THE DOCTOR TODAY IF

- the pain is accompanied by fever.
- the pain worsens over several hours.
- a sore throat accompanies the abdominal pain (a common sign of strep throat).
- the pain is accompanied by diarrhea that occurs more than twice.

Essential Facts

Children feel abdominal pain in several ways. They may have cramps or nausea. It may be intense or mild, sharp or dull, constant or occasional. The pain is usually concentrated in one area, but sometimes it travels from one part of the abdomen to another, or all the way through to the back. Often other symptoms are present, such as vomiting, headache, or fever. A child with abdominal pain may need to urinate or defecate more often than usual.

An infant can't tell you that her stomach hurts, of course, but she will probably show signs, such as a refusal to eat or drink, diarrhea, vomiting, and fussiness.

Causes

The possible causes of stomachache are as varied as the location and nature of the pain, ranging from minor infections to food poisoning, nervous tension to trauma. For 95 percent of children with abdominal pain, the cause is something simple and self-limiting, such as one of the following:

- *Stomach flu:* If your child's pain is intermittent and involves vomiting or diarrhea or both, she probably has a mild viral infection or an inflammation of the gastrointestinal tract, called gastroenteritis or the flu (see *Colds/Flu*). The flu usually lasts only 24 to 48 hours.
- *Constipation:* If your child's stools are very small and harder than usual, it may hurt her

to have a bowel movement. In that case, your child's stomachache is likely to be intermittent and feel like cramps. You can usually cure—and prevent—constipation simply by changing your child's diet: adding extra water and high-fiber foods such as grains, fruits, and vegetables (see *Constipation*).

- *Colic:* Colic is excessive fussiness in a newborn under 3 months old. The cause of colic is unknown, but a leading theory holds that the cause is an immature gastrointestinal tract, nervous system, or both (see *Colic*).

- *Urinary tract infection:* An infection in the urinary tract can cause abdominal pain, along with other symptoms such as the frequent urge to urinate and a burning sensation while urinating (see *Urinary Tract Infection*).

- *Strep throat:* This throat infection is sometimes accompanied by abdominal pain and a rash known as scarlet fever (see *Sore Throat/Strep Throat*).

- *Indigestion:* As with adults, abdominal pain in children can be caused by overeating or eating lots of sweets, such as chocolate.

- *Medication:* Some medicines, such as ibuprofen and antibiotics, can cause stomach upset.

- *Emotional distress:* Stomach pain is often a child's reaction to stress or anxiety (see *Anxiety Disorders*), such as a recent move, family turmoil, or pressure at school. This is one of the most common causes of chronic abdominal pain in children. Frequent stomachaches can also be a symptom of *depression.*

- *Injury:* A blow to the abdomen from a punch, sports play, a fall, or a car accident can cause abdominal pain and internal bleeding.

Less Common Causes

Though less common than the conditions previously described, several other conditions can cause abdominal pain in children. They include *appendicitis,* food allergies (see *Allergies*), food poisoning, lactose intolerance (problems with carbohydrate absorption), hernia (see *Hernia, Inguinal*), lead poisoning, *gastroesophageal reflux,* sickle-cell anemia (see *Sickle-Cell Disease, Anemia*), giardiasis (an infestation of the intestinal tract by the microorganism *Giardia lamblia*), pancreatitis (pancreatic tissue damage that occurs with several childhood illnesses, including mumps and *mononucleosis*), peptic ulcers (an open raw area inside the stomach or the first part of the small intestine), and intussusception (see What the Doctor May Do, below). In addition, some infections, including *hepatitis, pneumonia,* and *mononucleosis,* can cause abdominal pain.

What the Doctor May Do

If your doctor asks you to bring your child in for an examination, the nature of the exam will vary according to the age and sex of the child, as well as the location and type of pain. The doctor will first review your child's medical history, paying special attention to any recent injuries and symptoms such as vomiting, diarrhea, and fever. The doctor probably will then listen to your child's abdomen to make sure that the bowel sounds are normal. The doctor may also feel the abdomen for lumps and areas of tenderness that could indicate an infection or a blockage from a twisting of the bowel (called volvulus) or a telescoping blockage of the intestine (called intussusception)—both problems that frequently require emergency surgery. Some radiologists, however, can fix an intussusception by infusing radiocontrast material into the bowel, which moves the inner bowel wall away from the outer one, reducing the overlap.

For a newborn and infant, the doctor will assess the baby's health by checking that she has been gaining enough weight, seems well nourished, and isn't lethargic. For toddlers and older children, the doctor may ask about emotional difficulties in the child's life, from such things as a recent move or pressure at school, which might induce abdominal pain.

If the doctor suspects an infection, or if he cannot make a diagnosis based on a physical exam alone, he may perform other tests, including blood or urine tests. For example, lead poisoning, infectious mononucleosis, and sickle-cell anemia are diagnosed by a blood test. A urine test may indicate a urinary tract infection.

The doctor may conduct further tests, including X rays or sonograms (a painless imaging technique using sound waves) after the lab tests are evaluated to look for such things as kidney stones, an inflamed appendix, or gastrointestinal blockage. If your doctor suspects that pneumonia is causing the pain, he might order a chest X ray.

What You Can Do

If your child is vomiting or feverish, be sure to give her fluids to prevent dehydration. In addition, make your child as comfortable as possible by doing the following:

- *Burp your baby.* Infants under 2 months old need to be burped in the middle and at the end of every feeding so that air bubbles can move out of the stomach and esophagus (the tube that connects the throat to the stomach). Air that sits there can cause stomach pain. See page 73 for information on how to burp your baby.

- *Rest.* A little quiet time often can help relieve a stomachache.

- *Give acetaminophen.* Check with your doctor before giving *any* medicine for abdominal pain. If your doctor says it's OK, giving the correct dose of acetaminophen may help.

- *Apply heat.* Fill a hot water bottle with warm, not hot, water. Wrap it in a washcloth, and apply it gently to your child's abdomen to help soothe and relieve a stomachache.

- *Be understanding.* Stressful situations such as pressure at school or difficult relationships with friends can tie a child's stomach in knots. If your child often has stomachaches right before day care, school, or other stressful situations, take a few minutes to comfort her, hold her, and express understanding and sympathy.

Remedies to Avoid

Some remedies for pain and nausea can do more harm than good when a child has a stomachache. Don't give laxatives or substances to induce vomiting unless your doctor tells you to do so. And don't use acetaminophen for longer than 12 to 24 hours; otherwise, it might mask appendicitis or other conditions that require medical attention.

Prevention

You can reduce your infant's chance of picking up a stomach flu or other infections by breast-feeding instead of bottle-feeding. For all children, encourage frequent hand washing and other good hygiene methods described on page 366. In addition, you can prevent abdominal pain resulting from **constipation** by making sure that your child drinks fluids regularly throughout the day and eats high-fiber foods, such as fruits, vegetables, and whole-grain breads and cereals.

See also **Hernia, Umbilical.**

Abnormal Heart Rhythm (Dysrhythmia)

A steady, regular heartbeat is something most parents expect their infants to have, and the idea that your child's heart doesn't beat in a regular pattern, a condition called dysrhythmia, may be alarming. But different types of dysrhythmias (irregular heartbeats) occur often in children, and most are harmless and require no treatment.

Dysrhythmias (sometimes referred to as arrhythmias) that are either dangerous or cause symptoms are rare.

Signs and Symptoms

- Often, no symptoms
- Rapid heartbeat detected by feeling your child's pulse or heartbeat directly over the chest
- Pale or cold and sweaty skin
- Nausea and vomiting (along with other symptoms listed here)
- Chest pain
- Dizziness, fainting, light-headedness
- Listlessness or agitation and poor feeding in an infant
- Convulsions

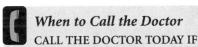

When to Call the Doctor
CALL THE DOCTOR TODAY IF
- any of the above symptoms appear.

Essential Facts

Although an irregular heartbeat can develop at any time, it is most common in newborns and young infants and usually corrects itself within the first year of life. Children between 8 and 12 years old may also develop dysrhythmias, some of which correct themselves with time. Dysrhythmias are less common in children of other ages.

Most children with dysrhythmias have structurally normal hearts, although children born with heart defects are more likely to have dysrhythmias, particularly after heart surgery. Only in rare cases does an irregular heartbeat indicate a serious heart disorder.

Types of Dysrhythmia

Sinus arrhythmia: a common, normal rhythm irregularity among young children. It is an increase in the heart rate when breathing in and a decrease when breathing out.

How the heart works: First the atria contract to pump blood to the ventricles. Then the atria relax, and the ventricles contract to pump the blood out of the heart. The steady rhythm that tells the heart muscle when to contract is maintained by a group of pacemakers, or specialized tissues within the heart that coordinate electrical impulses within the heart (which make up the sinoatrial [S-A] node and the atrioventricular [A-V] node), resulting in a regular heartbeat.

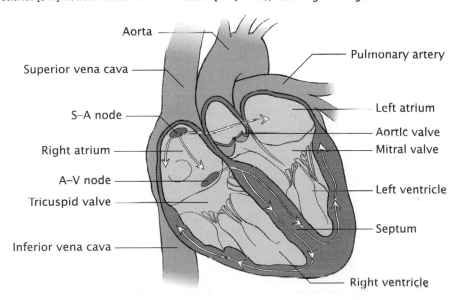

Bradycardia: a heart rate that is too slow. The definition of what's too slow depends upon the child's age and activity. For example, a newborn usually won't have a heart rate of less than 80 beats per minute. An athletically trained teenager may have a normal resting heart rate of 50 beats per minute. Rates below these may indicate bradycardia.

Tachycardia: a heart rate that is too fast. A fast heart rate originates in the upper heart chambers. As with bradycardia, the definition of "too fast" depends on the child's age.

Ventricular tachycardia: a rare and potentially fatal type of tachycardia rhythm that occurs when the lower heart chambers (ventricles) begin sending out their own chaotic, rapid beats. The most dangerous form of this condition is ventricular fibrillation, which can be fatal within seconds without emergency treatment (see CPR, pp. 380 and 383).

Causes

To understand dysrhythmias, you must understand how the normal heart beats. The heart muscle contracts and relaxes to pump blood through the heart's chambers to the arteries, which carry blood throughout the body. The steady rhythm that tells the heart muscle when to contract is maintained by a group of "pacemakers," or specialized tissues within the heart that coordinate electrical impulses within the heart, resulting in a regular heartbeat. The heart's principal pacemaker, a group of pacemaker cells at the top of the right atrium (the heart chamber), called the sinoatrial (S-A) node, generates tiny electrical impulses that spread throughout the heart to stimulate contraction of the heart muscle. The specialized fibers that carry the electrical stimulation throughout the heart are called the conduction system. A second pacemaker, the atrioventricular (A-V) node, may dictate the heart rate in case the sinoatrial node malfunctions. The atrioventricular node usually produces slower heart rates.

Your child's heart rate naturally changes as she grows. The resting heart rate of infants and young children, for instance, is much faster than the 60 to 100 beats per minute of the average adult (see box). A normal newborn's heart beats between 70 and 190 times per minute; a toddler's heart rate is between 80 and 130. The heart rate of a preschooler is between 80 and 120 beats per minute. After 6 years of age, a child's heart rate will level off between 75 and 115 beats per minute. Heart rate varies according to activity level, emotional state, and other conditions, such as whether the child has a fever.

Many conditions within the heart itself may cause dysrhythmias, as can several external factors. For example, heart defects present at birth or rheumatic heart disease (a heart valve and muscle infection) may cause dysrhythmias. Heart surgery can sometimes cause dysrhythmias as a complication of surgery. Many drugs taken in excessive doses also can cause dysrhythmias. These include antiasthma medications such as aminophylline, terbutaline, and other bronchodilators; cisapride; digitalis; some anesthetics; antidepressants; lithium; and cocaine. Certain household chemicals, including solvents, glues, and some hydrocarbons (such as gasoline), can also cause dysrhythmias when inhaled repeatedly (inhalant abuse). Stimulants, such as caffeine, cocaine, diet medications, and amphetamines, cause dysrhythmias in some children. Other causes include exercise, *fever, anemia,* anxiety (see ***Anxiety Disorders***), and hyperthyroidism (excessive function of the thyroid gland).

What the Doctor May Do

Because often no symptoms are present, your child's dysrhythmia may not be discovered until the doctor listens to her heartbeat during an exam. The doctor will then determine whether your child has any accompanying symptoms. Is

NORMAL HEART RATES FOR CHILDREN (in beats per minute)

Age	Average Rate	Lower and Upper Limits of Normal
Newborn	125	70–190
1 to 11 months	120	80–160
2 years	110	80–130
4 years	100	80–120
6 years	100	75–115
8 years	90	70–110
10 years	90	70–110

your child aware of her unusual heartbeat? If she is aware of it, what seems to bring on the dysrhythmia and does anything help stop it? If it is a fast rate, how fast? Does your child feel weak, light-headed, or dizzy? Has she ever fainted? The answers to these questions will help your doctor make a diagnosis. Your doctor may refer your child to a heart specialist (pediatric cardiologist) for expert consultation.

To properly identify a dysrhythmia, the doctor will probably order an electrocardiogram (abbreviated as either ECG or EKG), a test that records the heart's electrical activity and detects abnormalities of the heart's rhythm. In order to record the heart activity, the doctor or technician places small disks called electrodes on the child's body, one on each arm and leg, and usually six or more across the chest. Your child won't feel any pain, because the machine only records electrical activity and doesn't pass electricity into the body. For more information, the doctor may order a Holter monitor, which continually records the ECG over a period of hours. In other cases, the doctor may take an ECG reading while a child is exercising. Other tests include a type of transesophageal ECG reading (taken from an electrode placed in the esophagus) to supply more information about the dysrhythmia, a cardiac catheterization with an electrophysiological study (taken by catheters inserted into the heart through the blood vessels), or an echocardiogram (an ultrasound image of the heart).

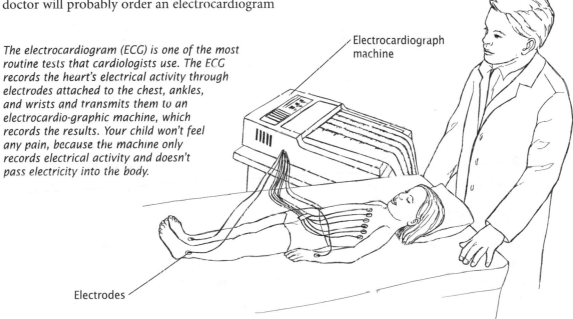

The electrocardiogram (ECG) is one of the most routine tests that cardiologists use. The ECG records the heart's electrical activity through electrodes attached to the chest, ankles, and wrists and transmits them to an electrocardio-graphic machine, which records the results. Your child won't feel any pain, because the machine only records electrical activity and doesn't pass electricity into the body.

Electrocardiograph machine

Electrodes

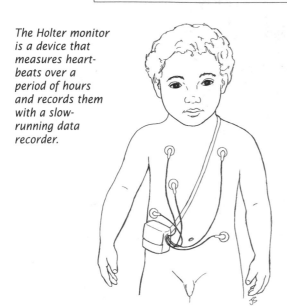

The Holter monitor is a device that measures heartbeats over a period of hours and records them with a slow-running data recorder.

In general, dysrhythmias will not require treatment unless the condition is dangerous or causes serious symptoms. Treatment is usually reserved for children with extremely fast or slow heart rates, shock or heart failure, or fainting spells and convulsions. Various available drugs, such as digitalis, beta-blockers, verapamil, and others, are quite effective, but because they may produce severe side effects if not taken exactly as directed, doctors administer them with caution.

If your child experiences severe episodes of certain types of tachycardia, she may be able to manage the attacks herself with the use of several techniques you can discuss with her doctor. These techniques include coughing, applying cold compresses to her forehead, or closing her mouth and nose and then forcing air up from the lungs (called the Valsalva maneuver). All these methods will slow down the heartbeat.

Some new techniques show great promise in the treatment of many forms of tachycardia. Radiofrequency ablation uses special electrodes inserted into the heart during cardiac catheterization. After the conduction system and the mechanism of the tachycardia are mapped, short bursts of radiofrequency energy are used to "short-circuit" the tachycardia.

If your child experiences severe bradycardia (slow heart rate), your doctor may administer drugs called anti-arrhythmics, which cause the heart to beat faster. Drug therapy for bradycardia is usually only temporary, however, because the drugs themselves may cause irregular heartbeat over time. Children who experience ill effects from severe, long-term bradycardia usually require an artificial pacemaker, which uses electrical impulses to stimulate a regular heartbeat.

What You Can Do

Work with your doctor and cardiologist to understand your child's condition and how to best treat it. If your doctor or nurse asks you to check your child's heart rate, you can learn to feel her pulse or listen to her heart with a stethoscope. If your child is taking medication to treat her dysrhythmia, you can make sure that she takes it on time. If your child has frequent episodes of fast heart rates, the doctor may show you and your child ways to slow the heart rate. If your child has an artificial pacemaker, your doctor or nurse will give you the information you need to check how it's working.

Prevention

Most cases of dysrhythmia in children cannot be prevented. Be sure, however, to learn if your child needs to avoid any medications or intense athletic activities in order to avoid worsening an existing dysrhythmia.

▌ *Abrasions*

See *Cuts and Scrapes.*

Abscesses

See *Boils.*

Acne (Pimples)

Although we tend to think of acne as an adolescent problem, even the soft, clear skin of an infant or a child can sometimes be marred by blemishes. Acne may develop in newborns (neonatal acne), for example, or in children 7 to 9 years old (when preadolescent hormones start flowing). Fortunately, most cases of acne can be treated at home and leave no permanent scars.

Signs and Symptoms

- Red, white, or black bumps, sometimes with yellow pustules, usually across the cheeks, forehead, and chin

When to Call the Doctor
CALL THE DOCTOR TODAY IF

- your child's acne is severe or does not respond to home treatment.

Essential Facts

Three main types of acne exist:

- *Neonatal Acne:* Neonatal acne, also known as infantile acne, occurs mostly in boys from 3 to 6 months old. A temporary condition, neonatal acne may appear on the forehead, cheeks, and chin and looks like white pimples, which usually disappear without a trace. Scarring is rare. Infantile acne may recur, but usually clears up within the first few years of life.

- *Acne Vulgaris:* This form of acne appears commonly in adolescence, but can develop in 7- or 8-year-old children. Somewhat more common in boys than girls, acne vulgaris usually occurs on the face, chest, and back. Several kinds of skin eruptions, including whiteheads, blackheads, and pimples, may be present.

- *Medication-Related Acne:* Several kinds of medications trigger childhood acne outbreaks. Most commonly, steroid acne can occur when a child receives cortisone medication for an illness or a disease such as arthritis. Eruptions usually appear 2 or more weeks after treatment begins: on the face, the neck, the chest, the shoulders, the arms, the upper back, and—rarely—the scalp.

Causes

Most cases of acne are due to collections of dead skin cells and hardened oils in the oil gland canals—the tiny glands contained in the hair follicles that secrete a fatty oil (called sebum) to lubricate your hair and skin. Acne occurs when these cells and sebum form a plug that closes off the pore, causing the follicle wall to bulge, thus creating a whitehead. If the pore stays open, the top surface of the plug may become darkened by dirt and oils, causing a blackhead. Pimples develop when whiteheads rupture the follicle wall and become infected.

The overproduction and collection of sebum is most often stimulated by hormonal changes that occur temporarily during infancy, puberty, or adolescence. These hormonal changes usually resolve themselves within a few months or a year, and when the hormonal fluctuations stop, the acne clears up as well. For reasons not yet understood, male hormones appear to trigger acne more often than female hormones, and thus more boys than girls have the condition.

What the Doctor May Do

Acne—especially infantile acne—usually doesn't require treatment. Your doctor will probably simply reassure you that the condition will clear up on its own within a few months. Medication-induced acne often clears up by itself once the medication is withdrawn. To alleviate the symptoms in the meantime, the doctor may sometimes suggest oral and topical medications, such as antibiotics and cleansers with benzoyl peroxide, a chemical that prevents the growth of acne-causing bacteria and helps unclog the oil ducts.

If your older child's acne vulgaris doesn't clear up after 2 or 3 months of home treatment with benzoyl peroxide, consult a doctor. The doctor may suggest one or more of the over-the-counter medications described here. In cases of moderate to severe acne vulgaris, the doctor may prescribe an oral antibiotic to reduce bacterial growth and the redness caused by the skin's reaction to the bacteria. She may also prescribe topical antibiotic creams or lotions.

For young women, estrogen (usually in the form of birth control pills) may help clear up acne because estrogen suppresses the hormonal activity that stimulates excess oil secretion. Two drugs, tretinoin (a topical formula) and isotretinoin (taken by mouth), are derived from vita-

QUESTIONS PARENTS ASK
Common Beliefs About Acne

Q: Does eating chocolate and french fries cause acne?
A: No evidence exists to support the old theory that candy or greasy foods trigger or exacerbate acne.

Q: Does acne develop because of poor hygiene and excessive dirt?
A: The cause of acne is more than skin deep. Hormonal activity triggers the production of excess oil that clogs oil glands below the skin's surface. No amount of cleansing will prevent or clear up an acne outbreak, but it is important to keep skin clean to reduce the chances of infection.

min A and can be effective in treating severe acne. These drugs may have side effects, such as dry skin, eye irritation, extreme sensitivity to the sun, and others, and require close medical supervision. They should not be taken by pregnant women, because they cause an increased risk of fetal abnormalities.

What You Can Do

Here are suggestions to help clear up your child's acne:

- *Apply benzoyl peroxide.* Available over the counter, acne lotions or gels containing benzoyl peroxide can help penetrate the skin with medication. Choose the lowest concentration of benzoyl peroxide (2.5 percent) to avoid skin irritation. Do not use such products on infant acne, which clears up by itself.

- *Test lotions before using.* To avoid a possible skin reaction to an acne preparation, rub a tiny drop of the product inside your child's forearm. Wait a day to make sure no redness or irritation appears, then use the lotion according to the package directions. If your child has a bad reaction, call his doctor for suggestions.

Acne occurs when dead skin cells and sebum form a plug that clogs the pore, causing the follicle wall to bulge. Pimples develop when whiteheads rupture the follicle wall and become infected.

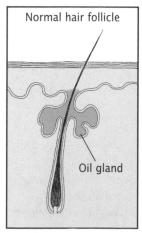

Normal hair follicle

Oil gland

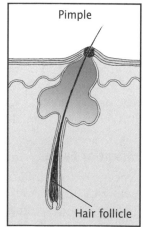

Pimple

Hair follicle

- *Buy "non-acnegenic" or "non-comedogenic" skin care products.* These are designed not to exacerbate acne. Steer clear of soaps and cosmetics that irritate and exacerbate acne—mainly those with heavy oils that clog the pores. Ask your doctor or dermatologist for suggestions.
- *Encourage a "hands-off" policy.* Picking at or squeezing pimples will only irritate them and encourage infection. Even hard scrubbing can worsen an outbreak. Encourage your child to wash his face—gently—two or three times a day and otherwise keep his hands away.

Prevention

It is not possible to prevent an outbreak of neonatal acne. But there are several steps you can take to reduce an older child's chances of an acne outbreak. Make sure your child avoids soaps and cosmetics that trap oil beneath the skin. Be aware that wearing helmets and hats that trap sweat and dirt along the forehead may also trigger or exacerbate acne. But make sure that your child wears a helmet during activities when this safety equipment is important.

See also *Rashes.*

Allergies

Does a waft of tree pollen make your child sneeze? Are his eyes set ablaze whenever he cuddles his cat? Does he get a stuffy nose or a skin rash, or does he wheeze after eating certain foods? If you've answered yes to any of these questions, your child may be one of 46 million people in the United States who experience allergies. Children of all ages can have allergies, and some are allergic to two or more substances (called allergens). While most allergic reactions are uncomfortable but pose no serious threat, some allergies to certain foods or bee stings can cause life-threatening reactions. See Allergic

Shock (Anaphylaxis) on page 390. That's why it's important to identify any allergies your child may have and take the precautions described in this section.

Signs and Symptoms

- Itchy, red eyes, nose, throat, or skin
- Runny nose and sneezing
- Wheezing or coughing
- *Hives*
- Swelling of the lips, throat, tongue, or other body parts
- *Vomiting* or *diarrhea*

When to Call the Doctor
CALL FOR EMERGENCY HELP IF
- your child has difficulty breathing and/or turns blue.

  For first aid information, see page 380 if your child is less than 1 year old and page 383 if your child is 1 year of age or older.

CALL THE DOCTOR IMMEDIATELY IF
- your child's lips or throat swell.
- your child is wheezing and complains of chest tightness.

CALL THE DOCTOR TODAY IF
- your child develops a rash, hives, or other symptoms.

TALK WITH THE DOCTOR AT YOUR CHILD'S NEXT CHECKUP IF
- your child has recurrent rashes.
- your child has a frequent runny nose or itchy, watery eyes.

Essential Facts

Allergies tend to run in families: If you have allergies, your child is more likely to have them. But even children without a family history of allergies can be affected. Allergens that cause little or no reaction upon first exposure can cause intense reactions on repeat exposures. Some allergies cause **asthma** episodes characterized by wheezing or difficulty breathing, which must be diagnosed and treated quickly.

Many children "outgrow" their allergies by adolescence—their airways mature and become less affected by irritants, or they learn to avoid allergens. Certain foods (nuts and shellfish) are more likely to cause lifelong allergies. But other foods that often cause allergic reactions in children (including milk, soy, peanuts, eggs, and wheat) are less likely to provoke allergic reactions as a child grows older.

Causes

An allergy is a disorder of the body's defense (or immune) system. An allergy occurs when the cells of the immune system unleash a chemical response against a normally harmless substance. In other words, an allergic person's immune system treats pollen (or other allergens) like a

deadly enemy that must be eliminated from the body at all costs. Histamine, one such chemical released by cells, causes itching and rashes in response to an allergen.

Allergy symptoms are side effects of the body's efforts to rid itself of the offending substance, also known as the trigger. In rare cases, the allergy may be so severe that the child goes into a kind of allergic shock (anaphylactic shock, see p. 390). When this happens, allergy symptoms such as hives, itchy skin, and swollen eyes rapidly progress to include coughing, nausea, difficulty breathing, increased heart rate, and a serious drop in blood pressure. Children allergic to bee stings and certain foods (particularly peanuts, other nuts, and shellfish) are more susceptible to anaphylactic reactions, which are true medical emergencies.

Other types of allergies include hay fever (runny, itchy nose and eyes) from inhaled pollen, and allergies to dust and animal dander. The skin rash that results from exposure to poison ivy, poison oak, or poison sumac is another form of allergic reaction. Some substances, such as tobacco smoke, act as irritants and although they don't provoke a true allergic reaction, the symptoms they cause are similar.

Common Allergic Triggers

- Animal dander
- Certain foods (most commonly milk, eggs, soy, peanuts, other nuts, fish, shellfish, wheat)
- Cockroaches
- Dust mites
- Stinging-insect venom
- Medication
- Pollen
- Latex

Common Irritant Triggers

- Smoke (tobacco and other kinds)
- Perfumes
- Detergents and disinfectants
- Cold weather

Common allergens: Normally harmless substances like pollen and dust mites can create allergic reactions in your child when the immune system treats them as deadly enemies, unleashing a chemical response.

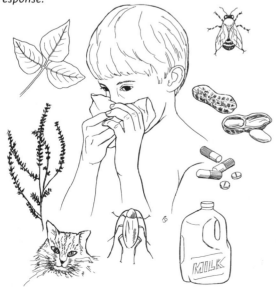

What the Doctor May Do

No simple diagnostic test can determine which trigger causes your child's runny nose, skin rash, or other symptoms. Instead, doctors diagnose allergies by asking you and your child about the timing and nature of symptoms—taking a thorough allergy history. Frequently, this history alone can identify an allergen. For example, if your child wheezes only when holding his cat, he's probably allergic to cats. If your child stops wheezing when he's at his grandmother's cat-free house or at school, this further confirms the diagnosis.

Allergy Testing

If your child's symptoms suggest allergies but you haven't identified the triggers, your doctor may advise visiting an allergist—a physician who specializes in diagnosing and treating allergies. Depending on your child's symptoms, history, and other factors, the specialist may perform one of the tests outlined below.

Skin Testing Skin testing involves introducing tiny amounts of extracts of various common allergens into your child's skin by one of two methods. In the prick test, the doctor or an assistant applies droplets of extracts on the child's arm using a device that applies eight drops at once in a grid pattern pricked on the skin. In the intradermal test, the doctor injects allergen extracts just under the skin of the upper arm, which causes tiny blisters to form. The number of allergens included in this test will depend on your child's symptoms and history. If the symptoms occur on a seasonal basis, for instance, your doctor may include the common pollens in your area. If the symptoms occur year-round, she'll add dust mites and molds, and if your child is around pets often, she'll add extracts of dander.

If your child is allergic to a substance, his skin will redden and develop a small hive at the site where the allergen was introduced. Skin test-ing can cause tingling and a bit of discomfort, and it requires a child to hold still and not rub or scratch the site for 10 to 20 minutes. Results are available right away.

Blood Testing Blood tests can measure the amount of allergic antibody (IgE) to specific allergens that is in the blood. But blood testing is a less sensitive method. It can miss allergies found by skin testing, for example, and it is more expensive. It also takes longer; you must wait about 2 weeks to get the results.

Food Elimination Diet If you and your doctor suspect that your child is allergic to something he's eating, the doctor may suggest that you remove the suspected foods from your child's diet for 7 to 10 days to see if symptoms disappear.

Allergy Medications

The best treatment for allergies is to keep whatever is causing the allergy away from your child as much as possible. But your doctor might also prescribe medications (see chart, p. 434). Also, if your child has a food allergy or another allergy that could cause the severe allergic reaction known as anaphylaxis (see Allergic Shock, p. 390), your doctor may give you an epinephrine autoinjector to use in case of emergency.

For milder allergy symptoms, if your child is over 6 years old, ask your child's doctor whether a prescription antihistamine may be useful. Over-the-counter medications that may help include diphenhydramine or medications containing chlorpheniramine or brompheniramine in syrup or pill form. Ask your child's doctor about using these medications.

For food allergies, if your child is having a mild allergic reaction that involves only the skin, choose an over-the-counter oral antihistamine such as diphenhydramine. If your child has any other food allergy symptoms, such as a runny or stuffy nose, itching or swelling of throat, wheezing or shortness of breath, coughing, nausea, or vomiting, administer an epinephrine injection and bring your child to the emergency room or a doctor's office immediately.

Occasionally, if your child is allergic to an unavoidable substance or has to take large amounts of medicine to control his allergies, the doctor may prescribe immunotherapy (allergy shots) to reduce or eliminate allergy symptoms. The shots may be needed for 3 years or more.

What You Can Do

Be alert for allergy signs in your child, especially if allergies run in your family. If the doctor diagnoses your child with an allergy, work with her to find the allergy triggers and then to eliminate them from your child's surroundings or diet as much as possible.

Watch for signs of food allergies, particularly those that might indicate a severe allergic reaction. For example, if your child is having a mild reaction, limited to itchy skin, you can use an oral antihistamine (see chart). But if you notice other symptoms, such as hives; itching or swelling of the lips, throat, or other body areas; wheezing; shortness of breath; difficulty breathing; coughing; nausea; vomiting; diarrhea; stomachache; fainting; or an increase in heart rate, administer the epinephrine injector prescribed by your child's doctor as soon as possible and call for emergency assistance or take your child

▬ ALLERGY MEDICINES AND THEIR ACTIONS

Medication	Actions	Form	Possible Side Effects
Antihistamines	Reduce itching; dry up runny nose	Pills, liquids	Drowsiness, delirium, dry mouth, irritability
Decongestants	Reduce nasal swelling	Pills, liquids	Irritability, high blood pressure, rapid heart rate, insomnia
Bronchodilators	Ease wheezing, asthma symptoms (e.g., bronchial spasms)	Pills, liquids, inhaler	Agitation, rapid heart rate, dizziness, headache, tremors
Cromolyn	Prevents symptoms of allergies and asthma; stabilizes cell membranes	Nasal spray, inhaler, eyedrops	Spray: Nasal irritation Inhaler: Cough Eyedrops: Eye irritation
Corticosteroids	Relieve severe allergies; limit inflammation	Pills, liquids, inhaler	Inhaler: Local irritation, yeast infection of mouth Pills, liquids: Fluid retention, weight gain, mood changes, and others with long-term use
Leukotriene blockers	Prevent or relieve inflammation for asthma	Pills	Nausea, headache
Epinephrine	Emergency treatment of anaphylaxis agitation	Syringe, autoinjector	Increased heart rate

to the emergency room. Children do die from food allergies, and a food allergy reaction, particularly to peanuts and other nuts, is a true emergency.

Prevention

If your child has a family history of allergy (parents or siblings with allergies), reducing exposure to allergens (see Common Allergic Triggers, p. 432) may help prevent allergies. Here are some tips for eliminating various allergens.

Dust and Dust Mites

- Encase pillows, mattress, and box spring in mite-proof covers—they are sold widely in medical supply stores.
- Vacuum or wipe clean the covers on pillows or mattresses once a week. A microlined vacuum bag or a vacuum cleaner that contains a high efficiency particulate air filter (HEPA) can screen out substances as small as 0.03 microns in diameter. Without such filters, vacuuming will only distribute dust more widely throughout the room.
- Wash sheets, blankets, and bedspreads in hot water once a week. Choose quilts or comforters that can be laundered frequently.
- Choose wood or tile floors, which are easier to keep clean than carpets (which harbor dust mites).
- Remove stuffed animals from your child's room. If your child insists on sleeping with one, choose one that you can launder in hot water often.
- Replace cloth curtains or blinds in your child's room with vinyl roller shades. Wipe the shades clean weekly, or wash the curtains in hot water frequently.
- Remove stuffed furniture and wall-to-wall carpeting from your child's room, if possible.
- Store unused shoes, clothing, toys, and books in easily dusted plastic containers with lids.

- Organize closets so that you can clean them weekly.
- Eliminate excess clutter and dusty books and objects from your child's room, and keep dusty objects away from your child.
- Thoroughly dust and mop your child's bedroom weekly.
- Clean the furnace annually. Damp mop heating grates. Have air ducts cleaned.

Molds

- If you live in a humid climate, use a dehumidifier in your child's room. Clean the dehumidifier regularly to discourage mold growth.
- Use mold and mildew cleaners. Clean the bathroom with white vinegar or diluted bleach weekly. Rinse well after cleaning. Install fans.
- Cover your walls with paint, not wallpaper. Mold can grow beneath wallpaper.
- Carefully clean and maintain window air conditioner units. Mold grows in pooled water. Change filters frequently.
- Have your child avoid outdoor areas with decaying vegetation, such as piles of dead leaves or compost bins.
- Don't let your child play in damp basements or cellars. Using a dehumidifier can reduce mold and mildew in these areas.

Pets

- If possible, find a good new home for your child's furred and feathered pets. If not, make the pet an outdoor animal, as much as is possible with that type of pet. Wash and brush the pet—outside—at least once a week. Never allow the pet in your child's bedroom.
- Encourage your child to wash his hands and, depending on the severity of the allergy, to change his clothes and bathe after playing with a furred or feathered pet.

Pollen

- Keep windows and doors shut during pollen season, especially in your child's bedroom.

- Consider running an air-cleaning unit in your child's bedroom if you don't have an air filter or cleaner in your home's heating system.

- Drive with the car windows shut and air conditioning on during pollen season to reduce exposure to outdoor allergens.

- Minimize outdoor playtime during the peak pollen seasons if your child is sensitive to pollen. If you have a lawn, mow it when your child is elsewhere.

- Try to keep your child indoors between 5 A.M. and 10 A.M., when pollen levels are highest.

- Have your child bathe and shampoo every night before going to bed during pollen season.

Foods

- Read labels carefully, and avoid products containing foods to which your child is allergic.

- Teach your child to ask questions about food ingredients when eating outside the home. Or better yet, have your child eat only food prepared at home.

- Teach your child not to share or trade food, utensils, or food containers.

- Alert your child's teachers, school cafeteria staff, bus driver, and school nurse to your child's food allergy, especially if it results in a severe reaction, such as allergic shock (see p. 390). With help from your doctor, instruct the staff precisely about what to do in an emergency.

General Measures

- Eliminate secondhand tobacco smoke, which worsens allergies and asthma.

- Avoid using vaporizers in your child's room. Mites and molds thrive in humidity. Or, if you must use one, scrub thoroughly with a mild bleach solution and rinse well daily.

- Eliminate house plants. They gather dust and harbor mold.

- Don't use a wood-burning stove if your child has asthma or is sensitive to smoke.

◾ Amblyopia and/or Strabismus

If you're like most parents, you can't stop staring at your new infant, adoring her wide-eyed wonder. Take the opportunity to observe whether her eyes are aligned properly and moving together at the same time. Although a newborn baby's eyes may normally wander and seem to move independently for brief periods, this pattern usually disappears within a few months. But some children are born with a problem known as strabismus ("cross-eyes"), in which the eyes continue this pattern of wandering independently (misalignment) over the long term. Strabismus can lead to subnormal vision, known as amblyopia, or "lazy eye." But if recognized and treated early, strabismus will usually leave no permanent vision problems.

Signs and Symptoms

- The crossing or drifting of one eye, or both eyes, after 4 months of age

- If both eyes are involved, eyes may "cross" at different times

- Symptoms may be more obvious if the child is tired, ill, or under stress

When to Call the Doctor
CALL THE DOCTOR TODAY IF

- your child's eyes are constantly crossed or misaligned.
- your child's eyes cross often after 4 months of age.
- your child's eyes don't seem to track together.

TALK WITH THE DOCTOR AT
YOUR CHILD'S NEXT CHECKUP IF

- you have questions about your child's vision.
- your child's eye appears to drift.
- your child has difficulty reading or seeing the chalkboard in school.

Most cases of strabismus result from an imbalance or incoordination of the muscles controlling eye movement. Seeing with both eyes when one is deviating would cause double vision, so the brain suppresses the image from the diverging eye.

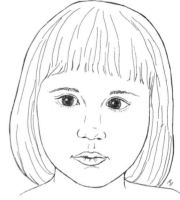

Essential Facts

Strabismus refers to a condition in which a child does not focus both eyes on the same object at the same time. While the child focuses on an object with one eye, the other turns either inward (esotropia), outward (exotropia), upward, or downward. In some cases, only one eye deviates (is misaligned with respect to the other). In other cases, the eyes take turns deviating. Strabismus can lead to amblyopia, when one eye always crosses, and the child no longer uses that eye to see. That eye, in effect, becomes "lazy."

Strabismus is fairly common. About 4 percent of children under age 6 years have the condition, and the incidence is much higher among children with developmental disorders. For instance, about half of children with cerebral palsy have some form of strabismus.

A child with strabismus may begin favoring the normal eye without ever realizing it, suppressing the vision in the deviating eye and enjoying relatively comfortable vision in the normal eye. Eventually, the lesser-used eye grows weaker and loses at least some of its ability to see. However, the outlook for a child with strabismus is excellent if a doctor detects the condition early and begins correcting it right away.

Causes

An imbalance or a lack of coordination of the muscles controlling eye movement is the cause of most cases of strabismus. Although the cause of this imbalance is mostly unknown, strabismus occasionally may develop if your child is injured, has another eye problem, or develops cataracts (a clouding of the lens due to inheritance or injury). Strabismus sometimes runs in families, and is more common in preterm infants and children with cerebral palsy. It may be present at birth or develop later.

Strabismus usually causes amblyopia, the condition in which one eye crosses or becomes "lazy," but any vision problem—including nearsightedness and farsightedness—affecting one eye may result in amblyopia. This condition causes more vision problems than all other eye diseases and injuries combined, and is usually treatable, if caught early. Other causes of amblyopia include cataracts, eye infections existing at birth, and eye injury (see *Eye Injuries*).

What the Doctor May Do

To diagnose strabismus, an ophthalmologist first performs a complete eye exam. He'll follow your child's eyes as they focus on nearby and distant objects and as she glances left and right, then upward and downward. A method of diagnosing strabismus in older children involves covering one eye at a time while your child stares at an object. If a child has strabismus, the deviating eye will then jump or move to focus on what the child is looking at when the straight eye is covered.

The goal of treatment for both strabismus and amblyopia is to develop the best possible vision in both eyes. To achieve that goal, your child needs to use the weaker eye to help it regain its vision.

If muscle imbalance and incoordination (strabismus) is causing your child's vision problem (amblyopia), the doctor will probably suggest placing a patch over the normally functioning eye. This process will require her to use her weakened eye, thus strengthening it over a period of several weeks to several months. Another option is to put prescription eye drops that blur vision in her good eye to encourage her to use the weak one.

To correct the alignment problem that may be causing her vision problems, the doctor may prescribe special glasses. But if glasses don't succeed in straightening her eyes, the doctor may use surgery to correct the alignment. In some cases, both glasses and surgery are necessary.

What You Can Do

If your child is being treated for amblyopia, possibly the most difficult challenge is getting your child used to the eye patch required to treat most cases. Follow these tips to help your child cope with wearing an eye patch:

- *Focus on the problem.* Your child will probably need to wear the patch for at least a few hours daily. If she is old enough, explain why she needs to wear the patch. You can show her by covering her "good" eye and asking her how it feels to look with the other. By seeing the dif-

ferences in vision between the two eyes, she'll understand the importance of strengthening her weak eye by wearing the patch.

- *Be consistent.* As the parent, it's up to you (with your doctor's advice) to make and maintain the rules. If your child needs to wear the patch for 3 hours, don't let her remove it unless it's urgent—and if she does, insist that she make up the time tomorrow. Create a system of rewards and consequences to encourage her to wear the patch.

- *Alert the school nurse, teacher, or day care administrator.* If your child must wear a patch at school or day care, make sure that her caregivers understand her condition and the importance of the patch.

- *Follow up.* Follow the schedule your doctor recommends for follow-up vision exams, which will help ensure that the condition is corrected. Routine vision screening is recommended for all children.

Prevention

Although you can't prevent these conditions from occurring, you can help prevent any damage by recognizing the signs and having the condition treated promptly. Alert your doctor if you suspect a problem with your child's eye movements or vision, then follow his advice carefully. Regular vision screening is the best way to detect these problems in older children.

See also *Vision Problems.*

▍ *Anal Fissures*

See *Constipation.*

▍ *Anemia*

Anemia, a low level of red blood cells, is a condition with few, if any, symptoms in children.

That's one reason to bring your child for regular checkups. Doctors diagnose the condition with routine blood tests. Anemia is more common than you might guess. About 700,000 toddlers in the United States don't get enough iron in their diets (the primary cause of anemia), and about a third of them are anemic because of it. If identified and treated early, most anemia cases respond well to treatment and have no lasting effects.

Signs and Symptoms

Mild cases of anemia:
- None

Severe cases of anemia:
- Pale skin, particularly on nail beds, inside the eyelids, and around the gums
- Fatigue and listlessness
- Poor attention span
- Shortness of breath on exertion
- Dizziness
- Fast heart and breathing rates

When to Call the Doctor
CALL THE DOCTOR IMMEDIATELY IF
- your child is listless.
- your child is short of breath or breathing very quickly.

TALK WITH THE DOCTOR AT YOUR CHILD'S NEXT CHECKUP IF
- you have any concerns about your child's diet.
- you have questions about whether your child may have anemia.

Essential Facts

Red blood cells contain hemoglobin, a protein that delivers oxygen from the lungs to the tissues everywhere in the body. When the body doesn't have enough red blood cells with hemoglobin, the blood cannot carry enough oxygen. This condition is called anemia, a blood disorder that, when severe or untreated, can cause dizziness, weakness, rapid heart rate, rapid breathing, and fatigue, as well as other health problems. Anemia can last for a long time (chronic) or occur and disappear suddenly (acute). The condition may also accompany chronic illnesses, such as kidney failure, or—in very rare cases—it may result from excessive blood loss, infection, or exposure to drugs or toxins.

More than 30 types of anemia exist, each with a different cause and treatment. Each type falls into one of two categories: problems producing red blood cells (most often from iron deficiency) or increased losses of red blood cells (due to bleeding or to the body's breaking down or damaging its own red blood cells).

Except for cases caused by bleeding, anemia results from the imbalance between the production and destruction of red blood cells. This balance is normally maintained by proper functioning of the bone marrow, which produces red blood cells. Constant production and destruction of blood cells is necessary because the cells naturally wear out after about 120 days. As a result, old blood cells are destroyed and new ones are produced to take their place. When this process is disrupted, anemia results.

Causes

There are many causes of anemia, including lack of dietary iron and excess bleeding. These two problems cause most childhood anemia cases. But there are other causes. Sometimes, for example, the body abnormally destroys its own cells. In other cases, the body doesn't produce enough red blood cells or produces red blood cells that don't have enough hemoglobin. In still other situations, **lead poisoning** interferes with the production of the iron-containing component of hemoglobin, leading to insufficient synthesis of hemoglobin, which results in anemia.

Iron-deficiency anemia is, by far, the most common type of anemia in children. It occurs when a child's body doesn't receive enough iron to produce sufficient red blood cells. Other, rarer forms of nutritional anemia include deficiencies of vitamin B_{12} and folic acid, which are also essential for hemoglobin synthesis and function.

Iron-deficiency anemia sometimes appears in newborns as the result of a lack of iron storage before birth—which is one reason that obstetricians urge pregnant women to eat lots of iron-rich foods. Iron-deficiency anemia in children over 6 months old is usually caused by insufficient dietary iron. Preschoolers grow rapidly and their blood volume increases; thus they are susceptible to iron deficiency because their bodies need large amounts of iron. After about 5 years old and until adolescence, children need less iron to meet the body's demands. Consequently, children over 5 years of age seldom become iron deficient as a result of insufficient dietary iron. At any age, iron-deficiency anemia can develop if children lose blood. Blood loss in children is often due to low-level, sometimes unsuspected, bleeding from the gut (the gastrointestinal tract).

Some types of anemia are inherited, such as when red cells are especially fragile because of their shape or internal structure. One example is **sickle-cell disease,** in which abnormal hemoglobin tends to congeal and deform red blood cells into the shape of a sickle (a crescent-shaped cutting tool). These deformed cells damage easily and do not carry oxygen efficiently. *Thalassemia* is the term describing two other forms of anemia resulting from the underproduction of certain proteins in hemoglobin. The resulting hemoglobin is fragile and inefficient at carrying oxygen, so that children with the disorders do not grow properly and have a range of medical problems.

In rare types of anemia known as *red cell aplasia,* the bone marrow produces too few red blood cells. In other instances, the body produces too few red blood cells, white blood cells (which fight infection), and platelets (which help blood clot after injury). When all three types of cells are affected, the condition is termed *aplastic*

anemia. This may occur after infection or exposure to certain toxins or medications. Aplastic anemia is rare, but may be life-threatening.

What the Doctor May Do

Since mild anemia usually has no symptoms, you may not know that your child is anemic until your doctor discovers it after giving your child a blood test during a routine exam. Or, if your doctor suspects that your child may be anemic, she may run tests to measure the components of his blood and to examine the size and shape of his red blood cells, to confirm the condition. Routine tests include the following:

- *Hemoglobin:* Taken to measure the amount of hemoglobin in red blood cells. Normal levels are 11 grams per deciliter or higher.

- *Hematocrit:* Taken to measure the percentage of total blood volume that the red blood cells occupy. Normal levels are 33 percent or higher.

- *Reticulocyte hemoglobin:* Taken to measure the amount of hemoglobin in the reticulocyte portion of the total red blood cell count. Normal levels are 28 picograms per deciliter or higher.

- *Blood lead:* Given to distinguish between anemia and lead poisoning. Normal blood levels are less than 10 micrograms per deciliter.

- *Stool analysis:* The doctor can analyze the child's stool to detect evidence of gastrointestinal bleeding. For sickle-cell anemia, a test called hemoglobin electrophoresis may be used to analyze hemoglobin. Tests may also be performed on siblings and parents if an inherited anemia is suspected. The doctor can also test for anemia caused by too much cow's milk by checking for small amounts of blood in the stool.

Iron-deficiency anemia treatment usually requires including more iron-rich foods in the child's diet or giving the child daily iron supplements. Mild cases of anemia usually respond well to simply increasing the amount of dietary iron (see the chart on iron-rich foods), but your doctor may prescribe iron supplements if dietary changes don't work. Infants and toddlers usually take liquid iron drops, while older children may take a liquid form or multivitamin tablets with iron. Iron supplements may cause slight constipation or mild stomach upset, and stools may be dark or black. Even after your child is no longer anemic, he may require iron supplements to build up his iron stores. Because vitamin C can enhance iron absorption, give iron supplements with a glass of orange juice. Giving iron with liquid also prevents the iron from staining the child's teeth.

What You Can Do

Follow your doctor's instructions carefully. If your doctor prescribes iron supplements, don't give your child more than the recommended dose: Iron supplements, when taken in excess, can cause poisoning. Keep your own iron supplement pills and vitamins out of reach of children. Store them in a locked cabinet. Iron is best given on an empty stomach about ½ hour before meals. If stomach upset occurs, reducing the dose or giving the iron with meals may help.

Give your child food rich in iron. Healthy infants and toddlers need about 1 milligram of iron per kilogram (about 2 pounds) of body weight every day. Premature babies, because they lack full stores of iron, may need even more iron in their diets. Older children require 10 milligrams a day. The best sources of dietary iron for children are lean red meat, poultry, and fish. Leafy green vegetables, whole grains, dried fruits, legumes, and molasses are also rich in iron, although the iron from these is less readily absorbed than iron from animal protein such as red meat. Iron found naturally in foods is more easily absorbed than that used to "fortify" foods. Nevertheless, iron-fortified foods, such as infant cereals for babies age 4 months and older, can be an important part of an iron-rich diet.

In addition, many factors influence how well the body absorbs iron. Vitamin C, for instance, enhances absorption. Milk and milk products, on the other hand, decrease the body's iron absorption.

IRON-RICH FOODS

Food	Serving Size	Iron Content* (milligrams)
High Iron Content		
Bran flakes, 40 percent enriched	¾ cup	8.1
Beef liver	3½ oz.	6.7
Oatmeal, fortified instant	1 pkg.	6.3
Moderate Iron Content		
Corned beef	3 oz.	3.7
Dried peaches	½ cup	3.3
Blackstrap molasses	1 Tbs.	3.2
Apricots, dried	½ cup (20)	3.1
Baked potato, with skin	1 medium	2.7
Steak, lean sirloin	2.5 oz.	2.4
Hamburger, extra lean	3 oz.	2.2
Raisins, seedless	⅔ cup	2.0
Spaghetti (iron in pasta)	½ cup, cooked	1.7
Roast beef, lean	1.8 oz.	1.6
Egg, fried or scrambled	2	1.4
Peanuts, roasted	½ cup	1.4
Tuna salad	½ cup	1.3
Green peas, frozen	½ cup, cooked	1.3
Broccoli	1 spear	1.3
Prunes, dried	5 large	1.2
Chicken, without skin	3½ oz.	1.2

Source: U.S. Department of Agriculture, 1990.
*Iron content does not reflect the amount of iron ultimately absorbed by the body.

Drinking cow's milk too early is probably the most common cause of iron deficiency in infants. Cow's milk contains too little iron. Breast milk or iron-fortified formulas contain all the iron most babies need. Also, cow's milk contains proteins that may irritate a baby's stomach and bowels, causing small amounts of blood loss daily, which can lead to anemia. Cow's milk should be avoided for children under 1 year old. Toddlers should drink plenty of milk, but only as part of a well-balanced diet.

Prevention

Iron-deficiency anemia is often preventable simply by providing your child with a healthy, balanced diet that includes iron-rich foods.

Animal Bites

See *Bites, Animal and Human.*

Anxiety Disorders

Although people think of childhood as a carefree and simple time, children often have worries and fears. These fears often recede as children mature, develop self-confidence, and learn to better understand the world (see Dealing with Fears, p. 188). But if your child's fears and worries begin to cause her problems in social situations, developmental achievements, or academic performance and she cannot function normally, she may have an anxiety disorder. Anxiety disorders are among the most common childhood mental health disorders. Fortunately, with treatment and loving support, most children with anxiety disorders can overcome their fears.

Signs and Symptoms

- Verbal expressions of fear and anxiety
- Nightmares
- Panic attacks
- Stomachaches
- Headaches
- Sleep problems
- Clinging and dependent behavior
- Reluctance to sleep or to attend school
- Chest pains

When to Call the Doctor

CALL THE DOCTOR IMMEDIATELY IF
- your child talks of suicide or hurting herself.
- you suspect that your child may be contemplating suicide.
Note: Suicide is rare in children but thoughts of suicide are a signal that the child needs help.

CALL THE DOCTOR TODAY IF
- your child's fears or worries are persistent and interfere with daily activities.
- you are concerned about your child's emotional well-being.
- your child has a panic attack.

TALK WITH THE DOCTOR AT YOUR CHILD'S NEXT CHECKUP IF
- your child has frequent nightmares.
- your child seems overly clingy and fearful.
- your child has frequent but short-lived stomachaches or headaches.
- your child withdraws from normal social activities and interests.
- your child is extremely shy.

Essential Facts

Some childhood fears are typical. Beginning as early as 7 months, and often continuing through 3 years of age, many toddlers fear strangers. Fear of the dark, monsters, witches, loud noises, and dogs or other animals is also common in preschoolers. School-age children often worry about injury, illness, death, problems with family and friends, and school performance.

A child with an anxiety disorder may exhibit a wider range of symptoms, including frequent tearfulness, nightmares, and verbal expressions of worry and fear. Withdrawal from normal activities and friends is another sign of anxiety, as well as its common—but potentially more serious—cohort, *depression.* Symptoms of an anxiety disorder may escalate into a full-blown panic attack, during which a child's heart and breathing rates increase and she begins to sweat and tremble with fear and anxiety. Panic attacks may be accompanied by dizziness, nausea, or a feeling of impending death.

Several types of anxiety disorders exist. Among those most commonly affecting children are the following.

Separation Anxiety Disorder

Separation anxiety and fear of strangers are normal phases of infant development. In most cases, these fears and anxieties will dissipate as your child ages and matures physically and emotionally. But some children are more affected by these fears than others. Discuss the matter with your child's doctor if you feel your child's anxieties have started to interfere with her participation in daily activities. Although most children overcome separation anxiety by 4 or 5 years of age, a few continue to have problems. Children with this disorder may refuse or be reluctant to be away from their parents—even to attend school or to spend the night at a friend's house. They avoid being alone, have nightmares about separation, and experience extreme distress or physical symptoms (such as stomachaches, headaches, or vomiting) before or during a separation from parents.

Phobias

Another type of anxiety disorder involves overwhelming fears of specific things (such as an animal) or situations (such as being in the dark). Phobias are very common among children.

According to the American Psychiatric Association, 43 percent of 6- to 12-year-old children have seven or more such fears, and most of these fears will eventually dissipate without the need for treatment. Again, as is true for most psychological problems, you need only be concerned about your child's phobia if her fears significantly affect her ability to enjoy and perform her everyday activities. If that's true for your child—if her fear of spiders or dogs keeps her from going outside at all, for instance, or if she becomes hysterical upon contact with them—discuss the problem with your child's doctor or a child psychologist or psychiatrist. Most simple phobias disappear on their own, but some may require treatment.

School Phobia

Separation anxiety often gives rise to school phobia, or "school refusal," in which a child refuses to attend school or becomes sick from anxiety about attending. Sometimes her anxiety stems from a fear of leaving her parents. In other cases, she fears the academic or social challenges of school. This behavior requires early action to find the right solution. Talk to your child's doctor or a child psychologist or psychiatrist.

Generalized Anxiety Disorder (GAD)

Also called "overanxious" disorder when it occurs in children, GAD involves extreme and unrealistic worries about the uncertainties of life in general—about school, about clothing, about anything and everything, but not necessarily centered on one object or situation, as is true for phobias. These worries are persistent and debilitating. A child with GAD fears for the future, worries about the past, and frets about her ability to cope with the present. She may suck her thumb, bite her nails, pull or twist her hair, or have trouble sleeping. If your child seems constantly worried and anxious, talk with your child's doctor or a child psychologist or psychiatrist.

Obsessive-Compulsive Disorder

Some children are troubled by persistent thoughts, such as fears of infection by germs and dirt, that make them act out repetitive rituals or acts—such as constant hand-washing; constant cleaning and ordering of the room; or elaborate, ritualized preparations for simple functions like eating or dressing—which can interfere with normal functioning. Obsessive-compulsive disorder is very rare in children and always requires medical attention.

Causes

Scientists now believe that an interplay of three major factors causes most cases of anxiety. Biological factors include the levels of brain chemicals called neurotransmitters, such as serotonin and dopamine. Psychosocial factors include stress triggered by an injury or emotional shock, such as a parent's death, a divorce, or a move. Behavioral factors include interaction with people at home, school, or play. Some children are naturally more anxious than others, and genetic influence may play a role. These children can usually learn, with help, better ways to deal with their anxieties.

What the Doctor May Do

If your child's anxiety is severe and prolonged, your doctor will recommend a counselor or therapist—usually a child psychologist or psychiatrist—to evaluate her further and, if necessary, provide longer-term counseling and additional support for you and your child.

Therapy Techniques

A therapist may use play therapy, behavioral techniques, or both to relieve your child's anxiety and help her better cope with her fears.

Play Therapy With this method, the therapist helps the child work out the anxiety by having her express it through play. If your child is terrified of dogs, for instance, the therapist may play a game with her using a stuffed dog so that your child can express her fears and gradually learn to feel comfortable with animals.

Behavior Therapy Through this method, a child learns to overcome fear through relaxation techniques, such as deep breathing and picturing peaceful settings, and through gradual exposure to the anxiety-causing object or situation. The child may watch someone touch the feared object; she may be rewarded for moving gradually closer to it. A child with a compulsion to constantly wash her hands may be asked to touch "contaminated" objects and refrain from hand-washing for successively longer time periods. The therapist may use biofeedback (which measures muscle contractions, body temperature, and heart rate changes) to let a child see her stress and anxiety if she doesn't recognize it and then learn to control it.

One exercise used to treat school phobia involves having a parent (or another loved one) attend school with the fearful child, first for an hour, then for 45 minutes, and so on. The time is gradually shortened until the child feels comfortable attending alone.

Older children—from about 9 to 14 years old—often benefit from participating in rope-climbing courses, outdoor challenge programs, and other well-monitored and directed activities designed to boost self-esteem and create a sense of mastery over the environment. Once a child starts succeeding in these areas, anxiety about the world and her place in it may gradually diminish.

Medication

For some children, medication may help relieve severe anxiety. In the hands of experienced medical professionals, the use of several types of medication can be effective in treating anxiety.

If your doctor prescribes medication, make sure that you understand fully what the drug is, how it works, what symptoms it is meant to treat, and how long it will take before you see any effect. Your doctor will monitor your child with care, and may suggest frequent follow-up appointments to evaluate her progress. These are very potent drugs with side effects that vary, depending on which drug is prescribed. Watch for side effects, and ask your doctor what to do if they occur.

What You Can Do

- *First, acknowledge your child's concerns.* Reassure her of her safety, and offer your help and support. Children rarely fake anxiety for other purposes—such as extra attention or goodies. Let her know you understand that her fear is real even if the source of her fear is unrealistic.

- *Let your child know you'll always be there.* Providing a sense of security, support, and consistency is the most important "medicine" you can give your child.

- *Establish and maintain a regular schedule.* What children with anxiety disorders often fear most is change and uncertainty. The more you can do to maintain a calm and stable routine, the better.

- *Plan ahead for major changes.* Anxiety disorders often develop after a major change in family circumstances. If you know you're going to divorce, move, have a baby, or even change jobs, prepare your child by explaining, in advance, the upcoming change and assure her that she will continue to be safe and well loved.

- *Maintain control and stability.* Remain calm when your child is scared or anxious; otherwise she may conclude that there is really something to fear. Make sure she tries to perform her normal activities as much as possible, despite her fears. For a school phobia, your best strategy may be to insist that your child attend school. Your doctor and school counselor can offer other techniques; ask them for advice.

- *Answer questions.* Whatever the concern, answer your child's fear-based questions briefly and honestly, letting her know that you understand her fears. If she catches you off-guard with a difficult question, tell her you need to think about it before you answer. Don't dismiss her fears by brushing them away with such statements as, "There's no such thing as monsters." Instead, let her know that you understand that her fear is real even though the monsters are not.

- *Safety-proof your home.* Although medications, razors, and poisonous substances should not be within reach of any child, take special care to keep them away from children with anxiety disorders, who are particularly vulnerable to hurting themselves. Guns should never be kept in a home where a child lives.

Prevention

Creating a stable and loving environment for your child may help diminish anxiety, but because the cause is often unknown, no surefire prevention method exists.

See also **Behavioral Problems.**

▌ Apnea

See *Infantile Apnea.*

▌ Appendicitis

If your child has a bad stomachache, how can you tell whether it's just a stomach flu or whether it's appendicitis—a medical emergency?

Appendicitis is an inflammation of a small pouch of tissue that extends from the beginning of the large intestine. Familiarize yourself with the symptoms of appendicitis so that if you see them, you can act quickly. The earlier appendicitis is treated, the quicker and more complete a child's recovery.

Signs and Symptoms

- Abdominal pain around the navel and/or lower right side that worsens over a few hours
- Fever
- Nausea and/or *vomiting*
- Loss of appetite
- Constipation
- *Diarrhea*

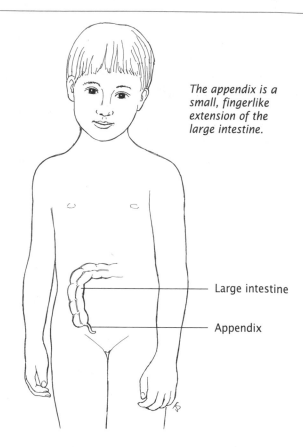

The appendix is a small, fingerlike extension of the large intestine.

Large intestine

Appendix

 When to Call the Doctor
CALL FOR EMERGENCY HELP IF

- your child shows symptoms of shock (dizziness, confusion, rapid pulse) (see p. 418).
- your child is doubling over with abdominal pain.

CALL THE DOCTOR IMMEDIATELY IF

- your child shows symptoms of appendicitis.

Essential Facts

About 4 out of 1,000 children under 14 years old get appendicitis every year. It is rare in babies under 1 year old and most common in teenagers. Appendicitis usually begins with pain around the navel, followed 1 or 2 hours later by nausea and sometimes vomiting. The pain grows more intense and often moves to the lower right portion of the abdomen. The entire area becomes extremely tender even to a light touch or a slight movement of any part of the body. Occasionally, the pain will radiate to the groin or down the leg. Sometimes your child will experience pain on the left side of the abdomen

or in the lower back. The child may have other symptoms, including loss of appetite, flushing or whiteness of the cheeks, mild fever, rapid heartbeat, occasional diarrhea, and the urge to urinate frequently. As the inflammation worsens, the abdomen may become rigid and distended.

Children under 5 years old don't always show the classic signs of appendicitis. Sometimes the pain isn't severe, or it comes and goes, then becomes more severe over several days. Call the doctor if your child's pain gets worse over the course of a day.

Appendicitis must be treated immediately, because it can lead to rupture of the appendix within 36 to 48 hours after the symptoms begin. When this occurs, the appendix can spill feces and bacteria into the abdominal cavity, resulting in a potentially life-threatening abdominal infection called peritonitis.

When Is a Stomachache Appendicitis?

Appendicitis can be difficult to diagnose—even for doctors—so it's no wonder that parents may worry that their children's stomachaches are something more serious than a stomach flu. The chart outlines some simple signs to help you differentiate between the two conditions.

Causes

The most common cause of appendicitis is a blockage of hardened feces inside the appendix, a small, fingerlike extension of the large intestine that secretes mucus to lubricate part of the intestinal tract. The blockage leads to inflammation and infection. Why the blockage occurs is unknown.

What the Doctor May Do

The doctor will note the location of the pain in the abdomen and other symptoms to determine if they might be caused by appendicitis. If so, she will probably test your child's blood or urine and take X rays, an ultrasound, or both to see whether the intestine or appendix is blocked or inflamed. She may admit your child to the hospital to see if the pain gets progressively worse with time, a sign of appendicitis.

If your child has the symptoms of appendicitis, he will most likely need exploratory surgery for the diagnosis to be confirmed. If your child has appendicitis, the surgeon will remove the appendix. Increasingly, the operation of choice is laparoscopic surgery, in which a long, thin instrument is inserted through a small incision in the abdomen to perform the procedure. It is less invasive than conventional surgery and recovery time is shorter. Most children need to take antibiotics after surgery to prevent infection. Complications include rupture of the appendix and peritonitis, an inflammation of the lining of the intestines usually caused by an infectious agent. Both of these conditions

■ DIFFERENCES BETWEEN STOMACH FLU AND APPENDICITIS

Stomach Flu	Appendicitis
Symptoms Vomiting, diarrhea, fever, lack of appetite.	Pain is on lower right side and may worsen with movement. Little or no diarrhea. Constipation, loss of appetite, vomiting, redness or whiteness of cheeks, fever, frequent urge to urinate.
Onset Vomiting, diarrhea, and abdominal pain start at about the same time.	Pain usually starts well before vomiting.
Location of Pain Throughout the abdomen.	Begins around the navel, then usually moves to the lower right side.
Duration of Pain As long as diarrhea and vomiting occur, but usually improves within 6 to 12 hours.	Usually builds and does not ease up, becoming more severe over time.

require hospitalization and intravenous antibiotics.

What You Can Do

If your child complains of a severe stomachache, or has stomach pain that seems to be getting progressively worse, call the doctor immediately. Children with appendicitis don't always have the classic symptoms.

Don't give your child any medicine. Enemas and laxatives can cause the appendix to break open or rupture. Painkillers, in relieving the

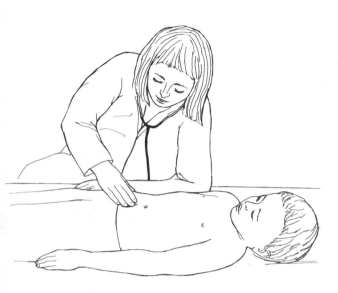

When your child is examined, the doctor will probably press her hand against your child's abdomen to test for appendicitis. Appendicitis usually begins with pain around the navel. Later, the pain grows more intense and often moves to the lower right part of the abdomen. The entire area becomes extremely tender to even light touches or slight movements of any part of the body.

discomfort, can mask the pain and make diagnosis difficult. Also, don't give your child anything to eat or drink on the way to the doctor's office or hospital. If he needs surgery, he will have general anesthesia, which is safest on an empty stomach.

See also *Abdominal Pain/Stomachache.*

Arrhythmia

See *Abnormal Heart Rhythm.*

Arthritis

See *Juvenile Rheumatoid Arthritis.*

Asperger Syndrome

See *Pervasive Developmental Disorder.*

Asthma

The sight of a child straining for breath is an alarming but common problem for many parents. Asthma is the most common chronic childhood disease, affecting about 4.8 million children in the United States. Asthma, an irritation or inflammation of the airways, is growing more common, particularly in children. Asthma in children has increased by 73 percent in little more than a decade. The word *asthma* comes from the Greek word for "panting," which probably doesn't surprise you if you've witnessed your child trying to breathe during an asthma episode. Fortunately, about half of children with asthma outgrow the condition by about 4 to 6 years of age. For those who don't, asthma is a serious but manageable condition that usually shouldn't impede your child's ability to participate fully in activities.

Signs and Symptoms

- Shortness of breath, wheezing, or difficulty breathing
- Nostrils flaring
- Cough
- Sucked-in appearance of skin around neck and between ribs, caused by the child's straining for breath
- Bluish color (lack of oxygen)
- Lack of stamina during exercise

When to Call the Doctor

CALL FOR EMERGENCY **HELP IF**

- your child has difficulty breathing and/or is turning blue.
- your child is straining for each breath, with nostrils flaring and chest heaving.

For first aid information, see page 380 if your child is less than 1 year old and page 383 if your child is 1 year of age or older.

CALL THE DOCTOR IMMEDIATELY IF

- your child has previously been diagnosed with asthma but is not responding to the usual measures.
- your child is wheezing hard and visibly tiring.

CALL THE DOCTOR TODAY IF

- your child is wheezing for the first time.
- your child's symptoms are accompanied by fever or chest pain.
- your child continues to wheeze and have difficulty breathing even while using prescribed medications.

TALK WITH THE DOCTOR AT YOUR CHILD'S NEXT CHECKUP IF

- your child's asthma is interfering with normal activities or sports.
- your child is missing a lot of preschool or school because of asthma.

Essential Facts

Although wheezing is the symptom most often associated with asthma, children with asthma don't always wheeze or cough. Instead they may experience rapid or noisy breathing, chest congestion, and chest tightness that may be overlooked or unidentified. Children with asthma may also have less stamina than their peers during playtime.

Asthma usually appears in children over 2 years old. The condition occasionally affects infants, but more often, asthmalike symptoms are actually caused by a cold or flu. Many babies under 2 years old wheeze because of a different condition, called **bronchiolitis.** Bronchiolitis, which is usually caused by a viral infection, sometimes precedes asthma.

The asthma patients who don't outgrow this condition by 4 to 6 years old continue to have asthma episodes and may go on to develop other allergy symptoms (see **Allergies**), such as hay fever. Asthma may be more common among city children because of greater air pollution rates in cities. Premature infants, especially those who required breathing assistance at birth, are more prone to develop wheezing than full-term babies because of problems with the growth of their lungs.

QUESTIONS PARENTS ASK

What Happens During an Asthma Episode?

An asthma episode involves several conditions:

- Spasms, or contractions, of the muscles surrounding the small airways in the lungs, which impede the air exchange necessary for normal breathing
- Inflammation (irritation and swelling) of the lining of the airways
- Mucus production that clogs the airways
- Increased reactivity of the lungs

The lining of the airways, the treelike pattern of thin-walled passages in the lungs, may swell during an asthma attack. When this happens, some of the air your child needs to exhale becomes trapped, leaving her unable to inhale enough oxygen. Feelings of suffocation can ensue, resulting in panic and even greater difficulty breathing.

During an asthma episode the treelike pattern of small air passages in the lungs constrict and become clogged with mucus, and the lining of the airways may swell. When this happens, some of the air your child needs to exhale becomes trapped, causing her to have difficulty inhaling.

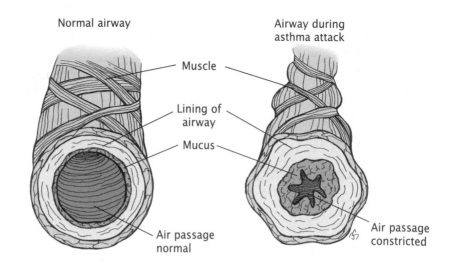

Normal airway

Airway during asthma attack

Muscle

Lining of airway

Mucus

Air passage normal

Air passage constricted

Severity and Complications

Not all cases of asthma have the same severity; some children have very mild conditions, whereas others experience life-threatening episodes. Some wheeze only infrequently when confronted with a particular allergen, such as animal dander, or when the pollen count is particularly high. Other children wheeze more or less every day, often without a known trigger, and require frequent emergency department visits and hospitalizations.

In children with moderate to severe asthma, two complications can be life-threatening. In the first, the high pressures generated in the lungs by the wheezing and struggling to breathe burst some alveoli (tiny air sacs in the lungs), allowing air to escape into the chest cavity, which causes chest pain and further breathing difficulties (pneumothorax).

A second complication is respiratory failure, as the child fatigues from the strenuous effort required to breathe in a prolonged, severe attack. When this occurs, the child will need to be hospitalized and given intravenous fluids, medications, oxygen, and possibly mechanical ventilation.

Causes

Triggered by either an upper respiratory tract infection, an allergy, or an irritant, such as cigarette smoke, asthma affects the airway system of bronchi and bronchioles—small air passages in the lungs, which constrict and become clogged with mucus. In babies and young children, the most common trigger is upper respiratory tract infections—colds and flu that attack the lungs and airways. Allergies to animal dander, feathers, pollen, and mold are also common triggers of asthma in this age group. Cigarette smoke, cockroach allergens, and dust mites may also provoke an asthma episode.

A variety of medical problems besides asthma can cause a young child to wheeze. The chart presents a list of childhood conditions that cause wheezing.

What the Doctor May Do

If your child is having trouble breathing when you bring her to the doctor, he may first have your child inhale a bronchodilator drug to open her airways and then start treatment with inhaled steroid medication to reduce the lung

CAUSES OF WHEEZING

Cause	Example
Infections	Bronchiolitis, bronchitis
Heart problems	Congenital heart failure
Objects in the airway	Aspiration of liquid, part of a peanut, small toy part
Anatomical abnormalities	Vascular ring (a rare constriction of airways), tracheoesophageal fistula (an abnormal opening between the trachea and the esophagus)
Inherited conditions	Cystic fibrosis
Allergies or toxic exposures	Animal dander, pollen, molds, pollution, other inhaled chemicals
Asthma	Allergic, exertional, nocturnal, cold, others
Masses or other obstructions	Bronchial cysts, benign tumors, cancers, bronchial web (a rare congenital airway obstruction)

inflammation clogging her airways. If the episode is more serious or difficult to treat, your doctor may admit her to the hospital, where higher doses of drugs can be safely administered.

Before making a diagnosis of asthma, however, your doctor must rule out breathing problems caused by other conditions (see chart). He may order a chest X ray to make sure that she doesn't have a respiratory tract infection or another problem. In an older child, pulmonary function tests can help evaluate the volume and mechanics of a child's breathing.

Once your doctor confirms a diagnosis of asthma, you, your doctor, and your child will work together to avoid future episodes and prevent the condition from interfering with her everyday activities. The first step is trying to identify asthma triggers. To see how these things relate to the onset of your child's asthma, the doctor may have you keep careful track of your child's behavior and habits, how much she exercises, and what she was doing when the asthma episode started. Sometimes, your doctor may use skin sensitivity tests to identify specific allergens that may be triggering her wheezing.

In very mild cases of wheezing triggered by a viral cold, the doctor may recommend plenty of rest and fluids. The wheezing often clears up in a few days as the virus disappears.

When wheezing is more frequent, but still mild, the doctor may prescribe medicines (to control the symptoms and open the blocked airways) to be used at the first sign of wheezing and continued for 3 to 5 days after wheezing has stopped to ensure a complete recovery. When wheezing is moderate to severe and episodes occur frequently and without much warning, the doctor may increase the intensity of treatment by prescribing inhaled corticosteroids (to reduce inflammation) and/or bronchodilators and instruct the child to use the medications daily rather than only during wheezing episodes.

Medications for Asthma

Depending on how chronic or severe your child's asthma is, the doctor will probably recommend medication. Most medications for asthma are inhaled. Two main types of medication are used to treat asthma.

Long-Term Controllers A child who has persistent asthma symptoms on a fairly regular basis will need a long-term controller medication. These medications are anti-inflammatory agents, that is, they help prevent airway inflammation.

- *Corticosteroids (inhaled and oral):* The strongest, most effective anti-inflammatory medications currently available, inhaled corticosteroids have become the most widely used treatment for asthma. These medications reduce inflammation in the airways and improve air flow to the lungs. Children using these medications should be monitored for reduced growth rate and other side effects. The lower the dosage, the lower the chance of growth reduction or other side effects. The dosage your doctor prescribes is related to the severity and persistence of the asthma. Some examples of these medications include beclomethasone, budesonide, flunisolide, fluticasone, and triamcinolone.

- *Cromolyn sodium and nedocromil:* Mild to moderate anti-inflammatory medications can be used daily or as a preventative treatment before contact with an unavoidable allergen (e.g., visiting a house where cats or dogs live).

- *Long-acting beta$_2$ agonists:* Bronchodilators for use with anti-inflammatory medication may be especially helpful for nighttime symptoms or as a preventative treatment before exercise. One example is salmeterol.

- *Methylxanthines (theophylline):* Mild to moderate bronchodilators used mainly with inhaled corticosteroids for nighttime symptoms.

Fast-Acting Asthma Medications These inhaled medications are not usually taken on a daily basis but are used to quickly relax the muscles around the small breathing passages, providing relief from moderate to severe asthma symptoms. Many people also use oral medications for quick relief.

- *Short-acting beta$_2$ agonists:* First choice for quick relief of acute asthma episodes; the most common is albuterol.

- *Leukotriene inhibitors:* Provide extra relief when used in combination with a beta$_2$ agonist in severe episodes. Can be used as an alternative to beta$_2$ agonists. Examples are zafirlukast and montelukast.

- *Oral corticosteroids:* Used for moderate to severe episodes to speed recovery, prevent recurrent episodes, and decrease inflammation and mucus. One example is prednisone.

What You Can Do

The first time your child experiences an asthma episode, don't try to care for her at home. Call your doctor immediately, or bring your child to an emergency room. If your child is in severe distress, call for an ambulance.

If your child's doctor has determined that your child has asthma, follow these suggestions in case of another episode:

1. Know the warning signs of an impending episode so you can begin treatment early.

2. Make sure that your child takes her medication as directed.

3. Place your child in a sitting position (rather than lying down flat) to allow her to breathe more easily.

4. Stay calm, and try to calm your child. The more upset your child becomes, the worse the episode will probably be.

5. Call your doctor if your child's symptoms are accompanied by fever or chest pain, if she continues to wheeze or have difficulty breathing for more than 2 hours after you administer medication, or if your child develops any side effects.

Do not . . .

- attempt to treat your child's first asthma episode yourself.
- give your child over-the-counter medications unless your doctor prescribes them.
- let any asthma attack go untreated.

If you are planning a trip with your child, call your doctor to obtain a refill of your child's medications. Make sure you have more than one refill with you when you travel.

Using Inhaled Medication Wisely

If your child uses a metered dose inhaler or a nebulizer to inhale asthma medication, you can do several things to make sure that as much medication as possible reaches her lungs rather than remaining in her mouth, where it can be swallowed. Delivering more medicine to the lungs will increase its effectiveness and reduce the possibility of side effects. Side effects, although uncommon, can include oral thrush (a fungal infection in the mouth), throat irritation, and voice changes.

The most common and most effective method for improving the delivery of medication to the lungs is the use of a spacer (also called a holding chamber) with the child's inhaler. If you do not have one, ask your doctor for one and ask how to use it. A spacer is a portable device that attaches to the inhaler, trapping the medication in the air inside the chamber and increasing the likelihood that it will reach the lungs. For children under 5 years old, a spacer with a mask attached may work even better.

Another variation that can help parents determine whether a small child is inhaling most of the medication is a spacer that comes with a collapsible bag, which allows the parent and child to see whether the complete dose has been inhaled.

Using a Spacer To make sure that most of the medicine reaches your child's lungs

- shake the inhaler thoroughly before use.
- make sure your child holds her breath for approximately 10 seconds after inhaling.
- always make sure your child rinses her mouth after using the inhaler. Have your child spit out the rinse water.
- wash the mouthpiece and spacer with water. Most spacers can be washed in the dishwasher.

Using a Nebulizer Children with severe asthma, particularly those under 5 years old, may benefit from using a nebulizer, a hand-held cup with a plastic mask attached by a hose to a compressor,

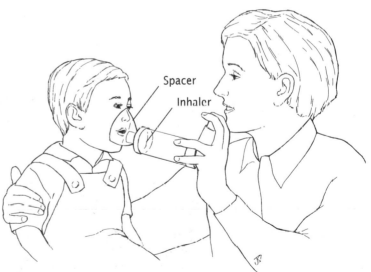

Spacer

Inhaler

A spacer—a portable device that attaches to the inhaler—is a common, effective method for improving the delivery of medication to the lungs. Using a spacer can reduce the amount of medication left in the mouth, making it more likely to reach the lungs.

which delivers medication in a steady stream. Nebulizers are less portable and convenient than a metered-dose inhaler with a spacer, but can be useful for young children who may find the mechanics of using an inhaler difficult.

If your child resists having the mask placed against her mouth, try using a plastic foam cup instead. Many infants and young children will not resist a cup. Here's how to do it:

1. Punch a hole in the end of a foam cup just large enough for the end or mouthpiece of the nebulizer inhaler to be inserted.

2. Place the proper dose of medication in the inhaler chamber.

3. Hold the cup as close as possible to the child's nose and mouth

4. Give the nebulizer treatment for 20 to 30 minutes or for as long as your doctor recommends.

Using a Peak Expiratory Flow Meter

In addition, you and your child can help better manage her asthma by using a peak flow meter, a small, easy-to-use instrument that measures how fast your child can blow air out of her lungs after taking a deep breath. This is called the peak expiratory flow rate, or PEFR. People with asthma cannot always feel the early changes taking place in their airways, because these changes occur gradually over several minutes or hours. By the time symptoms develop, these people can be experiencing a 25 percent or greater decrease in lung function. Monitoring the peak flow by measuring how much air your child can blow out of her lungs can help you and your doctor assess your child's lung function and the state of her asthma. Keep a diary, recording her PEFR daily or as often as your doctor suggests. Most children ages 6 years and above can successfully use a peak flow meter. The PEFR is

often valuable in making decisions about the following:

- Effectiveness of asthma medications
- Adding or stopping medications
- Seeking emergency care
- Controlling environmental triggers

Your doctor will help you and your child learn to use the peak flow meter correctly and will suggest how often you should monitor lung function based on your child's asthma pattern.

Prevention

It may be impossible to prevent asthma entirely, but you can probably eliminate many triggers of your child's asthma episodes. Controlling dust and avoiding animal dander are particularly important. (For more suggestions on eliminating allergens, see p. 435.) Exercise may help prevent asthma in later years. Poor fitness during the childhood years may be linked to asthma in adulthood. Exercise will also help your child better cope with a wheezing episode because it builds strength in the respiratory muscles and increases lung capacity.

A yearly flu (influenza) shot for your child and family may prevent influenza, which can trigger a wheezing episode. Allergy shots can desensitize children to the environmental allergens that trigger asthma episodes. Avoid exposing your child to secondhand tobacco smoke, which increases the frequency and severity of wheezing.

Consult your doctor about preventing asthma episodes. For exercise-related asthma, use of an inhaled bronchodilator or other medication recommended by your child's doctor before exercise can help prevent an episode.

See also *Allergies.*

Astigmatism

See *Vision Problems.*

Athlete's Foot

See *Ringworm.*

Attention Deficit Disorder (ADD, ADHD)

Preschoolers are often easily distracted and seem to have short attention spans. But when these qualities persist in a school-age child and his inability to concentrate or focus his attention begins to interfere with learning and social interactions, he may need to be evaluated for the signs and symptoms of attention deficit disorder (ADD). ADD, also known as attention deficit/hyperactivity disorder (ADHD), is the most common behavioral diagnosis in children. Estimates of the number of children affected by ADD range widely from 1.5 percent to 9 percent of children or even higher. About four times as many boys as girls are diagnosed with ADD, although experts believe that the condition may sometimes be overlooked in girls. ADD concerns parents, teachers, and doctors because it can threaten normal academic achievement and social development. With treatment, however, most children with ADD will thrive.

Signs and Symptoms

In children 5 years of age and older:

- Difficulty sustaining attention
- Inattention to what others say
- Impulsivity
- Trouble following instructions
- Frequent shifting of activities without completing tasks

- Frequent fidgeting or squirming when seated
- Difficulty taking turns
- Tendency to answer questions before they're completed
- Difficulty playing quietly
- Excessive talking
- Frequently interrupting or intruding on others

When to Call the Doctor
CALL THE DOCTOR TODAY IF
- your child is easily distracted, inattentive, or impulsive for more than a week or two.
- you or your child's teacher are concerned about your child's attention, behavior, learning ability, and social relationships.

Essential Facts

ADD is difficult to diagnose in children before 5 years of age because symptoms such as distractibility, frequent fidgeting, and impulsivity are common among preschoolers. Many children who display these symptoms at age 4 have learned to control these impulses effectively by age 7. As a result, ADD cannot usually be accurately diagnosed until a child is nearing or has reached school age and begins having problems in the classroom.

Attention disorders affect each child differently, and the symptoms listed above are just a few of the most common. Because many children have at least some of these symptoms, the diagnosis must be made carefully and the symptoms must usually be present before 7 years of age and last for at least 6 months for a diagnosis of ADD.

Types of ADD

Some children experience some but not all of the symptoms of ADD. Doctors identify three types of ADD:

- *Predominantly inattentive type:* Children with this type are distractible, but not very hyperactive or impulsive. They may exhibit no hyperactive symptoms. For unknown reasons, most children with this type of attention disorder are girls.

- *Predominantly hyperactive-impulsive type:* These children are hyperactive and impulsive, but more attentive. Once they settle down, they can concentrate better than their more inattentive ADD counterparts but not as well as a child without ADD.

- *Combined type:* Most children have this type of ADD and experience all three symptoms in varying degrees.

Whatever type of attention disorder a child has, he'll probably have trouble focusing on instructions, finishing tasks, and interacting socially.

Although children often show signs of ADD while in preschool, you may not notice the problem until your child enters the more structured setting of kindergarten or first grade. Classrooms require a level of self-control that children with ADD find difficult to maintain. Your child may find sitting still at a desk and finishing work, or even organizing it, virtually impossible. He might be disruptive and quick to anger, often picking fights or refusing to wait his turn.

ADD is considered a learning problem because it interrupts a child's potential to learn. He might be labeled bad or weird at school, and feel isolated. Having an attention disorder can cause *depression,* anxiety, low self-esteem, anger, and defiance.

Although by adolescence, many children experience fewer symptoms, especially those of hyperactivity, they still need special care to learn and develop. In some cases, ADD is a lifelong condition requiring consistent support and treatment. Although the symptoms of attention disorders may diminish over time, studies show that 50 to 70 percent of children with such a disorder in elementary school still exhibit symptoms as adults, although it isn't always a detriment: Many adults diagnosed with ADD as children achieve success in later life.

Various conditions—such as vision and hearing impairment (see *Hearing Loss*), sleep disorders, seizure disorder (see *Seizures*), *depression,* bipolar disorder, obsessive-compulsive disorder (see p. 444), *anxiety disorders,* and language disorders (see *Learning Disorders*)—can mimic ADD. As a result, careful evaluation and diagnosis becomes even more important.

Causes

No one knows what causes ADD. Children with low birth weight tend to have ADD more often than others. Attention disorders also run in families and, like learning disorders, may result from brain structure or functioning abnormalities. Twenty to 30 percent of children with an attention deficit disorder have a parent with ADD. Alcohol, drug, and tobacco use during pregnancy may also play a role in ADD. In rare cases, exposure to toxins such as lead (see *Lead Poisoning*); complications during pregnancy; and even brain infections such as *meningitis* may influence the development of the disorder. Negative family influences and early childhood experiences—a parent's death, childhood abuse, or neglect—probably don't trigger the development of an attention disorder, but may affect its severity and lessen a child's ability to cope with everyday stresses.

Despite extensive investigation, no data connects any particular foods, food additives, preservatives, or sugar to this disorder. In particular, the effects of sugar have been thoroughly studied and found to have no causal effect. Sugar doesn't cause hyperactivity or ADD.

What the Doctor May Do

If you or your child's teachers think your child might have an attention disorder, consult his doctor, who will try to rule out any physical or medical causes. If the doctor suspects an attention disorder, she may refer your child to a developmental pediatrician, a neurologist, or a mental health professional experienced in diagnosing the disorder. If your child is in school, a well-trained school counselor or psychologist may be able to begin the evaluation. Your child's doctor may recommend a multidisciplinary team approach involving educators, a child psychologist, and other mental health professionals.

The diagnosis of ADD should never be made casually. A diagnosis can only be made after a thorough and careful evaluation that will probably include an intelligence test and a physical exam with a vision and hearing screening, because other conditions may mimic ADD. Children with hearing loss, for example, may appear inattentive and hyperactive, when instead they're frustrated because their communication is affected.

If physical problems are ruled out, the health professional will assess your child's behavior at school and at home. She will discuss your child with you, and perhaps his teacher, and observe his behavior at her office and possibly at home or at school. She will consider intelligence test results and other academic measures, and she may perform tests designed to identify specific learning problems to pinpoint your child's difficulties. The evaluators may also give you questionnaires to gather information about your child's health history and family background and to identify behavior characteristic of ADD.

The management of attention problems usually involves education about the diagnosis, behavioral therapy, counseling, and—sometimes—medication. No evidence shows that special diets designed to improve a child's behavior or reduce hyperactivity are effective.

Counseling will help your child adjust to his diagnosis, cope with the demands of his disorder, and deal with self-esteem problems or mood disorders. Behavioral therapy provides social skills training, such as anger management, and works toward increasing your child's attention and self-control, helping him find new ways to learn to communicate and interact socially. A system of rewards for both home and school that recognizes small, positive changes is often effective. A trained clinician may show you and your child's teacher how to help your child with these skills.

Medications for ADD

Many children with ADD benefit from medication. Doctors primarily use three types of medication to treat children with ADD:

- *Stimulants:* The most commonly used medications for ADD include methylphenidate, pemoline, and dextroamphetamine. These stimulants help children with ADD focus and concentrate. Despite their name, these medications don't stimulate or increase hyperactivity or impulsivity.

- *Antidepressants:* If stimulants don't reduce your child's symptoms or if your child also has a mood disorder, your doctor may suggest tricyclic antidepressants (amitriptyline, nortriptyline, imipramine, desipramine), which help decrease the mood swings so often a part of the symptoms of ADD.

- *Clonidine:* This medication was first used to treat high blood pressure. Doctors have also found it effective in treating the hyperactive-impulsive symptoms of attention disorders.

If your doctor prescribes medication, be sure its effects and side effects are closely monitored, because these medications work differently on every child. Your doctor may try a few medications before deciding on the right one and the right dose. *But be sure that your child receives medication only as part of an ongoing treatment plan that includes counseling and behavioral therapy.*

What You Can Do

If your child is diagnosed with an attention disorder, work closely with his teacher, counselors, and doctors on the treatment plan you've created together. Consistently apply the rewards and consequences you and the team have created. For example, if your child has trouble sitting in his seat for more than 10 seconds at a time, have him try to sit for 13 or 15 seconds. When he does, give him some positive attention by saying how pleased you are or by setting up a sticker chart or another reward system. The idea is to pay attention to his successes rather than focusing on his difficulty sitting still. Keep the health

and education team informed of any changes—positive or negative—in your child's condition so treatment can meet his changing needs.

Various techniques can help your child cope with his symptoms. If you join a support group for children with ADD and their families, you'll receive many suggestions. In the meantime, try the following advice:

- *Be truthful with your child.* Whatever your child's development stage, he probably realizes that he's different from his peers. Ask your doctor for suggestions on how to explain ADD and its effects to him. Never try to hide, minimize, or exaggerate the problem. And make sure your child realizes that, with help, he can control his behavior now and in the future.

- *Provide structure.* Maintain a consistent schedule. If you need to change it, provide ample

---

THE RITALIN CONTROVERSY

No parent wants a child to be on medication long-term. Because the use of medications for ADD has increased dramatically in recent years, there is concern that they are overprescribed. An estimated 3 to 5 percent of U.S. schoolchildren take the stimulant Ritalin (methylphenidate). Children with ADD don't always need medication. Many can be treated with a combination of group or individual therapy and behavior modification techniques (a system of rewards and consequences). If a child's problem is severe enough that therapy and behavior modification don't work, medication may be worth considering. These medications are intended to help the child maintain his focus and attention on his schoolwork and his homework.

Ritalin and similar drugs, such as pemoline, seem to help a large majority of children who take them, according to a review of more than 200 studies. In addition to reducing symptoms,

such medications boost self-esteem and improve mood. With these benefits, children usually function better in school and have an easier time dealing with other children. Your child may also notice a difference in his ability to focus and organize himself.

Some common side effects (such as insomnia, reduced appetite, weight loss, and irritability) can often be decreased or eliminated if the doctor reduces the medication dose. There's no evidence that the medicine leads to addiction or growth problems.

Some children need to take ADD drugs throughout their school years. But if a child is doing well, he may, under his doctor's supervision, temporarily stop his medicine (take a "drug holiday") to see if he remains symptom-free. If symptoms do return, they may be less severe than before, allowing your child to discontinue the medicine completely or to use a lower dose.

warning and reminders. A daily schedule can reassure children with ADD and help them remember what to do and when. Use timers and alarm clocks to keep your child on track during the day.

- *Organize your home, especially your child's room.* Create clearly marked spaces for toys, schoolbooks, and clothes, and have your child put things away when he's done with them.

- *Set reasonable goals.* Your child will progress at school, at home, or in social situations by working toward modest, clearly defined goals. Encourage your child to finish the next homework assignment on time or to get a better grade on the next quiz, instead of suggesting that he get a B in his math class this quarter.

- *Accent the positive.* When your child meets a goal and receives praise, his self-esteem increases. Rein in any feelings of frustration and annoyance if he fails to achieve a goal, and reassure your child of your love, respect, and trust in him.

- *Work closely with your school system.* Inform your child's teachers of the behavioral techniques you're using, so they can participate in the process.

Prevention

You may not be able to prevent ADD, but recognizing the problem, finding assistance, and treating your child with love and consistency can reduce its effects. Although most cases of ADD do not have a known cause, there is some evidence that exposure to alcohol during pregnancy (fetal alcohol syndrome) or exposure to lead (in paint, water, and soil) during early childhood may later result in symptoms characteristic of ADD. Reducing exposure to alcohol and drugs during pregnancy and having your child's blood-lead level checked annually are important preventative measures.

▌ Autism

See *Pervasive Developmental Disorder.*

▌ Baby Bottle Tooth Decay

See *Cavities.*

▌ Back Pain

"Oh, my aching back!" is a complaint you hear far more frequently from adults than young children. Although back pain from poor posture, accidents, or sports injuries can certainly occur at every age, back pain in children under 10 years old is unusual. If your child complains of back pain, tell your child's doctor.

Signs and Symptoms
- Mild to severe pain, often in the lower back
- Stiffness or tightness

When to Call the Doctor
CALL FOR EMERGENCY HELP IF
- your child has seriously injured her spine or neck, such as in a motor vehicle accident or playing sports (see p. 419).
- your child has weakness, numbness, tingling, or pain in one or both legs.

CALL THE DOCTOR IMMEDIATELY IF
- your child is limping.
- your child has frequent or painful urination, or bloody or discolored urine.
- a fever accompanies back pain or stiffness.

CALL THE DOCTOR TODAY IF
- the back pain worsens instead of getting better.
- the back pain persists after several days.

Causes

The following sections describe the most common causes of back pain in children.

Muscle Strains Sudden twisting motions, such as those that occur during tennis and football, can cause muscle strains. Injury to soft tissue (muscles, tendons, and ligaments) may be accompanied by swelling and inflammation, both of which make pain worse.

Overexertion A sprain, a strain (see *Sprains and Strains*), or another injury caused by a specific motion or an activity, such as lifting a heavy object, can cause back pain. Injury resulting from poor posture or lack of fitness can also make a child's back hurt.

Stress As is true for adults, anxiety or stress can make children keep tightening the muscles supporting the back, head, and neck, causing pain in those muscles.

Sports Training If your child participates in sports or dance training, back pain may be due to a stress fracture of the lower back.

Accidents Fractures and dislocations of the spine can result from falls, car accidents, or other physical traumas. These injuries always require immediate medical attention. Falling on the tailbone can be very painful, causing aches that extend into the lower back.

Illness Back pain is often an uncomfortable side effect of the flu or another viral infection. Lower back pain or flank pain can be caused by bladder or kidney infections and occasionally even kidney stones. Rare causes of childhood back pain include the following: *juvenile rheumatoid arthritis;* ankylosing spondylitis, ruptured disks; cysts on the spine; structural abnormalities of the spine or hip; differences in leg length; diseases of the spine such as *scoliosis,* spinal tumors, and cancers; and certain nerve disorders.

What the Doctor May Do

Treatment of back pain depends on its cause. For most back strains, rest and over-the-counter pain relievers (follow the dosage instructions carefully) are the treatments of choice. Your child should feel better in 2 to 3 days.

If a fever or other symptoms are present, the doctor may test your child's blood or urine to determine the source of the infection. If he identifies a urinary tract infection, he'll prescribe antibiotics. If the back pain is related to a sports injury, car accident, or another physical trauma, the doctor might order an X ray to see if any spine abnormalities are present. An X ray might also be needed if the back pain isn't related to an infection or an injury, but nonetheless doesn't go away by itself. More detailed imaging tests, such as a bone scan or an MRI (magnetic resonance imaging), may also be necessary.

Less commonly, a stress fracture or another structural problem may be causing the pain. In this case, the doctor may recommend that your child wear a brace to stabilize the bones and tissues involved. How long the brace is needed depends on the severity of the child's condition. In rare instances, traction to immobilize the whole back may be necessary for healing. This treatment can be done at home, but it may be needed for weeks or even months, depending on the child's condition. Your child's doctor may also recommend physical therapy to correct any tightness or weakness contributing to the back pain.

What You Can Do

If you know that a minor muscle strain is causing your child's pain, you can relieve her discomfort with over-the-counter pain relievers, such as ibuprofen or acetaminophen. Immediately after an injury and for 2 to 3 days thereafter, apply ice or an ice pack wrapped in a towel to reduce pain, bleeding, and swelling. After 2 to 3 days pass, if the pain or swelling persists, heat from a warm water bottle or heating pad can relax the muscles.

Your child will probably require—or want—bed rest until the pain passes. To decrease the pain during this period, try tucking a pillow under your child's thighs. By flexing the child's hips and knees, the pillow will take strain off the back. You might also put a bed board beneath your child's mattress to make it firmer and better able to support the back muscles and joints during recovery.

Prevention

The best way to prevent back pain is to reduce the risk of back injuries by taking precautions against accidents.

- Use safety gates in the house to prevent toddlers from falling downstairs.

- Insist that your child use car seats or seat belts in the car.

- Carefully supervise young children in the kitchen and bathroom, where floors can be slippery. Don't let children climb on counter tops or other high surfaces: Falls onto a hard floor can cause injuries to the back and other body parts.

- Encourage your child to exercise regularly to strengthen and increase flexibility in the back, thereby reducing the risk of strains or sprains. Encourage her to do warm-up and stretching exercises before and after playing sports.

▌ *Bed-Wetting (Nocturnal Enuresis)*

It has a fancy name—nocturnal enuresis—but parents know it as simply "wetting the bed." One of the most common problems of childhood, bed-wetting affects up to 20 percent of 5-year-

old children who don't have bathroom accidents during the day. Fortunately, most children who wet the bed outgrow the problem naturally, without medical treatment.

Signs and Symptoms

- Nighttime bed-wetting in preschoolers on a regular basis despite full urinary control during the day
- Bed-wetting after 6 years of age

When to Call the Doctor:
CALL THE DOCTOR IMMEDIATELY IF
- a fever accompanies a sudden episode of bed-wetting.
- your child has a burning sensation when urinating.

CALL THE DOCTOR TODAY IF
- your child is drinking much more liquid than usual or has lost a lot of weight despite a normal appetite.
- your child is wetting the bed regularly after having been dry at night for a while.
- your child's urine stream is abnormal (spray, drizzle, or off to one side).

TALK TO THE DOCTOR AT YOUR CHILD'S NEXT CHECKUP IF
- your child's behavior is worse, or he seems troubled.
- you or your child is concerned about bed-wetting.
- your child is still wetting the bed and is 6 years of age or older.

Essential Facts

Doctors generally apply the term *enuresis* to bed-wetting that occurs in children over 6 years old, although any child who wets the bed after staying dry at night for several months may also be diagnosed with enuresis. About 75 percent of children who wet the bed have primary nocturnal enuresis (PNE), which means that they have never stayed dry at night on a regular basis. The others have secondary enuresis, which means that they have been dry for a while and then begin wetting their beds again, often following an emotionally stressful event or even a schedule change or a trip. Enuresis is three times more common in boys than in girls, and it tends to run in families.

Although physical long-term effects seldom occur, bed-wetting often has a psychological impact. A child who wets the bed is apt to feel shame and embarrassment about the problem, as well as anxiety about being accepted by his peers. Enuresis often affects school-age children when their social development is greatest, and they are starting to become more independent by sleeping over at friends' homes or attending overnight camps. A child who wets the bed is likely to avoid such situations out of embarrassment, and thus miss out on some important childhood experiences.

This condition is hard on parents as well because of the difficulties of dealing with wet bedding in the middle of the night and the feeling of disappointment over the child's inability to control his bladder. Despite this stress, be careful not to blame your child or convey anger or disappointment, but provide the loving support your child needs to deal with the problem.

Causes

Bed-wetting is not usually caused by an underlying physical disease but instead is the result of delayed physical maturity of the child's bladder control mechanisms. There are several reasons for this condition.

Genetic Factors Primary enuresis appears to have a genetic component—it tends to run in families. If both parents had the problem as children, their child has a 70 percent chance of

having it. If only one parent had the condition, their child has a 40 percent chance of having it. In fact, geneticists have located a gene believed to be at least partially responsible for most PNE cases. Secondary enuresis also runs in families.

Hormonal Factors New research indicates that some children with enuresis may have decreased levels of a hormone called antidiuretic hormone (ADH). These children may produce up to four times the normal amount of urine, thus making it difficult for them to control their bladders through the night.

Small Bladder Size One factor that may contribute to bed-wetting is a small bladder capacity. As children grow older, their bladders also grow larger; this may explain why the problem resolves itself with age.

Sleep Arousal Older children may wet the bed because they are not yet able to wake themselves up when their bodies signal a full bladder. These children often just need more time and practice.

Stress, Change, or Upset In children with previously good nighttime bladder control, enuresis can sometimes be caused by emotional anxiety, stress, or changes in routine. They can regress in some of their development as a bid for parental attention. A move to a new house, the arrival of a new baby, or even an exciting event like a birthday party or vacation can trigger periods of bed-wetting in some children.

Physical Illness Only about 5 to 10 percent of bed-wetting cases have a physical cause, such as a *urinary tract infection, diabetes mellitus,* or a neurological problem. *Sickle-cell disease,* kidney disease, and lower spine disorders are other potential physical causes.

What the Doctor May Do

The doctor will ask questions about your child's health history and do a physical exam. If the doctor suspects a urinary tract infection, diabetes, or another physical cause of bed-wetting, he will perform laboratory tests to confirm an underlying medical problem and begin treatment. Once the underlying cause is controlled, the bed-wetting will probably stop on its own. If the bed-wetting is not caused by an underlying disease or condition, the doctor will discuss options depending on the child's age, motivation, and desire to participate.

Bed-Wetting Alarm

If the problem persists and your child is 6 years of age or older and is motivated to try to correct the problem, the doctor may suggest using a bed-wetting alarm. The alarm has two parts, a moisture sensor that goes in the child's underwear and a buzzer that attaches to the pajama shirt. When the sensor detects any moisture, the buzzer sounds.

The first step when learning how to use an enuresis alarm is for the child to learn to awaken to the alarm. He can accomplish this by following a self-awakening program using imagery (see Six Steps to Self-Awakening, p. 464). After a time, the alarm will alert your child to the need to urinate, and he can get himself up and to the bathroom before his bladder is empty. Use the alarm for 3 to 4 weeks after dryness is achieved. This method is usually successful within about 2 to 3 months. One caution: This method only works if your child is old enough, motivated to help solve his problem, and willing and able to cooperate.

Medication

The doctor might prescribe medications, as well. One medication is desmopressin acetate nasal spray (DDAVP), an antidiuretic hormone that reduces the amount of urine released by the kidneys. The child inhales the spray through the nose at bedtime. Although desmopressin is usually effective in reducing the frequency of bed-wetting, the problem often returns after the child stops taking the medication. Because it hasn't been shown to be safe for long-term use, desmopressin is usually reserved for short-term use, sleep-overs, camp visits, and other special circumstances.

What You Can Do

First of all, don't despair. Children usually outgrow this problem with no medication or other treatment. Most children's bed-wetting difficulties resolve themselves between 6 and 10 years of age without treatment. Don't feel guilty: You're not a bad parent because your child wets the bed, and neither does it mean that your child has a behavior or psychological problem. Nevertheless, the situation may trouble you and frustrate and embarrass your child. Here are a few tips that may ease the situation for both of you:

- *Reassure your child.* Tell your child that you know he isn't wetting the bed on purpose and that you understand how difficult the problem is for him.

- *Tackle the practical.* Make the cleanup as easy as possible. Cover your child's mattress with a waterproof sheet. Another option is to place a waterproof mat (with a comfortable, cotton-like finish) on top of the bottom sheet. This way, when your child wets at night, you—or preferably, he—can simply remove the wet towel or mat rather than changing the entire set of bedding. Leave dry nightclothes out for him to change into should he wake up after wetting the bed.

- *Take special time.* If you think bed-wetting is a response to a stress, be open to your child's needs and concerns. For example, if the family is preoccupied with a new baby, set aside special time reserved for reading or playing with him instead of the baby.

- *Establish a morning routine.* Suggest, in a non-blaming way, that your child put wet sheets, towels, and pajamas in the hamper himself;

He'll feel more in control of the situation. This is not a punishment. Having him do some of the work will help motivate him. The success of this approach, like the others described here, depends largely on your positive attitude and your child's age and stage of development.

- *Limit nighttime beverages.* That extra glass of water or juice before bedtime will worsen any problems your child has with holding his bladder. Caffeinated beverages, such as cola and iced tea, are particularly bad choices because caffeine stimulates urination. Discourage him from drinking fluids for 2 hours before bedtime.

- *Encourage your child to do exercises.* Both bladder-stretching and stream-interruption exercises may be useful for children with enuresis. During the day, encourage your child to hold his urine for several minutes after feeling the urge in order to gradually "stretch" or increase the bladder's capacity. Another exercise is to have your child start urinating and stop midstream to improve muscle (urinary sphincter) control and increase nighttime awareness of a full bladder.

- *Establish nighttime bathroom breaks.* Tell your child that getting up at night to urinate rather than trying to "hold it" is okay. Leave the bathroom light on to guide his way, but don't wake him up at night to urinate. Your child needs to be the one to make this decision so that he can develop control.

Prevention

Most of the known causes of bed-wetting are beyond the child's control. Addressing areas of

---

SIX STEPS TO SELF-AWAKENING

If your child is using a bed-wetting alarm, be sure that he uses the following technique to learn to awaken at night and use the toilet when his bladder feels full. Have your child follow these steps:

1. Lie on the bed with eyes closed.
2. Pretend it is the middle of the night.
3. Pretend his bladder is full.
4. Pretend his bladder is trying to wake him up.
5. Run to the bathroom and empty his bladder.
6. Remind himself to get up during the night when he feels the need to urinate.

Chart your child's good behavior. A positive reinforcement system—such as a chart that identifies successful nights with a gold star or another reward—helps many children. Reserve this approach for children who have occasional dry nights. If he is wetting every night, reward him for helping with the cleanup in the morning.

Be patient. Solving a bed-wetting problem may involve a commitment from both you and your child, and it may take more than 6 months to achieve success.

Do not . . .

- shame or scold your child, or let any child or adult do so. Your child's bed-wetting isn't deliberate. Instead, be supportive and tell him how proud you are of him for trying.

- overly praise your child for a successful night. Be supportive, but don't imply that your child could continue this behavior if he tried harder. Making a big deal over dry nights may only make your child feel pressured and anxious, which can cause bed-wetting in some children.

stress and making an effort to spend special time with him may relieve his concerns and resolve his behavioral regressions. You can take steps toward a solution to chronic bed-wetting while helping him preserve his self-esteem.

■ *Behavioral Problems*

Young children often respond to stress or change with temper tantrums, physical aggression, and defiance. As difficult and upsetting as this behavior may be, it is usually quite normal in terms of your child's development and, thankfully, quite short-lived. However, serious behavioral disorders—those that cause physical harm, prevent full participation in normal activities, or are prolonged and uncontrollable—can sometimes develop. Early diagnosis and treatment can help prevent behavior problems from interfering with family life.

Signs and Symptoms

Less severe:
- Hair pulling
- Head banging
- Frequent temper tantrums and breath holding
- Stubbornness or hostility
- Lying, cheating
- Profanity (if used experimentally rather than aggressively)

More severe:
- Verbal aggression and hostile profanity
- Physical aggression to self or others
- Stealing
- Cruelty to animals
- Fire setting

When to Call the Doctor

CALL THE DOCTOR TODAY IF
- your child is injuring herself or others.
- the disruptive or damaging behavior is prolonged, constant, or uncontrollable.
- the behavior interferes with your child's participation in school, family, or social activities.

TALK WITH THE DOCTOR AT YOUR CHILD'S NEXT CHECKUP IF
- your child cannot control her behavior even with frequent time-outs.
- you are concerned about your child's behavior and development.

Essential Facts

If you're about to scream because of your child's behavior, you're not alone (see Coping with Stress, p. 212). In fact, about half of all preschoolers in the United States are brought to the attention of physicians because of destructive or disobedient behavior. The causes of this behavior vary. Your child may sometimes throw tantrums, hold her breath, or pull her hair in response to communication problems or upsetting events, such as a move to another community, the birth of a sibling, or even an exciting upcoming event like a birthday party. But in other cases, such behavior appears to be unrelated to specific events or family environments.

As is true for other psychological or behavior issues, whether your child's problem requires treatment depends on how long the behavior persists and how much it interferes with her ability to perform and enjoy her daily activities. An occasional temper tantrum—even a violent one—is usually nothing to worry about. If, on the other hand, your child often flies into uncontrollable rages that frequently upset her own or the family's routine, she may need help in resolving her struggle. Some of the more common troubling behavioral difficulties are described in the following sections.

Hair Pulling

Many young children play with their hair, especially infants who actually have hair. They appear to be comforted by twisting, pulling, twirling, or stroking strands of hair. Such behavior is perfectly normal and usually passes on its own by the time a child is about 6 years old. But a condition known as trichotillomania, or compulsive hair pulling, is rarer and more serious. A child with this condition pulls out her hair or breaks it off, sometimes causing bald patches on the scalp or removing the eyebrows or eyelashes. Usually resulting from extreme anxiety, anger, or sadness in response to long-term family problems or a recent crisis, hair pulling under these circumstances can be self-destructive and requires medical attention.

Head Banging

Head banging—repetitive banging of the head, usually at bedtime or upon awakening, against a mattress or the side of the crib—is common among infants and young children, occurring in about 5 to 15 percent of children in this age group. Although disturbing to parents, this behavior rarely causes physical harm. Like thumb sucking and rocking, head banging may be a self-comforting habit a child begins at about 1 year old and usually outgrows by 3 years old. In some cases, head banging may occur as part of a temper tantrum. Generally speaking, head banging does not persist for more than about 6 months. In rare instances, head banging may be due to headaches, earaches, or other pain that frustrates your child enough for her to try to drive away the pain in this manner. See your child's doctor if your child repeatedly exhibits head banging, or if the head banging is extreme or causes you concern.

Temper Tantrums

Temper tantrums are considered a normal part of childhood development, typically beginning at about age 15 months, peaking at 2 years old, and often continuing through 3 or 4 years old. Tantrums (which range from whining, negative, and demanding behavior to out-of-control screaming, kicking, and head banging) result from a child's growing sense of self and desire for independence and an inability to verbalize feelings, delay gratification, or control events or emotions. (See How to Handle a Tantrum, p. 188.)

Breath Holding

During a tantrum, your child may hold her breath purposefully, until she turns blue or faints. While the experience can be frightening, this kind of breath-holding spell is rarely cause for alarm. Your child's breathing will resume normally. Handle breath holding as you would any tantrum (see above), and talk to your child's doctor about it, especially if it happens more than once.

Keep in mind that some breath-holding episodes have nothing to do with behavior. Many children will have an involuntary breath-holding spell. This is more common between 12 and 18 months of age, but it can occur any time from 6 months to 6 years. In most cases, involuntary breath holding is harmless and the episodes will eventually cease on their own as your child's brain and body develop and mature. The thing to remember is that this kind of breath holding is an involuntary reaction caused by an as yet unknown neurological trigger. Usually, your child will start breathing on her own relatively quickly; uncommonly, she may pass out or have a seizure. If such an event occurs, bring her to a physician for an evaluation.

Lying

Lying is a behavior that children can learn by being lied to themselves. It usually starts emerging in response to fear of punishment. For instance, your son, who spilled his chocolate milk all over your white rug, may tell you that his brother did it out of fear that you'll be angry. The lie may seem harmless, but if you don't intervene, the lies will no doubt continue over more serious matters. You can help your child unlearn this behavior by teaching him to ask for help when a mistake or an accident occurs. Explain that when such problems arise, you would be happier to hear the truth, and invite your child to try the truth the next time. Be sure to follow through and continually show appreciation for his honesty. If your school-age child is habitually lying, use these tactics and seek the help of a child behavior specialist.

Cheating

It may be difficult for a younger child to resist the urge to move ahead a few spaces on the game board when no one is looking, out of fear that her opponent is going to take the lead. As with lying, this sly behavior may seem harmless, but if repeatedly allowed, cheating among the younger set could lead to more serious forms of cheating, such as academic cheating, in later years. It's best to explain to your young child that you understand her desire to win, but that cheating is not fair. You could then work with her to improve her winning strategies.

Academic or scholastic cheating in older children can have serious consequences. To curb academic cheating, be sure that your child understands that doing her best and getting help if needed are much better than cheating. You, of course, must also lead by example and be sure that no form of cheating occurs in your household.

Verbal Aggression and Hostile Profanity

Verbal aggression and hostile profanity are among the less common, more severe behavioral problems described here and in the next few sections. Verbal aggression and profanity are mostly learned kinds of behavior. If your child uses them as strategies to get what she wants and it works, she's likely to continue using them. To curb this behavior, remember that you set the example in your home and your child will model the behavior you exhibit. Be sure that you don't give in to your child's demands on a consistent basis. For example, if your child yells and swears, ignore the demand and warn her that yelling and swearing are inappropriate and won't work. Remember that praising your child when she chooses other appropriate avenues for dealing with her anger or distress is just as important as not rewarding her undesirable behavior.

Physical Aggression to Self or Others

A physically aggressive child bullies other children, hits, or destroys. Hitting and biting are more commonly exhibited in the preschool years, but by the time children reach school age, most have mastered the skills needed to control and manage the anger and frustration that can lead to aggressive behavior. If your school-age child is aggressive, you can help by strictly and consistently enforcing punishments in the form of consequences, for example, taking certain privileges away for a week (see What You Can Do, p. 469). Remember that spanking your child will only reinforce her negative behavior and rewarding your child when she does control her anger is as important as punishing her.

If your child has repeatedly tried to injure others or herself, you should also seek the help of a child behavior specialist who can offer effective strategies to curb the behavior.

Stealing

You can respond most effectively to stealing by your own example and by using teachable moments. For instance, if you find after leaving a store that your child has taken something, gently explain that it is not appropriate and walk back into the store with the child. The item can be replaced on the shelf together or handed to the clerk. Remember also to reinforce your message by rewarding your child for her honesty. It is important to use this as a nonpunitive teaching opportunity unless the stealing is repeated. If your child continues to steal despite these efforts, call your doctor or a mental health specialist.

Cruelty to Animals

It is important to distinguish between a young child who pulls a cat's tail too hard because she doesn't know any better or inadvertently hugs a puppy too tightly and the child who is intent on hurting an animal. The latter behavior can be indicative of a serious behavioral disorder, especially if the cruelty occurs more than once. If it appears that your child is trying to hurt pets or other animals, bring her to a physician for an evaluation.

Fire Setting

Most children under 10 who set fires do so out of curiosity—an important distinction from the child who sets a fire with destructive intent. The best way to prevent your child from playing with matches is to closely supervise her and keep any matches, lighter fluid, or other flammable materials out of sight. If you have caught your child playing with matches or a lighter, be sure to explain to her the dangers of setting a fire. You may want to call your local fire department and ask about appropriate educational programs.

Intentional fire setting is a learned behavior and is usually indicative of severe behavioral problems. Studies have shown that children who deliberately set fires are usually victims of neglect in their homes and most exhibit other aggressive behavior. If your child has set a fire, call your doctor, who will refer you to an appropriate specialist to evaluate your child.

Causes

Most children undergo a period of normal development when behavior problems are the rule, not the exception. Usually, such behavior is a way to test limits and to get attention from you and others. Indeed, behavioral problems can develop under various situations. Sometimes, emotional stress, triggered by a sudden change in the environment (separation, divorce, or relocation) or a family member's death or illness, causes children to develop more troubling or longer-lasting behavior problems. Some children with communication problems exhibit behavior problems because they are frustrated by their failure to communicate. When they acquire better communication skills, their behavior problems often disappear.

Behavioral problems can also develop in response to, or as a symptom of, a number of medical conditions. Certain genetic disorders, such as Prader-Willi syndrome and Klinefelter's syndrome, have associated behavioral and psychological problems. Children with developmental problems such as autism (see *Pervasive Developmental Disorder*) or *attention deficit disorder* often develop behavioral problems that require special parenting skills and patience.

What the Doctor May Do

In most cases, your doctor will reassure you that your child's behavior is not dangerous. If he's concerned about your child's physical, developmental, or emotional well-being, he may refer you to a neurologist, psychologist, or behavior therapist for an interview and further evaluation.

Your child's doctor or other health professional may suggest techniques to help change unwanted behavior through a system of rewards or consequences. For tantrums, for example, you may be instructed to remove her from the setting and give her a time-out: a 3- to 10-minute period in a restrictive area, such as a quiet corner. With this method, you can avoid reinforcing her negative behavior. Although this may trigger an even more intense tantrum at first, her behavior should improve with time. Another effective technique is to walk away and ignore the child's tantrum, thereby withholding the reward your child may be seeking—your attention. Instead, reward your child with your attention when she is behaving well. It is important to be as patient and as calm as possible throughout this often frustrating process. For most behavior problems, a health professional may advise you to record what happens right before the behavior occurs and how you respond, in order to figure out what situations trigger the behavior.

Hair pulling, twisting, or stroking usually requires no treatment. However, if the problem becomes serious, treatment combining psychotherapy and medication is usually necessary and successful. Since hair pulling is brought on by anxiety, anger, or sadness, the therapist will focus on alleviating that underlying stress.

Head banging is often best ignored unless your child is in danger of injuring herself, since intervening may cause her to increase the behavior. If head banging persists after 3 years of age, your doctor may suggest further developmental, neurological, and psychiatric evaluation. If your child has a bleeding or seizure disorder, or has developmental impairments and may hurt herself, your doctor might advise you to have her always wear a protective helmet. Children diagnosed with clinical depression or an anxiety disorder may benefit from antidepressant or antianxiety medications.

Children with developmental disorders need an integrated approach to treatment that includes counseling for the parents, therapy for the child, and special accommodations in the child's preschool or school. These, in a holistic manner, should address all of the child's and family's needs. Your child's doctor can coordinate this care with all the professionals involved.

What You Can Do

The best advice for parents in your situation is to remember one important fact: In all but the most stubborn situations, this phase will pass. In the meantime, remain as consistent and loving as possible. Here are some further tips:

- *Find the source of stress or worry.* Whenever possible, try to understand what's causing your child's negative behavior. You can avoid many temper tantrums and head-banging incidents, and some breath-holding spells, by avoiding the situations that trigger them.

- *Listen to your child.* Children often misbehave because they're frustrated or unhappy. Encourage your child to express her feelings and concerns openly, and listen to—but don't judge—your child's troubles, worries, and concerns. Acknowledge your child's feelings by telling her that you understand that she's upset.

- *Bolster self-esteem.* Build your child's strengths by providing opportunities for her to master various skills, such as running, reading, dressing, or being a good friend or sibling, and congratulate her on her progress. Catch your child being good: Reward good behavior with praise. In addition to receiving a self-confidence boost, your child will also find healthy new ways to assert her independence and maturity.

- *Take time-outs for temper tantrums.* Your child needs time and space to recover. Remember, children are often frightened by their own angry feelings, as well as by the intense feelings they arouse in their parents. Allowing your child the opportunity to recover and resolve her feelings will help you both through difficult periods. Time-outs work most effectively when used immediately, but sparingly. As a guideline, try using 1 minute of time-out for each year of age. Use a timer to monitor minutes. Simply withholding your attention for brief periods can also help reduce temper tantrums. Avoid rewarding the negative behavior.

- *Control yourself.* If you're like most parents, your child can "push your buttons" better than anyone else. Be sure to maintain control by appearing calm—even if you're furious inside. Often, taking a "time-out" yourself by leaving the room for a few minutes is helpful (see Toddler Discipline, p. 201). This will both set a good example for your child and keep you from battling in vain at your child's level.

- *Prepare for challenges.* Anticipate what situations trigger your child's behavior problems, build extra time into your schedule to deal with problem situations, and give your child time to respond to your requests. You'll be more relaxed if you aren't running late. Plan the consequences of misbehavior ahead of time to avoid punishing excessively out of anger. Be especially clear and consistent about rules and consequences (see Immediate Rewards and Consequences, p. 242), build more structure into daily routines, and prepare your child in advance if she will have to switch to a less enjoyable activity soon (see Routines and Rituals, p. 185).

- *Avoid sending the wrong message.* Some punishments, such as spanking or yelling, may teach children that violence is an appropriate response to anger. Such behavior may encourage behavior problems. Try to make the consequences fit the misbehavior, while demonstrating that you will continue meeting your child's basic needs. Never spank a child. Avoid locking your child in a room, hitting in anger, withholding food, or giving other punishments that, in effect, reduce a parent to the child's level of behavior.

Prevention

Providing a safe, calm, and healthy family environment and establishing a nurturing relationship with your child may prevent—or at least reduce the severity of—many behavioral problems.

Birthmarks

Although we tend to associate clear, soft skin with infancy, many babies are born with birthmarks (skin discolorations, either flat or raised) caused by a collection of small blood vessels or pigment just below the surface. Present at birth or appearing in the first months of life, most birthmarks are completely harmless. In rare cases, extensive pigmented birthmarks may be associated with problems of the skeletal system, eyes, teeth, or central nervous system or later skin cancer development. Some birthmarks, although harmless, may appear unattractive or disfiguring to a parent or child. If this is the case, ask your doctor whether the birthmark is likely to fade or whether corrective procedures are available.

Signs and Symptoms

- Flat or raised patches that appear around the time of birth and do not fade quickly

Essential Facts

Dark brown birthmarks, or moles, are circular or variable in shape and may be flat or raised. They may have hair growing out of them. The doctor may refer to these dark moles as nevi. They are usually permanent but harmless. In rare instances, moles may be precursors of melanoma, a skin cancer that may occur later in life. If your child has a large, dark brown mole, your doctor may suggest removing it to prevent skin cancer from developing.

Blue or gray spots (also called Mongolian spots) are very common among darker-skinned people. They may look like flat blue bruises in the skin, usually on the lower back or buttocks. They will fade over several years. Like most other birthmarks, they pose no health problems.

Café-au-lait spots are flat, tan areas of the skin that are present at birth or appear during infancy or early childhood. Although one to three café-au-lait spots are common in normal children, more than six may indicate a health problem. Be sure to ask the doctor about them.

Port-wine stains (flat hemangiomas) look exactly like their name—a reddish purple flat stain on the skin. These birthmarks may appear over much of the face and forehead or the limbs and won't disappear, although they may eventually fade. Port-wine stains are harmless, except in rare cases when they may indicate a neurological disorder called Sturge-Weber syndrome.

Stork bites (flat angiomata or salmon patches) appear as small, flat pink stains on the back of the neck, the upper eyelids, the nose, or the lower back. They usually disappear within a few years, but those on the neck may persist indefinitely. Stork bites are completely harmless.

Strawberry marks (capillary hemangiomas) are raised, bright red patches or bumps appearing during the first few weeks or months after birth on any part of the body. They may disappear by the time the child reaches 5 years old, but usually enlarge rapidly, growing darker or lighter before disappearing. They occur most commonly in girls and may bleed spontaneously.

Cavernous hemangiomas are very large, extensive collections of blood vessels that may cause disfigurement of the face, neck, or other areas of the body. These congenital defects may be complicated by infection, vision interference (if near the eye), blood-clotting abnormalities, and other associated defects. They may shrink during infancy and early childhood.

What the Doctor May Do

In most cases, no treatment is necessary. If your child's birthmark is unsightly and does not disappear as he gets older, your doctor may refer you to a dermatologist or plastic surgeon. Birthmarks, including port-wine stains, can be treated with many techniques, including laser therapy.

Hemangiomas that develop sores during their rapid growth phase usually require medical attention. If a hemangioma interferes with the functioning of body structures, your doctor may prescribe steroids or other medications, such as interferons, to hasten shrinkage. She may also recommend radiation treatments in select cases.

Moles should be examined by your child's doctor at regular checkups for size or color changes. Removal is rarely necessary, but may be appropriate if the mole is particularly large. Large moles are more likely to develop into skin cancer later in life.

What You Can Do

Ask your child's doctor what kind of birthmark your child has. Most birthmarks (including small moles, stork bites, or small hemangiomas) will need only to be monitored. In most cases, you won't need to give the birthmark a second thought.

If a strawberry mark bleeds, place a clean gauze pad or handkerchief over the mark; it should stop bleeding after a minute or two, but watch for signs of infection, such as swelling or redness around the mark.

Most importantly, try to help your child feel comfortable about his birthmark by relaxing. Know that if the mark doesn't disappear on its own, several safe, effective methods can remove or at least hide it. If you and your child decide against cosmetic surgery when he gets older, there are "camouflage" makeup preparations to cover the birthmark.

Prevention

There is no way to prevent birthmarks.

▌ *Bites, Animal and Human*

It can happen in an instant: Your child is patting her kitty gently at first, but then pulls the tail, and the cat responds with a quick but deep bite on her hand. Or a strange dog nips at your child's leg in the park. Even a spat between preschoolers can involve one child's biting another before adults can intervene. As alarming as they may seem, however, most bites (animal and human) are minor and heal without complications with appropriate treatment. But some animal bites can transmit disease, so call your doctor for immediate advice if your child has been bitten.

Signs and Symptoms

- Bleeding, redness, or swelling
- Irregular, jagged cut
- Tooth marks

When to Call the Doctor
CALL FOR EMERGENCY HELP AND BEGIN FIRST AID IF

- your child has been bitten by a venomous snake or wild animal and has
  - difficulty breathing and/or is turning blue.
  - signs of allergic shock (see p. 390).
  - throat tightness or *seizures.*

For first aid information, see page 380 if your child is less than 1 year old and page 383 if your child is 1 year of age or older.

CALL THE DOCTOR IMMEDIATELY IF

- your child's skin is broken (punctured or torn) by an animal or a human bite.
- the area around the bite becomes swollen and red.
- you notice swollen glands near the bite.
- your child is bitten by any wild animal or an animal that has not received rabies shots.
- your child is exposed to any animal at risk for carrying rabies (e.g., bat, fox, raccoon, skunk).

CALL THE DOCTOR TODAY IF

- you have any questions about the status of your child's tetanus vaccinations.
- you notice pus or drainage from the wound.

Essential Facts

Although most animal or human bites heal completely with time, any bite that breaks the skin is potentially dangerous, and some require stitches. An animal bite may become infected by bacteria from the animal's mouth, sometimes with rabies (a central nervous system disease that is fatal if left untreated), or with tetanus (which causes muscles to go into severe, constant contractions). Some bites can cause serious wounds, facial damage, and emotional trauma. Cat bites, for example, cause deeper, penetrating wounds (puncture wounds) that are more likely to become infected because of the long, needle-like teeth. Dog bites are often large and jagged and require stitches.

Human bites rarely cause serious disease or become infected. But in rare cases, human bites can transmit some diseases, such as the **HIV/AIDS infection,** hepatitis B or C (see **hepatitis**), or the herpesvirus (see **Cold Sores**), if the person doing the biting is infected.

With any animal bite, be sure to consider the possibility of rabies. The wild animals most likely to be infected with rabies include raccoons, skunks, foxes, and bats. Be aware that not all animal bites will appear as obvious bite marks. Bats, for instance, may not leave an obvious mark. If you suspect that your child has been bitten by a wild animal, contact your doctor or emergency room and seek treatment. Public health officials should be notified so that they can quarantine the animal to monitor it for rabies and make sure no other children are bitten. Domestic animals such as dogs, cats, and ferrets may also become infected with rabies.

QUESTIONS PARENTS ASK
Biting in Child Care and Blood-Borne Diseases

Q: If a child in my son's day care has a blood-borne disease, such as HIV or hepatitis B, should I be concerned?

A: Transmission of blood-borne diseases in child care settings is extremely rare, but it is not nonexistent. It is possible for a child infected with the hepatitis B virus (HBV) or HIV to transmit the disease through a bite that breaks the skin. However, the decision to admit an HIV- or HBV-infected child into a child care center is usually made after a team of qualified individuals, including the program director and the child's doctor, evaluate whether the child poses a significant risk to other children because she tends to bite, frequently scratches, or has bleeding problems.

Check to make sure that the child care center is following universal cleanliness precautions to help prevent the spread of infection, regardless of a child's health status (see Is the Facility Clean? p. 326). If your child is bitten, the provider should know to clean and disinfect the wound with peroxide or an over-the-counter antibacterial cream. These measures will prevent bacterial infection, though not infection from HIV or hepatitis. In case of doubt about a bite, the caregiver should call a doctor immediately.

What the Doctor May Do

Your doctor will begin treatment by washing the tissues around the wound thoroughly with soap and water. The doctor will also try to determine whether your child's tetanus immunization is up-to-date. If not, he will give your child a tetanus booster. He will also try to find out if there is any possibility that the animal had rabies.

If a threat of rabies exists, treatment will include a thorough initial cleaning and two other parts: The first part is a series of five vaccine injections given over 28 days. In addition, the doctor will inject a dose of human rabies antibodies into the tissues surrounding the wound and possibly into the buttocks as well.

Otherwise, the doctor will evaluate the wound's seriousness and determine whether stitches may be necessary. The doctor may also prescribe antibiotics for particularly large bites or those that appear infected, to prevent or fight infection.

What You Can Do

If your child is bitten, the first step is to isolate the animal (put it in a closed room or a cage) if possible, so it can do no further harm. If it is a wild animal, or even a neighbor's pet, call your local animal control officer or the police immediately. Report the bite to your doctor and the local health authorities. The animal may need to be captured and observed for signs of rabies. Don't attempt on your own to deal with a wild animal or any animal that is acting strangely. Most domestic animals are vaccinated for rabies, but if you have any doubt, tell your doctor. The animal may need to be confined and observed by a veterinarian for 10 days for signs of rabies. Wild animals may need to be killed and tested for rabies.

Meanwhile, calm and reassure your child. If the bite is bleeding, control the bleeding by putting pressure on the wound with a clean gauze, towel, or washcloth until it stops bleeding. Once the bleeding has stopped, wash the wound in warm water. Call your child's doctor. See *Cuts and Scrapes* for more on cleaning wounds.

Prevention

Never allow a pet, even a family pet with no history of aggression, to be alone in a room with an infant. Teach young children not to approach or pet unfamiliar animals, tease animals, or interfere when an animal is eating or sleeping. The key to safety around animals is adult supervision and common sense.

Help prevent human bites by teaching your child not to direct her aggressive impulses toward other children. Day care is one of the most common sites where biting occurs. Ask your day care providers about their policies regarding biting. Encourage them to take steps to discourage this and other aggressive behavior in your own and other children.

What is most important, keep your child's tetanus vaccinations up-to-date. She should have a series of them from the age of 2 months to 5 years and then booster shots every 10 years after that. (See p. 110 for a full immunization schedule.)

PREVENTING DOG ATTACKS

According to the Humane Society of the United States, about 3 million dog bites are reported each year. If you are a pet owner, be responsible about making sure that your animal's immunizations are up-to-date and that the rabies vaccination is recent. To help prevent a potentially emotionally and physically scarring event, teach your child not to inadvertently mistreat pet cats or dogs. Some children don't realize that tail pulling, holding an animal too tightly, or playfully teasing a pet can cause the animal to react.

Also, teach your child how to react if a dog threatens her.

- *Stay still.* If a dog approaches your child, have her stop in her tracks. Even a friendly dog will chase her if she runs.

- *Don't stare directly into the dog's eyes.* A dog feels threatened by direct eye contact and will be more likely to attack.

- *Give the dog a command.* Have your child say "sit" or "no" in a firm but low voice. If the dog obeys, your child can then slowly walk away.

- *Lie facedown on the ground.* If all else fails, teach your child to lie facedown on the ground and cup her hands behind her neck with her forearms and elbows covering her ears. This way, her face and head are protected in case the dog attacks. Usually, the dog will just sniff at your child and leave.

▌ Bites, Insect

See *Insect Bites and Stings.*

▌ *Bladder Infections*

See *Urinary Tract Infection.*

▌ *Bleeding Disorders*

See *Hemophilia.*

▌ *Blisters*

A blister is a common and usually quite harmless skin problem that takes the form of a buildup of fluid between skin layers. Eventually, the body absorbs the fluid within the blister and the outer layer dries out and peels away. However, if the blister breaks open and exposes the new, tender skin, the area may become sore and infected. A blister can be tiny—the size of a pinhead—or several inches in diameter. Most blisters are easily treated at home, but some more severe blisters or those caused by burns or exposure to toxic chemicals require medical treatment.

Signs and Symptoms

- Fluid-filled bubble of skin

When to Call the Doctor
CALL THE DOCTOR TODAY IF

- red streaks appear to be spreading from a blister.
- cloudy fluid appears in a blister, indicating an infection.
- your child has a blister larger than a dime.
- your child has blistering as the result of exposure to fire, a chemical, or a drug.
- your infant gets frequent blisters for no apparent reason.

Causes

Rubbing or chafing from ill-fitting shoes is the most common cause of blisters, but burns, allergic reactions to plants (see *Poison Ivy, Poison Oak, Poison Sumac*) or insect bites, and exposures to certain chemicals and medications can also cause blisters to appear on the skin. Some conditions that cause blisters include the following:

Allergies Common allergic reactions include the effects of plants such as poison ivy and poison oak. Stevens-Johnson syndrome, a severe allergic reaction to a drug or chemical, results in extensive blistering, mouth sores, bleeding, and life-threatening complications.

Medications In rare cases, many drugs, including phenobarbital, topical tretinoin, sulfonamide, penicillin, and another antibiotic (ciprofloxacin), can cause skin irritation with extensive blistering, a condition called toxic epidermal necrolysis.

Chemicals Some industrial chemicals, including kerosene, turpentine, caustic acids or alkaline agents and a strong bleach (sodium hypochlorite), can cause blistering of the skin.

Infection Certain strains of the bacterium *Staphylococcus aureus* produce toxins that cause extensive blistering. This condition, called scalded skin syndrome because it resembles an extensive burn, is sometimes complicated by an infection in the blood (sepsis) and usually requires hospitalization and intravenous antibiotics.

Inherited Conditions Inborn errors of metabolism can cause a blistering condition of the skin called epidermolysis bullosa. This rare condition requires careful monitoring and treatment by a dermatologist.

What You Can Do

First of all, don't prick or try to open a blister; that will increase the risk of infection. Instead, carefully dress it with a bandage to protect it from further damage. If it breaks open, wash the exposed skin gently with soap and water, then apply antibiotic ointment and a bandage.

If wearing certain shoes caused the blister, change your child's shoes. Replace the dressing often, and watch for signs of infection. Most blisters heal within a few days.

What the Doctor May Do

Only if the blistering is bigger than a dime, becomes infected, or is caused by something other than a minor chafing, burn, or exposure to poison ivy or oak do you need to take your child to the doctor. The doctor will treat the blistering according to its cause and degree of severity. The doctor might decide to burst a large blister and treat it with an antibiotic cream, such as bacitracin, as a protective measure. If it is already infected, she may prescribe oral antibiotics. If the doctor suspects the blistering may be caused by exposure to a drug or chemical or by an infection, she will try to determine the cause, eliminate the exposure, and treat the skin condition accordingly.

Prevention

You can take the following steps to reduce your child's chances of developing blisters:

- *Buy your child shoes that fit.* Make sure that no more than one half to 1 inch of "growing room" is left at the toe, and that heels don't slip up and down easily when your child walks. If your child plays sports, provide shoes appropriate to the sport.

- *Protect your child from exposures to blistering agents.* Keep all household chemicals and medications locked up and out of reach of your child. When outdoors, protect him from exposure to excess sunlight and poisonous plants.

See also Burns (p. 394).

▌ *Blood Pressure*

See *High Blood Pressure.*

▌ *Body Piercing*

See *Ear and Body Piercing Infections.*

▌ *Boils (Furuncles)*

It may be unpleasant to think that your baby's or child's soft, sweet skin could be marred by something as ugly as a boil, but these are not uncommon. Boils are often painful, red lumps that are treatable and short-lived. Resembling oversized pimples, boils are bacterial infections that form in the lower skin layers. They appear as red lumps, pea-sized or larger, that eventually fill with pus, come to a head, and may break and drain, or be reabsorbed by the surrounding tissue. Boils are sometimes called furuncles, and your doctor may refer to them as abscesses, although not all abscesses are boils.

Signs and Symptoms
- A large, painful, red lump
- Increasing tenderness and throbbing as pus builds up inside the lump

When to Call the Doctor
CALL THE DOCTOR TODAY IF

- a boil is in an awkward or a sensitive location (face, armpit, or buttocks).
- red streaks or swollen glands (signs of infection) appear near the boil.
- a drained boil does not seem to heal after 2 to 3 days.
- your child experiences multiple, persistent, and recurrent boils.
- your child has a boil and/or other signs of general illness, such as fever, lethargy, or vomiting.

Essential Facts

Although they can erupt anywhere on the body, boils most commonly appear on the face, neck, buttocks, and upper back. In most cases, only one boil at a time forms on a child's skin, and with proper care, it usually disappears within a week. Ignoring a boil completely may increase the chance of further infection. Complications involving boils usually result from improper treatment. Squeezing a boil, for instance, may cause scarring and force pus into uninfected areas or into the bloodstream, spreading infection. Puncturing or squeezing a boil near the nasal area may spread the infection to other areas of the head.

Causes

A boil forms when bacteria (usually *Staphylococcus aureus)* invade an opening in the skin, such as a hair follicle or scratch, and cause an infection. Conditions that cause breaks in the skin—insect bites, cuts, and dermatitis—also increase a child's risk of developing a boil. Certain long-term systemic conditions, including **diabetes mellitus,** some immune deficiencies, and malnutrition, may trigger boils. Some children may be chronic carriers of staphylococcal bacteria, which results in occasional eruption of boils.

What the Doctor May Do

If your child has a boil, see your doctor for an evaluation. If the boil is in a difficult position or has not begun to heal in a few days, the doctor may surgically lance (open) the boil in a procedure called an incision and drainage (I & D). She may analyze pus from a boil to determine the cause of the infection and will prescribe antibiotics. Usually boils clear up within 1 to 2 weeks.

What You Can Do

Keep the skin around the boil clean and dry. If the boil is located on the shoulder or a place where clothing might rub it, bandage it lightly to protect it from friction.

You can help bring the boil to a head by soaking it with warm, wet compresses for about 3 minutes, several times a day. After the boil opens and drains, wash the area thoroughly with soap and water, and apply antibiotic cream to prevent further infection. In some cases, the boil may not break and drain, but gradually fade as the fluid is reabsorbed by the surrounding tissues.

Prevention

The recommended way to prevent boils is to practice good hygiene. Regular use of antibacterial soap may keep bacteria-sensitive skin as clean as possible and prevent the carrying of staph bacteria. In addition, treat skin irritations correctly and promptly.

Bone Tumors

See *Cancer.*

Botulism

See *Food Poisoning.*

Bowlegs and Knock-Knees

As their names imply, bowlegs are legs that bow, or curve out, below the knees, and knock-knees are knees that turn inward when a child is standing. These conditions are usually a normal part of physical development and require no treatment.

Signs and Symptoms

- The ankles touch, but the knees don't touch when the child is standing (bowlegs).
- The knees touch, but the ankles don't touch when the child is standing (knock-knees).

When to Call the Doctor

CALL THE DOCTOR TODAY IF

- your child is in pain.

TALK WITH THE DOCTOR AT YOUR CHILD'S NEXT CHECKUP IF

- the condition worsens after 2 years of age.
- the condition persists past 4 years of age.
- the condition interferes with normal physical activity.
- the curvature is extreme or present in only one leg.

Essential Facts

Bowlegs, which may show up as early as 10 weeks of age, are sometimes the lingering result of the flexed position the hips maintained in the uterus. Standing and walking help the legs straighten out, and the legs usually assume a normal shape by 2 years.

Knock-knees may develop in a child whose posture has been normal up until around 3 or 4 years of age. Knock-knees are often caused by the child's attempt to keep her balance by bending her knees as she walks. Overweight children are most likely to develop knock-knees, because their developing bones and joints have trouble

supporting their weight. The problem usually goes away on its own between 5 and 8 years of age, when the structure of the knee matures.

Causes

These conditions occur most often as a normal part of a young child's physical development, and they usually disappear without treatment. Other, rarer, causes include infections, tumors, and the following conditions:

Blount's Disease This bone disease involves asymmetrical bone growth that makes the upper part of the shinbone bow out just below the knee. It usually affects just one leg, making the child's posture look uneven. Although it is most common in children between 1 and 3 years old, Blount's disease can also occur in children 9 years and older.

Rickets This disease is caused by a vitamin D deficiency that weakens bones and can cause the legs to bow out. Black infants are especially prone to rickets, because their skin doesn't manufacture vitamin D from sunlight as easily as white skin does. Although rickets was once common, the ready availability of vitamin-D-fortified milk and other foods has significantly reduced the incidence of the disease in the United States.

Congenital Bone Malformation Bowlegs or knock-knees can be the result of an underlying bone malformation present at birth.

What the Doctor May Do

Your child's doctor will examine your child, observing her legs while she stands and walks. For a baby, the doctor may hold her in a standing position on the examining table. Depending on your child's age and the severity of the condition, the doctor may suggest that your child see an orthopedic specialist (bone doctor) for further evaluation. In severe cases, an orthopedic specialist may recommend corrective shoes, braces, or even surgery, depending on the cause of the problem.

What You Can Do

Unless the doctor tells you otherwise, the only thing you can do for your child with bowlegs or knock-knees is wait. The problem usually passes on its own as the child's growing muscle strength helps straighten out the legs. If the condition is caused by an underlying problem, you and your child's doctor will discuss treatment options.

Prevention

You can take the following steps to reduce your child's chances of developing knock-knees or bowlegs:

- *Maintain a normal weight.* You can help prevent knock-knees by helping your child stay at a normal weight.

- *Prevent vitamin D deficiency.* Make sure that your child gets at least 400 international units (IUs) of vitamin D every day. If she spends time outdoors every day, her skin will manufacture vitamin D naturally. But she will also need vitamin D in her diet from such sources as vitamin-D-fortified milk, as well as eggs, liver, and fish.

- *Encourage good posture.* Discourage your child from sitting with her feet behind her and her knees splayed out to the sides, a position that can harm knee posture. Instead, encourage your child to sit either cross-legged or with her knees drawn up in front of her.

QUESTIONS PARENTS ASK
Should Infants Stand?

Q: Does holding a young infant often in a standing position cause bowlegs?

A: Holding an infant who has not yet begun to walk

in a standing position is harmless. In fact, many infants enjoy being held so that some of their weight is on their feet. It allows them to exercise and strengthen their leg muscles, which they'll use more when they begin walking soon. Be sure always to support the head and neck when holding a newborn or young infant.

▌ *Brain Tumors*

See *Cancer.*

▌ *Bronchiolitis*

Your infant is wheezing, and his breathing is quick and labored. You can see the muscles under his ribs and in his neck working to bring in more air. Other family members have a simple cold, but your baby is worse. He's having trouble sucking his bottle or pacifier and hasn't eaten anything today. Chances are that he has a bout of bronchiolitis. Bronchiolitis is a common illness that causes inflammation of the bronchioles—the small airways of the lungs.

Signs and Symptoms

- Difficulty sucking, swallowing, eating, and/or drinking
- Rapid breathing, sometimes with high-pitched wheezing
- Persistent coughing
- *Fever*

When to Call the Doctor

CALL THE DOCTOR IMMEDIATELY IF

- your child is struggling to breathe or has blue or gray skin around his lips, face, or fingernails.
- more than 15 seconds go by between your infant's breaths.
- you cannot wake your child.
- your infant under 6 months of age has a fever above 100.2°F.
- your baby's cold symptoms worsen, and his breathing becomes labored.
- your baby shows signs of dehydration (dry mouth, listlessness, decreased or dark-colored urine).

CALL THE DOCTOR TODAY IF

- your infant is wheezing.
- your child is over 6 months and has a fever (102°F or above).
- his coughing is accompanied by vomiting.

Essential Facts

Bronchiolitis tends to affect babies under 2 years old. Symptoms such as high-pitched wheezing, a constant hard cough, and eating problems due to difficulty sucking and swallowing are often signs of bronchiolitis. As the amount of oxygen in your baby's bloodstream decreases, a bluish tint may appear around his mouth and fingertips. Your infant may dilate his nostrils and contract the muscles under his rib cage, attempting to breathe more air. He may grunt, and you may see his stomach rising and falling as he breathes.

Usually, bronchiolitis clears up in about the same time as a case of the common cold—and often without medical treatment. But when the lining of the bronchioles (the smallest airways of the lungs) swells and fills with mucus, it may block an infant's tiny air passages, causing breathing problems. Although most infants recover completely, bronchiolitis sometimes results in long-term medical problems such as asthma or continued wheezing in childhood.

Infants exposed to other children through day care or siblings have an increased risk of developing bronchiolitis. More severe disease

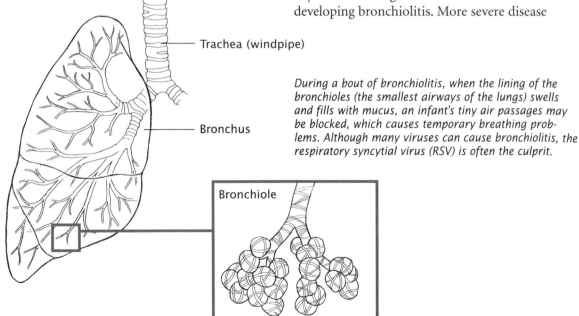

During a bout of bronchiolitis, when the lining of the bronchioles (the smallest airways of the lungs) swells and fills with mucus, an infant's tiny air passages may be blocked, which causes temporary breathing problems. Although many viruses can cause bronchiolitis, the respiratory syncytial virus (RSV) is often the culprit.

Trachea (windpipe)

Bronchus

Bronchiole

Alveolar sacs

may occur in premature infants or those with a chronic disease, such as cystic fibrosis, heart disease, or immune problems.

Causes

Most babies who develop bronchiolitis have been exposed to someone with a cold or flu. Although many viruses can cause this condition, the respiratory syncytial virus (RSV) is often the culprit—especially between October and March, when RSV is most common. A vaccine for RSV is under development.

What the Doctor May Do

In order to diagnose bronchiolitis, the doctor will thoroughly examine your child, especially his nose, chest, and lungs. She may also take a mucus sample from the back of your child's nose in order to identify the virus causing the infection, and she may take a chest X ray. As with all viral illnesses, antibiotics are ineffective. Therefore, your doctor will attempt mainly to treat your baby's symptoms and keep him comfortable until the virus runs its course.

The doctor may suggest saline nose drops and a bulb syringe to help clear out the baby's nose. Less commonly, the doctor may have your child use a bronchodilator (a type of medication that opens the breathing tubes) in her office through a device that passes air through a liquid medicine and turns it into a mist that can be breathed into the lungs through a face mask (nebulizer). In some cases, the doctor may have you use the device at home, as well. Not all cases of bronchiolitis are helped by this treatment, so your doctor will first assess whether it will benefit your baby before recommending it.

If your baby's oxygen level is low, the doctor will hospitalize him, usually for a day or two, to give him extra oxygen until he can keep his oxygen levels up. If the baby is dehydrated, he may need intravenous fluids until he can drink enough to maintain body fluids. New therapies

to treat bronchiolitis, such as steroids or antiviral medications, are being investigated for their effectiveness.

Children hospitalized with bronchiolitis usually recover completely within a few weeks. But younger infants, premature infants, and infants with chronic illnesses—such as heart disease, *HIV/AIDS infection, cystic fibrosis,* immune deficiency, and premature infants with lung disease (see *Prematurity*)—who are more likely to be hospitalized, may have more severe cases of bronchiolitis and take longer to recover.

What You Can Do

Keep your baby as comfortable as possible to help him rest. If your baby's condition doesn't improve within a day or two, call your doctor. If your baby is struggling for breath at any time, bring him to the nearest emergency room immediately.

- *Give plenty of fluids.* Try breast-feeding or bottle-feeding more often than usual, both to soothe your child and to keep his fluid levels up. A baby with enough fluids should wet his diapers at least every 4 hours.
- *Treat the fever.* Treat your child's fever with acetaminophen or ibuprofen. You can also place a lukewarm cloth on his forehead to cool his fever (unless it makes him shiver).
- *Clear the breathing passages.* Suction your baby's nose with a bulb if it seems to be blocked with mucus, or insert saline nose drops to loosen mucus for easier removal.

Prevention

To protect your child from the viruses that cause bronchiolitis, be sure that you and your baby's other caregivers practice proper hygiene, including regular hand-washing and the other methods described on page 366.

Whenever possible, keep your infant away from people with colds or the flu, especially in the winter, when more people are sick. If your child is at high risk for bronchiolitis, your doctor may advise you not to bring your child to day care during the winter season, to avoid exposing him to the viruses that cause bronchiolitis. If your infant is premature and at high risk for severe RSV or for bronchiolitis, the doctor may recommend preventative therapy between October and March of the child's first year. This therapy involves monthly injections of palivizunab, an immune antibody directed toward the RSV virus. The doctor will usually make this recommendation only after consulting with a pediatrician who specializes in neonatology, intensive care, or pulmonology.

Another way to prevent your child from developing bronchiolitis is to protect him from secondhand tobacco smoke. The presence of secondhand smoke in the baby's environment puts your baby at higher risk for many respiratory symptoms.

See also *Colds/Flu; Cough; Croup; Epiglottitis; Pneumonia.*

Bruises

All parents of an active child are familiar with the purplish marks that appear on the skin after a bump or fall. Most bruises disappear with no treatment in a few days. A bruise is a mark in the skin, usually the result of a blow or bump that ruptures the small blood vessels near the skin's surface. Most bruises need no special attention unless the injury is severe.

Signs and Symptoms

- Purple-red mark on the skin that fades to black and blue, then green or yellow
- Tenderness for a day or two
- Swelling, if the bruise is over a bone

 When to Call the Doctor
CALL THE DOCTOR IMMEDIATELY IF

- the pain gets worse after 24 hours (an underlying bone could be broken).
- multiple bruises appear without injury and in unusual spots, such as the trunk or back, which may indicate a bleeding disorder.
- multiple bruises appear and the child has a fever.

Essential Facts

A bruise is a collection of blood that has escaped from broken blood vessels because of injury or, rarely, disease. The blood settles in a space between muscle and skin and is visible through the skin's surface. Some people tend to bruise more easily, for reasons not yet fully understood. Fair-skinned people tend to show bruises more obviously than darker-skinned people.

You can distinguish a bruise from a rash or another skin discoloration by watching what happens after you apply gentle pressure: If it doesn't appear lighter after you press it gently with a finger, the mark is a bruise. All other purple-red marks on the skin blanch (look pale) under pressure.

Causes

Toddlers sometimes get bruised foreheads as they learn to walk, whereas preschoolers commonly have bruises on the fronts of their legs from jumping and climbing. Bruises on the back or buttocks are unusual in children, and although sometimes caused by rare blood diseases, they may be signs of child abuse. If you notice unexplained bruises on your child's back or buttocks or other areas of the body, have your doctor examine your child.

Less commonly, excessive bruising and bleeding may indicate a bleeding disorder such as *hemophilia* or other clotting abnormalities; leukemia (see *Cancer*); or idiopathic thrombocytopenic purpura (ITP), a deficiency of blood platelets. With ITP, patches of bruises are the only visible sign that an underlying purpura exists. In some cases, diseases produce pinpoint-to pinhead-sized bruises called petechiae. Contact your child's doctor if you notice unusual bruising or prolonged bleeding.

What the Doctor May Do

Bruises themselves need no medical treatment, but if your child has a very painful bruise or several that occur without explanation, bring her to your doctor. If your doctor suspects that an underlying disease may be causing the bruises, he may recommend a complete physical examination, including blood tests and other diagnostic examinations. If he suspects a fracture or another serious injury, he will take appropriate steps to diagnose and treat the injury.

What You Can Do

Apply a cold compress or an ice pack for $1/2$ hour or so, as soon after the injury occurs as possible, which will help to contain the bruise.

Do not . . .

- apply ice directly to the skin. Instead, use a commercial ice pack, or make one by placing ice cubes in a plastic bag and then wrapping the bag in a towel.

Prevention

While avoiding all minor bruises is impossible, you can take steps to protect your child from injury. Watch your infant or toddler carefully to protect her from falls, and take the measures described on page 141 to make your home safe for a small child. Your infant or toddler should be secured with a safety strap when in a carriage, a stroller, an infant seat, or any other baby equipment. Make sure that your older child wears protective gear, such as a helmet, while participating in athletic activities and biking (see Playing It Safe, p. 274), and make sure that your child's activities are appropriate for her age and skill level.

Some infectious causes of bruising can be prevented. The pneumococcal vaccine (see p. 112) will prevent petechiae. Another vaccine prevents infection by certain types of meningococcal bacteria, which can cause fever and purpura, but is recommended only for children in certain high-risk groups. Children exposed to meningococcal infection should receive antibiotics. Consult your doctor about this, and ask him to make sure your child's vaccination schedule is up-to-date (see Childhood Immunization Schedule, p. 110).

See also Fractures (Broken Bones) on page 409.

▌ *Bruxism*

See *Tooth-Grinding.*

▌ *Burns*

See page 394.

▌ *Cancer*

Cancer comes in many forms and has a wide array of symptoms. That's why parents sometimes suspect cancer when their children have unexplained symptoms. But fortunately, cancer among children is very rare—on average 1 to 2 children in 10,000 are diagnosed with cancer in the United States each year—and, thanks to recent advances, more children than ever are cured after treatment. Early diagnosis and treatment offer the best approach for children with any form of childhood cancer.

Signs and Symptoms

Because there are so many kinds of cancer, each with a variety of symptoms, this section will not list them all. Common general symptoms include fatigue, unexpected weight loss, malaise, frequent headaches, fevers, and irritability and other changes in behavior. If parents make sure that children have regular checkups and report any unusual symptoms to the child's doctor, early diagnosis is more likely.

Essential Facts

Many different types of cancer exist. All types share one common characteristic: uncontrollable cell growth. Unlike normal young cells, which mature to form the various organs of the body, cancer cells multiply rapidly, destroy normal cells, and interfere with growth and development. Cancer cells keep dividing and do not stop, forming tumors or spreading to other parts of the body.

Many cancer types produce no symptoms until the disease is quite advanced. Others cause nonspecific symptoms that can be mistaken for ordinary viruses and are difficult to detect and diagnose. General signs may include fatigue, loss of appetite and weight, and recurrent fevers. Some cancers produce obvious swelling or pain. Your doctor will probably attempt to rule out more common conditions before considering cancer as a serious possibility. Cancer does not develop overnight, and minor delays in diagnosis do not usually affect the ability to cure cancer.

Although cancer in adults develops most commonly in the lung, breast, and colon, cancer in children generally affects other areas, such as the blood and the lymphatic systems, the brain, the nervous system, and bones. Many different types of cancer can affect children, but almost half are either leukemia or brain tumors.

Leukemia

Leukemia, although rare, is the most common childhood cancer. A person with leukemia has too many immature white blood cells in the blood and bone marrow. These immature, underdeveloped white blood cells may clog healthy body tissues and organs, leading to organ dysfunction. In addition, these cells don't fight infection as mature white blood cells do, and they prevent normal blood cell production. Because the normal blood cells in the bone marrow are crowded out by leukemia cells, the normal blood cell and platelet levels can become dangerously low.

The two most prevalent types of childhood leukemia are acute lymphoblastic leukemia (ALL) and acute myelogenous leukemia (AML). ALL, the most common type, causes the production of too many cells called lymphoblasts. In AML, cells called myeloblasts are overproduced. Leukemia treatment, which can last months or years, involves chemotherapy (anticancer drugs) and sometimes radiation. Many complications are associated with therapy. In recent decades, better treatment strategies for both types of leukemia have dramatically improved the outlook for children with leukemia. Over 90 percent of children with ALL can be cured.

Brain Tumors

A brain tumor is an abnormal growth of cells forming a tumor inside the brain. A tumor can affect any of the brain's complex functions. It can exert damaging pressure on delicate tissue, interfering with virtually any function controlled by the brain. The outlook for a child with a brain tumor depends on the tumor's location and its type. Not all brain tumors are cancerous (malignant). Tumors are considered malignant if they grow rapidly and consist of certain types of cancer cells. But even a benign tumor can be life-threatening, depending on its location and how large it grows. Brain tumors are the second most common childhood cancer, but only about 3 cases per 100,000 children are diagnosed each year.

Other Solid Tumors

Other solid tumors are also rare. These masses can arise in any organ, and symptoms depend on where the tumor occurs.

Lymphoma The third most common cancer in children, lymphoma is a cancer of the lymphatic system, that is, the body organs and tissues that produce and transport lymphocytes (infection-fighting white blood cells). The first sign of lymphoma is often a painless, progressive swelling of a lymph node or group of lymph nodes in the neck, armpits, or groin. However, swollen lymph nodes are a common sign of infection and do not usually indicate cancer. Lymphoma occurs in only 1 to 2 children out of 100,000 each year.

Bone Tumors These are malignant skeletal tumors. The most common childhood cancers starting in the bone and skeletal connective tissues are osteosarcoma (osteogenic sarcoma) and Ewing's sarcoma. Both usually occur in older children or adolescents. Although potentially life-threatening, both are very treatable, especially if they haven't yet spread to other parts of the body. Osteosarcoma usually begins at the end of a leg bone, but can be found in any bone. Only about 2 to 3 out of 1 million children (usually adolescents) are diagnosed with osteosarcoma each year. Ewing's sarcoma usually develops in the middle of long bones, but can also occur in any bone and sometimes in muscle, as well.

Wilms' Tumor Wilms' tumor is the most common type of kidney cancer among children. It grows rapidly, often swelling the abdomen. Other symptoms can include abdominal pain, poor feeding, and blood in the child's urine. Wilms' tumor appears most often in children between 1 and 5 years old, and is treated successfully in over 90 percent of cases.

Other solid tumors that occur in childhood include *neuroblastomas* (tumors of the adrenal glands or the part of the nervous system that monitors automatic body systems), *rhabdomyosarcomas* (rare, malignant muscle tumors), and *retinoblastomas* (malignant eye tumors usually diagnosed in very young children; they often run in the family). In general, solid tumor treatment involves surgery or radiation to the tumor, or both, and then usually chemotherapy.

Causes

No one knows what causes childhood cancer. Although it might result from a genetic predisposition or an infectious disease—perhaps caused by a virus—no one knows what causes cancer to develop in any one individual. A combination of factors is probably involved, including genetics and environmental factors (such as radiation, medications, toxins, and infectious agents). Cancers caused by environmental agents such as asbestos, cigarette smoke, and other pollutants occur more in adults than children, after many years of exposure to these substances, which probably began in childhood. Cancer is never contagious.

What the Doctor May Do

A physician who suspects cancer may refer the child to a childhood cancer specialist (a pediatric oncologist) at a cancer center or hospital. After recording the illness history and symptoms, an oncologist performs a careful physical examination, seeking specific abnormality or disease indicators. He will probably perform a series of laboratory examinations, beginning with blood tests and perhaps X rays. Depending on what type of cancer he suspects, other tests may be necessary. If the doctor sees abnormalities, he may take a biopsy, in which tissue or cells from the abnormal area (which may be a mass in the skin, bone, bone marrow, muscle, or other organs) are removed to be examined under a microscope. The entire evaluation process may take from a day to a week or more. Your child may be hospitalized while the medical team performs and evaluates the tests, or she may visit the hospital or clinic as an outpatient.

If the doctor confirms a cancer diagnosis, he and the parents or guardians decide together on the best treatment options. Because some treatments for childhood cancer are complicated, the doctor may recommend that treatment take place at a regional cancer center or teaching hospital where specialists are available. Before treatment begins, the medical team obtains consent from the parents or guardians by discussing the options with them and explaining the benefits and risks of the proposed therapy. The goal of therapy is to create and sustain a remission—the disappearance of cancer cells and symptoms. Cancer treatment changes constantly as research provides more effective therapies.

The kind of treatment provided varies according to the cancer type. Most cancer patients receive either surgery, radiation therapy, or chemotherapy or a combination of these therapies.

- *Surgery:* Surgically removing the cancerous tumor is usually recommended for children with solid tumors, like those in the brain or bone.

- *Chemotherapy:* This treatment uses a combination of anticancer medications to kill cancer cells or prevent their division. Anticancer medications affect not only cancer cells, but also other rapidly dividing normal cells, such as those in the hair follicles, bone marrow, and gastrointestinal tract. As a result, certain side effects, such as hair loss, nausea, vomiting, and low blood counts (see *Anemia*), are often unavoidable.

- *Radiation therapy:* Radiation involves the use of high-energy X rays or other ionizing radia-

tion sources. The radiation rays strike cell tissue, damaging DNA within. Cancer cells are more sensitive to radiation than normal cells because radiation tends to kill cells that divide rapidly, leaving most surrounding healthy tissue relatively unaffected. Although radiation is painless, the side effects can include fatigue, skin sensitivity, and rashes. Radiation side effects vary according to the part of the body being irradiated. Radiation is usually given daily for up to 5 weeks.

- *Bone marrow transplantation:* This treatment involves eradicating all of the cancer cells in the marrow along with all of the normal marrow cells. Then, new marrow cells from a matched donor are injected to repopulate the cancer patient's marrow with normal cells.

What You Can Do

If your child is diagnosed with cancer, you and your family will work closely with a medical team to treat the disease and to limit its effects, both mental and physical. With your help, the team can help your child through uncomfortable and sometimes anxiety-provoking procedures. You can also follow these suggestions:

- *Seek help.* Join a support group for families of children with cancer. Parents who have had similar experiences can provide information, practical suggestions, and emotional support. Consider counseling for family members who need help coping with the emotional demands of caring for a child with cancer.

- *Answer questions.* Be honest about any pain your child will experience, and let her ask questions or cry. If you feel you need a few minutes to cope, let someone else take over until you are calmer. When you talk to your child about her illness and the treatments she must undergo, first try to allay any misconceptions she may have. If she catches you off-guard with a difficult question, tell her you need to think about it before you answer. "Humanely tempered truth" and age-appropriate explanations are often your best bet. Prepare yourself to deal with questions about death, even if they are difficult to answer.

Also be sure to discuss your child's illness with her siblings. They need to know what is happening with their sister or brother, and to know that cancer is not contagious and was not caused by anything they did.

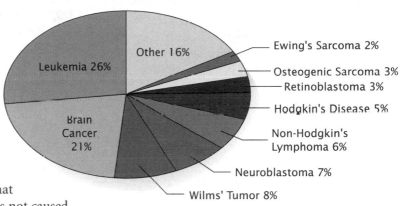

CHILDHOOD CANCERS

- Other 16%
- Leukemia 26%
- Brain Cancer 21%
- Ewing's Sarcoma 2%
- Osteogenic Sarcoma 3%
- Retinoblastoma 3%
- Hodgkin's Disease 5%
- Non-Hodgkin's Lymphoma 6%
- Neuroblastoma 7%
- Wilms' Tumor 8%

Source: National Cancer Institute SEER Program.

- *Inquire about adequate pain relief.* Before your child undergoes her first medical procedure, ask her doctor whether the procedure will be uncomfortable and how he can minimize the discomfort. Sufficient pain relief is especially important for children undergoing their first painful medical procedure; otherwise the effects of pain relief measures in later treatments may be reduced.

- *Bring personal items to the hospital.* When your child is hospitalized, she will feel more comfortable if she has a favorite blanket, stuffed animal, or video and some books and toys.

- *Provide a sense of security, support, and consistency.* This is especially important for a child who knows she has a serious illness. Your child will probably need frequent reassurance that she hasn't done anything wrong and that the disease is not a punishment for being bad. Remind her often that she is loved.

Some parents of children with cancer find it easier to avoid introducing many changes into their lives. Job, housing, and marital changes can all add unnecessary stress to a family already coping with cancer.

- *Treat your child naturally.* That means establishing rules. Although your instinct may be to pamper your child because she has cancer, a child with cancer—like any child—benefits from consistent, loving rules and expectations.

- *Take breaks.* Take time to do the things you enjoyed before your child became ill. If your child is hospitalized, ask relatives or friends to visit so you can take a break.

Prevention

Because the causes of childhood cancer are often unknown, preventative measures are not often available. But, over the long term, you can reduce the risk that your child will develop cancer as an adult by discouraging her from using tobacco products and encouraging her to eat a healthy and balanced diet (including plenty of fiber), to use sunscreen, and to exercise regularly.

■ *Canker Sores*

The bad news is that a canker sore feels as raw and irritated as it looks. The good news is that it poses no permanent health risk and clears up by itself within several days. Also known by its medical name, *aphthous stomatitis*, a canker sore is a painful area or eruption of the skin and tissues that line the mouth and tongue. Canker sores are extremely common, affecting more than 20 percent of people at one time or another. They are usually minor, if painful, irritations.

Signs and Symptoms

- Small, shallow ulcers in the lining of the mouth or tongue or on the gums, covered by a gray membrane and surrounded by a bright red circle
- Pain and soreness on contact

When to Call the Doctor
CALL THE DOCTOR TODAY IF
- your child's canker sore has not healed within a few weeks.
- your child's canker sores are preventing him from eating.

Essential Facts

Most people have their first bout with canker sores between 10 and 20 years of age. But children as young as 2 years old may develop them as well. Canker sores tend to return again and again, but the frequency of recurrences varies greatly. Some children experience only one or

▄ MOUTH ULCERS

Symptoms	Cause	Incubation	Duration	Recurs?	Treatment
Canker sores (aphthous stomatitis)					
Ulcers anywhere inside the mouth, lips, and cheeks	Several causes, including stress, viruses, bacteria, sensitivity to food, allergic reactions, hormonal factors, abrasions caused by biting the inside of the mouth	Variable	7 days	Yes	Acetaminophen or ibuprofen, ice chips or ice pops, topical creams
Cold sores (gingivostomatitis)					
Fever, drooling, refusal to eat, ulcers on cheeks, lips	Herpes type 1 virus	2–14 days	5–7 days	Yes	Acetaminophen or ibuprofen, ice chips or ice pops, topical creams
Hand-foot-and-mouth disease					
Low-grade fever, headache, mouth ulcers, rash on fingers and toes	Coxsackie A virus	3–5 days	5–8 days	No	Acetaminophen or ibuprofen, ice chips or ice pops
Herpangina					
Fever, drooling, ulcers on palate and back of throat	Coxsackie A virus	2–14 days	7–10 days	No	Acetaminophen or ibuprofen, ice chips or ice pops

two episodes during their childhood, whereas others may experience a continuous series of outbreaks.

Causes

No one knows exactly what causes canker sores. Several causes probably exist, even within the same person. Possible triggers include the following:

- Mouth abrasions, such as those caused by biting the inside of the cheek or lip
- Stress
- Viruses and bacteria
- Extreme sensitivity to certain foods (particularly sweets, nuts, and citrus acids)
- Allergic reactions and toxic drug reactions
- Hormonal factors

What the Doctor May Do

No cure exists for canker sores, but your doctor will suggest some home remedies and over-the-counter medications to relieve the pain.

What You Can Do

If your child develops a canker sore, you can help relieve the symptoms by following these hints:

- *Reduce inflammation.* Over-the-counter pain relievers—acetaminophen or ibuprofen—will ease the pain of a canker sore by reducing the inflammation.
- *Avoid irritating foods.* Citric acid (found in citrus fruits, pineapples, grapes, plums, and tomatoes) aggravates canker sores. Substitute bland foods until the sore clears up.
- *Rinse with water.* Encourage your child to rinse his mouth with lukewarm water. This process will help keep the sore clean and free of bacteria and ease the pain.
- *Give ice pops.* Sucking on ice pops can help relieve the pain and inflammation of a canker

sore. Avoid pops made with orange juice, which is highly acidic and may irritate the tissue.

Prevention

There are no known ways to prevent canker sores.

▌*Cavities (Caries)*

More parents than ever before hear, "Look, Mom and Dad, no cavities!" after their children's dental checkups. Indeed, dental cavities, also called caries, are far less common than they used to be, thanks largely to advances in preventative care, such as fluoridated water, toothpaste, sealants, early dental visits, and dietary supervision. Still, protecting youngsters' teeth from cavities and their complications takes teamwork on the part of parents, children, and their dentists.

Signs and Symptoms

- Pain in the jaw or tooth
- Sensitivity to hot, cold, or sweet foods or drinks
- Visible dark spots or discolorations on teeth
- In infants, staining or discoloration of the upper front teeth, particularly around the gum line and back surfaces of the teeth

When to Call the Doctor or Dentist
CALL TODAY IF

- your child complains of tooth pain or general mouth pain.
- there is unusual discoloration of part or all of a tooth.
- there is redness, pus, or swelling of the gum around a tooth.
- the face or jaw is swollen, warm, or red (often with fever).
- painful, tender bumps appear on the child's neck.

Causes

Cavities occur when acids, produced by bacteria in the mouth, break down tooth enamel—the outer shell of a tooth. The breakdown exposes the softer, living tooth parts (such as the dentin, which lies beneath the enamel, and the pulp) to damage and decay. The good news is that with prompt and proper treatment, the tooth can remain healthy and strong even if it starts decaying. If decay extends too far into the tooth, however, inflammation of the pulp may occur, which can cause pain, infection, and irreversible damage. Over time, such decay can result in the loss of the tooth.

Tooth decay begins when bacteria that live in the mouth and make up most of the plaque (a gelatinous mat of bacteria) begin to digest sugars and other carbohydrates. The bacteria produce acids from the sugars your child eats, and this acid begins to dissolve the tooth's enamel.

Three conditions are necessary for tooth decay to occur:

1. *Bacteria in the mouth.* It is normal for bacteria to live in the mouth. One particular bacterium *(Streptococcus mutans)* is primarily responsible for tooth decay.

2. *Food for bacteria.* Sugar, in particular, promotes tooth decay.

3. *Teeth that are susceptible to decay.* This susceptibility can be due to low fluoride levels in the teeth or physical characteristics of the teeth.

At first, decay just weakens the enamel and makes it more porous. Eventually, however, it breaks down the enamel and begins to affect the dentin. If the dentist doesn't remove the decay and fill the cavity, the decay will spread into the tooth's pulp, where blood vessels and nerve tissues are present. Once the bacteria reach this area, inflammation, pain, and eventually an abscess (infection with pus) can result.

Certain teeth are more susceptible to decay than others. Teeth with structural irregularities

Cavities occur when bacteria in your child's mouth start digesting sugars and other carbohydrates from the food she eats and produce acids, which break down tooth enamel and expose the softer, living tooth parts, which contain nerve tissue, to damage and decay. (A) Healthy tooth; (B) tooth with decay penetrating enamel; and (C) tooth with decay penetrating dentin.

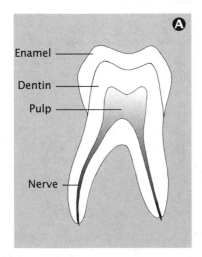 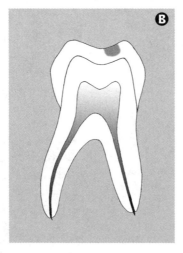 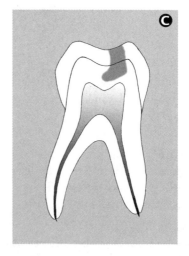

are particularly vulnerable. Irregularities include incompletely closed pits or fissures (depressions in the top or side of the tooth formed by the joining of the cusps of the crown), enamel defects, and irregularly shaped teeth. Restored (filled), irregularly shaped teeth, or teeth with braces are more difficult to clean, and thus are more likely to have decay.

Cavities can be problematic in children with certain medical conditions, such as acquired immune deficiency syndrome (see *HIV/AIDS Infection)* and other immune system diseases; acute rheumatic fever (see *Sore Throat/Strep Throat*); other heart diseases; and *sickle-cell disease.* Bacteria from a cavity can invade the bloodstream or organs in children with these conditions.

Early Childhood Caries (Baby Bottle or Nursing Tooth Decay)

Even infants and toddlers are susceptible to tooth decay. Both breast- and bottle-fed babies are susceptible to tooth decay as soon as their first teeth come in. Nursing bottle caries (also known as baby bottle tooth decay) typically appear in children who go to bed with a bottle of formula, juice, or milk. The sugar in the milk or juice sits in the mouth all night (or for several hours during nap time), allowing the bacteria in the mouth to produce acid from the sugars in the juice or formula and eat away at the baby's soft tooth enamel. Even breast-fed babies are susceptible, if they feed frequently throughout the night. Baby bottle decay usually affects the top front teeth, the top molars, and the canines (eye teeth).

What the Doctor or Dentist May Do

If your doctor suspects that your child has a cavity during a regular checkup or if your child complains of a toothache, the doctor will x-ray the affected tooth and, usually, the surrounding teeth as well.

QUESTIONS PARENTS ASK
Mercury in Silver Fillings

Q: Does the mercury in silver fillings pose any risk to my child's health?

A: There is no scientific evidence that supports the theory that mercury, which chemically binds the components of silver fillings, poses any health risk, except in the rare case that the recipient of the filling is allergic to mercury. The American Dental Association recommends silver over white fillings sometimes when the cavity is particularly large, because silver has been found to be more durable. There is no evidence that mercury fillings cause a *pervasive developmental disorder,* an *attention deficit disorder,* or *juvenile rheumatoid arthritis.*

Filling Cavities

A cavity appears on the X ray as a gray or black mark on a tooth's surface. The dentist will remove the decayed portion of a tooth with a dental instrument (drill) and replace it with a filling made of amalgam (silver) or composite (white plastic). For larger cavities, the dentist may inject a local anesthetic (usually lidocaine). But the use of newer filling materials and dental sealants has enabled dentists to make smaller fillings that require less drilling, and as a result, anesthesia is needed less often.

Applying Dental Sealants

The dentist can limit the damage to your child's teeth by coating them with plastic sealants to prevent decay. Dentists apply sealants most often to permanent molars—the 6-year molars, and later, the 12-year molars. Less commonly, a dentist may apply a sealant to a baby tooth—when the tooth looks particularly susceptible to decay.

Applying a sealant takes only 5 minutes per tooth—and costs only about half of what it would cost to fill a similar cavity. Most dental plans cover the cost. Using sealants is one of the most effective ways of preventing cavities from developing. But few families take advantage of this method: Less than 20 percent of U.S. school-age children have dental sealants on their permanent molars. The dentist will check the child's sealants every 6 months to see if follow-up maintenance is needed.

What You Can Do

Cavities and tooth decay can only be treated by dental professionals, but you can help prevent tooth decay and identify problems early by taking your child for a dental checkup and cleaning every 6 months.

Prevention

The number of school-age children without cavities in their permanent teeth has doubled (from 26 to 55 percent) in the last two decades. You can help prevent cavities from developing in your child's teeth using the following tips.

Prevent Baby Bottle Tooth Decay

If your baby has teeth, don't put her to bed with a bottle. Don't prop the bottle (always hold your baby while feeding), or if breast-feeding, avoid continual breast-feeding throughout the night.

It is important to protect your infant's baby teeth from decay because loss of these primary teeth before the secondary teeth are ready to replace them can cause the remaining primary teeth to shift position to fill in the gap. When her permanent teeth are ready to erupt, there's no room, and they may become impacted beneath the gums or come in crooked. This may cause an improper bite (a malocclusion), which may require orthodontic treatment (braces) and the removal of one or more permanent teeth.

Cavities in the baby teeth can also interfere with the development of the permanent teeth below the surface of your baby's gums. Follow your doctor's or dentist's suggestions to reduce your child's chances of future dental problems.

See a Dentist

Take your child to a dentist for her first visit within 6 months after the appearance of her first tooth or at least by her first birthday. Visit a dentist every 6 months beginning at 3 years of age.

Use Fluoride

Use a fluoridated toothpaste, and, depending on the fluoride level in your local water supply, use a fluoride supplement (tablet or drop form) that your dentist or physician prescribes. These supplements can cause staining on the teeth, usually in the form of mild white spots, if too much fluoride is consumed. Don't allow your child to swallow toothpaste.

To determine if your child needs to take a fluoride supplement and how much she needs, ask your local health department what level of fluoride is in your tap water so that you and your doctor can determine what dose of supplement is right for your child (see chart). Most likely, if your public water supply is fluoridated, your child won't need fluoride supplements. If the water your child drinks is mostly bottled or is processed by a home water treatment system (e.g., filters), talk with your doctor or dentist about her fluoride needs. Such water may or may not contain optimal levels of fluoride. If your drinking water comes from a private well, have your well water tested for fluoride content.

Supervise Tooth Brushing

Until your child is 6 or 7 years old, help with or supervise your child's brushing. Your dental hygienist may provide dye tablets that help show which teeth are not adequately brushed.

Introduce Flossing Early

As soon as your child has two back teeth that touch, start daily flossing. Until your child is old enough (probably at 7 or 8 years old) to perform the tricky maneuvers, you'll have to handle the job yourself. The easiest way to floss your child's

▬ *FLUORIDE SUPPLEMENT: DAILY DOSAGE NEEDED* (milligrams of fluoride)

	Birth to 6 Months	6 Months to 3 Years	3 Years to 6 Years	6 Years to 16 Years
If your tap water has 0–0.3 ppm of fluoride*	0.00	0.25	0.50	1.00
If your tap water has 0.3–0.6 ppm of fluoride	0.00	0.00	0.25	0.50
If your tap water has more than 0.6 ppm of fluoride	0.00	0.00	0.00	0.00

From "Oral Health Care Programs for Children and Adolescents: Policy of Pediatric Dentistry," special issue of *Pediatric Dentistry: Journal of the American Academy of Pediatric Dentistry* 18:24 (Reference Manual 1996–97). Reprinted with permission.
*ppm = parts per million.

teeth is to sit on a chair behind her while she is standing or kneeling, then have her lean back until her head is in your lap—a position similar to the one she would have in a dentist's chair. That way, you will be able to see and reach your child's teeth more easily.

Ask Your Dentist About Sealants

When your child is about 6 years old, her dentist will evaluate whether her newly erupted permanent molars will benefit from a plastic coating to prevent plaque from entering the deep grooves and pits of the biting surfaces.

Limit Sugary, Sticky Snacks

These foods tend to stick to the teeth and remain there a long time, encouraging tooth decay. Sticky, sugary foods such as candies and fruit rolls are the worst, but even the carbohydrates found in crackers and breads cause tooth decay if not brushed off the teeth shortly after eating. Sticky dried fruits, such as raisins, also promote tooth decay, because they stick to the teeth. Don't allow your child to snack or drink sugary drinks (including fruit juice) frequently. Limit snacks to specific times of day. Do not give them in the hour or two before bedtime.

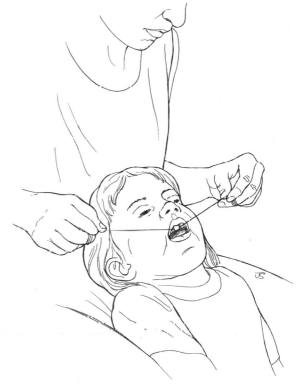

The easiest way to floss your child's teeth is to sit on a chair behind her while she is standing or kneeling, then have her lean back with her head in your lap—a position similar to the one she would have in a dentist's chair. Wind the floss around your middle fingers, and use your thumb and forefinger to manipulate it.

Encourage Drinking Water After Sweet Foods

The water will wash much of the sugar off her teeth. When drinking soda or fruit juice, encourage her to use a straw, which will minimize contact between the liquid's sugar and her teeth.

Give Sugarless Chewing Gum

Research shows that chewing sugarless gum after eating sweets reduces the likelihood of cavities developing.

AVOID THE WORST OFFENDERS

The following foods should be eaten only occasionally and then followed by thorough brushing and flossing:

- Sticky, gooey candies, such as gummies, caramels, and taffy
- Fruit rolls and similar chewy "fruit" snacks
- Gum with sugar
- Raisins and other sticky dried fruits
- Sugary breakfast cereals
- Hard candies, lollipops

■ *Cerebral Palsy*

"Cerebral" refers to the brain, and "palsy" to weakness and stiffening of the body. Cerebral palsy (CP) is a disorder of the part of the brain that controls body movement. It is a chronic, nonprogressive condition that is not contagious and usually not inherited, although a small number of conditions that cause CP are inherited. About 9,000 babies and infants are diagnosed with CP each year. CP does not always cause profound disability. Many children with CP learn to cope and thrive despite the challenges. Movement problems are often accompanied by other difficulties (including language, vision, and learning disorders, as well as

seizures). No cure exists for CP, although the symptoms can be managed, and some of the diseases that cause CP can be prevented.

Signs and Symptoms

- Physical and developmental delays
- Difficulty crawling or walking (lopsided crawling, dragging one arm or leg, heel tightness and persistent toe-walking)
- Weakness or poor motor control of the arm and leg on the same side of the body
- Reaching with one hand while keeping the other in a fist
- A floppy or stiff feeling in a child over 2 months of age when picked up

When to Call the Doctor
CALL THE DOCTOR TODAY IF
- you are concerned about your child's development.
- your child exhibits muscle weakness or poor motor control.

Essential Facts

Cerebral palsy is a term that describes a group of disorders that impair control of movement. Depending on where the brain injury is and how large an area is damaged, children with CP may have muscle tone that is too tight, too loose, or a combination of both. Children with CP cannot change their muscle tone smoothly and evenly, so their movements may be jerky or wobbly. The severity of the condition varies tremendously, ranging from mild muscle weakness and awkward movements to severe speech difficulties, an inability to walk, and *mental retardation.* CP does not cause mental retardation, but the same conditions that caused the brain damage leading to CP may also cause intellectual impairment.

The main types of CP are *spastic,* characterized by stiff and difficult movement; *athetoid,* characterized by involuntary and uncontrolled movement; *ataxic,* characterized by poor coordination and a disturbed sense of balance; and a *mixed* type, a combination of the other types. By far, spastic CP is the most common, affecting about 70 to 80 percent of people with the disorder. CP can affect one or both limbs on one or both sides of the body. A child with CP may also have some of the following symptoms:

- *Speech difficulties:* Most children with CP have a speech problem called dysarthria, a difficulty controlling and coordinating their muscles for speaking.

- *Learning disorders:* About one-fourth to one-half of children with CP also have a learning problem (see **Learning Disorders**).

- *Seizures:* About half of children with CP have **seizures**. Seizures usually last a few seconds to a few minutes and usually require medication to be controlled.

- *Failure to thrive:* Children with moderate to severe CP may grow and develop slowly. A baby may gain weight too slowly. An older child may be abnormally short, and a teenager may be short and have impaired sexual development (see **Failure to Gain Weight**).

- *Impaired vision or hearing:* Many children with CP have strabismus (see **Amblyopia and/or Strabismus**), in which the eyes are not aligned because of the differences in strength between the eye muscles. Hemianopia, experienced by some children with CP, is defective vision or blindness that impairs the normal field of vision in one eye. Impaired hearing (see **Hearing Loss**) is also more common among those with CP than in the general population.

Causes

Many causes of brain injury or damage during pregnancy, delivery, or in the period immediately after birth can result in cerebral palsy. Often, doctors cannot pinpoint the cause. But about 5 to 10 percent of children with CP acquired the disorder after birth, usually due to a brain infection, head injury, or childhood stroke (the blockage or rupture of an artery in the brain). Most cases, however, occur in the womb or during birth.

Because no cure exists, doctors have focused on preventing CP. One cause that has been almost completely eliminated by prenatal screening is brain damage caused by Rh blood factor incompatibility between mother and fetus. Another common cause, premature birth, sometimes can be prevented (see **Prematurity**). A third cause, lack of oxygen to the infant's brain during labor and delivery (fetal hypoxia), may be prevented by better monitoring of the fetus during labor and the use of cesarean section (surgical delivery of the baby through the abdominal wall) to avoid the complications of a difficult delivery.

What the Doctor May Do

If your doctor suspects CP, she will thoroughly examine your child and take a complete medical and developmental history. She may refer your child to a neurologist, an otolaryngologist (ear, nose, and throat doctor), an orthopedic surgeon, and other specialists. If your doctor diagnoses CP, she will probably also suggest that you enroll your child in an early intervention program designed to maximize his development. Among the special areas covered in such programs are the following:

- *Physical therapy:* To help your child learn better ways to move and maintain balance.

- *Speech and language therapy:* To help your child develop clearer speech, learn new words and grammar, and improve his listening skills. If your child has severe speech problems, the therapist may acquaint your child with assistive communication aids, which often employ symbol, letter, or word charts, to help him communicate. Technology that translates words typed by a child into words spoken by a computer is also available.

- *Occupational therapy:* An occupational therapist can help your child find ways to write, draw, brush his teeth, dress and feed himself, and control his wheelchair. She can also suggest special equipment to make everyday tasks like dressing and grooming easier for your child to perform alone. Once daily living tasks are mastered, an occupational therapist will find ways to ensure that your child is participating in leisure activities and school as independently as possible.

Depending on the severity of your child's condition, health care personnel may recommend orthotic appliances, surgery, or medication to treat symptoms of spasticity and loss of muscle tone. Your doctor may also prescribe medications to increase muscle tone.

What You Can Do

Participate in your child's treatment plan by learning appropriate exercises to improve his muscle tone and strength. You may need to help him with daily tasks he finds difficult, such as eating, bathing, and brushing his teeth. Your child will also need your emotional support, unconditional love, and reassurance to cope with his disability.

Many parents find support groups for parents of children with CP valuable. The groups allow people having the same difficulties to share their experiences and knowledge. For help finding support groups and financial assistance for children with disabilities, see Appendix: Parent Resources, Disabilities/Special Needs; Medical/Financial Assistance.

Prevention

Living a healthy lifestyle before and during pregnancy (see A Healthy Pregnancy, p. 3) may reduce your child's risk of developing CP, as may taking precautions to protect your child from head trauma (e.g., using a seat belt, wearing a helmet). But since the cause of CP is often unknown, it generally cannot be prevented.

See also ***Developmental Problems.***

▌ *Chest Pain*

The words "Mom, my chest hurts" might alarm you, but rest assured that chest pain is common during childhood and adolescence and only rarely indicates a heart problem or any serious disease. However, it can sometimes indicate that an injury or a disorder is present and a trip to the doctor is warranted.

Signs and Symptoms

Symptoms unrelated to the heart:
- Painful, persistent coughing
- Pain when breathing
- Stabbing pain in the lower front chest during strenuous activity (goes away during rest)
- Pain with movement

Symptoms that may be related to the heart:
- Severe chest pain that travels from behind the chest bone to the left shoulder and down the arm
- Skin color is bluish or very pale

When to Call the Doctor

CALL FOR EMERGENCY HELP IF

- your child has severe, constricting chest pain and a rapid and faint, or an irregular heartbeat.
- your child loses consciousness even briefly.
- your child has severe chest pain, accompanied by fever, breathing difficulty, or both.
- your child cannot catch her breath.
- your child's skin is blue or very pale and sweaty.
- your child is in shock (look for pallor, dizziness, confusion, or unconsciousness—see p. 418)

For first aid information, see page 380 if your child is less than 1 year old and page 383 if your child is 1 year of age or older.

CALL THE DOCTOR IMMEDIATELY IF

- your child has nausea or vomiting, along with the chest pain.
- your child's chest pain is rapidly becoming worse.
- your child complains of dizziness.

CALL THE DOCTOR TODAY IF

- your child has injured herself.
- a cough and fever are accompanied by chest pain.
- your child cannot take deep breaths.
- pain persists over several hours or is accompanied by breathing problems.
- your child has unexplained chest pain.

Causes

The following are the common causes of chest pain among children:

- *Severe coughing:* When a severe cough makes the lungs work hard, the chest muscles become sore. The diaphragm (the dome-shaped muscle that separates the chest from the abdomen) may also hurt from a child's coughing, and a child may experience tenderness around the lower edge of the rib cage.

- *Physical overexertion:* Your child might feel chest pain when she is physically active, especially if the activity is new or is not one she has recently been involved in. This pain, commonly called a "stitch in the side," feels like a stabbing pain in the lower front chest, usually on the left side. If your child rests for a minute or two, the pain disappears.

- *Injury to chest structures:* Injuries to the chest or abdominal area often cause chest pain. For example, muscle bruises or fractures of the breastbone or ribs cause chest pain, which is aggravated by breathing or chest movement.

- *Costochondritis:* This common inflammation of the ribs and surrounding cartilage is similar to other types of joint pain and is usually harmless. The cause is often unknown.

Less common causes of chest pain in children include the following:

- *Asthma:* Children with **asthma,** especially if it is undetected, may have significant chest discomfort or tightness from the effort needed to breathe.

- *Lung infections:* **Pneumonia** is a common cause of chest pain, accompanied by fever. Pleurisy (inflammation of the membrane surrounding the lungs) may occur with pneumonia and cause chest pain, fever, cough, and shortness of breath.

- *Drug abuse:* Many commonly abused drugs can affect the heart and coronary blood vessels that supply it with oxygen. Cocaine, for example, can cause both arrhythmia (see **Abnormal Heart Rhythm**), and constriction of the coronary arteries, which inhibits the flow of oxygen to the heart and causes chest pain (angina) and even heart attack. Smoking crack cocaine can cause inflammation of the lungs. Inhaling glues or solvents can cause arrhythmia, chest pain, and other conditions.

- *Lung rupture:* Also known as pneumothorax, lung rupture causes air to escape into the chest, causing pain. The escaped air compresses the lung and eventually leads to its collapse. Children with severe asthma are susceptible to pneumothorax, but this condition may arise without an apparent cause. Pneumothorax develops quickly, often with a sharp pain, and causes shortness of breath. Emergency medical care is required.

- *Anxiety:* Occasionally, children experiencing severe anxiety develop chest pain. Blood pressure, heart rate, and breathing rate increase and the child may feel faint or dizzy. This pain differs from that of broken ribs or sprained muscles. It's more of a discomfort or "funny feeling."

- *Heart attacks:* Children can have heart attacks (in which the heart muscle doesn't receive enough blood and oxygen). These are extremely rare and usually occur only in those born with a heart abnormality or whose arteries become narrowed due to inflammation caused by disease or unusually high cholesterol.

- *Other heart problems:* In rare cases, a child with other heart problems experiences chest pain, such as with pericarditis, the inflammation of the membrane (pericardium) surrounding the heart. Other causes of chest pain include structural defects in the pericardium; narrowing of the valve leading to the main artery of the heart, known as aortic stenosis; and certain abnormalities of the main artery in the body (the aorta), which cause it to tear or rupture. Myocarditis (inflammation of the heart muscle) and congestive heart failure also cause chest pain.

What the Doctor May Do

Your doctor will try to identify the cause of chest pain based on the location of the pain; your child's present health, medical history, and symptoms; and the results of a complete physical examination. In some cases, the doctor may request X rays of the chest, lungs, heart, or abdomen to detect possible injury or illness. If necessary, the doctor may use an electrocardiogram (ECG), an examination that electronically records the heart's actions, or an echocardiogram, a test that uses sound waves to form a picture of the internal structures of the heart and associated blood vessels to detect heart and lung problems.

Treatment will depend on the cause. Warm compresses on the chest or over-the-counter pain relievers can help relieve chest pain caused by aching muscles. Cough suppressants may help relieve chest pain caused by coughing. Ask your doctor about using these over-the-counter medicines for chest pain, and make sure to call your doctor if your child continues to have chest pain for more than 2 or 3 days while using these medications. For chest pain caused by bacterial pneumonia, your child's doctor will prescribe antibiotics. For chest pain caused by anxiety, the best treatment is calm reassurance.

What You Can Do

In most cases, you'll be able to determine what's causing the chest pains based on your child's recent activities. If the cause is not apparent or if the pain is persistent or severe anywhere in the chest or abdomen, call your doctor.

If your child's pain is caused by a muscle spasm or overexertion, it will quickly fade once your child rests, although it may recur once your child resumes the activity. A warm heating pad, hot-water bottle, compress, or bath or shower may relax sore muscles.

If you think your child's chest pain is caused by an injury to the chest (possible rib fracture, for example), consult your doctor so that he can examine your child for signs of a broken rib that could puncture her lung.

Prevention

Regular exercise and physical conditioning can help prevent chest pain from overexertion. Prevention of chest pain depends on the cause.

▮ *Chicken Pox*

Chicken pox is a highly contagious viral infection that most children contracted until the mid-1990s, when an effective vaccine became available and widely used. Until then, 95 percent of American children suffered the itchy rash of chicken pox before 18 years of age. Fortunately for those who get chicken pox, most cases resolve by themselves within a week or two with no lasting effects. But the disease poses serious health risks, and all children—except those with certain health problems such as an impaired immune system—should be immunized.

Signs and Symptoms

- Mild, flulike symptoms
- Low *fever*
- Rash (red pimples, usually on the trunk, with new lesions appearing each day)

When to Call the Doctor
CALL FOR EMERGENCY HELP IF
- your child has convulsions (see *Seizures*).

CALL THE DOCTOR IMMEDIATELY IF
- your child has lethargy, is vomiting, or has an unsteady gait (in older children).
- your infant has signs of chicken pox and is under 3 months of age.
- your infant under 6 months of age has a fever above 100.2°F.
- your child's rash becomes very red, warm, or tender (indicating cellulitis, a bacterial infection).
- your child with chicken pox complains of ear pain.

CALL THE DOCTOR TODAY IF
- you suspect that your child has chicken pox.
- your child has a fever that lasts longer than a few days.

Essential Facts

Chicken pox is contagious from a day or two before the rash appears until the blisters form scabs. Your child may become infected by coming into contact with another child who has the virus, even though that child may not yet have a rash. The incubation period (the period between exposure to the virus and onset of symptoms) can be as long as 14 to 21 days. Once your child has had chicken pox, she won't get it again, although the virus can remain dormant in the body and may reappear in adulthood as herpes zoster (shingles).

Chicken pox can spread like wildfire through a family, day care center, or classroom. It is infectious until the rash has completely scabbed over and no new rash has appeared in 24 hours—a process that can take from 5 days to 2 weeks. In most cases, fever accompanies the rash and is at its highest when the rash is at its peak, subsiding when scabs form over the broken blisters.

Although chicken pox is usually not serious, your child may feel uncomfortable because the infection can cause extreme itchiness. The rash often appears first on the trunk and face, then on the rest of the body. The rash develops into small blisters called vesicles, which easily burst when scratched. After they break open, the sores form an itchy crust on top of the skin. This crust falls away after about 5 to 10 days. Your child may have just a few spots, or the spots may cover her body. The most common complication is bacterial infection (see *Impetigo*) of the rash, often caused by scratching. If left untreated, this infection can cause permanent scars. Other complications of chicken pox include pneumonia, sore throat, ear infection, arthritis, muscle aches, or neurological symptoms such as shakiness and unsteady gait. Children with cancer or those whose immune systems are depressed run special risks from chicken pox. If your child has not had chicken pox and hasn't been vaccinated, discuss with your doctor the possibility of having her immunized.

In rare cases, the chicken pox virus may cause encephalitis, an inflammation of the brain.

A CHICKEN POX TIMETABLE

Day 1: On the day your child is exposed to the varicella-zoster virus, the virus infects the respiratory tract through contact with saliva or respiratory droplets.

Day 1 to 9: The virus incubates, but is not contagious until 2 days before the rash appears—your child may not appear ill or may have mild cold symptoms at this stage.

Day 10 to 20: Rash develops, along with fever, aches and pains, and other symptoms. Red spots appear and remain for 3 to 7 days. Blisters appear steadily and may break, oozing fluid. New crops of spots appear daily.

Day 13 to 17 (depending on severity of infection): Sores crust over completely and no new spots appear, signaling the end of the infection. The child may return to school when all lesions are crusted over and no new lesions are noted.

In other equally rare cases, children recovering from chicken pox sometimes develop Reye syndrome, a severe illness characterized by brain disease and deterioration of liver function. Reye syndrome is linked to aspirin use in children with chicken pox or other viral illnesses, and almost never occurs otherwise.

Causes
Chicken pox is caused by the varicella-zoster virus.

What the Doctor May Do
Your doctor will probably be able to diagnose chicken pox by hearing you describe the symptoms over the phone. In fact, most doctors prefer a telephone diagnosis for chicken pox in order to protect other patients in the office from infection. Only if your child's blisters become infected or if other complications develop will the doctor need to see her. If so, the doctor will evaluate the severity and perhaps prescribe an antibiotic medication. He may suggest using an antihistamine, such as hydroxyzine or diphenhydramine, to relieve itching.

What You Can Do
Keep your child home from day care or school until all the sores are crusted over—usually about 6 to 7 days after they first appear. Also keep your child away from adults who have never had chicken pox, especially pregnant women, who are at risk for severe disease.

You can also take the following steps to help your child feel as comfortable as possible.

- *Avoid direct sunlight.* Sun exposure can worsen the rash, making your child uncomfortable.
- *Rest and isolation.* Although your child needn't stay in bed, she may feel run-down and out-of-sorts, so encourage quiet play. Because the virus is so contagious, insist that she avoid

those who haven't had chicken pox until her blisters break and crust over completely—about 6 to 7 days after her rash first appears.

- *Give oatmeal baths.* If your child is itchy and uncomfortable, give her frequent lukewarm baths using an over-the-counter oatmeal or colloidal bath preparation. When you take her out of the tub, dry her by patting rather than rubbing, to reduce the chance of infecting the blisters.

- *Cut fingernails short.* This will help discourage scratching.

- *Offer ice chips or ice pops.* If your child has sores in her mouth, the cold can relieve the pain.

- *Reduce fever and inflammation.* Use acetaminophen or ibuprofen to reduce fever and alleviate any aches and pains that accompany the infection.

Do not . . .
- give your child aspirin if she has chicken pox or may have been exposed to chicken pox.

Prevention

Vaccination is the most effective way to prevent chicken pox. If your child is older than 1 year and has not yet had chicken pox, ask your child's doctor about vaccinating her. Otherwise, you can help prevent your child from contracting chicken pox by keeping her away from other children who have the virus and by encouraging frequent hand-washing and other good hygiene methods described on page 366.

QUESTIONS PARENTS ASK
Chicken Pox Vaccine

Q: Is the chicken pox vaccine safe? Should my child get it?

A: The American Academy of Pediatrics, the American Academy of Family Physicians, and the Centers for Disease Control and Prevention all recommend that healthy children receive the chicken pox vaccine, which is safe and effective. Booster shots may be recommended in future years, just as measles boosters are recommended today. Discuss this matter with your doctor. Most children receive their chicken pox vaccine between 12 and 18 months of age, when they receive their first measles, mumps, and rubella (MMR) vaccine.

The vaccine was approved for use by the Federal Drug Administration in 1995. While some parents question the need for the vaccine for an illness that is usually mild with no complications, experts recommend that all children be vaccinated because of the rare but potentially serious complications discussed earlier in this section. In the United States, about 100 deaths and 6,000 hospitalizations a year result from infection with the chicken pox virus—more than half of them in children.

The vaccine will also spare your child the uncomfortable, itchy rash and fever as well as the possibility of small, permanent scars that sometimes appear after the lesions heal. It also will prevent your child from missing a week of school and parents from missing a week of work.

▌ *Childhood Disintegrative Disorder*

See *Pervasive Developmental Disorder.*

▌ *Cleft Lip/Cleft Palate*

A cleft lip is a congenitally (present at birth) split upper lip that may involve one or both sides of the lip. A cleft palate is a congenitally split palate (roof of the mouth). In either case, the cleft (split) results from an incomplete fusion of skin, muscle, or bone during fetal development. The condition is usually apparent at birth but may be identified during pregnancy through a sonogram (ultrasound) exam. As unfortunate as any birth defect is, surgical treatment of cleft lip and palate is usually quite successful in repairing these abnormalities, achieving a result that functions well and looks good.

Signs and Symptoms

- A defect in the upper lip that may be small or may be a complete separation of the upper lip
- A V-shaped or U-shaped defect in the roof of the mouth, which can vary in width and length but usually extends from behind the front teeth or gums back to include the soft palate
- Double or W-shaped uvula (the small, dangling mass of tissue visible at the back of the throat)

When to Call the Doctor
CALL THE DOCTOR TODAY IF
- you have any questions or concerns about your child's cleft lip or palate.
- your child with cleft lip or palate has difficulty eating, breathing, or swallowing.

Essential Facts

About 1 in 750 white children born in the United States is born with a cleft lip, a cleft palate, or both. The condition is more common in people of Asian descent and less common in people of African descent. Although a cleft lip and cleft palate often occur alone, they sometimes occur together or accompany other conditions such as outer ear anomalies, cardiac anomalies, and various other syndromes. Rarely, a partial cleft of the soft palate (the fleshy area near the back of the roof of the mouth) may be discovered in later childhood. Cleft lip (alone or with a cleft palate) is more prevalent in boys. Cleft palate alone is more prevalent in girls.

Apart from cosmetic irregularities, cleft palates (and to a much lesser extent, cleft lips) may result in several problems. Both a cleft lip and a cleft palate interfere with the natural functioning of the mouth, which must close and be intact to perform normal speaking, eating, drinking, and breathing functions. The open palate (and sometimes the surgically repaired palate) may make speech sound nasal. Another speech problem results when the palate and the muscles used for speech are not fully developed. If these muscles cannot work properly, children find it difficult to build up enough pressure in the mouth to make the necessary explosive speech sounds for the letters *p, b, d,* or *t.*

Chewing problems may result from potential dental problems of children with clefts, especially a cleft palate. The teeth may be out of position, misshapen, or rotated, and there may be more or fewer teeth than normal. The lips, cheeks, tongue, and saliva may not clean the teeth as they do normally, resulting in tooth decay.

Children with a cleft palate also tend to experience recurrent or persistent ear infections and temporary hearing loss due to middle ear fluid. This occurs because malformations or malfunction of the palate muscles causes a dysfunction of the eustachian tube, allowing bacteria and viruses from the back of the nose to enter the space behind the eardrum.

The cleft (split) results from an incomplete fusion of skin, muscle, or bone during fetal development. Both conditions can be repaired surgically.

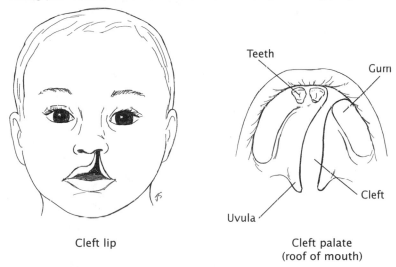

Cleft lip

Cleft palate
(roof of mouth)

Causes

Scientists still don't know the cause of clefts. In a few cases, a family history of the condition is present, suggesting a genetic cause. But often the cause is unknown and no family history exists. What is known is that something goes wrong with the way the fetus develops: In the case of cleft lip, the three parts of the lip—two tabs that grow in from the sides of the face and a central tab that grows down from the tip of the nose— don't fuse together normally during the fourth to sixth week of fetal development. In the case of cleft palate, which normally forms during the first 8 to 12 weeks of development, the bone and tissue that make up the palate don't grow together properly; an opening (or cleft) between the roof of the mouth and the inside of the nose results.

What the Doctor May Do

Surgery is the only way to correct cleft lip and cleft palate. Depending on the severity of the condition, many specialists may be involved in treatment, including a surgeon; an ear, nose, and throat specialist; specialized dentists (an orthodontist to straighten teeth, a prosthodontist to fit the child with special appliances); a speech-language pathologist; a feeding specialist; and mental health professionals to help children and their families cope with the effects of the condition. Another pediatric specialist or genetics counselor may be involved to rule out syndromes sometimes associated with cleft lip and cleft palate. Your doctor will most likely refer you to a surgeon first. The surgeon may be associated with a craniofacial center, which pulls together all the specialists that your child will need under one roof.

The primary goal of surgery is to establish proper functioning of the lip and/or palate and nose to enable the child to breathe, eat, and speak normally, although normal speech isn't always the result. Surgery is also aimed at creating a symmetrical appearance and providing a normal structure for the development of functional and attractive teeth. Surgery will not make cleft lip or cleft palate look completely normal, but approximates what would be normal. The result is often quite acceptable.

Typically, the surgeon performs a surgical closure of the cleft lip when the baby is about 1 to 3 months old, as long as the baby weighs enough and is otherwise healthy. Follow-up surgeries are often necessary. Because most cleft lips involve the nose, your doctor may recommend surgery to correct any nasal deformity when your child becomes a teenager.

The age at which a cleft palate is corrected depends on the size, shape, and degree of the defect, but surgery usually takes place between 8 and 12 months of age. Further surgery of the palate may be needed to correct speech defects. Bone grafting may be needed to improve dental function and appearance.

What You Can Do

If your baby is born with a cleft lip and/or palate, talk with your doctor about ways to make sure your baby gets adequate nutrition. Infants with unrepaired clefts often cannot feed in the usual way (by sucking) and require feeding with a special syringe, called a cleft lip feeder. Following cleft lip/palate surgery, you'll probably continue to feed your baby with a cleft lip feeder until the palate is repaired. As your child grows older, your doctor and other health professionals will advise you on how to work with your child's teachers and speech-language pathologist (if necessary) in order to help develop his speech to his full potential.

Prevention

Because children are born with these conditions, and because the cause is occasionally hereditary or, more often, unknown, cleft lip and cleft palate cannot be prevented. However, the condition is often diagnosed on a prenatal ultrasound, so that you can be prepared to seek the appropriate help and information at or before birth.

See also *Hearing Loss.*

▌ Clubfoot

Clubfoot is a common congenital (appears at birth) malformation of the foot and ankle that causes the foot to twist inward and downward. With prompt medical treatment, a child born with this condition will be able to walk, run, wear regular shoes, take part in sports, and lead a full, active life. Treatment should begin within a few days after birth.

Signs and Symptoms

- One or both feet turn downward or inward at birth
- Calf muscle may be shortened and under-developed

Essential Facts

Clubfoot, known medically as *talipes equinovarus,* appears twice as often in boys as in girls, occurring in about 1 in every 1,000 births. Clubfoot is not a painful condition and doesn't bother a baby unless the condition goes untreated until the child begins to walk. Untreated, the ankle and foot remain twisted and the foot cannot move up and down as it normally does. The heel cord is tight, making it impossible to bring the foot into a normal position. About half of the time, the condition appears in both feet. Infants born with this condition usually have no other abnormalities. But occasionally, the condition may be associated with other medical complications, such as a dislocated hip (see *Dislocations*). When only one foot is affected, the foot usually remains permanently smaller than the normal foot, even after treatment.

Another common but less serious foot malformation, *calcaneovalgus,* occurs when the foot is angled sharply at the heel, causing the foot to point sharply upward and outward. Often, the top of the foot can touch the shin bone. This mild deformity usually corrects itself without treatment when the child begins to walk. Vertical talus (rocker-bottom foot) is the more severe form of this foot deformity and requires treatment and surgery.

Clubfoot can be detected by prenatal ultrasound examination. There is no prenatal treatment for this condition, but consultation and discussion with a pediatric orthopedic surgeon may be beneficial.

Causes

The cause of clubfoot is not fully understood. Doctors used to think it was caused by the position of the developing fetus in the womb. But although some minor foot malformations result from this problem, the cause of clubfoot is now thought to be a combination of heredity and other factors such as infection, drugs, or disease, which may affect prenatal growth. No one knows exactly what factors cause it.

What the Doctor May Do

A doctor can usually diagnose the condition at birth or early infancy during a physical examination. The doctor will immediately refer your infant to an orthopedic specialist, and treatment can begin within the first week of life. The usual treatment of clubfoot is a series of corrective plaster casts intended to place the foot gradually into proper position. The doctor turns the foot

With prompt treatment, clubfoot can be corrected over time.

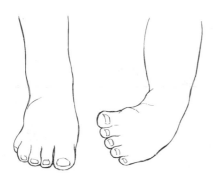

forward as far as it can go without pain and puts a plaster cast on it to hold it in position. The cast is changed every week. The process usually takes about 3 months, sometimes followed by full-time or nighttime use of braces or splints. Your doctor will probably refer you to a physical therapist, who will assess the movement and function of the child's foot and begin exercises to improve muscle tone, restore function, and maintain flexibility.

Treatment with casts does not always work. Sometimes the heel cord and other tendons and muscles of the ankle and foot are too tight to be stretched by a cast. If the foot fails to reach normal positioning within 3 to 6 months, an orthopedic surgeon will operate to lengthen the tendons and correct the bone deformity. For several years after treatment, follow-up visits to the doctor will be necessary to see if the foot remains fully corrected. If not, further treatment will be needed.

What You Can Do

Work with your child's doctor to see that your child gets the medical attention he needs. During the casting process, you will need to keep the cast dry and the skin around it dry to help prevent sores that sometimes develop where the cast rubs the child's skin. Skin lotion or petroleum jelly applied to the skin can help prevent chafing. Once the initial treatment is completed, bring your child to the doctor for regular checkups. You will also begin to do regular massaging and stretching of your child's feet to improve tone and flexibility. Ask the physical therapist for exercises you can do at home with your child each day.

Prevention

Because the cause of clubfoot is not fully understood and is at least partly due to genetics, there is, as yet, no prevention strategy.

▌*Cold Sores*

Cold sores, also known as fever blisters, seem to appear at the worst moments. Just in time for a party or the first day of school, this unsightly viral infection erupts on your child's lip. The good news is that cold sores are harmless and will pass on their own in time. The bad news is that they can be painful and unsightly and may often reappear, especially during times of illness or stress. To understand the difference between cold sores and other mouth ulcers, see *Canker Sores.*

Signs and Symptoms

- A blister or cluster of blisters around the outside of the mouth or nostrils
- Tingling, itching, burning, swelling at the site of the blister
- Fever, irritability, difficulty eating and drinking (upon initial infection)
- Sores inside the mouth

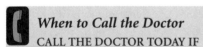

When to Call the Doctor
CALL THE DOCTOR TODAY IF
- the cold sore is near the eye.
- the sore becomes redder and spreads beyond about ¹/₂ inch in diameter.
- your child can't eat or drink adequately.

Causes

The virus that causes cold sores (usually herpes simplex virus type 1) is very common. This virus is related to, but different from, herpes simplex virus type 2, which causes most cases of genital herpes. Since herpes virus type 1 is transmitted in saliva, children usually contract the virus through direct contact with siblings, parents, or other adults.

Infection commonly occurs before 4 years of age, sometimes without symptoms. After the virus causes infection, it becomes dormant, but can be reactivated at any time, causing blisters. Many factors, including sunburn, fever, general ill health, emotional stress, and colds, can trigger a reactivation of the virus.

Before the sores appear, your child may feel a tingling, itching sensation. Blisters can be sore and uncomfortable and may itch or burn. Blisters often recur at the same location. Within 7 to 10 days, the blisters dry and form scabs, which heal within 1 to 2 weeks.

What You Can Do

Lip blisters will heal by themselves, with no need for medical intervention. Do not use over-the-counter cold sore preparations without your doctor's advice.

Over-the-counter pain relievers (not aspirin) can help relieve your child's pain or discomfort. Cool compresses or ice packs can also help relieve the pain. Encourage your child to get plenty of rest, to leave the cold sore alone, and to wash her hands often to avoid inadvertently spreading the virus to another spot on her body or passing it on to someone else. If she stops eating and drinking as much as she used to because the cold sore is tender, supplement her diet with sports drinks or liquid diet supplements that she can drink through a straw.

What the Doctor May Do

If the sore doesn't heal within a week or two, consult your doctor. He may examine the sore to rule out other causes. If the infection is severe or painful, your child's doctor may prescribe a medicated mouthwash to help numb the pain or an antiviral cream. The ointment acyclovir may also be prescibed to speed healing in persistent or severe cases.

Prevention

Herpes outbreaks are often chronic and are not easy to prevent. However, these tips may help:

- *Protect your child from overexposure to the sun.* Sunlight can trigger a cold sore outbreak. To prevent it, make sure that your child wears a hat and often applies lip balm that contains a sunscreen with a sun protector factor (SPF) of at least 15.
- *Help your child stay healthy.* Cold sore outbreaks can occur at any time, but children are particularly vulnerable when they're ill. Make sure that your child washes her hands frequently, eats a balanced diet, gets plenty of rest, and exercises on a regular basis to stay as healthy as possible.

Colds/Flu

Every parent dreads the onset of cold or flu symptoms in a small child. The congestion, fever, and other symptoms can make a child uncomfortable and irritable and disrupt the family's sleep and work schedules. During the winter and spring—the so-called flu season—children seem to get one cold or flu after another. Indeed, the average child may have 8 to 10 colds and one or more bouts of flu in his first 2 years alone. Although a cold or flu is rarely serious, be sure to watch your child for symptoms that might warrant a call or visit to the doctor.

Signs and Symptoms

- Congested nose, runny nose, or both
- Sneezing
- ***Cough***
- Sore throat
- Red, watery eyes
- Aching muscles
- Swollen lymph glands in the neck
- ***Fever***, chills
- ***Vomiting, diarrhea***

When to Call the Doctor

CALL FOR EMERGENCY HELP IF

- your child has difficulty breathing and/or is turning blue.

For first aid information, see page 380 if your child is less than 1 year old and page 383 if your child is 1 year of age or older.

CALL THE DOCTOR IMMEDIATELY IF

- your infant (under 6 months of age) has a fever higher than 100.2°F.
- your child (6 months or older) has a fever of 102°F or higher.
- a fever brings on a convulsion.

CALL THE DOCTOR TODAY IF

- your child's symptoms progress instead of improving after 3 to 5 days.
- your child develops an earache.
- your child has a persistent sore throat.
- your child vomits more than once a day (or for several days in a row), has diarrhea, or is becoming dehydrated.

Essential Facts

Viruses cause both colds and flu. The viruses, which can live in the environment for more than 3 hours, easily spread from person to person through casual contact or sneezing and coughing. Your child can catch a cold or flu virus from an infected person's hands or from contaminated objects—toys, books, telephones, drinking cups, used tissues, tables, and so forth. Children do not catch cold from being outdoors in the cold or being caught in a rainstorm or other such conditions.

Once transmitted to the nose or eyes, the virus moves into the breathing passages, causing these tissues to become inflamed and filled with mucus. Although the signs and symptoms of colds and flu are similar, the flu tends to be more debilitating, as the chart reveals.

All types of influenza and the common cold are highly contagious, especially because the virus is transmitted easily by person-to-person contact, often in droplets of mucus produced by coughing or sneezing. Other sources of infection include contaminated clothing, bedding, personal possessions, and household articles.

One to three days after exposure to a virus, a child starts to feel ill with symptoms that may include fever, a runny nose, or a scratchy throat. The child is infectious from 1 day before to up to 3 weeks after symptoms begin.

The condition may last from 3 days in mild cases to as long as 2 weeks. The flu usually starts with a sudden, high fever and many signs and symptoms of the common cold. Earaches, vomiting, and diarrhea are common signs of the flu during early childhood, although earaches can also occur with a cold. Older children and adolescents with the flu usually complain of chills or a cold sensation all over, fever (101 to 103°F), a

sore throat, coughing, a headache, red and watery eyes, a runny nose, and muscle aches. Less often, they complain of dizziness, eye pain, vomiting, and wheezing.

As if these symptoms weren't bad enough, cold and flu complications, including lung infections such as *pneumonia* and *bronchiolitis,* may also occur. Very young children with the flu can develop heart inflammation (called myocarditis) or Reye syndrome, a rare, life-threatening disease affecting the liver and brain.

Causes

At least 200 types of viruses can cause colds. The flu, also known as influenza, has two major types, A and B, each with several mutating (changing) strains. Both types most commonly affect children from 5 to 14 years old.

What the Doctor May Do

Usually, the doctor or nurse practitioner can diagnose a common cold or flu just by hearing you describe the child's symptoms over the

▬ COLD OR FLU? KNOWING THE DIFFERENCE

Symptom	Cold	Flu
Aches and pains	Slight	Often severe
Chest discomfort	Mild to moderate	Common, sometimes severe
Chills	Not severe	Often severe
Cough	Common	Severe
Diarrhea or vomiting	None or mild	Common, severe
Exhaustion	Not severe	Early, common
Fatigue, weakness	Mild	Common, lingering (up to 2 weeks)
Fever	Low	High (102–104°F)
Headache	Uncommon	Common
Sneezing	Common	Occasional
Sore throat	Common	Common
Stuffy nose	Common	Occasional

phone. This is especially true if the health professional knows a flu with particular characteristics, such as diarrhea or vomiting, is "going around." Should your child's condition become worse, or if his fever exceeds 102°F (or 100.2°F in an infant under 6 months old), you may need to bring your child in for an examination. The doctor will look for signs that the cold or flu has developed into or triggered a more serious infection, like pneumonia.

Because both colds and flu infections are caused by viruses, antibiotics aren't effective. Antiviral drugs to combat the flu are being developed by pharmaceutical companies. These drugs, if taken early, may cure or shorten the duration of the flu by blocking the release of the newly made virus from infected cells. These drugs, however, are new and are not yet widely used. Ask your doctor about them and other medications to treat the symptoms, which include over-the-counter remedies such as decongestants, antihistamines, and cough syrups (see **Cough**).

If your doctor diagnoses a bacterial infection, such as pneumonia or strep throat (see **Sore Throat/Strep Throat**), she may prescribe antibiotics.

What You Can Do

Follow your child's lead. Normally active children may become tired and quiet at this time. If so, let your child rest and don't expect him to maintain a normal, busy routine. If your child barely slows down—take that as a good sign—he's not that sick. Let him play, but limit strenuous activity such as sports or roughhousing. He may not have much of an appetite, but as long as he gets plenty of liquids, he can skip a few meals without risk.

Help him blow his nose if he has trouble doing it himself: Blowing one nostril at a time while holding the other closed often works best. If your baby is under 1 year old, try to keep his

QUESTIONS PARENTS ASK
Catching a Cold; Avoiding Milk During a Cold

Q: Do more colds occur in the winter because children play in the snow without gloves, or stay outside with wet or inadequate clothing?
A: None of those events cause a cold to develop or even make a child more vulnerable to a cold. The reason that winter is "cold and flu season" is that people tend to congregate indoors, with windows closed, leaving viruses to circulate easily.

Q: Is it true that one must feed a cold, starve a fever?
A: The recommended advice is to follow your child's lead when it comes to eating. If he's hungry, by all means feed him unless he has nausea or vomiting. In fact, take care to provide nourishment and fluids to a child with a fever, because fever raises the metabolism, the rate at which the body burns calories.

Q: I've heard that drinking milk creates mucus and should be avoided when you have a cold. Is this true?
A: No evidence shows that drinking milk—or eating ice cream or other dairy products—triggers mucus production or exacerbates congestion. If your child wants a glass of milk or a bowl of ice cream, feel free to give it to him, unless he has recently vomited or has stomach pain.

nasal passages clear by sucking the mucus out with a nasal syringe, especially before he nurses or goes to sleep.

Monitor your child's temperature. If your infant under 6 months old is running a fever above 100.2 °F, call his doctor right away. After 6 months of age, however, don't be alarmed if your child develops a mild fever. If it climbs above 102°F, call your doctor and try to reduce it using the methods described on page 567.

Do not . . .
- use nose drops or sprays for more than 3 days, because they can cause nasal tissues to

thicken, become irritated, and further block the nasal passages.

- give your child aspirin. Use acetaminophen or ibuprofen.
- give your baby under age 2 years a decongestant or an antihistamine without your doctor's advice.

Prevention

The viruses that cause these illnesses are highly contagious, especially in settings like child care and school, where many children come into close contact with one another. However, some commonsense measures may decrease your child's chances of catching a virus.

Teach your child to wash his hands frequently. Have him also cover his nose and mouth with a tissue when he sneezes or coughs to avoid spreading the cold or flu virus.

When it comes to the flu, vaccination can be highly effective—if the vaccine matches the particular influenza virus going around. Doctors usually vaccinate only toddlers and school-age children who have chronic diseases, such as heart, lung, and kidney disorders, or when public health officials anticipate a particularly severe strain of flu.

See also *Croup; Earache/Ear Infection; Sinusitis.*

▌ *Colic*

All babies cry, but babies with colic cry more than most. The usual strategies for soothing a crying baby, like rocking or carrying her, often don't work with colic. Trying to comfort a colicky baby is one of the most frustrating experiences of parenthood. Colic itself is not an illness or a symptom of an illness; most colicky babies are perfectly healthy. But if your baby cries excessively, be sure to tell the doctor, for two reasons. First, your doctor can make sure that her crying fits don't indicate a medical problem. And second, if the condition is colic, the doctor will probably have some suggestions for helping your baby—and you—feel better.

Signs and Symptoms

- More than 3 straight hours of intense crying on most days
- Crying with hands clenched and arms and legs pulled close to the torso, then extended
- Flatulence or a bowel movement at the end of a long bout of crying

When to Call the Doctor
CALL THE DOCTOR IMMEDIATELY IF

- you think the baby's crying might be related to a medical problem.

CALL THE DOCTOR TODAY IF

- you are concerned about your child's bouts of intense crying, and nothing you do is helping.

Essential Facts

About 20 percent of babies have colic, which means regular, long periods of crying. It usually begins around the third week of a baby's life and ends by 3 to 4 months of age.

Colicky crying is different from normal crying in several ways. First, it comes on more suddenly: The baby can be calmly feeding one minute and burst out crying the next. Second, it lasts longer. Although it's normal for babies under 3 months old to cry for up to 3 hours a day every now and then, babies with colic cry for longer periods nearly every day. These crying fits tend to start in the late afternoon or early evening. Parents try feeding and burping, diapering and patting, cajoling and playing, walking and rocking—and nothing helps. Third, colicky babies may look as if they're in pain, drawing in their arms and legs, clenching their fists, and grimacing.

Causes

Many causes of colic have been suggested over the years, including allergies to particular formulas, excess abdominal gas, or something a nursing mother ate that got into her milk and disagreed with the baby. But none of these factors have been found definitively to cause colic. Switching formulas usually does not solve the problem, although many people try this as a solution. Even though colicky babies frequently pass gas while crying, gas is an unlikely cause of colic. Instead, the gas may be caused by the excess air swallowed by a colicky baby as she cries. No evidence shows that foods in a breast-feeding mother's diet actually cause colic, although one study found that certain foods can make colic worse: cabbage, cauliflower, broccoli, cow's milk, onions, and chocolate.

It is now believed that there is no single cause of colic. In some cases, it may be an immaturity of the baby's digestive tract, which causes abdominal pain. In others, it may be an immaturity of the nervous system, which makes the baby exceptionally sensitive to (and bothered by) things like bright lights and loud noises or voices. According to this theory, it's no coincidence that colic tends to occur in the late afternoon and early evening, when Mom or Dad is rushing to make dinner or deal with older siblings who are tired and cranky. Colic may be a sensitive baby's way of responding to the increase in the overall stress level around her.

What the Doctor May Do

If you consult your baby's doctor, he first will make sure that nothing is physically wrong with your baby: that she's gaining weight properly and shows no signs of an infection or another medical problem that might cause long periods of inconsolable crying. If the diagnosis is colic, the doctor will advise you on how to comfort your child and manage your own stress until the condition goes away. If you bottle-feed, he may suggest changing formulas on the chance that it might ease your baby's discomfort. If you breast-feed, he may suggest that you avoid milk, broccoli, onions, caffeine, and other foods that may upset your baby's digestive system.

What You Can Do

Relieving colic is a matter of trial and error. Parents and doctors have found the following techniques to be helpful some of the time for some babies, but nothing works on every child. Even if something works one day, it won't necessarily work the next.

- *Swaddle your baby.* Being wrapped closely in a thin blanket may quiet a baby by making her feel warm and secure. (See p. 83 for instructions on swaddling.)

- *Carry your baby.* Often, the best medicine for a case of colic is the comfort your baby receives from being held upright, either in your arms or in an infant carrier on your back or front. If your baby's crying spells tend to coincide with dinner preparation, carry her in an infant carrier while you work. (To prevent accidental burns, put your baby in a safe place when you are at the stove or draining pasta.)

- *Try an infant swing.* The rhythmic motion helps some colicky babies calm down and fall asleep. However, babies shouldn't be put in a swing until they can hold their heads steady. Nor should they be left in a swing for hours on end, lest they miss out on opportunities to interact with you and other caregivers.

- *Burp your baby.* Burp her in the middle and at the end of every feeding to help eliminate air bubbles in the esophagus and stomach, which can cause abdominal pain. Also make sure that you hold your baby in a slightly upright position while she breast-feeds or takes a bottle, to minimize the amount of air that she swallows.

- *Use a hot water bottle.* Placing a warm (not hot) hot water bottle wrapped in a towel against your baby's abdomen can sometimes relieve abdominal pain.

- *Maintain a regular schedule.* The more predictable your baby's daily routine is, the better, because colicky babies appear to be sensitive to schedule changes. So try to feed your baby and put her down for naps at the same times every day.

- *Change the environment.* Take your baby for a walk to the park, even if she's in the middle of a colicky fit. Don't let the screaming embarrass you. A change of scene can work wonders, for her and for you. Even taking her into another room or out onto the deck or balcony may help.

- *Don't overstimulate her.* Dim the lights and turn down the music to avoid overwhelming your baby. If you've tried rocking and playing with your baby and you still cannot get her to stop crying, leave her alone for 10 minutes or so in a quiet, dim, safe place. The lack of stimulation might help her relax and fall asleep.

- *Try white noise.* The "white noise" of a vacuum cleaner, a car engine, or an automatic washer can sometimes calm a crying baby. (Do not, however, put the baby on top of the washer. Some parents feel that the vibration is soothing, but this can be dangerous.)

- *Take breaks.* Don't try to cope with this problem by yourself. Ask relatives and good friends to give you a break from your cranky baby. While they look after her, take a nap, or go to the movies or a ball game. Even some quiet time reading magazines at the local library can

help. Chances are, the more relaxed you are when you return, the calmer your baby will be.

Prevention

Carry your baby as much as possible in your arms or in an infant carrier on your back or front. Research suggests that the more time babies spend being carried, the less likely they are to become colicky.

See also ***Abdominal Pain/Stomachache.***

Conjunctivitis

See ***Pinkeye.***

Constipation

Unless a child has a daily bowel movement, parents may find themselves wondering, "Is my child going often enough?" There is a wide range of normal, with some children having two or three bowel movements a day and others having just one every 3 days. As long as your child has no discomfort, all is well. But if your child has hard, dry stools that cause pain when he tries to pass them, he's constipated. In general, the longer a child goes between bowel movements, the greater the chance of constipation. Though it can be uncomfortable, constipation usually isn't serious. In most cases, all it takes is having your child drink more fluids and eat more high-fiber foods.

Signs and Symptoms
- Hard, dry stools
- Pain on defecation
- Abdominal cramps or stomachache relieved by bowel movement
- Loss of appetite
- Possibly, blood in the stool

When to Call the Doctor
CALL THE DOCTOR TODAY IF
- your child regularly complains of pain when moving his bowels.
- blood is in his stool.
- your child frequently soils his underpants after being fully toilet trained.

Essential Facts

Constipation is fairly common, affecting at least 5 to 10 percent of children at some point. The tendency to be constipated seems to run in families. Though a single bout of constipation isn't serious, don't ignore it, because it may lead to more episodes and medical problems, such as encopresis. This chronic, treatable condition usually develops when school-aged children withhold stools and then develop a loss of muscle tone in the bowel. As a result, unexplained accidents occur at various times of the day.

The longer that stools are held in, the larger and harder they become, increasing the chance that, during a bowel movement, they will cause small tears in the anus (anal fissures). Anal fissures can be extremely painful and cause bleeding from the area. Fissures can prolong constipation by making bowel movements so painful that the child holds in his stools to avoid the pain. Abnormally large stools can also cause the large intestine to get stretched out of shape. When this happens, the intestine can lose muscle tone, and the reflexes that normally signal the need to have a bowel movement no longer function. Muscle tone and reflexes return when the constipation is treated.

Causes

The cause of constipation is often unknown, but diet certainly plays a role. A lack of fluids or fiber (fruits, vegetables, and whole grains) and an excess of fats and proteins can lead to hard, dry stools that pass slowly through a child's digestive system. A sudden change in a child's diet or the introduction of a new, constipating food can also cause the problem. Some infants become constipated when cereal, other solid food, or cow's milk is added to their diet. Rarely, cow's milk allergy (from infant formula or regular milk) can cause constipation.

Constipation can also be related to toilet teaching. Some toddlers or preschoolers resist having bowel movements at first as a way of rebelling against the process. The longer children hold in their bowel movements, the more likely the bowel movements will become impacted in the rectum and intestines. Such behavior is most common when parents push their children too early or too zealously to make the transition from diapers to the potty, or when children experience other stressors during the toilet teaching process, such as the birth of a sibling or a death in the family. (See the tips for successful toilet teaching on p. 199.) Older children may become constipated if they refuse to use a strange toilet and hold in their bowel movements when they're away from home—at school or when traveling, for example. Recurrent soiling of underwear is a symptom of encopresis, or chronic constipation. Encopresis may be difficult to treat and requires a special approach by you and your child's doctor.

Relatively rare conditions, including celiac disease (a chronic digestive disorder), **lead poisoning,** an underactive thyroid, and congenital problems with the rectum or colon (Hirschsprung's disease), can cause constipation as well. Constipation is also a side effect of some medications, including antihistamines and codeine. Consult your doctor if your child takes any medicine.

What the Doctor May Do

If your child has only been constipated for a day or so and has no other symptoms, he need not see a doctor. Chances are, all he has to do is make the simple dietary changes described later in this section. But if your child has severe pain or rectal bleeding, bring him to a doctor.

The doctor will ask about your child's symptoms, how long they have lasted, and what kinds of foods your child is eating. Then, she will examine your child's abdomen for signs of tenderness or abnormal swelling and examine his rectum and anus for tears. X rays or other tests are sometimes needed to confirm the diagnosis. The doctor may prescribe stool softeners and some dietary changes, such as an increase in fiber and increased liquids, to help relieve constipation. If these changes do not solve the problem, your doctor may recommend changing formulas (for an infant) or eliminating cow's milk from your child's diet to determine if cow's milk allergy may be the cause of constipation.

What You Can Do

The first thing to do is increase the amount of fluids and fiber in your child's diet. Fruits, vegetables, and whole grains are good sources of fiber. Fruits such as apricots or peaches are a particularly good choice, because they contain pectin, which can help relieve constipation. These changes should relieve your child's constipation in a day or so. In addition, examine your child's daily diet to see if he's eating an overabundance of constipating foods, such as bananas, milk, and white rice. If your child is eating these foods and is also constipated, cut back on them.

Encourage your child to be physically active. Daily exercise promotes normal bowel function by toning the abdominal muscles and stimulating bowel movements. Limit your child's time in front of the television, and encourage him to play outdoors with other children if the weather permits. Sign him up for sports or dance classes.

Prevention

A high-fiber diet with plenty of fluid and regular exercise can help prevent constipation. Mix in bran cereal with other cereals or when baking foods like muffins and breads. Make sure your child drinks plenty of liquid when he eats bran-containing foods.

See also ***Abdominal Pain/Stomachache.***

▌ *Cough*

No one likes a cough, particularly small children whose sleep can be disrupted for much of the night when a persistent cough sets in. But coughing is one of the body's most helpful defense mechanisms, protecting the throat, windpipe, bronchi, and lungs from infection and invasion from harmful substances or even small objects. Coughing is not an illness but the symptom of an illness. Fortunately, coughing usually clears up on its own and is not usually cause for alarm. If a cough persists, be sure to have your child examined by the doctor. Usually, a persistent cough is simply a postviral irritation and will subside by itself, but be sure to have the doctor rule out other possible causes.

When to Call the Doctor
CALL FOR EMERGENCY HELP IF

- your child is having difficulty breathing and/or is turning blue.

  For first aid information, see page 380 if your child is less than 1 year old and page 383 if your child is 1 year of age or older.

Essential Facts

A cough may be a passing occurrence or one sign of an underlying problem. Sometimes coughing begins suddenly when a child inhales a small piece of food or a foreign object. Other times, coughing can develop slowly over several days as a cold or flu grows worse. A cough is the use of the muscles surrounding the chest and the diaphragm to create an explosion of air traveling up the airway while carrying dust, mucus, and other debris in its path.

Coughing related to colds or flu (see *Colds/Flu*) may bring up fluids (called mucus) from the respiratory tract. If severe and continual, a cough can be tiring, even exhausting. Your child may vomit or become dizzy with the effort, and her chest muscles can become sore.

Most coughs start to subside as soon as the underlying problem clears up or responds to treatment, although a cough may persist for a few weeks even after the underlying infection has subsided. However, since some cough-producing lung infections develop into **pneumonia,** it is important to report a cough that lasts more than a few days to your child's doctor.

Causes

Many types of infections and irritations can cause your child to develop a cough.

Most Common Causes

- Viral infections, including the common cold, **croup,** and **bronchiolitis**
- Bacterial infections that lead to **sinusitis, pneumonia,** or whooping cough (see Preventable Childhood Diseases, p. 111)
- *Allergies* to various substances, including pet dander, molds, plant material, and certain foods
- **Asthma,** a chronic irritation of the airways
- Chemical irritants, such as chemical fumes, cigarette and cigar smoke, and gases
- Small objects or food particles inhaled into the windpipe or lungs (see Choking and Suffocation, p. 397)
- Reflux of the stomach fluids into the esophagus, with small amounts entering the airways (see **Gastroesophageal Reflux**)

Uncommon or Rare Causes

- Tumors of the lung or bronchial passages
- Heart disease and disease of the blood vessels
- Congenital defects of the connection between the esophagus and the airway
- Congenital defects of the trachea and bronchiole tubes
- **Cystic fibrosis**

What the Doctor May Do

Many coughs will go away by themselves. If the cough is persistent or severe, your doctor may ask you to bring your child in so he can try to track down the underlying cause of the cough. He'll start by asking questions about your child's symptoms and performing a clinical exam, concentrating on the respiratory tract. He may order an X ray of the lungs or sinuses, or take a culture (a swab of mucus or other secretions) of the nose or throat to identify a bacterial infection. Additional diagnostic tests vary according to other signs and symptoms.

If the cough is the result of a bacterial infection, your doctor may prescribe antibiotics, which should bring relief within 24 to 48 hours. If the cough is the result of a viral infection, antibiotics won't help—but the virus should run its course within several weeks. If the cough is chronic and persistent, your child may have an underlying allergy or asthma. Your doctor may prescribe decongestant, antihistamine, or bronchodilator medication depending on the underlying cause (see *Allergies* or *Asthma*). Or, your doctor may refer your child to an allergist for diagnosis and treatment. For children who have had several cases of unexplained pneumonia, the doctor may order a sweat test for cystic fibrosis, an uncommon, chronic illness that affects the lungs.

Your doctor may prescribe cough medicine. Over-the-counter medicines are probably over-

---

COUGH AND COLD MEDICINE GUIDE

- *Decongestants:* These medications open the air passages by shrinking the surrounding tissues and relieve the feeling of heaviness in the chest by reducing secretions, thereby clearing fluid from breathing tubes.

- *Expectorants:* Expectorants typically include an ingredient that loosens mucus, helping children bring it up and spit it out.

- *Suppressants:* Some cough suppressants are narcotic; they work by reducing the nerve impulse that triggers the cough.

- *Antihistamines:* These antiallergy drugs decrease the secretions and swelling of the mucous membranes. The active ingredient acts to combat a strong reaction in the body (the release of a powerful chemical called histamine) provoked by contact with an allergy-causing substance. As an antihistamine takes effect, coughing and other allergy signs slowly subside.

- *Throat soothers:* Soothers, such as the old-fashioned honey and lemon remedy, coat an irritated throat and relieve pain temporarily. Don't give cough drops to children under 3

years old, because of the possibility of choking. And don't give honey to children under 12 months of age, because of the possibility of botulism.

- *Bronchodilators:* Available only by prescription, bronchodilators relax and soothe the tissues surrounding the airway. As a result, the child has an easier time clearing mucus and debris from her airway, has fewer airway spasms, and suffers less constriction.

Because so many cough medicines containing so many different ingredients and strengths are available, be sure to consult your doctor about choosing the right medication at the right strength for your child. Dosages will vary by the age and weight of your child. Read the label for dosages carefully. For example, the active ingredients in over-the-counter medicines for adults may cause adverse reactions, including drowsiness, irritability, hallucinations, and high blood pressure, in small children. Some cough medicines contain alcohol and shouldn't be given to children. Others may contain ingredients that have no beneficial effect.

rated as reliable sources of relief. Temporary coughs resulting from mild irritation don't generally warrant treatment. Some cough medicines may reduce discomfort and rest an overburdened respiratory system for a few hours, but such medications aren't guaranteed to work. Ask your doctor whether he recommends any prescription or over-the-counter cough relief medications.

What You Can Do
Until the underlying cause of the cough is resolved, you can't do much to cure the cough. However, you can help your child feel more comfortable by following these tips:

- Make sure that your child drinks plenty of liquids, especially if she's running a fever.

- If your child is coughing a lot at night, prop her up with pillows to make swallowing the mucus or nasal discharge easier.

- Use a cool-mist humidifier in your child's room. Clean it often and thoroughly to avoid recirculating infectious particles and other irritants, such as dust, pollen, and mold, through the air.

- Keep your child away from airborne irritants like cigarette smoke as much as possible.

- If your child's cough is caused by allergies or asthma, try to protect her from environmental irritants and triggers as much as possible.

- Encourage your child to cover her mouth with a tissue when she coughs to prevent spreading the infection to others.

Prevention
Because most coughs are caused by highly contagious bacterial or viral infections, you probably cannot prevent your child from developing a cough. However, you can keep your child's lungs as healthy as possible by keeping her away from tobacco smoke, exhaust fumes, and smog, which can irritate the respiratory tract. You can also reduce the number of coughs and colds your child gets by teaching her good hygiene—washing her hands frequently and not sharing eating utensils, drinking cups, or tissues.

See also *Earache/Ear Infection; Sore Throat/Strep Throat.*

▌ *Cradle Cap*

Despite its sweet-sounding name, cradle cap is a rather unpleasant and stubborn—but quite common and harmless—skin condition of infancy and toddlerhood. It consists of thick, yellow skin patches on the scalp and forehead and behind the ears. Cradle cap is not contagious, but it may recur. Also known as seborrheic dermatitis of the scalp, cradle cap often appears within the first month of life and affects mostly infants, but it may appear periodically in children up to 5 years old.

Signs and Symptoms
- Yellow, scaly, or crusty patches on the scalp
- Red, scaly areas on the scalp

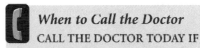

When to Call the Doctor
CALL THE DOCTOR TODAY IF
- the cradle cap is accompanied by red, scaly areas elsewhere on the body, including the face or neck.

Essential Facts
By itself, cradle cap is relatively harmless. But because the condition makes the skin more vulnerable to infection, it can lead to a yeast or bacterial infection if the area is not kept clean. It may be unsightly and itchy or irritating to your

infant or toddler. Sometimes the condition may appear on other parts of the body, such as the creases in the neck, the armpits, and the diaper area; behind the ears; and on the face. Most cases appear in early infancy and slowly disappear over several weeks or months. It is not usually uncomfortable or painful.

Causes

No one knows what causes cradle cap.

What You Can Do

You may choose to do nothing except keep your baby's scalp clean by washing it daily with mild baby shampoo. Cradle cap will often go away without treatment. Or, you can shampoo your child's hair once a day with a shampoo recommended by your child's doctor. Watch to make sure the shampoo does not cause further redness and irritation.

Do not . . .

- apply oils to the scalp, which can worsen the condition.
- scrub the scalp too hard while shampooing.
- shampoo too frequently. Once a day is plenty; washing overly often can have a drying effect that aggravates cradle cap.
- apply hydrocortisone cream without first checking with your doctor.

What the Doctor May Do

The doctor may recommend a medicated shampoo to clear up the problem.

Prevention

Cradle cap contracted during early infancy cannot be prevented. Daily hair washing with mild shampoo will help prevent recurrence.

■ Croup

Once you've heard it, you'll never forget the sound of a baby with croup: a cough resembling the bark of a seal. Croup is a common infection that inflames the upper airway and sometimes also affects the medium and smaller airways of the lungs. Also known as acute laryngotracheobronchitis (LTB), croup makes breathing noisy and sometimes difficult and—unlike bronchitis, which usually affects adults—most often affects children under 5 years old. About 5 out of 100 children in their second year of life experience croup. Of those, only 1.3 percent require hospitalization. Generally, the younger the child is, the more severe the symptoms. But croup is not usually serious and often can be treated at home.

Signs and Symptoms

- Barking cough
- Noisy, high-pitched breathing
- Fever, often low-grade
- Cough that starts out dry, but brings up mucus within several days
- Symptoms worsen at night
- Wheezing (in rare cases)

When to Call the Doctor
CALL FOR EMERGENCY HELP IF

- your child is struggling to breathe.
- your child is using the muscles of his rib cage to breathe, or his neck muscles appear to be sucked in with each breath.
- your child's lips become bluish or grayish.

For first aid information, see page 380 if your child is less than 1 year old and page 383 if your child is 1 year of age or older.

- your infant under 6 months old has croup or a persistent cough or fever of 100.2°F or higher.
- your infant is listless and very sleepy.
- your child has difficulty swallowing.
- your child shows signs of dehydration (dry mouth, sunken eyes, listlessness, confusion, decreased urine output, or dark-colored urine).

CALL THE DOCTOR TODAY IF

- your older child's fever climbs above 102°F or doesn't respond to medication.
- your child has a persistent, barking cough.
- your child cannot sleep because of croup symptoms.

Essential Facts

Young children have narrower and more collapsible air passages than adults do. The inflammation of croup narrows the air passages even further and causes the cough and/or the noisy, high-pitched breathing (stridor) of croup. The croup sound is caused by a narrowing of the windpipe just below the voice box.

Croup is uncommon in babies under 1 year old (who can catch an unrelated but similar illness called *bronchiolitis*). Croup, which usually lasts from a few hours to up to a week, is typically worse at night. Croup occurs most often in the fall and winter and is usually preceded by a mild upper respiratory viral infection with a runny nose, mild cough, low-grade fever, and perhaps a sore throat. A few days later, a croup attack may begin suddenly—usually in the middle of the night—as the child awakens with a seal-like cough and respiratory distress. Symptoms usually wax and wane.

With severe croup, you may hear the stridor whenever your child breathes. If your child's croup causes severe coughing, she may vomit from the coughing. If the upper airway continues swelling, breathing may be difficult. Be sure to monitor your child closely because, in rare instances, croup can be life-threatening.

Croup can also resemble *epiglottitis,* a rare but life-threatening bacterial infection. If a child with no prior cold suddenly starts drooling and gasping for air and gets a high fever, she may have epiglottitis. Call the doctor immediately.

Causes

Croup is triggered by viruses. Because some of these viruses cause upper respiratory tract infections as well, many children develop croup during or just after a bout with a cold. The virus attacks the airways, causing swelling and breathing difficulties.

What the Doctor May Do

Most croup cases can be managed at home. But call your doctor immediately if your child is having problems breathing—your doctor may advise taking him to an emergency room to determine the cause. The doctor will try to distinguish croup from other causes of respiratory distress, such as epiglottitis, bronchiolitis, and *pneumonia,* sometimes taking chest and neck X rays to examine your child's breathing passages. If your child becomes dehydrated, the doctor may give intravenous fluids or supply cool, moist air for him to breathe, perhaps with extra oxygen (possibly in a "croup tent," if he is an infant).

If your child has significant airway inflammation, the doctor may give a medication called racemic epinephrine by mist to decrease the swelling in the airways and help him breathe better. Because epinephrine can sometimes have a rebound effect and worsen the symptoms a few hours after the treatment, a child is usually hospitalized, or at least observed in the emergency room for a while (usually around 6 hours) after he is given this medication. The doctor may also give your child an injected or oral steroid medication to lessen the inflammation and open the air passages for easier breathing.

What You Can Do

First of all, stay calm and reassure your child. If he is old enough to understand, remind him to breathe as slowly and evenly as possible, which will help him relax. The tenser he is, the faster and harder he will breathe, which will narrow his airway further and cause more coughing.

A child with croup will probably be uncomfortable during the acute phase, but you can soothe him in the following ways:

- *Serve liquids.* If your child is not in significant distress and wishes to drink, try giving him sips of whatever liquids he'll drink. If the child is having problems breathing, do not give him anything to eat or drink, and seek medical help immediately.

- *Prop your child up, even during sleep.* Place pillows or books under the end of his mattress to raise it a few inches to help him breathe more easily.

- *Turn on the steam; try a blast of cold.* Some children improve with steam, others with cold air. You can try using a vaporizer in your child's room, or hold him in a sitting position on your lap in the bathroom with the hot shower running and the door closed, allowing him to breathe in the misty, humid air. This can decrease the airway swelling and make breathing easier. Or, try stopping the croup attack with moist, chilly outdoor air. If it's cold outside, bundle your child up and carry him outside for a few moments of fresh, cold air. Or drive for a few minutes with the car windows open. This can decrease swelling and help clear mucus.

- *Treat the fever.* If your child can swallow, give him the appropriate dose of liquid acetaminophen or ibuprofen to reduce the *fever*.

Prevention

You can help prevent croup by encouraging frequent hand-washing and the use of good hygiene methods, as described on page 366. Help your child avoid exposure to other people with colds, the flu, or other infectious illnesses. Also, protect your child from tobacco smoke, which may contribute to the development of respiratory infections.

See also *Colds/Flu; Cough.*

Cross-Eyes

See *Amblyopia and/or Strabismus.*

Cuts and Scrapes

Young children take lots of tumbles. Almost any childhood activity, from skateboarding to simply climbing the steps, for a toddler, can result in a fall and a cut or scrape. Cuts may look painful and scary, but most are easily treated at home. More serious cuts result from the use of knives or other sharp tools or from accidents involving bikes and motor vehicles. For a large or gaping cut that might need stitches (see p. 521), bring your child to the doctor or emergency room immediately—the sooner the cut is treated, the better it will heal.

Signs and Symptoms

- *Cuts:* injuries that break the skin and injure underlying tissue, causing bleeding
- *Scrapes:* injuries that scrape the top skin layer, causing bleeding

When to Call the Doctor

CALL THE DOCTOR IMMEDIATELY IF

- the wound is large ($1/4$ to $1/2$ inch or longer) and/or deep and bleeding.
- bleeding continues even after pressure has been applied for 15 to 20 minutes.
- a wound that is 1 to 3 days old shows signs of infection (redness, warmth, pain, swelling).
- the cuts are on the palm, neck, face, or genitals.
- your child has a fever or swollen glands near the wound (neck, underarms, groin).

CALL THE DOCTOR TODAY IF

- dirt, glass, or debris is embedded in a large scrape—the doctor should remove this.
- you are unsure whether your child's tetanus immunization is up-to-date.

Causes

Cuts

Cuts (lacerations) are wounds caused by sharp objects like knives, scissors, and ragged pieces of metal that break through the skin and into the tissues beneath. Because a cut is deeper than a scrape, the damage can be worse and more bleeding may occur. A cut can sometimes cause damage to the underlying nerves and tendons. One type of cut particularly prone to infection is a puncture wound made by a sharp object such as a pencil, animal or human teeth (see *Bites, Animal and Human*), or a splinter.

Scrapes

Scrapes (abrasions) tend to be caused by friction, usually a fall against a rough surface like a sidewalk. A scrape occurs when the outer skin layers have been rubbed off. Scrapes can be bloody, especially if they cover large areas, although the amount of blood lost is usually minimal.

What the Doctor May Do

If the cut is deep or the scrape is large, dirty, or infected, a doctor will clean the wound and, if necessary, stitch (suture) it under local anesthesia. Depending on the site and the type of wound, the doctor will use either self-absorbing stitches or stitches that must be removed later. Self-absorbing stitches disappear into the tissues and needn't be taken out after healing. Stitches that must be removed require another trip to the doctor or health clinic within 5 to 7 days for removal. *Do not try to remove stitches yourself.*

Stitches may be necessary under these conditions:

- The edges of the wound cannot be held together in another way long enough to permit healing to begin, and the cut is $1/4$ to $1/2$ inch or longer.
- The wound is located somewhere on the face or neck, where a scar may be disfiguring.
- The wound is located on a part of the body (such as the knee or elbow) where limb movement could prevent proper healing.
- Fat tissue (a white, soft substance) is protruding from the wound.

What You Can Do

Your first step is to determine the severity of the wound. Many cuts and most scrapes can be treated at home and will heal completely in a week or two. Call your doctor if you can't get the wound clean, if the wound is severe, or if you notice signs of infection (see When to Call the Doctor). Otherwise, you can treat the wound yourself.

Treating Cuts

If the cut is not severe enough to require medical attention, follow these steps:

1. Apply pressure. You can stop cuts from bleeding by applying direct pressure. Take a

clean cloth or piece of gauze, and press it directly over the wound for at least 5 minutes. Taking the pressure off too soon may cause more bleeding. If bleeding starts again after 5 minutes, reapply pressure.

2. Wash the cut with plain water, then pat the skin dry. Apply an over-the-counter antibacterial ointment or cream, then cover the wound with a sterile bandage.

3. Change the dressing daily, or whenever it gets wet or dirty, checking for signs of infection (redness or swelling around the wound, or pus emanating from the wound) that might warrant a trip to the doctor for treatment.

4. If the cut gapes, cover it with a sterile bandage and call your doctor.

Do not . . .

- apply a tourniquet, which cuts off circulation to the limb and ultimately causes more problems than it solves. If you can't get the cut to stop bleeding, apply direct pressure with a washcloth or bulky dressing and keep it on until you get your child to a doctor—as soon as possible (see Bleeding, p. 392).

Treating Puncture Wounds

Deep puncture wounds (such as those caused by stepping on nails) are more prone to infection than other wounds, despite their innocent appearance. Here is how you can prevent infection in these types of wounds:

1. Carefully clean and soak your child's foot with warm, soapy water.

2. Cover the wound with a clean bandage.

3. If the pain persists for more than a day or the area looks reddened or puffy, call your child's doctor.

Treating Scrapes

By definition, scrapes are superficial, and as long as you clean and dress them well, they should heal within a few days. Follow these tips:

1. Wash the wound with soap and water, then examine it carefully for dirt and debris. Scrub the area gently until no dirt remains.

2. If the wound bleeds, place a gauze sheet over it and gently apply pressure until it stops.

3. Apply an over-the-counter antibiotic cream, then bandage the scrape. Reapply frequently until the wound heals.

4. If you notice redness or red streaks coming from the wound, or if the wound begins to ooze or swell, take your child to the doctor. It may have become infected (cellulitis).

Most scrapes scab over quickly and heal with no further treatment. If you have used a dressing, change it daily or whenever it becomes dirty or wet. Once a firm scab has formed, a covering is no longer necessary. Discourage your child

---

TETANUS IMMUNIZATION

Keep your child's tetanus immunizations up-to-date. (See p. 110 for a full immunization schedule.) By the time your child enters kindergarten, she should have five tetanus shots. The DTP and DTaP immunizations both include tetanus immunization.

If your child has a cut or scrape, she should receive a tetanus booster if the following conditions apply:

- She has had three or fewer tetanus immunization shots.

- Her last tetanus shot was more than 5 years ago, and she has a puncture wound or a severe wound contaminated with dirt or feces.

- Her last tetanus shot was more than 10 years ago, and your child receives any injury.

from picking at the scab, which will only prolong healing time.

Prevention

To reduce the likelihood of cuts and scrapes, follow the childproofing methods described on page 143 and the sports safety precautions on page 275. Teach your about safety around sharp items like scissors or knives. To prevent puncture wounds, survey your child's play area for old boards and protruding nails, broken glass, and other hazards.

▮ *Cystic Fibrosis*

Cystic fibrosis (CF) is a serious genetic disease that affects many of the body's systems, particularly the lungs, pancreas, liver, and digestive tract. Although no cure is yet available for children born with cystic fibrosis, improved treatments have increased life spans to a median age of 31 years. A few people with cystic fibrosis now live into their forties and fifties. Cystic fibrosis is often detected within the first few months of life. Most cases are detected by the time a child is 2 years old but, rarely, symptoms may not appear until late childhood or adolescence.

Signs and Symptoms

- Very salty-tasting skin
- Persistent coughing or wheezing
- Pneumonia
- Excessive appetite but poor weight gain
- Bulky, foul-smelling stools
- Poor growth

Essential Facts

Cystic fibrosis is one of the more common genetic diseases, occurring in 1 in every 2,500 births in the United States. It is most common among Caucasian populations, in which 1 in every 20 people is a carrier of the disease. Since the gene for CF was discovered in 1989, the pace of CF research has accelerated rapidly, providing new hope for effective treatments.

To have the disease, a child must inherit two CF genes, one from each parent. People who inherit only one gene are carriers of the gene and can pass it on to their own children, but will not have the disease themselves. People who have a history of CF in their families can be tested to find out if they carry the gene, although the test cannot detect every case. A fetus can also be tested, but the test may not predict every case accurately.

The basic defect caused by the CF gene is the faulty transport of sodium and chloride (the component elements of table salt) within the epithelial cells that line the organs, such as the lungs and pancreas. Children born with this defect develop thick mucus in their lungs, which blocks the lungs' normal ability to clear themselves and instead allows bacteria to thrive. The result is infection. The thick mucus also harms the pancreas, preventing it from making enzymes needed for the absorption of food and causing weight loss or insufficient weight gain.

What the Doctor May Do

If your child's doctor has reason to suspect that your child has CF, she will diagnose the condition with a "sweat test," a quick, painless procedure that measures the amount of salt in a child's perspiration. A high level of salt indicates that the child has CF. Newborn screening for CF is routine in some states.

Treatment of CF depends on the stage of the disease and which organs are involved. Generally, treatment has two main parts: controlling lung infections and improving nutrient absorption when necessary. Occasionally, other conditions, such as asthma, sinusitis, nasal polyps, or arthritis of the joints, complicate the child's condition. Forceful coughing and infection can rupture the blood vessels in the lungs, causing the child to cough up blood. Forceful coughing can also break the air sacks in the lungs, leading to a condition in which air gets trapped in the chest (pneumothorax).

To help keep the lungs clear of infection your child's doctor may recommend a combination of chest physical therapy (a rhythmic drumming on the back using cupped hands to loosen mucus) and antibiotics administered orally or intravenously, or inhaled. The doctor may also recommend mucus-thinning drugs to be inhaled to help clear the lungs. In advanced cases, lung transplantation may be an option for some patients.

If the digestive system is affected, treatment will include an enriched diet, vitamins, and enzymes to improve absorption of nutrients. Regular physical examinations are important, and periodic hospitalizations may be necessary if your child is experiencing breathing difficulties or other complications.

What You Can Do

As a parent of a child with CF, your job will be to help ensure that your child gets the medical care he needs but also to help him lead as normal a life as possible. Restrict your child's activities only when necessary, according to your doctor's advice. You will meet with a physical therapist who will help you with therapies for your child, a nutritionist, and a social worker knowledgeable in helping families cope with the effects of CF.

Home treatment of CF will involve regular physical therapy to promote coughing and clearing the lungs, and administration of antibiotics or other medications. Your child will need to take vitamin supplements and nutritional supplements if weight gain is a problem. Avoid exposing your child to hot sun, and prevent dehydration by making sure your child drinks

adequate fluids. Children with CF are more prone to heat exhaustion or heat stroke than other children. Your child should receive a flu shot each year to help protect against potentially dangerous influenza infections as well as a vaccine for pneumococcal pneumonia.

Prevention

CF cannot be prevented, but couples who have a family history of the condition can be screened genetically with a test that detects most but not all genetic mutations that cause the disease. For more information on cystic fibrosis, see Cystic Fibrosis Foundation in Appendix: Parent Resources, Medical Conditions.

▍ *Dehydration*

People often think of dehydration as merely extreme thirst. But dehydration (a lack of adequate fluids) can be a medical emergency. It is the second leading cause of hospitalization of children under 5 years old, after respiratory infections. It is most likely to develop in infants and young children who have severe or prolonged *vomiting* or *diarrhea*.

Signs and Symptoms
- Decreased fluid intake
- Diapers dry more often than usual or decreased frequency or quantity of urination
- Sunken eyes
- Pale, dry skin
- Few tears when crying
- Dry mouth or tongue
- Lethargy or abnormal sleepiness
- Excessive irritability
- Rapid pulse
- Recent, rapid weight loss, especially for children under 2 years old

Judging the Severity of Dehydration

The chart below can help you determine the severity of your child's dehydration.

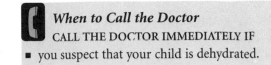

When to Call the Doctor
CALL THE DOCTOR IMMEDIATELY IF
- you suspect that your child is dehydrated.

■ SIGNS OF DEHYDRATION

Infants	Children
MILD DEHYDRATION (0–5 Percent)	
Increased thirst	Increased thirst
No bubbles in mouth	Dry mucous membranes
Dry lips	Dry lips
Fewer wet diapers	Decreased urination
Eyes slightly less glistening	Urine appears very yellow
MODERATE DEHYDRATION (5–10 Percent)	
Parched, cracked lips	Parched, cracked lips
Fontanel (soft spot) sunken	Sunken eyes
Eyes look dry, dull	Eyes look dry, dull
Dry diapers	No urination for 6–12 hours
No tears	Dry mucous membranes
Irritable, hoarse cry	Irritable, sluggish, tired
Skin dry, doughy to touch	Skin dry, doughy to touch
Weight loss	Weight loss (5–10% of previous weight)
SEVERE DEHYDRATION (10–15 Percent)	
Parched lips	Parched lips
Dull, filmed, sunken eyes	Dull, filmed, sunken eyes
Pale, dry skin	Pale, dry skin
Skin forms a "tent" when pinched	Skin forms a "tent" when pinched
Severe weight loss	Severe weight loss (>10% of previous weight)
Decreased blood pressure	Decreased blood pressure
Increased pulse	Increased pulse
Labored breathing	Labored breathing
Weak or inconsolable crying alternating with sleeping	Vacant stare
	Lethargic or irritable

Essential Facts

Dehydration is a lack of water in the body for metabolism, which is the conversion of food into energy. Infants and toddlers are more vulnerable to dehydration than older children, because their metabolic rate is much faster and they require proportionally more fluid. Because of their small size, even a relatively small fluid loss (through diarrhea or vomiting) can cause dehydration.

For children of any age, dehydration can impair metabolism. Body salts and minerals, such as sodium, potassium, calcium, and magnesium, are sometimes washed out along with the fluids. Depending on the problem's severity, dehydration can affect the central nervous system, the heart and circulatory system, the kidneys and urinary tract, and the respiratory system. Severe dehydration can be life-threatening, but fortunately, mild to moderate dehydration usually doesn't cause permanent damage, as long as it's treated adequately. The symptoms of dehydration can develop quickly in a child with severe diarrhea, repeated vomiting, and a high fever. Babies with these symptoms can become severely dehydrated within hours after diarrhea starts.

Causes

The most common cause of dehydration in infants and children in the United States is prolonged or severe diarrhea, often caused by a virus. Vomiting and excessive sweating connected with fever and hot weather can also cause a loss of fluids and lead to dehydration.

What the Doctor May Do

If your child has mild or moderate dehydration, the doctor may give her oral rehydration therapy (drinks of liquids with the right combination of essential salts and nutrients) in the office while observing her for several hours. If your child is severely dehydrated, the doctor will probably refer her to the emergency department of a nearby hospital, where she'll be given intravenous fluids, salts, and nutrients. After a few hours, the doctor may switch to an oral rehydration solution. Oral rehydration solution (such as Pedialyte and Ricelyte) can be purchased over-the-counter at most drugstores.

What You Can Do

If you notice any of the symptoms of dehydration, call your doctor right away. In the mean-

HOW MUCH LIQUID DOES A CHILD NEED EACH DAY?

Body Weight (Pounds)	Liquid Needed (Ounces)*
6	10
11	16
22	33
26	36
33	42
40	47
60	55
75	60
90	64

* Amount of any liquid required by a healthy child.

time, continue nursing or bottle-feeding your baby. If your child is older, encourage her to drink extra fluids. Even if she feels nauseated, she should be able to take small sips of oral rehydration solution. She should have about a tablespoon 20 minutes after vomiting, then 2 tablespoons about 10 or 15 minutes later, and 3 tablespoons 10 to 15 minutes after that, until she can drink about a cupful of fluid every hour. If your child vomits, start the process again. If she vomits a second time, call the doctor. Do not give sports electrolyte drinks. Those fluids are made to replace the salts lost with exercise and excessive sweating, not those lost from diarrhea. Instead, choose an oral rehydration solution prepared especially for infants and children, available at drugstores. If you have any questions, ask your doctor or pharmacist.

Once your child is no longer dehydrated, she can begin eating again. Follow the feeding guidelines for managing diarrhea.

How Much Liquid Is Enough?

The chart at left gives you an idea of the *minimum* amount of fluid most children need to stay healthy. A child with no signs of dehydration can get the necessary fluids from her normal diet (breast milk or formula for infants, and water or other caffeine-free, low-sugar liquids for older children).

Prevention

In young infants, you can prevent dehydration by increasing the amount of fluids (breast milk or formula) when a child has a fever or diarrhea. If the baby has diarrhea more than four times in a day, give her oral rehydration solution in addition to regular fluids. To prevent dehydration in older children, make sure they drink plenty of water or other noncaffeinated fluids when they have fever or diarrhea, and oral rehydration solution when they have repeated bouts of diarrhea or vomiting.

Depression

Your child doesn't seem like himself. He's withdrawn, doesn't eat right, and seems sad. He has trouble sleeping, or conversely, you have trouble getting him out of bed in the morning, and he doesn't want to go to school. He acts out aggressively or destructively or won't play with friends. Your child may be experiencing depression. Although relatively uncommon in children (and rare in children under 5 years old), depression can and does occur in childhood, becoming more common as children enter puberty.

Children generally bounce back remarkably well after an emotional setback, but those who are clinically depressed probably won't "snap out of it" without additional support and professional treatment. As is true for other kinds of psychological problems, think of your child's symptoms of depression on a continuum: If he feels down and withdraws from his friends for a few days after the death of a pet or even for no identifiable reason, but springs back to his normal self soon, you needn't be alarmed. If his depression is persistent—lasting for more than 2 weeks and involving not only a depressed mood but other changes in behavior (such as appetite changes, changes in sleep patterns, guilty feelings, and a diminished ability to concentrate, among others), then medical attention is probably warranted.

Signs and Symptoms

- Depressed or irritable mood most of the day for 2 weeks or more
- Poor hygiene, increasingly unkempt appearance

- Fatigue, loss of appetite, weight loss, or *failure to gain weight*
- Apathy, boredom, loss of interest in previously satisfying activities
- Problems in school, grades slipping
- Withdrawal from family and friends
- Thoughts of suicide (rare in young children)
- Excessive sleepiness or insomnia
- Symptoms with no medical cause (especially stomachaches and headaches)
- Low self-esteem or excessive or inappropriate guilt
- Aggression

When to Call the Doctor

CALL THE DOCTOR IMMEDIATELY IF

- your child talks about suicide—not wanting to live, "ending it all," and so forth.
- a teacher or another professional is concerned about your child's risk of self-harm.
- your child dwells on morbid subjects, such as suicide, death, disaster, or grisly accidents.

CALL THE DOCTOR TODAY IF

- your child hasn't "seemed himself" for more than a few days.
- a teacher or another professional has serious, ongoing concerns about your child's performance or behavior in school.
- your child experiences sadness accompanied by irritability or aggressive behavior and does not recover in a few days.
- for more than a few days, your child hasn't seemed to enjoy or hasn't participated in his usual activities.

Essential Facts

Depression is a mental illness usually characterized by intense feelings of worthlessness, unhappiness, and despondency. Depressed children cannot see a way out of their problems and are in despair. Unlike adults, whose symptoms usually include withdrawal and lack of interest, children's symptoms may include hyperactivity, defiant actions, aggression, and other negative behavior, as well as poor school performance. But these feelings and their symptoms are very different from those related to recent setbacks or disappointments or even a traumatic experience, like a family move, divorce, or death—although these situations can trigger depression. Depressed children usually develop changes in eating and sleeping patterns. Irritability and behavioral disturbances are also common symptoms. Guilt, anger, and feelings of low self-esteem often occur, although young children can't usually communicate those emotions and therefore express only general unhappiness. Depression in infants and toddlers is extremely rare.

The symptoms of depression usually develop gradually over days or weeks. In both children and adults, the course of depression may be quite variable: It can be mild and last only a few weeks or months, or severe and chronic and last more than a year. Working with a qualified health professional will help reduce both the severity and the length of your child's depression. Early intervention may also make later recurrences less likely.

Although distressing to parents and children, depression can be successfully treated, leaving a child to mature in a healthy, normal fashion. But because a depressed child may lag behind in school, in social skills, or in both, be sure to discuss with your child's doctor any concerns you may have about your child's mental health.

Suicide in children, although possible, is extremely rare. However, thoughts of death and suicide are not uncommon and should always be taken seriously.

Causes

Although scientists still aren't sure what causes depression, they have identified a number of potential triggers for the disorder, including the following:

- *Genetic and biochemical factors:* Most scientists now agree that depression tends to run in families. The inherited problem may be a vulnerability to a chemical imbalance in the brain, specifically in the levels of serotonin, dopamine, and norepinephrine. These substances, called neurotransmitters, are chemical messengers that carry information about mood and behavior to, from, and within the brain.

- *Physical illness:* Depression among children 5 to 9 years old may be prompted by a serious physical illness that requires the child to be bedridden for a long period, for example. Disruptions in the normal functioning of the endocrine system, resulting in too much or too little of certain hormones, such as thyroid hormone, may also cause depression.

- *External factors:* Major stress in the family, especially events that involve loss, such as a divorce, death, or even a move that takes a child away from friends and familiar surroundings, can trigger depression. Also, feelings of being unloved or unvalued can contribute to depression.

What the Doctor May Do

If you're worried about your child, take him first to his medical doctor, even if you think his problems are psychological. That way, his doctor can rule out any possible physical causes. If appropriate, your child's doctor can help you decide on a mental health professional—a child psychiatrist, psychologist, or social worker.

The mental health professional will meet with you, your family, and your child separately and together, to gather information to help her diagnose and treat your child. She will ask you about your child's physical and social development, family mental and medical history, and any changes, additional stresses, or upsetting events in your child's life. Your observations and insights are the key to this process—no one knows your child better than you. The more open you can be about your family situation, the better.

In addition, the professional will meet with your child alone to discuss his feelings—about the visit and about his health. She may also conduct further physical and psychological tests in order to more deeply understand your child's physical and emotional health. These tests will help assess the level of impairment and interference with normal activities the depression is causing, as well as evaluate the possibility that a learning disability may be involved. Following this evaluation, which could take up to four visits to complete, the health professional will make a specific treatment recommendation. The most common treatment for childhood depression is psychotherapy, which requires a series of meetings between your child, a professional, and—almost always—you and other members of your immediate family. Through various means, including play, artwork, and the special relationship your child develops with the therapist, your child can express his feelings, develop stronger coping techniques, and, finally, feel better about himself and the future. Depressed children especially need to learn to challenge their pessimistic beliefs and low self-esteem.

In some cases, a doctor may prescribe an antidepressant medication to alleviate your child's symptoms. The regular use of antidepressants in children remains controversial, mainly because guidelines on appropriate types and dosages for children are still being developed and have not yet been specified. However, if your doctor has experience in treating depressed children with medication, your child may benefit from antidepressants, especially if his depression is severe. Be sure to ask about potential side effects (which can range from a dry mouth to sleepiness and irritability), and inform your doctor as soon as possible about any that your child experiences. If your child is extremely depressed or suicidal and doesn't respond to treatment or he feels he may hurt himself, the therapist may recommend a brief or extended hospitalization in a mental health facility.

What You Can Do

The pain and sadness your depressed child feels is real, and what he needs from you most is your attention and love.

- *Let him know that you understand.* The most helpful support you can give your child is your understanding. By telling him, "I understand how you feel, and it's okay to feel that way," you'll be giving him a dose of the most powerful medicine available—your love and support. Depressed children commonly have parents who are also depressed. So if you (or your spouse) have clinical depression, explain to your child what depression is and that he didn't cause your depression.

- *Do away with guilt.* Although it's natural for you to blame yourself for your child's emotional difficulties, feeling guilty will only prevent you from interacting with your child with the honesty and openness necessary to help him get well.

- *Keep the lines of communication open.* One of depression's most common symptoms is withdrawal—a difficult reality for parents who want desperately to communicate with their child. Although forcing the issue is likely only to cause your child to retreat further, tell him directly that you're always there to listen to whatever he wants to tell you.

- *Keep alert for signs of a relapse.* Studies show that boys and girls who become depressed in childhood are at greater risk for developing later episodes of depression.

- *Try to bolster your child's self-esteem.* Because many depressed children have low self-esteem due to unreasonably high expectations, be sure to compliment your child when he achieves a goal, such as making a new friend or improving or maintaining school grades.

- *Safety-proof your home.* Keep dangerous items, such as razors, poisonous substances, and medications, out of the reach of all children. Guns should not be kept in a home with children or teenagers.

Prevention

Creating a warm and loving household, one in which your child feels valued and respected, is the best defense against depression. However, the development of depression depends on many factors, including genetic factors and physical illness, that may be beyond your control.

If you or your spouse has experienced depression, remain especially alert for the signs and symptoms of the problem in your child. Understand that this is a biological disorder and thus nothing to feel guilty about. Consult a family doctor or a mental health professional if you need further help in understanding the disease or in explaining it to your child.

Dermatitis (Atopic and Contact)

Dermatitis is a general term for skin irritation or rash. There are two main types: atopic (or allergic) and contact (or irritant). Atopic dermatitis, a noncontagious rash that is also known as eczema, appears as a red, itchy rash that never seems to go away. Contact dermatoses, on the other hand, are rashes that develop upon contact with a specific substance—poison ivy, for example, or a belt buckle or piece of jewelry containing nickel. Eczema tends to be chronic, while contact dermatitis is an acute condition that clears up as soon as the offending substance is removed.

Signs and Symptoms

Eczema:
- Red, itchy skin that becomes moist, oozing, and scaly
- Small bumps on the cheeks, forehead, or scalp
- Circular, slightly raised bumps and thickened, dry skin in older children

Contact (irritant) dermatitis:
- Red, itchy skin where skin makes contact with an irritating substance

When to Call the Doctor
CALL THE DOCTOR TODAY IF
- your child has any of the above symptoms.

Causes

Each type of dermatitis has a different cause. But there are six conditions that may make the problem worse:

- *Dry skin:* Often caused by excess washing or dry winter heat
- *Irritants:* For example, substances in cosmetics, tight or scratchy clothing
- *Heat and sweating:* Hot showers, baths, sunbathing, exercise
- *Emotional upset:* Family stresses, other upsetting changes in normal routines
- *Infections:* Bacterial skin infections
- *Allergens:* Foods such as peanuts, shellfish, eggs, milk, wheat

Eczema (Atopic Dermatitis)

Eczema is caused mainly by dry, highly sensitive skin—a condition that can be aggravated by certain allergies to foods, pollen, house dust, and other allergens. This condition frequently, but not always, runs in families. It appears in babies from 2 to 18 months, but may develop at any age. It often appears first on an infant's cheeks as red patches, which may spread to the rest of the face, neck, wrists, and hands. The rash may also appear on the skin behind the knees and inside the elbows. The rash is often itchy, and your baby may be fussy and irritable because of it. Older babies and children may try to scratch the rash. It may become worse when new foods are introduced into an infant's diet or when an infant comes into contact with inhaled allergens such as animal dander or pollen. Foods that most often contribute to eczema are eggs, milk, wheat, and soy. These foods often are used as ingredients in other foods, and your child may eat them daily without realizing it. Shellfish and peanuts also may trigger an outbreak.

Contact Dermatitis (Irritant and Allergic)

Allergic dermatitis is a condition that often appears if a child's skin touches a substance that causes allergy (such as latex or poison ivy), whereas irritant dermatitis is caused by any substance that irritates the skin (such as detergents). *Diaper rash* is a common type of irritant dermatitis caused by the skin's being irritated by damp, soiled diapers. Frequent contact with saliva, either from drooling or the constant licking of the lips, is the most common cause of irritant dermatitis on the face. Poor hygiene, such as infrequent diaper-changing or failure to properly clean a child's diaper area after a bowel movement, can also lead to irritant dermatitis.

Common causes of contact dermatitis are metal alloys found in inexpensive jewelry and buckles containing nickel, substances found in shoe rubber, tanned leather, shoe and clothing dyes, fabric finishers, and cleaning solutions. Certain medications and preparations applied to the skin, such as antihistamines, anesthetics, and preservatives, are also common irritants. Nail cosmetics, which can contain formaldehyde, toluene, and other chemicals, may also cause contact dermatitis.

The rash that appears after contact with poison ivy and similar plants (see *Poison Ivy, Poison Oak, Poison Sumac*) is also a form of contact dermatitis, caused by an allergic skin reaction to urushiol, an oily substance in the leaves of these plants. Urushiol is also found in the skin of mangoes and the shells of cashews, which can cause a similar rash.

What the Doctor May Do

Your doctor will work with you to identify the triggers that may be causing your child's condition. If your child has contact or irritant dermatitis, your doctor will advise you to keep the irritating substance (laundry detergent, for example) away from your child. Similar advice holds if it is an allergic response—to a pet, for example. The treatment is to keep the animal confined to places where your child won't be spending time, or if this fails, to find a new home for the animal.

In addition, your doctor may prescribe an oral antihistamine or a corticosteroid cream to apply to the skin if the dermatitis is chronic (as in the case of eczema) or severe. Your doctor will decide whether your child needs medication based on the extent of the rash, your child's discomfort, and whether the rash has appeared in particularly sensitive places, such as on the face or genitals. Both antihistamines and corticosteroid creams reduce inflammation and itching, usually within a few hours. In severe chronic cases the doctor can refer your child to a pediatric dermatologist (a doctor specializing in skin conditions).

Because certain ultraviolet light (UVB) appears to help clear up some cases of eczema, the doctor may recommend light therapy. In that case, your child would be exposed to a controlled amount of UV light a few times a week until the condition improves. Light therapy is generally not recommended for fair-skinned children who may sunburn easily.

What You Can Do

You can help in two ways. First, work with your doctor to identify and eliminate the cause of the rash if possible. Also, if your child has a rash, help her relieve the discomfort, as described in this section, and avoid irritating the skin further.

Identify the Cause

To identify the triggers that may be causing the condition, observe what your child is doing, eating, or wearing when outbreaks occur. If you can identify the triggers, teach your child to avoid them as much as possible. Check your child's diet. Children with eczema are often allergic to one or more of these substances: eggs, milk, wheat products, tomatoes, nuts, fish and shellfish, citrus and tropical fruits.

For contact dermatitis, see whether anything has touched your child's skin that could be causing the rash, including wet or soiled diapers for babies or poison ivy or poison oak for older children. Jewelry, laundry detergents, and perfumed or harsh soaps or lotions are also causes. Also consider other allergens that might be aggravating the condition, such as animal dander, pollen, and latex.

If you still can't find the cause of the dermatitis, consider this: Puzzling dermatitis cases are sometimes traced to one of the thousands of herbal and natural remedies and dietary supplements on the market. Herbal creams and ointments and herbal teas and vitamin supplements, particularly if taken in large doses, can cause

skin reactions. Some herbal remedies contain a dozen ingredients, any of which might trigger a rash. If your child has an unexplained skin reaction, tell your doctor of any herbal or natural remedies (including lotions, pills, or teas) your child may be using. Just because something is labeled "natural" doesn't mean it is harmless.

Reduce Discomfort

Once an outbreak occurs, you can use several strategies to limit its course and lessen the symptoms:

- *Keep the skin moist.* Moisture is important for treating eczema, so soothe the rash with emollient creams—products designed to trap moisture under the skin. If the eczema is severe, the doctor may recommend that you wrap the skin in a cloth wet with water and lotion overnight.

- *Install a humidifier.* If your house is dry, a humidifier can moisten dry air, which contributes to itchiness.

- *Keep the area clean.* Use a gentle cleanser such as a lotion containing aloe vera, which helps prevent skin from drying.

- *Choose cotton clothing,* which is less irritating to the skin than wool or acrylic. Some parents worry that sleepwear treated with fire-safe coatings might cause dermatitis, but this has not been shown.

- *Keep your child's fingernails short.* If your child is scratching the rash, try using mittens or gloves so that she won't break open the skin when she scratches.

- *Relieve itchiness* by applying an over-the-counter hydrocortisone ointment (1 percent concentration) to the rash, after checking with your doctor. For severe itching, your doctor may prescribe an anti-itch medicine such as hydroxyzine.

Prevention

You can reduce the number of dermatitis out-breaks if you can identify the cause and eliminate your child's exposure as much as possible.
See also ***Allergies.***

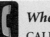

> ### When to Call the Doctor
> CALL THE DOCTOR TODAY IF
> - your child is not achieving some of the developmental milestones listed in the age-by-age chapters of this book.

▌*Developmental Problems*

Watching your child develop is one of the most rewarding aspects of parenthood. Children mature at different rates, even within the same family. But although every child develops at his own pace and normal development varies widely, it is wise to watch for signs of developmental problems.

If you're concerned about your child's development, review the developmental milestones in the earlier chapters of this book. Remember that minor differences in development are not significant: You needn't be concerned unless your child lags far behind or is not making progress toward achieving a particular milestone. If you or your child's doctor notice a problem, ask the doctor about having the appropriate specialist evaluate your child. The earlier a problem can be diagnosed and treated, the better the chances that it can be corrected, diminished, or improved.

Signs and Symptoms

- Your child isn't achieving some of the developmental milestones in the age-by-age chapters of this book.
- Your child is behind other children in his age group in language, learning, or motor development areas.
- Your child seems withdrawn socially, fails to respond to his name, or avoids looking at people.

Essential Facts

Children's development varies almost as widely as the differences in children themselves. Even siblings develop along different time lines, with boys often differing from girls in their developmental pace. But some developmental problems are well known, including these:

- *Cerebral palsy:* an abnormality in the brain area that affects movement and muscle tone (see ***Cerebral Palsy***)

- *Mental retardation:* a condition in which a child's intelligence is significantly lower than most of his age group and his ability to adjust to surroundings is diminished (see ***Mental Retardation***)

- *Learning disorders:* an impairment in one or more learning areas, such as reading, writing, speaking, or physical development (see ***Learning Disorders***)

- *Pervasive developmental disorders:* a group of conditions characterized by an impairment in communication and interaction. One of the best-known examples is autism (see ***Pervasive Developmental Disorder***).

All developmental disorders can vary widely in severity. For example, a child with cerebral palsy may have muscle impairment but no intellectual disability, while another child with cerebral palsy may experience intellectual impairment as well as muscle impairment. Some children have developmental problems specific to a certain area, such as hearing, language or speech delays, or motor development problems.

Causes

The causes of developmental problems are wide-ranging. Some problems are genetic, caused either by genes inherited from a parent or by genetic mutations. Causes before birth include chromosome damage, such as the chromosome abnormality that causes Down syndrome; birth injuries, especially those in which oxygen is denied to the brain for a period of time; and prenatal exposure to infection or toxic substances, such as drugs and alcohol. Other causes occur after birth and include head injuries and accidents, such as near-drowning. Often, however, the cause is undetermined. If this is the case with your child, you can best help your child by focusing on appropriate treatment rather than worrying about the cause or blaming yourself for your child's problems.

What the Doctor May Do

When you report your concerns about a developmental problem to the doctor, be wary of advice to "wait and see if he outgrows it." The earlier a problem is diagnosed and treated, the better. Your doctor's first step when you report a developmental concern will likely be a medical review to rule out physical causes: Speech delays, for example, can be caused by hearing loss.

The physical exam may be followed by a developmental evaluation, possibly with a developmental specialist. Depending on the results, your doctor or the specialist may recommend speech, language, occupational, or physical therapy or other evaluations, such as hearing and vision testing. Your child's doctor will continue to assist in the early detection of problems and in coordinating medical referrals. In addition, your doctor can coordinate family counseling.

Ask about the early intervention program in your area. Federal law requires that states provide therapy for infants and toddlers with developmental problems. Local school systems are required to provide help to children 3 years of age and older.

What You Can Do

Bring any concerns about your child's development to your doctor's attention. You may decide to find a doctor with special child development training for consultation, although developmental pediatricians are not available in all geographic areas. Be persistent about finding help for your child's needs. You know your child best, and your instincts about how well your child is developing are probably the most accurate. The following tasks summarize the most important steps you can take to help your child with developmental problems:

- *Seek advice* from doctors and therapists.

- *Use state and federally mandated help,* through the early intervention program in your area if your child is under 3 years of age and the local public school system if your child is over 3 years of age.

- *Follow up.* Follow the suggestions of your child's doctors and therapists. The treatments and therapies they recommend are important in stimulating your child's development. They may not cure the problem, but they may help your child catch up to his peers.

- *Seek counseling.* Ask your child's doctors and therapist how to contact support groups or counselors experienced with developmental problems. Parents who have had similar experiences, or experienced counselors, can give you practical advice and emotional support.

Prevention

Although developmental problems are usually not preventable, you can take steps to encourage healthy development.

- *Pregnancy:* Seek early prenatal care, and avoid the use of tobacco, alcohol, and drugs during pregnancy (see A Healthy Pregnancy, p. 3).

- *Child safety:* Avoid accidents by childproofing your home, and always use car seats properly (see p. 369). Encourage the use of helmets and other sports safety equipment.

- *Health care:* Bring your child to the doctor for regular checkups, and keep his immunizations current (see p. 110).

- *Play:* Create enriched learning experiences for your child. Talk and play with him as much as possible. Give him various child-safe toys and the freedom to explore a child-safe area (for more on ways to stimulate development at each age, see Chapters 4–7).

▌ *Diabetes Mellitus*

Diabetes mellitus is one of the most common chronic diseases in children, adolescents, and adults. More than 16 million people in the United States have diabetes; about 125,000 of them are under 19 years old. Although diabetes is a serious disease, children with diabetes can live healthy lives if they follow the treatment plan their physicians prescribe.

Signs and Symptoms

- Constant thirst
- Frequent urination
- Unexplained weight loss
- Fatigue, listlessness
- Increased hunger
- *Bed-wetting*
- Yeast infections in the vaginal area

When to Call the Doctor
CALL FOR EMERGENCY HELP IF

- your child exhibits symptoms of rapid, deep breathing.
- your child has severe, progressive abdominal pain.
- your child is pale and cold, with dry, mottled skin (see symptoms of shock, p. 418).
- your child shows signs of confusion, lack of coordination, drowsiness, or unconsciousness, or has a seizure (see *Seizures*).

For first aid information, see page 380 if your child is less than 1 year old and page 383 if your child is 1 year of age or older.

CALL THE DOCTOR IMMEDIATELY IF

- your child with diabetes has sunken eyes and appears dehydrated.
- your child with diabetes is nauseous and vomiting and/or has abdominal pain.

CALL THE DOCTOR TODAY IF

- your child with diabetes has decreased appetite for more than a day.
- your child shows signs of increased fluid intake; increased frequency or quantity of urination.
- your child with diabetes has a fever and signs of infection.

TALK WITH THE DOCTOR AT
YOUR CHILD'S NEXT CHECKUP IF

- you have questions about diabetes or its treatment.

Essential Facts

The signs and symptoms of childhood diabetes can begin suddenly at any age and may become dramatically evident within a few days to a couple of weeks. Diabetes in children under a year old is rare. The condition is diagnosed most commonly between 10 and 14 years of age. The most common signs are constant thirst and increased frequency and quantity of urination, which are most noticeable at night, when children with undiagnosed diabetes frequently awake with an urgent need to urinate or start wetting their beds. Some children begin to lose weight despite a normal or increased appetite.

Diabetes mellitus disrupts metabolism (the cell's chemical processes that convert food into energy) and is characterized by high blood sugar (glucose) levels. Normally, the blood sugar level is tightly regulated by the body metabolism. But when diabetes is present, consistent medical care is required to keep levels normal or near normal. Without treatment, high blood sugar levels and other metabolic disturbances of diabetes can, over time, damage small and large blood vessels, thus causing kidney, eye, nerve, and heart damage, which are all complications of diabetes.

Two main types of diabetes exist:

- *Type 1 diabetes:* Sometimes called juvenile diabetes, childhood diabetes, or insulin-dependent diabetes mellitus, this type of diabetes most often develops in children and young adults. Each year, nearly 12,000 children are diagnosed with type 1 diabetes. These children depend on daily injections of insulin (a hormone essential for glucose metabolism) in order to stay healthy.

- *Type 2 diabetes:* Sometimes called non-insulin-dependent diabetes, this disease mainly affects overweight adults over age 40, but is occurring more frequently in overweight adolescents. Type 2 diabetes is more common in African American and Hispanic adolescents.

Why Do Blood Sugar Levels Rise in Children with Diabetes?

Foods that contain proteins, fats, and carbohydrates are normally broken down into simple, easily absorbed chemicals. One of these is a form of simple sugar, glucose, which fuels many important body activities. The pancreas (a large gland behind the stomach) produces insulin, which helps glucose enter the cells. Normally, the pancreas produces the amount of insulin needed for glucose to enter body cells. In people with type 1 diabetes, however, the pancreas produces little or no insulin. As a result, glucose builds up in the blood and urine and exits the body unused and the body loses an important fuel, even though the blood contains large amounts of glucose. Because glucose cannot enter cells normally, it accumulates in the blood, a condition known as hyperglycemia. Insulin also allows the body to store glucose as glycogen (a carbohydrate composed of long chains of glucose) and converts excess glucose into fat, which is an efficient form of storing fuel.

Severe insulin deficiency resulting in high blood sugar levels causes frequent urination and increased thirst, eventually leading to an excessive breakdown of stored fats. This results in the formation of large amounts of ketones (water-soluble products of fatty acid oxidation produced by the liver) and the breakdown of protein. This condition is known as ketoacidosis. It can lead to diabetic coma and is an emergency situation that can develop within 24 hours if a child has severe insulin deficiency. That is why it is important that a child with diabetes never goes off her prescribed dose of insulin. Symptoms of ketoacidosis include a flushed face, dry skin, a dry mouth, headaches, nausea, vomiting, abdominal pain, drowsiness, blurry vision, fruity-smelling breath, a rapid heartbeat, and rapid, deep breathing. Without immediate treatment, a child with ketoacidosis can lose consciousness and die.

Causes

Scientists believe that type 1 diabetes is an autoimmune disease, in which the body's

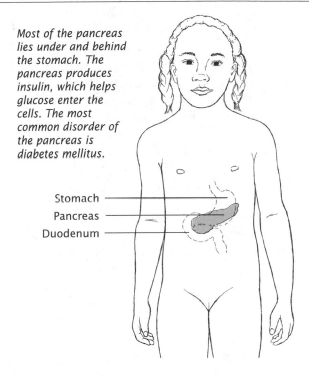

Most of the pancreas lies under and behind the stomach. The pancreas produces insulin, which helps glucose enter the cells. The most common disorder of the pancreas is diabetes mellitus.

Stomach
Pancreas
Duodenum

immune system has destroyed the insulin-producing cells, called beta cells, of the pancreas. So far, no one knows why the body attacks its own beta cells. One theory is that exposure to certain common viruses or other environmental factors in susceptible individuals may also increase a child's risk of diabetes. Such exposure may trigger the destruction of insulin-producing pancreatic cells in a genetically susceptible child. Diabetes sometimes runs in families.

What the Doctor May Do

If your child's doctor suspects diabetes, he will examine your child and take a detailed medical and family history. A child who has a family member with the disease is at higher risk of developing it. Your doctor may use a urine test to detect sugar and ketones in your child's urine and a blood test to measure the amount of sugar in the bloodstream. Because children with newly

diagnosed diabetes may be quite sick, treatment may first take place in the hospital, where doctors can monitor the child's electrolyte balance (including sodium, potassium, calcium, and phosphorus levels). Dehydration and ketoacidosis can be treated promptly with insulin and intravenous fluids. Regular doses of insulin can stabilize the child's body chemistry. In the hospital, the child and family will be educated on diabetes management and self-care.

Diabetes requires constant attention and daily care to keep blood sugar levels close to normal. Management of the disease focuses on five major practices:

- *Insulin injections:* Parents learn how to inject insulin under the skin to return a child's blood sugar to a nearly normal level. A child's pancreas may still make small amounts of insulin, becoming more deficient over a period of months until it makes no insulin at all. As a result, the insulin dosage may gradually increase. Finding the right insulin dose is one of the trickiest parts of diabetes management, and the dose will change depending on the child's age, weight, diet, and activity levels. Insulin injections are necessary two to four times a day, depending on the child's age, the severity of diabetes, and the success of the therapy. Once the child is old enough to handle the task herself with supervision—usually around 12 years old—she will work with her diabetes treatment team (doctor, diabetes nurse, dietitian) to determine the correct doses.

- *Diet:* Your physician, with the help of a nutritionist or dietitian specializing in diabetes treatment, will prescribe a meal plan for your child. Fortunately, a "diabetes diet" is really a healthy, nutritious way of eating for the whole family. Generally, your child should receive about 55 percent of her daily calories from complex carbohydrates (especially bread, pasta, rice, fruits, and vegetables), 30 percent (or less) from fat, and 15 to 20 percent from protein. See Using the Food Pyramid, page 236, for more information on nutrition. Your goal should be to have your child eat three balanced meals a day, with three snacks interspersed. It is important that these be eaten at about the same time each day.

- *Physical fitness:* Regular exercise will increase the body's sensitivity to insulin and assist in maintaining a desirable body weight, which may help keep diabetes under control. Individual and group sports can promote fitness and overall good health for children with diabetes.

- *Blood sugar testing:* Your doctor will explain to you and your child (depending on her age) how to measure her blood sugar at home with a glucose monitoring system by placing a drop of blood on a chemically treated strip and inserting it into a meter for a blood sugar reading. You will probably need to test your child's blood sugar levels frequently, before meals and at bedtime each day and between midnight and 3 A.M. once a week.

- *Managing side effects:* Achieving control over diabetes means balancing diet, exercise, and insulin injections on a day-to-day basis. The balance is easily thrown off if you forget an injection or if your child exercises or eats more or less than usual, or if your child has a fever, an infection, or surgery. Two diabetic emergencies can occur: hypoglycemia (low blood sugar), which results from too much insulin and/or insufficient food, and ketoacidosis, which can result from insufficient insulin or an infectious illness.

Mild symptoms of low blood sugar, or insulin reaction, occur fairly often. Symptoms such as crankiness, confusion, inattention, and drowsiness may appear within minutes after a child takes excess insulin or exercises too much without eating additional carbohydrates, or when a child using insulin eats too little food or the normal meal or snack is delayed. This condition must be treated immediately with sugar or sugary foods (e.g., fruit juice, glucose tablets). If your child doesn't receive enough sugar, she may lose consciousness. Your doctor will describe how to treat the condition quickly.

What You Can Do

Having a child diagnosed with diabetes is a major event that will affect the whole family. Fortunately, a large support network exists in the form of medical professionals and parent support groups. You can rely on these sources of help as you take the following steps to help manage your child's condition.

- *Learn all you can.* Managing diabetes is a complicated task. Ask health professionals about devising healthy meal plans, giving insulin shots, boosting your child's self-esteem, and managing side effects.

- *Be on the lookout.* Stay alert for signs of infection in your child, such as fever, lethargy, congestion, headaches, or stomachaches, and report them promptly to your child's doctor.

- *Encourage participation.* Managed properly, diabetes should not prevent your child from playing, learning, and exploring with her peers—and that includes participation in sports and other physical activities. The more active your child is, despite the need to take insulin and control her diet, the better off she'll be emotionally and physically.

- *Take care of yourself.* Especially at the start, coping with your child's diabetes may become a full-time job. If you're not careful to take time out for yourself, you risk developing a stress-related condition. Ask your doctor or fellow support group members about finding qualified child care so that you can take some time away from your child and her illness.

■ *Inform school or day care personnel.* Be sure to inform your child's day care providers or teachers about your child's condition, how to treat it, and what to do in an emergency.

Prevention

You cannot prevent type 1 diabetes, but you can reduce the risk of long-term complications by helping your child learn to manage the condition carefully to maintain blood glucose levels close to normal as much as possible. Helping your child practice healthy weight control measures can reduce the risk of developing type 2 diabetes.

■ *Diaper Rash*

No matter how carefully you care for your baby, he'll probably have diaper rash at some point during his infancy—most babies do. The good news is that diaper rash is almost never serious, can almost always be treated at home, and usually looks far worse than it feels. Often treatment is simply a matter of keeping the skin dry by changing your child's diapers more frequently and allowing his skin time to air-dry between changings.

Signs and Symptoms

■ Red, sometimes scaly or rough skin in the diaper area

■ Pimples in the diaper area or near the belly button

When to Call the Doctor
CALL THE DOCTOR IMMEDIATELY IF
■ your child has rashes elsewhere on his body or if a fever accompanies the rash.
■ the rash is getting worse by the hour.

CALL THE DOCTOR TODAY IF
■ the rash lasts more than a few days (indicating a potential yeast infection).
■ the rash is extensive.

TALK WITH THE DOCTOR AT YOUR CHILD'S NEXT CHECKUP IF
■ your child gets diaper rash frequently.

Essential Facts

Although diaper rash is easily treatable, make sure to take steps quickly to prevent the condition from worsening. Most cases of diaper rash are caused by irritant dermatitis, a rash that appears when the skin touches an irritating substance—in this case wet or soiled diapers. But when diaper rash lasts more than a few days, or occurs frequently, then a yeast infection, an allergy, or another underlying illness may be the cause.

Causes

Diaper rash occurs because the diaper traps urine, feces, chemicals from the diapers, and other material close to your baby's skin, causing irritation and inflammation. But not all rashes in the diaper area are diaper rashes. *Chicken pox, impetigo,* and yeast infections (see *Thrush*) produce rashes that may appear around the genitals and buttocks, but are quite different in cause and treatment from diaper rash. If you use cloth diapers, the rash could be a reaction to your laundry detergent.

What the Doctor May Do

Your doctor will try to determine the cause of the rash. Most cases are caused by contact with soiled diapers. If the rash is infected, the doctor may prescribe an antibacterial ointment, or if it is severe, the doctor may advise you to use a cortisone cream to reduce inflammation.

What You Can Do

The best thing you can do for your baby is to keep him dry and clean by changing his diapers frequently—every 2 or 3 hours, or as soon as he has a bowel movement. But be cautious about changing and wiping your child too frequently, which can rid the skin of its natural protective oils.

Until the rash clears up, wash your child's diaper area with warm water during each changing. Pat it dry gently but thoroughly. Whenever possible, allow his skin to dry for 10 to 15 minutes before putting diapers on. Apply lots of barrier cream, such as zinc oxide, vitamin A & D ointment, or petroleum jelly. If the rash does not clear up after 3 to 4 days, your baby may be allergic to a chemical used to clean or manufacture the diapers. Try changing diaper brands. Or switch from cloth to disposable diapers. Change laundry detergent if you use cloth diapers.

Do not . . .

- use talcum powder or scented lotions on a diaper rash. They often cause more irritation.
- use baby wipes containing alcohol, perfume, or soap that can irritate. One alternative to wipes is a washcloth with water and mild soap.
- use plastic pants over a cloth diaper. They will only trap in the moisture and make the rash worse.

Prevention

Most babies will have an episode or two of diaper rash, but you can prevent or reduce the problem by changing your baby frequently and allowing his skin to dry between changes. If it's warm outside, you may also want to let him play in the backyard without a diaper.

See also **Rashes.**

Diarrhea

A child's bowel movements normally vary in number and consistency. On some days they're looser than on others. But a loose stool doesn't necessarily mean diarrhea. A child has diarrhea if her bowel movements increase in frequency, liquidity, and volume. Most cases of diarrhea in childhood aren't serious and don't warrant a trip to the doctor. They go away by themselves within a day or so.

When to Call the Doctor

CALL THE DOCTOR IMMEDIATELY IF

- your child shows signs of dehydration.
- diarrhea is accompanied by abdominal pain traveling from the navel to the lower right side of the abdomen (a possible sign of appendicitis).
- blood is in the stool.
- your child has severe abdominal pain.
- diarrhea is accompanied by a high fever or lasts longer than 48 hours.
- a rash or jaundice accompanies the diarrhea.

CALL THE DOCTOR TODAY IF

- you suspect that your child has food poisoning (e.g., she has eaten seafood, undercooked hamburger, raw milk, or unpasteurized juice).
- your child is less than 6 months old and has symptoms of diarrhea.
- your older child's diarrhea lasts longer than 2 or 3 days, or she has other symptoms of illness, such as fever, rash, or vomiting.
- your family recently returned from a camping trip or foreign travel, and your child has symptoms of diarrhea.

Essential Facts

Diarrhea is common, especially during the first 3 or 4 years of life. The only illnesses that appear more often in young children are colds and other upper respiratory infections. Most cases of diarrhea last 2 to 4 days and are related to a mild infection such as a gastrointestinal virus.

Diarrhea affects children in different ways, with younger children tending to have more frequent, more watery stools. Stools may vary in color, from light brown to yellow to green. Bleeding can occur when frequent loose bowel movements irritate the rectum. If any blood is visible, call the doctor immediately.

Causes

By far, the most common cause of diarrhea in children is a viral infection of the gastrointestinal tract. Viral infections are usually spread from child to child. The most common virus is known as rotavirus.

Bacterial infections, which account for about 15 percent of cases of gastroenteritis (stomach or intestinal flu or infection), can be caused by *food poisoning* or drinking contaminated water or coming in contact with an infected person. Though they're not as common, other organisms, including fungi and parasites, can also infect the intestinal tract (see *Worms: Pinworm and Other Parasitic Worms*). Intestinal infections aren't the only cause of diarrhea. Respiratory infections, like the common cold, can cause it, too (see *Colds/Flu*). In fact, infection anywhere in the body can alter gastrointestinal function, resulting in diarrhea, or sometimes in *constipation.*

A condition sometimes called toddler's diarrhea appears in some toddlers and preschool children. The child may have frequent, loose stools over a period of months or even years. The condition is not caused by any infection or other illness. In this case, when diarrhea isn't related to an illness, it could be a sign that there is a problem with your child's diet, such as an overconsumption of fruit juice or caffeinated beverages, which tend to cause loose stools.

Frequent or ongoing diarrhea episodes can also be a symptom of a food allergy or intolerance (see *Allergies*). For example, some children (especially those of African, Asian, or Mediterranean origin) are lactose intolerant. That is, they get diarrhea after drinking milk and eating milk products because they have a deficiency of lactase, an enzyme needed to digest lactose (a sugar in milk). Milk products can also cause diarrhea in children who are allergic to the protein in milk. Another cause of frequent diarrhea is celiac disease, an allergy to gluten (a complex protein found in wheat).

Other causes of diarrhea in children include medications. Diarrhea can be caused by laxatives, stool softeners, or mineral oil, for example. Antibiotics, such as amoxicillin, often change the normal bacteria present in the bowels and change the character of the stool so that it is looser and more frequent. Sugar, caffeine, and nicotine all can cause diarrhea in young children. *Cancer* treatments and radiation poisoning can injure the lining of the bowels, causing severe diarrhea.

Uncommon causes of childhood diarrhea include such chronic conditions as *cystic fibrosis;* ulcerative colitis, an inflammatory disease of the colon characterized by diarrhea with discharge of mucus and blood and cramping abdominal pain; or Crohn's disease, a chronic inflammation of the gastrointestinal tract (esophagus, stomach, and intestines). Both ulcerative colitis and Crohn's disease result in the swelling of mucous membrane lining and are characterized by diarrhea with discharge of mucus and blood and abdominal cramping. Other uncommon causes of diarrhea include *HIV/AIDS infection,* immune deficiencies, and some tumors.

What the Doctor May Do

If your child has a mild fever and vomiting that doesn't seem to be related to a particular food, the doctor will probably assume that she has a stomach virus, meaning gastroenteritis. The doctor will advise you about how to keep your child comfortable and prevent *dehydration* until the illness passes.

If the doctor suspects food poisoning or a nonviral infection, the doctor may take a stool sample to identify the bacterium or parasite responsible, then prescribe antibiotics. If a food allergy or intolerance is causing chronic diarrhea, the doctor will suggest eliminating the offending food from your child's diet. If your child has chronic diarrhea caused by a physical defect, she might need surgery or long-term medical care.

What You Can Do

The most important thing to do when your child has diarrhea is to make sure that your child drinks enough water or other fluids to prevent dehydration. If she doesn't ask for something to drink regularly, give her sips of oral rehydration solution every 10 to 15 minutes, even if she feels nauseous.

You can feed your child a normal diet, as long as she's hungry and is not vomiting. Don't withhold formula, breast milk, or cow's milk, unless your doctor advises you otherwise. Though milk products were long thought to make diarrhea worse, children who drink milk and eat other foods actually improve half a day faster than those on a limited diet. Dairy foods also help children with diarrhea by restoring nutrients lost through diarrhea.

If your child is still in diapers, pay special attention to her diaper area, which may become irritated. Change soiled diapers promptly, then wash and dry your child's bottom. Spread petroleum jelly on her diaper area to protect it from diaper rash.

Don't give over-the-counter antidiarrheal products. They can mask ongoing symptoms that enable your doctor to diagnose the cause of the diarrhea. Also, by making fluids and salts build up in the intestines, these medications can prevent you and your child's doctor from monitoring your child's fluid loss. Thus your child could become seriously dehydrated without the usual sign—frequent diarrhea—to alert you of the danger.

Prevention

From birth, you can reduce the chance of diarrhea by breast-feeding your baby, because ingredients in breast milk reduce the risk of infections and food allergies. Getting your older child into the habit of washing her hands on a regular basis will help stop the spread of viruses. If your child is in day care, encourage her caregivers to wash their hands after diapering each baby and before handling food. Also try limiting the amount of juice and sweetened beverages, like soda and juice drinks, because they can cause loose, frequent stools. Don't give your child caffeinated beverages (many colas and sodas contain caffeine), because they cause fluid loss.

■ Dislocations (Arm, Hip)

You quickly pull your toddler out of a car's path or jerk his arm to keep him from falling. He cries out in pain and then protects his arm by holding it close to his side with the elbow slightly bent. What's occurred is elbow dislocation, or "nursemaid's elbow," a common injury in children under 4 years old. Nursemaid's elbow and most other types of dislocations—including developmental dislocations that show up soon after birth—aren't usually serious and won't cause permanent damage, as long as they are diagnosed and treated promptly by a medical professional.

Signs and Symptoms

- Sudden pain, weakness, or immobility in a joint
- Unusual appearance of a joint or a bone beneath it (e.g., a knee bent backward)
- Your child is cradling an arm

When to Call the Doctor
CALL THE DOCTOR IMMEDIATELY IF

- you suspect that your child has dislocated a joint.

Essential Facts

A joint is the meeting of two or more bones to form a movable part. Whenever a bone slips from its normal position in a joint, a dislocation occurs. Virtually any joint in the body can become dislocated, but in children under 4 years old, the elbow is most vulnerable because young children are most likely to have their arms yanked as their parents or baby-sitters try to keep them out of harm's way. Older children may dislocate a knee or shoulder as the result of a sports injury. Some playground equipment, such as merry-go-rounds, can also cause dislocation injuries. Dislocations may also show up at birth or soon thereafter. Such developmental dislocations usually affect the hip and are often diagnosed at birth.

Dislocations can be painful and may take several days to several weeks to heal. If your child experiences a dislocation, bring him to a doctor right away; dislocation can lead to long-term problems that prevent the joint from functioning properly. For example, the nerves and ligaments may be permanently weakened, or injury of the joint cartilage may lead to arthritis.

Your older child may dislocate a knee or shoulder as the result of a sports injury. If your child experiences a dislocation, bring her to a doctor right away to avoid long-term problems that prevent the joint from functioning properly. (A) Normal shoulder; (B) dislocated shoulder. Note the change in the normal contour of the shoulder near the areas of dislocation.

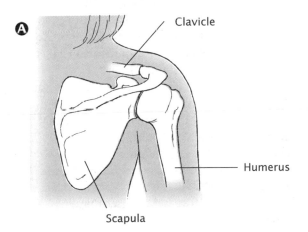

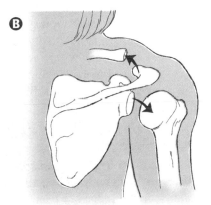

Causes

These are the most common causes of dislocations:

- *Injuries:* All joints are held together by tough, fibrous bands called ligaments. When a joint is forced to move beyond its normal range, ligaments can be torn. If the tearing is serious enough, the bone can slip out of place, becoming dislocated. Injury-related dislocations of the shoulder, fingers, toes, and other joints are most commonly caused by sports activities, and tend to occur in schoolchildren and adolescents. They are usually quite painful.

- *Congenital (present at birth) hip dislocation:* About 1 out of every 100 babies has a hip dislocation that becomes apparent soon after birth. In most cases, the dislocation is caused by either genetic factors or a loose ligament connecting the hipbone socket to the head of the thighbone. A hip dislocation is painless to an infant and is rarely obvious. It can only be detected by a physical examination and certain tests. Pediatricians routinely look for signs of these dislocations during a newborn's physical exams. If the doctor suspects a dislocation, an ultrasound exam or X rays may be needed to confirm the diagnosis. The problem often resolves itself within the first few days of life, as the ligament grows stronger. Of the cases that need a doctor's treatment, about 90 percent can be cured completely within about 2 months. The treatment involves keeping the hip stable in a special harness or cast. If not diagnosed or treated within a few months, this condition may lead to poor posture, walking difficulties, and chronic pain.

- *Congenital (present at birth) lax ligaments:* Some children are born with loose tendons and ligaments, which predispose them to dislocations. A congenital connective tissue condition, Ehlers-Danlos syndrome, also predisposes children to dislocations.

What the Doctor May Do

If you suspect that your child has dislocated a joint, call the doctor immediately, even if it appears to have slipped back into place. The doctor will conduct a physical examination (which is sometimes all that is needed to diagnose a dislocation) and might also order X rays to confirm the diagnosis and to see whether any fractures exist.

Treatment depends on the joint affected, as well as the cause of the dislocation. For nursemaid's elbow, a doctor usually can relocate it by bending the arm at a 90-degree angle and, while holding the forearm near the elbow, twisting the wrist and forcing the palm to face upward. If done within a few hours of the injury, the child usually feels a click near the elbow, and within minutes, the pain subsides and movement returns to normal. In fact, the elbow often slips back into place while it's being positioned by a technician for an X ray. If treatment is delayed for more than a few hours after the injury, however, the repositioning procedure is more difficult and the discomfort longer-lasting, and the child may have to have her arm held in position with a sling for a few days. Occasionally, nerves or blood vessels or other structures can become trapped when the joint snaps back into place. Your child's doctor can examine for such a complication and treat it if necessary.

Sometimes the doctor will relocate the joint and then hold the affected limb in place with a cast or sling until the injured tissues heal. Doctors try to keep recently dislocated joints in slings or casts for as little time as possible so that the joints don't become too stiff. During the recuperation period, the doctor may suggest that the child perform some exercises that involve strengthening the muscles around the joint.

Unfortunately, a child who dislocates his shoulder or elbow once has a good chance of dislocating it again within a month, because the ligaments are still loose. Your doctor may teach you how to diagnose an elbow dislocation and how to reposition the elbow yourself if the problem becomes chronic. But never try to pop any joint back into place without proper training. If a certain joint becomes dislocated frequently, surgery may be required.

Treatment of congenital hip dislocation depends on the age of the child and the severity of the dislocation. It usually involves relocating the joint manually, then stabilizing it with a special brace, harness, or splint.

What You Can Do

Call the doctor immediately if you think your child has dislocated a joint. You'll probably have to take him to a hospital emergency room. Don't attempt to relocate a joint yourself, unless a doctor directs you to. But you can reduce your child's discomfort and swelling by applying ice to the joint. Follow the doctor's directions about care, including the use of pain relievers to ease your child's discomfort and physical therapy exercises to strengthen the muscles around the affected joint.

Prevention

Congenital dislocations cannot be prevented, but early detection and treatment are crucial if you wish to avoid future problems and disabilities. In addition, you can prevent problems by being careful how you hold and play with your child. Twirling children around by the arms is a frequent cause of nursemaid's elbow, as is suddenly pulling on their arms or picking them up by their hands. To reduce the chance of injury-related dislocations, encourage your child to warm up before strenuous exercise and wear protective equipment during competitive sports

such as football.

See also *Sprains and Strains.*

▌ *Dizziness*

We've all experienced dizziness: the feeling that either the room is spinning or our bodies are whirling. Sometimes, the symptoms include nausea and even vomiting. Also called vertigo, dizziness results from a disturbance of the body's balancing mechanism and—despite some discomfort—usually clears up without treatment.

Signs and Symptoms

- Spinning sensation
- Light-headedness, faintness
- Pallor, nausea, or *vomiting*

When to Call the Doctor
CALL FOR EMERGENCY HELP IF

- your child loses consciousness or has a seizure (see *Seizures*).

  For first aid information, see page 380 if your child is less than 1 year old and page 383 if your child is 1 year of age or older.

CALL THE DOCTOR IMMEDIATELY IF

- a high fever or a stiff neck accompanies symptoms.
- your child is delirious.
- your child has a severe headache.
- your child cannot stand and walk or is acting very sick.
- your child has vision or hearing problems.

CALL THE DOCTOR TODAY IF

- dizzy spells recur frequently or last several hours.
- ear pain or hearing loss is also present.
- your child is taking medication that may be causing the dizziness.

Essential Facts

Many routine activities can cause dizziness or light-headedness. Bending backward or standing up suddenly, for example, can temporarily affect blood flow to the head and produce a dizzy feeling or light-headedness. Several minor illnesses and a few serious ones can also cause dizziness.

Causes

The body's balance mechanism is located in the inner ear, and anything that disrupts that mechanism can cause dizziness. Usually this balance returns to normal within a few minutes or seconds—the body is good at making minor adjustments quickly—but, if not, dizziness may lead to nausea and a bout of vomiting or, rarely, a *fainting* episode. Here are some common triggers:

- *Physical activities:* The most common causes of dizziness in children are physical activities involving spinning. Once the spinning stops and balance returns, dizziness passes. Many older children become light-headed when rising suddenly from a lying or sitting position.

- *Motion sickness:* Your child may become dizzy and nauseous while traveling in a car, a boat, or an airplane. *Motion sickness* occurs when movement disrupts the child's inner balance mechanism located in the inner ear.

- *Emotional triggers:* Some children may feel dizzy or nauseated—or may even faint briefly—after seeing something that frightens them (e.g., blood, a scary movie scene). This is caused by overstimulation of the vagus nerve and blood vessels, which leads to a momentary fall in blood pressure, producing the symptoms. The sensation usually disappears within a minute or so.

- *Infections:* Ear infections (see *Earache/Ear Infection*), fevers, the flu, and headaches are common causes of dizziness, because they, too, can affect the balance mechanism.

- *Head injury:* A trauma to the head (e.g., from a fall or a blow) can disrupt a child's sense of balance and lead to dizziness. See Head Injuries, page 410.

- *Migraine:* Migraine headaches (see **Headaches**) are accompanied by dizziness, light-headedness, or spinning vertigo in 10 to 15 percent of patients. Episodes of dizziness—even without headache—can be a symptom of migraine.

- *Hypoglycemia:* Going too long without food can produce low blood sugar (hypoglycemia), which can cause light-headedness and a dizzy sensation in some people.

- *Dehydration:* Going too long without fluids can cause blood pressure changes that cause a child who changes position suddenly to feel dizzy. (See **Dehydration**.)

In very rare cases, dizziness may signify a brain tumor (see **Cancer**), another problem affecting the brain, or, in some cases, an **abnormal heart rhythm.**

What the Doctor May Do

If your doctor is concerned about your child's dizziness, he will examine her and take a history of the symptoms, paying special attention to inner ear problems or infections that might be triggering the spells. He will take your child's blood pressure, before and after she rises suddenly, to determine whether a drop in blood pressure occurs. If so, he will suggest that your child rise more slowly from a sitting or lying position. If he cannot find an obvious cause, he may suggest that you visit a neurologist (brain and central nervous system specialist) or an otolaryngologist (ear, nose, and throat specialist) for further evaluation. Diagnostic tests may include noninvasive procedures such as vision and hearing exams, neurological exams, and brain diagnostic tests such as an EEG (electroencephalogram), an ECG (electrocardiogram), a CT (computed tomography) scan, and an MRI (magnetic resonance imaging).

What You Can Do

If your child becomes dizzy, have her sit or lie down until the episode passes. If she is seated, have her put her head between her knees to increase blood flow to the brain and help keep her from fainting. If she lies down, elevate her legs for the same reason. The episode should pass within a few minutes.

Prevention

Treating the underlying cause may help eliminate the problem. For example, eating will resolve the light-headed feeling of low blood sugar. Giving your child plenty of fluids will reduce the dizzy sensation that accompanies dehydration. If your child is affected by the sight of blood or scary movies, avoiding such triggers may be the ounce of prevention you need. If dizziness usually occurs after the child rises suddenly, help your child learn to rise more slowly.

Down Syndrome

See *Developmental Problems.*

Dysrhythmia

See *Abnormal Heart Rhythm.*

Earache/Ear Infection

When most parents talk about ear infections, they usually mean infections of the middle ear (called otitis media)—one of the most common afflictions of infancy and toddlerhood. About 75 percent of children in the United States experience one or more such ear infections before they enter first grade. But the middle ear isn't the only part of the ear that can become infected. Fungi or bacteria can cause an infection of the external ear (also known as otitis externa or swimmer's ear) and ear canal. A virus can also attack the inner ear, although this type of ear infection is quite rare. Although often quite painful and sometimes accompanied by temporary hearing loss, earaches and ear infections are usually easily treated and cause no lasting damage.

Signs and Symptoms

External Ear Infections (Otitis Externa)

- Initial itchiness
- Pain when outside of ear is touched
- Red, swollen ear canal
- Red, swollen auricle (the visible, outer part of the ear)
- Discharge of pus
- Hearing loss

Middle Ear Infections (Otitis Media)

- Ear pain; child pulls at the ear
- Ear drainage
- Fever
- Dizziness
- Hearing loss
- Vomiting; loss of appetite
- Ringing or buzzing in the ear

Inner Ear Infections (Labyrinthitis)

- Severe dizziness
- Spinning sensation
- Vomiting
- Ear pain
- Ear drainage
- Hearing loss

When to Call the Doctor
CALL THE DOCTOR IMMEDIATELY IF

- your child has a seizure.
- your child is in severe pain that does not lessen after you give him acetaminophen or ibuprofen.
- your child is extremely dizzy.
- your child seems lethargic.
- your child is vomiting.

CALL THE DOCTOR TODAY IF

- you suspect that your child has an ear infection.
- there is liquid coming out of your child's ear.
- your child has difficulty hearing.
- your child hears a buzzing or ringing.
- your child seems off balance.

Essential Facts

External Ear Infections

An external ear infection occurs when the normal ear canal "flora" (bacteria and fungi that live in the ear canal) overgrow as a result of moist conditions. Excess earwax may contain or trap the bacteria or fungi, leading to swelling of the ear canal. The swelling may extend to the outer ear and cause severe pain. If hair spray or other chemicals enter the ear canal, the irritation can also make the ear canal skin more vulnerable to infection. Also, the skin of the outer ear canal can become stretched or injured by insertion of a foreign object—even a cotton swab—and bacterial or fungal infections may develop.

Of the two external ear parts, the auricle is the least likely to become infected, although ear piercing or other injuries to the ear can sometimes lead to infection of the auricle. (See *Ear and Body Piercing Infections.*)

Middle ear infections (otitis media) are the most common causes of earaches. When a middle ear infection occurs, the eustachian tube becomes swollen and then blocked, causing the buildup of fluid and pressure in the middle ear.

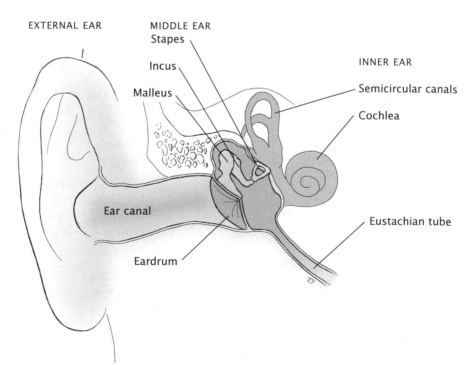

Middle Ear Infections

Children under 6 years old are the most susceptible to middle ear infections, which are the most common cause of earaches. The peak age for these infections is from 6 to 24 months. That is because a youngster's eustachian tube, which connects the back of the nose to the ear, is short and horizontal, and thus able to pass along bacteria or viruses from the back of the nose to the middle ear. Most middle ear infections are associated with a cold or the flu. (See *Colds/Flu.*)

Boys are slightly more susceptible to middle ear infections than girls. Other factors that may increase a child's risk of getting middle ear infections are attending day care, a family history of middle ear infection, and bottle-feeding rather than breast-feeding. A child's habit of falling asleep with a bottle in his mouth may also be a contributing factor, although there is no definitive scientific data linking this to ear infections.

When a middle ear infection occurs, the eustachian tube becomes swollen and subsequently blocked, causing the buildup of fluid and pressure in the middle ear. The eardrum appears pink or red from inflammation; it may be stretched tight or even bulging. That's why the pain of a middle ear infection can be made worse by chewing, swallowing, nose-blowing, or lying down, all of which affect pressure inside the middle ear. In most cases, fluid buildup in the middle ear can also result in temporary *hearing loss.* This type of hearing loss is generally reversible with appropriate therapy.

Untreated, a middle ear infection can lead to serious complications, including damage to the small bones and other structures in the middle ear, resulting in hearing loss. The delicate membrane of the eardrum may stretch and burst, leaking pus, which can lead to infection of the outer ear. A less common complication of long-standing, repeated or chronic ear infections is a buildup of cells and debris in the middle ear into a large mass called cholesteatoma, which pushes against and damages other structures in the middle ear. Uncommonly, an acute ear infection may spread to deeper tissues and to the mastoid bone behind the ears, resulting in an infection called acute mastoiditis.

Inner Ear Infections

This very rare kind of ear infection causes inflammation of the membrane structures of the inner ear (which consists of the cochlea—where the hearing nerve is—and the labyrinth, where the balance mechanism is). Inner ear infections can also result from either viral or bacterial sources.

The viral form, viral labyrinthitis, can occur when a virus—such as one that causes measles, mumps, or the flu—invades the inner ear. Subsequent inflammation may cause significant dizziness and hearing loss, which is sometimes permanent. However, viral labyrinthitis usually resolves without any long-term complications.

Bacterial labyrinthitis develops when an acute middle ear infection spreads to the inner ear or when *meningitis* (inflammation of the protective covering of the brain and spinal cord) spreads to the inner ear. Bacterial labyrinthitis usually results in significant and permanent hearing loss, and possible damage to the structures on the infected side. The infection is now very uncommon, thanks to the use of antibiotics to treat middle ear infections, although it still sometimes occurs as the result of bacterial meningitis.

What the Doctor May Do

External Ear Infections

If your doctor suspects that your child has an external ear infection, the doctor will look for signs of swelling, redness, or debris in the ear canal. If she determines that your child has this infection, she will first clean the ear canal. Debris often needs to be removed. She will then prescribe ear drops that may contain antibiotics (to kill bacteria causing the infection) and steroids to reduce swelling. She may also place a "wick" in the ear canal, a device that carries medicated drops all the way down the ear canal. For severe external ear infections, your doctor may prescribe oral antibiotics as well.

Middle Ear Infections

If your doctor suspects that a middle ear infection is causing your child's discomfort, she'll examine your child's ears with an otoscope (a lighted instrument for examining the interior of the ear). She'll also inspect your child's nose and throat. If your child has otitis media, the doctor will probably see a bulging, sometimes red eardrum, a sign of increased middle ear pressure, or fluid in the middle ear. She will also use a bulb attached to an otoscope to push air through the ear canal so that she can assess whether the eardrum is mobile. Normally, air would cause the eardrum to move. However, if the eardrum is markedly thickened or there is middle ear fluid, or if both conditions exist, then eardrum mobility is significantly diminished.

Your doctor may prescribe antibiotics to relieve inflammation and lessen the chances of complications. Over-the-counter antihistamines and decongestants are not effective in treating this condition, although they may help relieve other cold and flu symptoms that sometimes accompany a middle ear infection.

For severe or recurrent cases of otitis media, an ear, nose, and throat specialist may recommend making a small incision in the eardrum (a procedure called myringotomy), then placing a tube through it. The tubes reduce the likelihood of repeated infection and usually improve hearing while they are in place. General anesthesia is usually required for the placement of ear tubes, particularly for small children, who cannot hold still during the procedure. The insertion of ear tubes, a common procedure nowadays, takes less than one half hour and requires no hospital stay. The tubes will generally remain in place for 9 months to a year, at which time they usually fall out by themselves. While the tubes are in place, children are free to bathe, shower, and swim, but some doctors recommend using earplugs during these activities to keep the ears dry. If the ear tubes fall out too soon, they may need to be replaced.

Follow-up care after a middle ear infection is an essential part of treatment. Make sure to give your child the full course of antibiotics, and keep your follow-up appointment (usually 3 to 4 weeks later) so that the doctor can make sure that the infection has resolved. Your child may need a hearing test once the infection is completely gone. Most children experience some temporary hearing loss during the infection, but hearing should return completely within 4 to 6 weeks after the infection clears. Sometimes, however, the middle ear fluid does not resolve even if the acute symptoms of otitis media do. In that case, there may be continued hearing loss and you may then be referred to an ear, nose, and throat specialist for further hearing evaluation and the possible placement of ear tubes. Infants and young children with repeated middle ear infections should have their hearing screened frequently, because hearing loss can impede speech and language development at this crucial age.

Inner Ear Infections

Treatment of bacterial labyrinthitis requires systemic antibiotic therapy. If the inner ear infection occurred as a result of a middle ear infection, the middle ear may be need to be surgically drained. The doctor may also prescribe medicine to alleviate symptoms of dizziness.

What You Can Do

Once your doctor diagnoses an ear infection and prescribes treatment, you can help your child by

If your child has frequent ear infections, his doctor may suggest the insertion of a small drainage tube into the eardrum to allow fluid to drain.

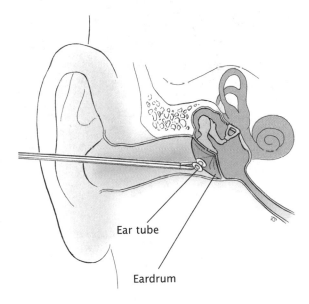

Ear tube

Eardrum

making sure he takes all his medication and then by making him as comfortable as possible. Fortunately, oral antibiotics generally provide pain relief within 12 to 24 hours.

- *Relieve the pain.* While you're waiting for the antibiotics to work, over-the-counter pain relievers can help alleviate the pain and reduce any fever that accompanies the infection. (For middle ear infections, the doctor may also recommend topical anesthetic eardrops unless your child has ear tubes or a hole in the eardrum. Don't use eardrops without first consulting your doctor.)

- *Warm the ear up.* Many children with ear infections find that a warm—not hot!—hot-water bottle held against the ear helps relieve the pain. Fill the bottle with warm water, wrap it in a dry towel, then have him hold it against his ear or lay his ear against the bottle while he rests in bed.

- *Keep the ear dry.* Be sure to keep your child's ear canal dry (except, of course, for any eardrops his doctor prescribes). Keep water, shampoo, hair spray, or bubble bath from getting into the ear until the infection clears. For external ear infections, place cotton in the ear and cover it with petroleum jelly to make a watertight seal whenever your child bathes or showers. Also, if your child has swimmer's ear, don't let him swim or submerge his head while bathing for 2 to 3 weeks until the infection is completely gone.

Prevention

Like the common cold and flu that often precede or exacerbate ear infections, the bacteria and viruses involved are common, so you probably cannot avoid the problem altogether. Check to be sure your child's immunization schedule is up to date (see p. 110). The pneumococcal vaccine will prevent some forms of bacterial middle ear infections (see p. 112). In addition, the following tips will help you reduce the chances that your child will be infected.

Preventing External Ear Infections

- Keep your child's ears as dry as possible during swimming by having him use earplugs.
- After he swims, dry your child's ears with a towel or hair dryer on a low setting.
- Ask your doctor about eardrops that may prevent swimmer's ear.
- Avoid using cotton swabs, bobby pins, or anything besides a soft, damp cloth to clean the ears.

Preventing Middle Ear Infections

- *Don't smoke around your child or let others do so.* Studies show that children of smokers have more colds and ear infections than children of nonsmokers.

- *Breast-feed your baby.* As your doctor may have told you, breast-feeding offers your child extra immunity against certain types of infections. Breast milk also contains a substance that appears to help prevent bacteria from sticking to the mucous membrane of the throat. If your child uses a bottle, don't let him fall asleep with it in his mouth.

Ear and Body Piercing Infections

Pierced ears are now a common sight among children of almost any age. Piercing of other body parts for decorative purposes has also become common among adolescents. When performed properly and maintained with care, pierced earlobes are a harmless decoration. But all piercing, including ear piercing, carries the risk of infection. Earlobes are usually safe for piercing when the procedure is done correctly; piercing other body parts, including the ear cartilage, is more likely to lead to infection and complications. Ear cartilage, for instance, has lower blood flow, and therefore bacteria cannot be flushed away easily to other parts of the body. The American Academy of Dermatology strongly recommends against piercing any part of the body other than the earlobe. If an infection occurs at the site of a piercing, you must act quickly to avoid unpleasant scarring, pain, and even the development of a creeping infection of deeper tissues called cellulitis.

Signs and Symptoms
- Redness, tenderness
- Tenderness or pain at the piercing site
- Yellow discharge
- Swelling of the earlobes or other pierced body tissue

When to Call the Doctor
CALL THE DOCTOR IMMEDIATELY IF
- the earring clasp becomes embedded in the skin and you can't remove it.
- there is severe pain at the pierced site.

CALL THE DOCTOR TODAY IF
- an unexplained fever occurs.
- the lymph node in front of or behind the earlobe swells.
- swelling or redness spreads beyond the pierced area.

Causes
The most common causes of infection are the use of unsterile equipment or posts or frequent touching of the pierced area with dirty hands. Another frequent cause is wearing earrings and body jewelry that are too tight because the posts are too short. Tight earrings and jewelry don't allow air to enter the channel through the earlobe, and the pressure reduces blood flow to the earlobe. Inexpensive posts sometimes have rough areas that scratch the channel and allow infection to enter. Posts containing nickel can also cause an itchy allergic reaction.

Piercing any part of the ear other than the lobe can lead to infection with complications and the need for surgical removal of infected tissue, possibly leaving the ear permanently disfigured. Do not pierce the cartilage of your child's ear. Ear cartilage infections are generally caused by bacteria different from and more difficult to treat than those that commonly cause earlobe infections. Cartilage has fewer blood vessels and therefore takes longer to heal. Pierced body parts other than the ear are less exposed to the air, are more likely to become infected, and take longer to heal.

What You Can Do

If your child has a tendency to bleed easily or form thick scars called keloids, or if she tends to get staphylococcus skin infections, such as frequent episodes of impetigo or boils, your best choice is to avoid piercing her ears, and discourage an older child from having any body piercing done.

If signs of infection appear, remove the jewelry and cleanse the post with rubbing alcohol. Swab the skin of the affected area with rubbing alcohol as well. See your doctor for treatment, and begin a program of regular cleaning with soap and water. Apply an over-the-counter antibiotic ointment. Continue using the antibiotic ointment for 2 days beyond the time the infection seems cleared. Most mild infections will clear up within 1 to 2 weeks. Remove the jewelry during the healing process.

What the Doctor May Do

If the infection doesn't clear up with home treatment, the doctor may have you remove the jewelry. He may prescribe a strong antibiotic cream or a course of oral antibiotics. In more severe cases, the doctor may need to remove infected tissues surgically.

Prevention

You can reduce your child's chances of infection by taking these steps:

- Do not have any part of your child's body pierced except the earlobe.
- Find a qualified jeweler or dermatologist who understands sterile techniques and uses only sterile equipment.
- Use jewelry with 14-karat (or higher) gold or stainless steel posts (at least at first).
- Do not remove the posts for 6 weeks after piercing.
- For the first couple of weeks after the piercing, clean both sides of the earlobes or other skin area with rubbing alcohol, then turn the posts three rotations at least twice a day.
- Refrain from touching the earrings or lobes, except when removing or inserting earrings.
- Wash your hands before touching the pierced area.
- Polish or discard any post with rough spots.

TATTOOING

Another method of body adornment that also poses the risk of infection is tattooing. Tattooing is the injection of permanent colors under the skin's surface. Even when performed by trained professionals, tattooing is dangerous and poses the risk of bacterial infection, as well as infection with **hepatitis** or HIV/AIDS (see **HIV/AIDS Infection**). Tattooing is permanent and not recommended for children.

Ear (Object Lodged in Ear)

Most parents enjoy their children's limitless curiosity, until it leads to trouble, like when a child puts an object in his ear just to see what happens! From time to time, various unexpected objects—especially small and round ones, such as seeds, beans, nuts, dried corn, raisins, beads, or small wads of paper—may find their way into a child's ear.

Fortunately, these objects are usually too large to get far into the ear canal, and you'll be able to remove them easily. If an object becomes deeply lodged in the canal, however, pain and irritation—even temporary hearing loss or eardrum damage—may result.

Signs and Symptoms

- Pain and itching around the ear
- Discharge from the ear
- Hearing loss
- Swelling of the ear

☎ *When to Call the Doctor*
CALL THE DOCTOR IMMEDIATELY IF
- an object is lodged in your child's ear canal.

Essential Facts

While most objects can be easily dislodged, an object that becomes trapped and goes unnoticed (e.g., a wad of tissue, a raisin) can cause bacterial infection. A bacterial infection may also develop if the walls of the ear canal are injured by a foreign object, exposing tissue to bacteria and fungi. With prompt attention, foreign objects rarely cause permanent damage to the ears or to hearing. Even when an object punctures an eardrum, the injury usually will heal spontaneously in 2 to 3 months or can be corrected surgically.

What the Doctor May Do

Your doctor will try using special instruments and a small suction apparatus to remove the object. If this technique fails, your doctor will probably recommend that your child see an ear, nose, and throat specialist, who will remove the object.

What You Can Do

If the object is visible and not lodged in the canal, you may be able to remove it at home. Be careful, however, not to push the object further into the ear canal as you attempt to remove it. Follow these steps:

- Have your child point the affected ear toward the floor.

- Grasp the top of the outer ear and pull up and out. This will straighten the ear canal.

- Have your child shake his head. The object should fall out.

- If the object remains in the ear, call your doctor right away.

Do not . . .

- try to remove the object with your fingers or with any pointed object. This may either push the object further into the ear canal or cause injury to the ear.

Prevention

The best thing you can do is to keep small objects out of your child's reach, and teach him never to put anything in his ear.

See also *Earache/Ear Infection.*

▪ *Epiglottitis*

Epiglottitis generally refers to an uncommon but serious bacterial infection of the epiglottis (the little flipper valve over the voice box). Epiglottitis occurs most often in children 2 to 4 years old. The infection requires immediate emergency treatment, because it can obstruct breathing.

Signs and Symptoms

- Gasping for air or severe difficulty breathing
- Drooling
- *Fever* (103–105°F) that may come on suddenly
- Irritability and restlessness
- Tilting the head forward, with the jaw pointed out, the mouth open, and the tongue protruding
- A severe sore throat
- Refusal to eat or drink

When to Call the Doctor
CALL FOR EMERGENCY HELP AND REFER TO *WHAT YOU CAN DO* BELOW IF

- your child sits with her head forward, mouth open, and tongue partly out and is having difficulty breathing.
- your child's skin turns pale or bluish gray.
- your child loses consciousness.

For first aid information, see page 380 if your child is less than 1 year old and page 383 if your child is 1 year of age or older.

CALL THE DOCTOR IMMEDIATELY IF

- your child is drooling, has a fever, and is refusing to drink.

Essential Facts

The symptoms of epiglottitis usually begin suddenly and include an extremely sore throat and a fever of 103°F or greater. A child with epiglottitis feels extremely sick and makes a harsh or raspy sound when she breathes in (stridor). She may sound as if she is choking, although an older child may still be able to talk, with difficulty. A child with epiglottitis will have problems speaking and swallowing and may drool. She may sit with her head forward, mouth open, and tongue partially out. Epiglottitis is most common from December to May. In rare cases, it may lead to complications, such as *pneumonia, meningitis,* arthritis, or fluid in the lungs. With treatment, your child will probably recover completely within 2 weeks. But because epiglottitis

can cause life-threatening respiratory distress and an inability to breathe and other life-threatening conditions, you should seek emergency treatment immediately if you notice the symptoms.

Causes

Haemophilus influenza type b (Hib) bacteria was the most common cause of epiglottitis before the Hib vaccine was required. Now, other bacteria, such as those that cause pneumonia, sometimes cause epiglottitis by infecting the epiglottis. When the epiglottis swells from an infection, it can block the windpipe and obstruct breathing.

Epiglottitis is generally caused by a serious bacterial infection of the epiglottis (the little flipper valve over the voice box). When the epiglottis swells from an infection, it can block the windpipe and obstruct breathing.

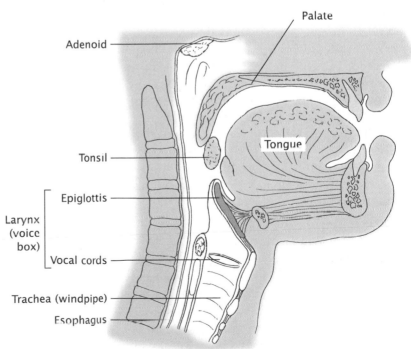

What the Doctor May Do

In the emergency room, every effort will be made to keep your child calm. Generally, no invasive or painful procedures are performed, as this might possibly cause the child to get upset and develop more obstructed breathing. If epiglottitis is considered a possible diagnosis and the child is clinically stable, an X ray of the child's neck will be taken in the emergency room to evaluate the epiglottis. If the X ray suggests epiglottitis, or if the child's breathing is so obstructed that there is no time for an X ray, the child will be taken to the operating room.

In the operating room, the child will undergo general anesthesia and then the airway will be evaluated. If epiglottitis is diagnosed, the doctors will insert a breathing tube into the child's trachea, usually through her mouth, bypassing the airway obstruction. The doctor will then take a culture of the epiglottis. In rare cases, when the breathing tube cannot be inserted because the swelling is too severe, the doctor may surgically create a temporary airway (tracheotomy). The breathing tube or temporary airway will be kept in until the swelling recedes, usually within 2 to 3 days. Usually, the doctor provides extra humidified oxygen through the tube or airway, especially during the acute phase of the infection.

To treat the infection, antibiotics are always given, usually for 10 days, first intravenously, and then orally. Family members may also receive antibiotics to help them avoid getting the infection.

What You Can Do

Epiglottitis is an acute emergency. If your child exhibits symptoms, stay calm and immediately call for emergency help. While you are waiting for the ambulance, encourage your child to breathe slowly and evenly and do your best to help her remain as calm and relaxed as possible.

Do not . . .

- try to look down your child's throat using a tongue depressor or other instrument.
- make your child move her head.
- try to open the airway with your finger.
- make your child vomit.
- insist that your child lie down.
- give your child food or water.

These actions could instantly block your child's airway. Instead, encourage your child to breathe slowly and evenly until the doctor sees her.

Prevention

One of the best ways to prevent epiglottitis is to be sure your child receives her Hib vaccine at her 2-month, 4-month, and 12- to 15-month checkups to help prevent infection with the bacteria that cause epiglottitis. Even if your child has been vaccinated, consult your doctor if she has been exposed to someone else with epiglottitis. The doctor may give her and all family members preventative antibiotics, because epiglottitis is transmitted by close contact.

To protect your child from the bacteria that cause epiglottitis, encourage frequent handwashing, and practice the other good hygiene methods described on page 366.

■ Eye Injuries

A child's eyes can be injured in countless ways—scratched by a speck of sand or bruised during active play. Fortunately, most such injuries are relatively minor and cause no lasting eye or vision damage. But about a third of the cases of child blindness are due to eye injury, so be sure to take safety precautions and respond quickly and correctly should an injury occur.

Signs and Symptoms

- A watery eye
- Pain, irritation, and redness
- Bruising around the eye or cheekbone
- Blurry or double vision
- A visible object or particle in the eye
- Sensitivity to light

When to Call the Doctor
CALL FOR EMERGENCY HELP IF

- the eye is out of its socket or appears displaced in the socket.
- the eye seems severely damaged by a sharp object or from trauma.

For first aid information, see Eye Injuries, page 407.

CALL THE DOCTOR IMMEDIATELY IF

- the pupils of the eyes are unequal in size.
- blood appears in the pigmented portion of the eye.
- an object becomes embedded in the eyeball or sits on the eye's surface.
- pain persists for more than one half hour.
- your child experiences blurry vision, loss of vision, or severe eye pain or tenderness, especially after an injury.
- your child cannot open his eye after an injury.
- the eyelid or eyeball is cut or scraped.
- toxic chemicals have touched the eye.

CALL THE DOCTOR TODAY IF

- your child persistently complains of light sensitivity.
- your child persistently complains of blurring or double vision.

Causes

- *Foreign bodies:* The most common cause of pain in a child's eye is the presence of an irri-tant, such as sand, grit, or dust. If something scratches the transparent membrane (conjunctiva) covering the inner surface of the eyelid and the white of the eyeball, blood may pool on the eye's surface. Grit or other matter can become embedded in the eyeball, damaging the cornea (the surface of the transparent membrane over the eyeball) and causing further pain and irritation. A scratch or a slight indent on the cornea may also feel as if there is something in the eye, especially when the eyelid moves over it. Toxic chemicals may cause pain if they splash in the eye.

- *Eyeball cuts or punctures:* These injuries are always serious; even small wounds can be a problem. Such injuries can damage all parts of the eye, including the cornea, the white of the eye (sclera), the retina (the rear portion of the eye that receives light rays), or other membranes.

- *Cuts on the eyelids:* The cuts may involve the eyelid margin (near the eyelashes) and the tear duct openings, which may require surgery. Such cuts can usually be repaired, if they are not too extensive.

- *Blunt force injuries:* Eye injuries can occur when an object, such as a ball or even an elbow, forcefully strikes a child's eye. Blunt blows to the eye can tear tissue or cause bleeding inside the eye, making the eyelid blacken and swell. The eye socket bones can be chipped or fractured. This type of injury may also affect your child's vision. If an injury damages the eye nerves as well, the lid may droop, and your child may not be able to raise or lower it.

What the Doctor May Do

In most cases, eye injuries heal by themselves or with the self-help measures described here. Nevertheless, be sure to ask your ophthalmologist or

Eyeball cuts or punctures can damage all parts of the eye, including the cornea, the sclera (the white of the eye), the retina (the rear portion of the eye that receives light rays), and other membranes. Fortunately, most such injuries are relatively minor and cause no lasting eye or vision damage.

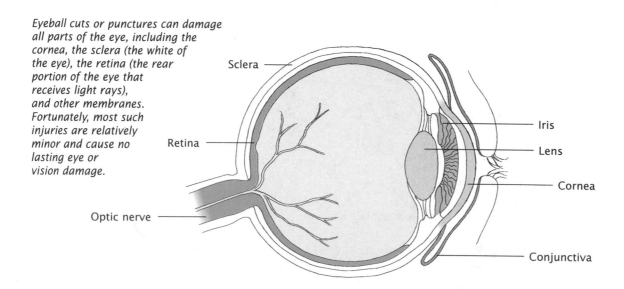

your child's doctor for advice whenever your child's eye is injured. Eye injuries that seem minor should be watched closely, because underlying injuries may not be obvious.

The doctor may prescribe antibiotic eyedrops or ointment to prevent infection, or she may recommend an eye patch if the cornea has been scratched. An eye patch will keep your child from constantly irritating the scratch by moving his eyelid across it. The doctor may also touch a paper strip with fluorescein (a type of temporary fluorescent dye) to the film of tears covering the eye, so that she can detect scratches on the cornea more easily. If there is an injury, tears will pool in the scratch or crater on the eye's surface, making the defect more noticeable. She may also rinse the eye, if she suspects the presence of a chemical or a foreign object.

In rare instances, your child may need surgery for the repair of lid, eyeball, or eye socket injuries. Internal bleeding in the eye may require close observation by a physician and hospital treatment—occasionally even surgery.

What You Can Do

If your child receives a serious cut or a blow to the eye, call for emergency help and see page 408 for emergency treatment information. For minor irritations, bumps, or blows, follow these suggestions. (Always wash your hands before touching the eye or eye area.)

- *Foreign objects:* If a speck of dust, an eyelash, or another tiny object has landed on the surface of your child's eye and he can open the eye, look for the object. If it doesn't appear to be embedded in the eyeball, try to wipe it away with a clean handkerchief or cotton swab. If that fails, flush the foreign object out by pouring a glass of water or eyewash across the open eye. See the illustration on page 559 for instructions on rinsing the eye.

- *Cuts:* Any cuts to the eyelid or eyeball require immediate medical attention. Cover the eye with a gauze pad, and go to an emergency room immediately.

- *Nontoxic irritants:* If your child gets soap in his eye, have him tilt his head over the sink so that the irritated eye is open nearest the sink, and pour a glass of water or two over the irritated eye. Alternatively, you can position him face up in the shower, allowing the water to pour over the open eye. You can also try splashing water into the open eyes. Call a poison center for advice if you are unsure of how a chemical can affect the eye.

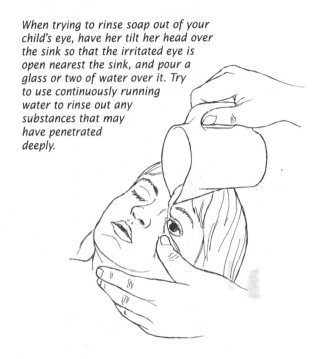

When trying to rinse soap out of your child's eye, have her tilt her head over the sink so that the irritated eye is open nearest the sink, and pour a glass or two of water over it. Try to use continuously running water to rinse out any substances that may have penetrated deeply.

- *Blunt force injuries:* If your child receives a severe blow to or near the eye, call your doctor for advice. If your child can easily open his eye, examine it carefully. Do you see blood coming from the eyeball itself? (Check to see if the blood in the eye is from an outside wound on the nose or forehead.) Are your child's pupils the same size in both eyes? Does he have blurry vision or feel nauseated? Is his eye sensitive to light? If not, and he is not in pain, chances are that no serious injury occurred. Your doctor may suggest the following tips to reduce the discomfort of bruising of the eyelids and the possibility of swelling:

  1. *Apply cold.* During the first 24 hours, use an ice pack or crushed ice wrapped in a towel. Never apply ice directly to the eye, as it could damage the delicate eyelid skin. Apply the cold pack every 5 to 10 minutes, for about 5 to 10 minutes each time, to shrink blood vessels and decrease bleeding into the surrounding tissue.

  2. *Switch to warm.* After about 48 hours, your doctor may have you apply a warm washcloth to the injury to avoid infections in the eyelids. By doing so, you may also help the body reabsorb blood.

Do not . . .
- touch or try to remove anything embedded in the eye.
- rub at any speck in the eye.
- apply ice directly to the eye.

Prevention

Your child's vision is precious. You can help protect your child against injuries with the following strategies:

- *Insist on protective eye gear.* Most eye injuries occur during physical activities such as basketball, baseball, swimming and pool sports, and racket and court sports. Make sure your child wears safety glasses or a helmet with a brim, or both, when playing sports involving a stick, a thrown or hit ball or puck, or close aggressive play (see Sport-by-Sport Safety, p. 275). Swimmers can protect their eyes with swim goggles.

- *Provide adequate supervision and instruction.* Discourage your child from playing with potentially dangerous items such as pencils, scissors, or knives. Even common household articles, such as paper clips, elastic cords, wire coat hangers, rubber bands, and fishhooks, can cause serious eye injury.

- *Select appropriate toys and games.* Don't let your child play with projectile toys, such as darts and bows and arrows, or air-powered rifles, pellet guns, or BB guns. These three types of guns, in particular, are so dangerous that the U.S. government reclassified them as firearms and banned them from toy departments. Various projectile toys still available in toy stores, such as suction-cup darts, may also pose risks; use your judgment when deciding what to allow your child. But soft toys, such as foam balls, are unlikely to cause harm.

- *Prohibit fireworks.* Never allow your child near fireworks. Bottle rockets, in particular, cause more than half of fireworks-related eye injuries.

- *Provide sunglasses with UV protection.* The harmful ultraviolet (UV) rays that can cause skin disorders may also burn the surface of the cornea, leading to eye damage. For this reason, children of all ages should wear sunglasses. The American Academy of Ophthalmology and the American Optometric Association both recommend wearing sunglasses that block out at least 99 percent of UV light. But even with sunglasses, your child should never look directly into the sun.

- *Keep chemicals out of reach.* Many household chemicals, including ammonia, the contents of spray cans, and cleaning fluids, can injure a child's eyes. Lock these products out of reach.

- *Beware of lawn-mowing accidents.* Lawn mowers can lift and throw pebbles and twigs that can hit your child in the face and eye. Keep children away when mowing. If you allow your older child to mow, you may want to consider having him wear protective eyewear.

Failure to Gain Weight

Everything about your child is unique, including her growth rate. Nevertheless, at your child's regular checkups your doctor will monitor your child's growth and weight gain in order to catch any nutrition or growth problems early. With early intervention, such problems needn't lead to long-term complications.

Signs and Symptoms

- Your child doesn't gain weight at a rate appropriate for her age
- Physical skills (rolling over, sitting, standing, and walking) develop slowly
- Your infant's length or child's height do not increase at the expected rate

When to Call the Doctor
CALL THE DOCTOR TODAY IF
- you are concerned about your child's weight, height, feeding, or overall development.

Essential Facts

At your child's regular checkups, your child's doctor will weigh and measure her length (or height for toddlers), weight, and head circumference. He will compare your child to normal standards (see Appendix: Growth Charts) and plot her growth rate. You needn't worry unless your child deviates significantly from her previous growth pattern, appears to stop growing, or is not gaining weight.

Most children who fall below normal growth standards have slow weight gain or are underweight. Children with poor weight gain typically are not getting enough nutrition to sustain normal growth, because of an underlying medical problem, feeding problems, or an inadequate diet. The problem usually becomes evident before 18 months of age. The outlook for children with poor weight gain depends on the underlying cause, the duration and severity of the problem, and the child's age at which the problem develops and is identified. The earlier the problem is diagnosed and treated, the better the outlook for complete recovery.

Causes

Usually when a child stops growing, it is due to a feeding problem that prevents her from getting enough calories. A fussy newborn may refuse to eat much, for example, or a sleepy infant may not be feeding frequently enough or long enough at each feeding. (For information on breast-feeding, see page 62. For information on bottle-feeding, see page 70.) Your child's doctor will monitor your child's growth pattern to make sure that, overall, she is gaining weight at a healthy rate.

Various problems can contribute to poor weight gain. An infant who is withdrawn, hypersensitive, or colicky (see *Colic*) is more likely to have trouble gaining weight. Also, anything that impairs the parents' response to their baby's emotional or physical needs, including health problems, depression, and stress, increases the risk of poor weight gain. Poor growth is also more likely if a parent is unprepared for or uneducated about child care responsibilities. Food struggles, which often emerge in the toddler years along with a child's independence, can also result in problems gaining weight. In rare cases, emotional deprivation can cause poor weight gain.

Chronic illness may also affect her growth and development. Diseases that lead to poor weight gain include malabsorption, a gastrointestinal disorder that interferes with food absorption; *cystic fibrosis*, which causes an inability to absorb nutrients; sickle-cell anemia, an inherited blood disease (see *Sickle-Cell Disease*); other chronic anemias (see *Anemia*);

recurrent infections; kidney disease; acquired heart disorders; congenital heart disease; and, in rare cases, hormone deficiencies, such as those caused by an underactive thyroid gland.

Physical problems, such as a severe nasal obstruction or a cleft palate (see *Cleft Lip/Cleft Palate*), may also cause difficulty in feeding and receiving adequate nutrition. Children with neurological conditions, such as *cerebral palsy*, or *developmental problems* may have difficulty with the actions required for eating, such as sucking, chewing, and swallowing. Other conditions that may result in a failure to gain weight include recurrent *vomiting, gastroesophageal reflux*, and a hyperactive or irritable temperament that makes feeding a child difficult. Chronic gastrointestinal diseases, such as celiac disease, ulcerative colitis, or Crohn's disease, can also cause failure to gain weight. The root of the problem may also lie in continuous use of certain medications intended for some inflammatory and autoimmune diseases.

What the Doctor May Do

If your child is having problems with weight gain, your doctor will first examine her and ask questions to try to find out when your child stopped gaining weight and why. He may also watch you feed your child to see how she reacts and how much she eats.

The doctor will conduct a detailed analysis of your child's diet to determine the total calories, amount of protein, and other essential nutrients. The first step in treating problems with weight involves meeting a child's nutritional needs. An underweight infant must get extra calories and adequate protein to catch up to the standard weight.

If your doctor is unsure why your baby isn't gaining weight, he may suggest a short hospital stay to further investigate various diagnoses. If an underlying medical or social problem is causing your baby's growth problems, your doctor will treat that condition or refer you to a specialist. You and your doctor will also need to discuss ways to improve your child's home feeding regimen.

If you have problems feeding your baby, the doctor may suggest that you participate in parent-child therapy designed to strengthen your feeding regimen with your baby or child. Typically, the therapist watches a parent and child interact during mealtimes, identifies problems, and offers the parent suggestions.

What You Can Do

First, try to relax. As long as you follow the doctor's advice about your child's growth, you can probably keep her on track. In the meantime, here are some tips to help your infant or child gain weight.

Helping a Baby Gain Weight

Here are some ways to help your baby gain weight.

- *Feed your baby at will.* Whenever your baby seems hungry or is willing to eat, feed her. Don't refrain from feeding her to stay on a schedule.

- *Focus on the feeding.* Make sure the room is quiet, and avoid distractions when giving your baby the bottle or breast. Turn off the TV and the telephone ringer. Find a comfortable chair and a footstool. Surround the chair with everything you might need: juice, water, books, munchies, and extra diapers. Try soft, calming music. Place a pillow behind your back. Take your time. Create a warm atmosphere for the feeding.

- *Sleep with your baby.* Breast-feeding during naps and at nighttime can help you further increase the frequency of feedings.

If your baby seems to fall asleep during feedings, you can try these tips:

- Undress your baby before feeding. Bundling and swaddling may encourage a sleepy baby to sleep through feedings. Undressing her allows skin-to-skin contact, and the cooler air may help stimulate her. Depending on the temperature of the room, you may loosely cover her with a blanket so that she isn't too cold.

- Burp her frequently. You'll want to do this each time her sucking diminishes and she starts to look sleepy.

- Rub the baby's forehead with a cool, yet not cold, washcloth.

- Change her diaper before feeding her or if she falls asleep during a feeding.

- If you are breast-feeding, switch her back and forth from one breast to the other to help keep her awake. Try to make sure that she feeds at least twice on each breast.

- Try, try again. After feeding your baby, keep her upright on your lap or in her infant seat instead of laying her down to sleep. Burp her, and then feed her again 10 to 20 minutes later.

Another important thing to remember is to avoid power struggles. As early as late infancy, from around 7 to 9 months, when solid foods are being introduced, your baby will begin to discover her independence and may refuse meals or want to feed herself. The best thing you can do is maintain a relaxed attitude. If she doesn't want to eat, pack up the meal and try again later. If she wants to feed herself, give her her own spoon, and continue to feed her with another spoon. Try as best as you can not to be unduly anxious about her intake.

For information on feeding infants, see pages 103, 126, and 161.

Do not . . .

- jiggle your infant or play active games with your baby after she eats. Allow the milk to settle in her stomach.

- reduce or replace feedings with a pacifier. Otherwise, your baby may get upset, expecting to find milk on the other end of the nipple, and have trouble eating next time.

- give your baby juice in a bottle. The sugar in the juice can depress the appetite.

- add extra water to formula or substitute water for formula to try to save money. Instead, ask your doctor about special programs that can help you buy formula for your baby. For more information on the Women, Infants and Children Program, see Appendix: Parent Resources, Financial/Medical Assistance.

Helping Your Child Gain Weight

For older children, use these tips to help them gain weight:

- Enrich calorie intake by serving high-calorie meals and snacks. Be sure to pack the most calories into every bite. For instance, top graham crackers with peanut butter. Add grated or melted cheese to vegetables and pasta. Finger foods are excellent for toddlers who enjoy the freedom of feeding themselves.

- Establish eating strategies that help form good eating habits (see the Feeding and Eating sections in the age-by-age chapters).

- Serve a midmorning and midafternoon snack, in addition to three meals, and if your child isn't interested in eating, or pushes the food away, give her permission to leave the table.

- Serve small portions, and allow your child to ask for seconds.

- Restrict eating and drinking to meal and snack times. Do not allow food or beverages, except water when thirsty, in between planned meal and snack times.

Do not . . .

- use food for rewards, punishment, or bribes. For example, dessert should not be withheld if your child refuses to "clean her plate."

HIGH-CALORIE FINGER FOODS FOR TODDLERS AND YOUNG CHILDREN

▌ Protein sources:
Cheese, cut into cubes or strips
String cheese
Lunch meats, cut into strips
Small meatballs made from ground beef, veal, or turkey
Breaded chicken nuggets
Fish sticks
Graham crackers or cookies topped with peanut butter

▌ Fruits:
Avocado slices
Banana slices
Papaya and mango slices
Pitted prunes

▌ Vegetables:
French-fried zucchini, mushrooms, or onion rings
Cooked pumpkin or squash cut in squares
Zucchini, pumpkin, or squash bread
Soft, cut-up vegetables, such as cucumbers dipped in sour cream

▌ Starches and grains:
French fries
Muffins, rolls
Wheat germ (add to cereals, salads, and yogurt or mix into cookie batter)
Granola (add to cookies, muffins, bread batters, yogurt, pudding, and ice cream)

HIGH-CALORIE TOPPINGS

Maximize caloric intake by adding these toppings to your child's favorite foods.

- Granola: Sprinkle into yogurt, pudding, and ice cream.
- Wheat germ: Add to cereals, salads, yogurt, and meat dishes.
- Mayonnaise: Use on salads, vegetables, and sandwiches. (It has twice as many calories as salad dressing.)
- Cheese: Add grated cheese or melted cheese to vegetables, fish, meats, eggs, pasta, rice, and sauces.
- Peanut butter: Spread on toast, bread, crackers, cookies, waffles, and fruits.
- Sour cream: Add to potatoes, beans, and squash. Use with salad dressing as a vegetable dip.
- Butter, margarine, oils: Add to soups, gravies, mashed potatoes, cooked cereals, rice, noodles, spaghetti, other pastas, and sauces.
- Powered instant breakfast: Add to drinking milk.
- Fortified milk: Use as a beverage replacing milk and substitute for water when making cooked cereals, soups, and instant cocoa.

Prevention

By feeding your baby whenever she seems hungry and by taking her to regular doctor checkups, you can reduce the likelihood that she will have problems gaining weight. Regular, relaxed and cheerful mealtimes without pressure to eat will encourage good nutrition.

See also **Short Stature.**

Fainting (Loss of Consciousness)

Fainting, or loss of consciousness, is uncommon in small children. But occasionally, a child may experience dizziness or a brief loss of consciousness because of factors ranging from injury to emotional upset, such as a reaction to the sight of blood. Fainting is generally a symptom of a harmless illness or upset. In rare cases, however, it may signal a more serious illness. So be sure to report any fainting episodes to your child's doctor.

Signs and Symptoms

- Dizziness
- Loss of consciousness
- Nausea or vomiting

When to Call the Doctor
CALL FOR EMERGENCY HELP IF

- your child loses consciousness for a prolonged period.

  For first aid information, see page 380 if your child is less than 1 year old and page 383 if your child is 1 year of age or older.

  CALL THE DOCTOR IMMEDIATELY IF

- your child faints and regains consciousness within seconds to a minute or so but doesn't seem right (lethargic, slurred speech, not thinking clearly, confused).

  CALL THE DOCTOR TODAY IF

- your child faints frequently or faints without an obvious cause.

Causes

Many causes of fainting exist, including a sudden high fever, a head injury, or any movement that reduces blood flow to the brain, such as standing too fast or exercising vigorously. Many children feel faint in response to certain triggers, such as an injury, extreme heat, an illness, or strong emotions. In extremely rare cases, a brain infection (such as encephalitis), heart disease, seizures, dysrhythmia (see **Abnormal Heart Rhythm**), or a brain tumor can cause fainting.

What the Doctor May Do

Unless your child faints frequently or has other symptoms, your doctor will simply tell you what to do in case of another spell. If another one occurs, she will probably examine your child and take a thorough history, especially noting the events precipitating the fainting spells (a fall or another physical trauma or an upsetting emotional event). Your doctor may take blood tests to rule out possible causes, such as infection. Or, she may refer your child to a cardiologist for a heart evaluation. An electrocardiogram (ECG), a test that measures the electrical impulses of the heart, may also be necessary.

If your doctor doesn't know why your child faints, she may have you consult a neurologist (a brain and nervous system specialist) for further evaluation. Sometimes, no cause for fainting will be found, and thus no treatment—except for learning how to cope with future spells—will be necessary.

What You Can Do

Monitor fainting spells, and consult your doctor when they occur. If your child becomes dizzy (see *Dizziness*), help him sit down and put his head between his knees, which will help the dizziness pass. A cold washcloth on his forehead may comfort him if he feels faint. Reassure him and have him rest for about 10 minutes after fainting or until he feels well.

Prevention

Often fainting cannot be prevented, especially if it happens suddenly. If your child knows the warning signs (dizziness, nausea, and sweating) and he places his head between his knees or lies down, he may avoid fainting. What may appear to be fainting can sometimes turn out to be an underlying seizure disorder or other neurological condition. Treatment of an underlying neurological or cardiac problem will often prevent further fainting.

▌ *Fever*

The first thing to understand about fever is that it is a sign of illness—not an illness itself. A fever is an increase in body temperature of at least 1 degree above normal. A fever is usually higher than 100°F but can be as low as 99°F, depending on the child's age. Most illnesses that cause fever are minor ones, but some are more serious and require medical attention. It may help you to think of fever as a warning signal that lets you know that your child's body is fighting an infection—usually bacterial or viral—and is therefore helpful. Unless the fever is high, long-lasting, or both, you treat a fever mainly to help your child feel better. Your child's doctor can evaluate whether to treat the underlying cause.

Signs and Symptoms

- Sweating, with hot, moist skin
- Elevated body temperature
- Flushed, warm appearance
- Often accompanied by lethargy, fatigue, loss of appetite, or chills

When to Call the Doctor
CALL THE DOCTOR IMMEDIATELY IF

- your infant under 6 months has a fever of 100.2°F or higher.
- your child over 6 months old has a fever of 102°F or higher.
- your child has a fever and is unusually drowsy, has a loss of mental alertness, labored breathing, a newly spreading rash, abdominal pain, joint pain, or any other symptoms.
- your child has a stiff neck, cannot bend her head forward, and complains of sensitivity to bright light (signs of a brain infection called meningitis).

(continues)

CALL THE DOCTOR TODAY IF

- your infant under 6 months has a fever.
- your toddler under 2 years old has a fever for more than 12 hours.
- your child over 2 years old has a fever that persists for more than 2 days.
- your child suffers from recurrent fevers without explanation.

Essential Facts

Normal body temperatures can range from 97 to 100.5°F, depending on the child. A child's normal body temperature can also fluctuate quite a bit throughout the day. Depending on the season, time of day, activity level, emotional state, and other factors, body temperature can vary by a degree or so in a healthy child. Body temperature usually peaks between 6 P.M. and 1 to 2 A.M. These fluctuations do not indicate fever (a sign that the body is fighting infection).

Most fevers in children are caused by mild, self-limiting viral infections and last only a few days. They range from about 100.4°F to 104°F or higher. For information on how to take your child's temperature, see page 352. Fever stimulates the immune system to destroy viruses and bacteria, and the higher body temperature also kills germs. Therefore you need to treat a fever only if your child is uncomfortable or the fever is high. Your doctor may recommend treating a fever with acetaminophen or ibuprofen if it is 101°F or higher to help your child feel better.

Fortunately, children generally handle fevers well. Fever may begin slowly or develop in a matter of hours. The speed with which it comes on and the height it reaches, however, do not necessarily indicate the seriousness of the underlying cause. Your child's fever may rise as her overall condition grows worse, then subside as she improves. Her fever may spike to a high point, or it may remain steady throughout the course of the illness.

Febrile Seizure

One potential complication of fever is a febrile seizure (see *Seizures*). The faster a fever rises, the more likely that a febrile seizure could develop. About 4 percent of children experience these usually harmless seizures with a high temperature (usually above 105°F) that begins suddenly or rises rapidly. They occur most often in children between the ages of 6 months and 3 years. A seizure may also accompany certain infections, including shigella, a bacterial infection from contaminated water or food that causes diarrhea. Ask your doctor for an evaluation if your child has a seizure, especially the first time, so that she can rule out any serious medical problems.

Causes

Many things cause fever—most often, a viral or bacterial infection. The causes can be divided into two kinds: acute (usually of short duration with a definite end) and chronic or recurrent (occurring repeatedly over time).

Causes of Acute Fevers

- Viral infections, such as colds, influenza, chicken pox (see *Colds/Flu*)
- Bacterial infections, such as earaches, urinary tract infections, *pneumonia*, meningitis, sepsis, and rickettsial disease (Rocky Mountain spotted fever)
- Poisoning (if a child inhales a hydrocarbon chemical, such as those in furniture oil or gasoline, a chemical pneumonia accompanied by fever may result)
- Heatstroke, in which a high, life-threatening fever occurs (see p. 412)
- Some antibiotics, antihistamines, and other medicines, which can produce fever as a side effect

Causes of Chronic Fevers

- Routine viral infections occurring in sequence (e.g., one common cold's following another)
- Chronic inflammatory diseases (e.g., *juvenile rheumatoid arthritis*)
- Chronic or relapsing infections, such as tuberculosis, malaria, or typhoid
- Endocrine gland disorders, such as hyperthyroidism (excessive secretion of thyroid hormone)
- Heritable conditions such as acute Mediterranean fever
- Cancers (see *Cancer*)

What You Can Do

When your child has a fever, be sure to take your child's temperature every 4 to 8 hours. Call the doctor according to the guidelines on page 565, and keep her quiet and calm. Give her plenty of fluids to avoid dehydration. Report any fever in an infant age 3 months or younger.

Encourage Your Child to Drink Fluids

Water and watered-down fruit juices are best, but as long as the beverage doesn't contain caffeine (which is a diuretic and will cause your child to lose fluids), let your child enjoy whatever quenches her thirst. Caffeine is an ingredient in many soft drinks, as well as coffee and tea. If your child suffers from vomiting and diarrhea at the same time as the fever, you can give her a pediatric rehydration solution, which you can purchase without a prescription, to restore proper mineral balance in the body.

Lower Your Child's Temperature

You needn't always reduce your child's fever. In fact, tracking the course of an illness by monitoring the pattern of the fever can be helpful. However, if the fever is making your child

---

UNDERSTANDING A FEVER OF UNKNOWN ORIGIN

Rarely, children develop persistent fevers for which a doctor cannot easily find an underlying cause. A fever designated as an FUO (fever of unknown origin) has three general characteristics:

- An elevation of more than 100.5°F, measured several times a day over several days
- A duration of 2 or 3 weeks
- A cause that remains unidentified even after investigation in a hospital or clinic

In most cases of an FUO, doctors eventually find an underlying cause. These causes fall into three broad categories: viral and bacterial infections (most common), autoimmune diseases such as lupus or juvenile rheumatoid arthritis (uncommon), or cancers (rare).

In children under 6 years old, the cause of an FUO is usually a viral or bacterial infection. For older children, an inflammation of connective tissue is more often the culprit. Your doctor will advise you on how to handle an FUO should your child develop one.

---

uncomfortable, you can try one or more of these methods of lowering a child's temperature.

- *Dress your child in light clothing.* Although your instinct may be to bundle up an ill child, this may be the wrong approach when it comes to fever. A diaper and a short-sleeved shirt for an infant or summer pajamas for an older child may be more comfortable.
- *Cool with a lukewarm sponge bath.* If a child's temperature remains above 103°F for more

than an hour, a lukewarm-water sponge bath for 15 to 20 minutes can help. Test the water first, as water that is too cold can cause your child to cry or shiver, which may drive up her fever. The water should feel comfortably warm. Have your child sit in navel-deep water, and use a washcloth to wash the water over the skin continuously. If the child begins to shiver, or her lips turn bluish, add warm water to the tub. After the bath, dry your child and dress her. Then, take your child's temperature again after 30 minutes. If the fever has not dropped by a degree or two, repeat the tub bath in an hour.

- *Give medication to reduce the fever.* If the fever does not begin to go down after you have cooled your child by removing clothing or giving her a sponge bath, give acetaminophen or ibuprofen according to the dosage instructions on the package. Your doctor may direct you to give your child one or another of these medications or to alternate them. Follow the dosage instructions on the package carefully.

Do not . . .

- give your child aspirin to reduce a fever unless the doctor specifically recommends it.

- use rubbing alcohol to reduce the fever. Alcohol can irritate the skin.

- attempt to "starve a fever." If your child is hungry, encourage her to eat and drink. The body uses more calories with higher temperatures, and she needs the energy to fight off infection.

What the Doctor May Do

If your child's doctor asks to see her, the doctor will try to determine the cause of the fever. Because fevers are symptoms of another illness or condition, reducing the fever won't cure the underlying cause. Be prepared to answer the following questions:

- How long has your child had a fever?

- How high is it now? How high has it been?

- Does the fever follow a particular pattern during the day?

- Does your child have any other signs or symptoms, including diarrhea, vomiting, coughing, or just not acting like herself?

In many cases, your health professional will reassure you that your child probably has a common viral infection that will resolve itself in a day or two and recommend acetaminophen, ibuprofen, or a sponge bath to lower the fever. If the doctor diagnoses a more serious underlying cause, he will take the appropriate steps, including medications and other treatments to treat the condition. Otherwise, he'll probably just advise you on keeping your child comfortable until the illness runs its course.

Prevention

You cannot completely prevent fevers or the infections that cause them, but you can reduce the frequency of infection by encouraging frequent hand-washing and practicing the good hygiene methods described on page 366.

▌ Fifth Disease

If your child has had a mild fever for several days when a bright red rash suddenly appears on his face, which looks as if someone has slapped his cheeks, fifth disease (erythema infectiosum) may be the cause.

Signs and Symptoms

- High fever for several days before the appearance of rash
- Bright red rash on both cheeks for 1 to 3 days followed by a pink, lacelike rash on arms and legs and sometimes a runny nose, fever, sore throat, headache, muscular aches and pains, and fatigue

When to Call the Doctor
CALL THE DOCTOR TODAY IF

- your child has a high fever.
- you notice the symptoms of fifth disease.
- your child develops a rash and is taking medication.

Essential Facts

Fifth disease is so named because it is was the fifth of several common childhood viral infections (including rubella, measles, chicken pox, and roseola) found to produce a rash and sometimes mild symptoms such as a fever. The facial rash, which is often followed by a lacelike pink rash on the arms and legs, may come and go for several weeks before it finally disappears with no treatment. Fifth disease is usually a minor but highly contagious illness.

Causes

Fifth disease is caused by a virus (Parvovirus B 19) that spreads from child to child by direct contact. The disease is no longer contagious when the rash appears (about 4 to 14 days after exposure). By the time you and your doctor realize that your child has fifth disease, your child may have exposed his entire play group to the disease. After 5 to 10 days, the rash fades, with the face clearing first, followed by the arms, and then the trunk and legs.

What You Can Do

Call your doctor to report the symptoms. If your child suffers uncomfortable symptoms, you can provide relief by giving him acetaminophen or ibuprofen to reduce his mild fever and a decongestant to relieve his stuffy nose, especially if congestion disrupts his sleep. Keep your child home until the fever and rash subside.

What the Doctor May Do

Although fifth disease is a minor illness that passes on its own with no need for treatment, its symptoms resemble other, more serious infections. So be sure to have a doctor confirm the diagnosis whenever possible. After you call your doctor, you may need to bring your child in for examination. Although the doctor can reassure you with this diagnosis, she can do nothing to shorten the course of the infection, which lasts a few weeks.

Prevention

You cannot completely protect your child from fifth disease, but encouraging frequent hand-washing and practicing the good hygiene methods described on page 366 will help protect your child from this illness and other infections.

Flat Feet

Slap, slap, slap. Anyone who has heard a baby walk barefoot knows this sound: It's the sound of little feet—feet without arches—hitting the floor. Both the noise and the flatness of the baby's feet are perfectly normal.

Signs and Symptoms

- The entire sole of the foot touches the floor when your child is standing or walking.

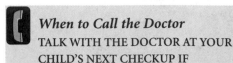

When to Call the Doctor
TALK WITH THE DOCTOR AT YOUR
CHILD'S NEXT CHECKUP IF

- your child appears flat-footed after several years of walking.
- your child experiences foot pain or muscle spasms.
- your child has difficulty walking or running.

Causes

All babies have flat feet, because they are born with a thick padding of fat on their soles. The padding starts to disappear when babies begin to walk. Walking strengthens and shapes the foot's tendons, ligaments, and bones to form an arch, and by 3 or 4 years old, the arch is fully formed. Sometimes, however, loose ligaments cause the front of the foot to turn outward and the feet to remain flat. Rarely, a child will have truly rigid flat feet and have trouble moving the feet up and down or from side to side. The cause is a structural abnormality and may require surgery.

Another congenital (present at birth) abnormality, called a vertical talus (anklebone), gives an infant rounded, rocker-bottom feet and also requires surgical correction.

What the Doctor May Do

Most small children's flat feet are normal and need no treatment. If your doctor thinks that your child's condition needs further evaluation, he may do an examination and take X rays to determine the extent and cause of the condition. Your child's doctor will observe your child's gait and examine her feet, checking their mobility and strength.

If the condition is severe and painful, the doctor may recommend techniques for repositioning the foot bones so that they can develop a normal arch, or he may refer your child to a physical therapist, who will prescribe walking exercises to help straighten the foot bones and strengthen and tighten the ligaments. Your child's doctor may recommend arch supports, but special shoes are rarely needed.

What You Can Do

In most cases, your child's feet will gradually develop a normal arch during her first few years of life. Otherwise, follow the instructions given by the doctor or the physical therapist.

Prevention

Flat feet cannot be prevented. For example, there are no particular types of shoes that a child can wear to prevent flat feet.

Food Poisoning

One of the most important things parents can do is protect their children from food poisoning, known medically as food-borne disease. When your child has diarrhea, vomiting, or general abdominal upset, don't assume that your child has the flu. Think about whether your child has recently eaten any food that might have been contaminated by inadequate cooking or refrigeration. Uncooked or partially cooked meats, poultry, and eggs (and products made with raw eggs) are among the most common sources of the bacteria that cause food poisoning.

Signs and Symptoms

- Nausea, *vomiting*
- *Diarrhea* (possibly bloody) or abdominal pain or cramps
- *Fever*
- Signs of *dehydration*, including cool, dry, pale skin; a dry tongue; thirst; a rapid pulse; and sunken eyes in infants

When to Call the Doctor

CALL FOR EMERGENCY HELP IF

- your child suddenly becomes weak, confused, or restless and is having difficulty breathing.
- your child shows signs of allergic shock (see p. 390).

For first aid information, see page 380 if your child is less than 1 year old and page 383 if your child is 1 year of age or older.

CALL THE DOCTOR IMMEDIATELY IF

- your child shows signs of dehydration.
- your child has severe diarrhea or is vomiting repeatedly.
- your child has bloody diarrhea.
- you have any reason to suspect that your child has consumed poisonous mushrooms or contaminated, infected, or spoiled food.

Essential Facts

Children are particularly susceptible to the wide array of food-borne illnesses caused by improper food handling. Although food poisoning usually passes relatively quickly without treatment, some cases are serious and life-threatening. Food poisoning is a major cause of pediatric illness. Public health officials attribute as many as 6.5 million cases of illness and 9,000 deaths annually in the United States to food-borne disease. The number of food poisoning cases may actually be five or six times higher than the number of reported cases, because food poisoning often goes unrecognized, masquerading as a common virus or stomach flu.

Causes

Food poisoning occurs after a person eats food contaminated by bacteria or other tiny organisms that cannot be seen, smelled, or tasted. The most common organisms that cause food poi-

soning are *Staphylococcus* and *Salmonella,* but more than a dozen others can cause disease.

Common Bacterial Causes

Staphylococcus aureus
- Incubation period: 1 to 6 hours
- Duration of illness: 1 to 3 days
- Sources: cooked meats and fish, cold foods, cream or custard fillings, dairy products, salads, vegetables, fruit
- Signs and symptoms: explosive diarrhea, severe abdominal pain, vomiting

Salmonella
- Incubation period: 5 to 72 hours
- Duration of illness: 2 to 5 days
- Sources: eggs, poultry, cheese, water, foods made with raw eggs, raw meats, or foods contaminated with fecal matter
- Signs and symptoms: fever, diarrhea (possibly bloody), nausea, vomiting, abdominal pain

Shigella
- Incubation period: 24 to 96 hours
- Duration of illness: 5 to 7 days
- Sources: water and food contaminated by fecal matter
- Signs and symptoms: high fever, diarrhea (possibly bloody), dehydration, severe abdominal pain, seizures

Clostridium perfringens
- Incubation period: 8 to 12 hours
- Duration of illness: 1 day
- Sources: cooked meats sitting at room temperature, stews, meat pies, dried foods
- Signs and symptoms: cramps, watery diarrhea, possible fever and vomiting

Campylobacter jejuni
- Incubation period: 48 to 120 hours
- Duration of illness: 4 to 7 days
- Sources: raw meat or poultry, raw milk, water
- Signs and symptoms: diarrhea (possibly bloody), abdominal pain, fever

Bacillus cereus
- Incubation period: 1 to 5 hours
- Duration of illness: 6 to 24 hours
- Sources: cooked or fried rice, cereals, dried foods, spices, herbs
- Signs and symptoms: abdominal cramps, nausea, vomiting

Bacillus cereus
- Incubation period: 8 to 16 hours
- Duration of illness: 12 to 24 hours
- Sources: puddings, meats
- Signs and symptoms: watery diarrhea

Listeria monocytogenes
- Incubation period: 1 to 70 days
- Duration of illness: variable
- Sources: raw milk, uncooked meats, pâté, shellfish, cheese, coleslaw
- Signs and symptoms: flulike illness, meningitis, stillbirth

Escherichia coli 0157:H7
- Incubation period: 3 to 4 days
- Duration of illness: less than 7 days
- Sources: contaminated meats, raw milk, unpasteurized apple cider, roast beef, salami, salad dressing
- Signs and symptoms: bloody diarrhea, abdominal cramps, headache, nausea, vomiting, renal failure, anemia

Escherichia coli (traveler's diarrhea)
- Incubation period: 12 to 72 hours
- Duration of illness: 1 to 3 days
- Sources: many raw foods, salads, meats
- Signs and symptoms: abdominal pain, cramps, watery diarrhea, weakness

Vibrio parahaemolyticus
- Incubation period: 12 to 24 hours
- Duration of illness: 48 hours
- Sources: raw or undercooked shellfish (including crabs, oysters, clams, and shrimp)
- Signs and symptoms: watery diarrhea, cramps, vomiting

Common Nonbacterial Causes

Hepatitis A
- Incubation period: 3 to 6 weeks
- Duration of illness: variable
- Sources: shellfish, including mussels, oysters, and clams; contaminated, unwashed soft fruits (fresh or frozen berries); water
- Signs and symptoms: mild diarrhea, weakness, jaundice, liver disease

Giardia
- Incubation period: 1 to 3 weeks
- Duration of illness: 3 to 6 weeks
- Sources: contaminated water from streams or lakes, foods containing contaminated water
- Signs and symptoms: greasy diarrhea, flatulence, bloating

Cryptosporidium
- Incubation period: 6 days
- Duration of illness: 6 days
- Sources: water, cider
- Signs and symptoms: diarrhea, weakness, vomiting

Three Common Types of Seafood Poisoning

Scombroid Poisoning
- Duration: 3 to 4 days
- Source: flesh of spoiled fish of the scombroid species (bluefish, tuna)
- Signs and symptoms: flushing, feeling of warmth, nausea, vomiting, headache

Ciguatera Poisoning
- Duration: complications may last from weeks to months
- Source: spoiled reef fish (jade, snapper, barracuda, dolphin)
- Signs and symptoms: headache, dizziness, changed sensations of hot and cold, memory loss, paralysis, coma

Paralytic Shellfish Poisoning (PSP)
- Duration: 3 to 4 days
- Source: contaminating toxin, known as "red tide," which filters through shellfish beds (clams and mussels)
- Signs and symptoms: weakness, headache, paralysis or even coma

IS IT THE MAYONNAISE?

If you're like most Americans, you've been told since childhood that mayonnaise can cause food poisoning. The truth is, commercially prepared mayonnaise— any mayonnaise that you buy in a jar from the store— is usually safe. The real danger lies in homemade mayonnaise made with contaminated raw eggs. Common picnic foods such as egg salad and chicken salad can pose a risk, not because of mayonnaise, but because the poultry or eggs contain bacteria, which multiply when left unrefrigerated for too long. Pack these foods in coolers with ice packs for up to 2 hours, and don't remove them until it's time to eat.

What the Doctor May Do

If you suspect food poisoning, call your doctor immediately. She'll ask what symptoms your child is experiencing, what foods he has eaten recently, and where they were obtained, and if anyone else who has eaten the same food feels ill. Laboratory tests to identify a specific toxin or organism are complicated, but sometimes needed.

While botulism and mushroom poisoning are medical emergencies and frequently require hospitalization, most other forms of food poisoning resolve themselves within a few hours or days. If your child is dehydrated because of severe vomiting and diarrhea, the doctor will suggest fluid replacement with rehydration solutions. If the condition is severe, hospitalization and intravenous fluids may be necessary. Rarely,

and only if the doctor identifies the specific bacteria involved, she may prescribe an antibiotic to resolve the infection more quickly. Antibiotics usually do not help cure the illness, because most food poisoning is due to the toxins produced in the food by the bacteria.

What You Can Do

If your child suddenly begins to vomit or experience severe diarrhea, watch his condition carefully for signs of dehydration. Infants tend to become dehydrated faster than older children, and at all ages, dehydration is more likely to develop when vomiting and diarrhea occur together. If your infant or child doesn't urinate at least three times a day, show tears when crying, and have a moist mouth, call the doctor or poison control center.

Once a doctor or poison control center has advised you about your child's condition, the best thing you can do for him is to try to keep him comfortable. Here are some tips to help you do so:

- *Guard against dehydration.* If your child is hungry, allow him to eat, but actively encourage him to drink fluids, at least several sips of water or a rehydration solution every hour.

- *Reintroduce food slowly.* As soon as he starts to feel better, offer small meals of bland food for the first 24 to 48 hours after symptoms abate. Soups, yogurt, and nonfatty foods are easiest to digest.

- *Consult your doctor about testing suspicious food.* Your doctor may test the food that may have made your child ill. If it was commercially prepared and is found to contain harmful bacteria, contact the local health department.

Prevention

The best way to protect your family from food-borne diseases is to practice good hygiene and cooking practices.

Cleanliness Is the Key

- Wash your hands thoroughly before preparing food.

- Prepare meats and poultry with care by first rinsing them thoroughly, then washing your hands again with soap and water before continuing with food preparation.

- Keep raw meats and their juices far from other foods in the refrigerator and on counter tops.

- Use smooth cutting boards made of hard maple or plastic and free of cracks and crevices. These kinds of boards can be cleaned easily. Avoid boards made of soft, porous materials. Wash cutting boards with hot water, soap, and a scrub brush to remove food particles. Then sanitize the boards by putting them through the automatic dishwasher or rinsing them in a solution of 1 teaspoon of chlorine bleach in 1 quart of water. Consider using one cutting board only for foods that will be cooked (such as raw fish) and another only for ready-to-eat foods (such as bread, fresh fruit and vegetables, and cooked meat, poultry, and fish).

- Always wash and sanitize utensils after using them for raw foods.

- Wear gloves if you have a cut or scrape on your hand.

- Wash and rinse your hands and equipment frequently during preparation and cooking.

- Wash kitchen sponges frequently in a solution of hot water and bleach, or put them through a cycle in the dishwasher regularly. Replace them often.

- Avoid preparing food when you are sick, particularly if you have nausea, vomiting, abdominal cramps, or diarrhea. Or, if you must prepare food for your family, wash your hands thoroughly with soap before and after handling food.

Cook and Store Foods with Care

- Always refrigerate prepared foods within 2 hours. Don't allow these foods to cool to room temperature. Slow cooling and incomplete heating give *Salmonella* bacteria time to multiply.

- Heat food thoroughly before serving it.

- Cook thawed meat and poultry immediately. Make sure to thoroughly cook food. Use a meat thermometer for large cuts of meat, pork, roasts, or turkeys. The Food and Drug Administration (FDA) suggests cooking until the center of the meat cut or roast reaches the following temperatures:
  Beef: 165°F
  Pork: 160°F
  Whole poultry: 180°F
  Poultry breasts: 170°F
  Ground chicken or ground turkey: 165°F

To make sure seafood is well cooked, follow these suggestions:

- *Fish fillets and fish steaks:* Slip the point of a sharp knife into the cooked fish and pull aside. Make sure the edges are opaque and the center slightly translucent, with flakes beginning to separate.

- *Shrimp, scallops, and lobster:* Check the color. Shrimp and lobster turn red, and the flesh becomes pearly opaque when cooked. Scallops turn milky white or opaque and firm.

- *Clams, mussels, and oysters:* Cook until the moment their shells open. That means they're done. Throw out those that stay closed.

- *Stuffed poultry:* Stuff raw poultry just before cooking it. Better yet, cook your poultry and stuffing separately. Store leftover stuffing in a separate container in the refrigerator.

- *Marinades:* Marinate raw meat and poultry in the refrigerator, not on the counter. Don't baste your food with or serve marinade that has been in contact with the raw meat unless you cook it first: Otherwise, if the meat was contaminated, the marinade will be, too.

- *Eggs:* Buy only refrigerated eggs. Keep them refrigerated until you are ready to cook and scramble them. Cook eggs thoroughly until both the yolk and white are firm—not runny—and cook scrambled eggs until no liquid is visible. Use cooked recipes for hollandaise and similar sauces, and do not eat raw eggs or serve food with raw eggs in it, such as homemade eggnog, Caesar salad dressing, or mayonnaise. Cook egg dishes or casseroles with eggs to an internal temperature of 160°F. Don't eat or allow your children to eat uncooked cookie, cake, or brownie batter containing raw eggs.

- *Refrigerator storage:* Make sure your refrigerator temperature is 40°F (5°C) or lower, and that your freezer is 0°F (−18°C) or lower.

- *Freezer storage:* Store raw ground meats in the freezer for no more than 3 to 4 months; cooked meats for a maximum of 2 to 3 months.

Choose What Your Children Eat with Care

Guard against food-borne diseases by avoiding certain high-risk items.

- Never purchase or serve foods from damaged, dented, or cracked containers.

- Do not serve unpasteurized milk, milk products, juices, or ciders.

- Do not serve rare meats. Hamburger should be cooked all the way through.

- Do not give honey to a baby under 1 year old.

- Warn your child never to sample even a small part of any wild mushroom or other fungus, no matter how harmless it appears.

- Always buy shellfish from reputable, well-known dealers, and never go clamming or shellfish harvesting on beaches or tidal flats closed because of a red-tide warning. If you have any doubts about the area, call the local Coast Guard or health department.

- Check food labels for "Use by," "Sell by," or "Best if used by" dates, and do not buy the product beyond this date. Once you purchase a product, make it your goal to use it by that date.

- Only buy frozen foods that are frozen solid and show no signs of product leakage. Leakage could indicate that the product has been thawed in the past.

- Take fresh meats, poultry, and fish—as well as all frozen food—home as soon as possible. Do not store the food in the car while you do other shopping.

- Don't purchase raw, pre-stuffed turkeys or chickens. Stuff poultry immediately before cooking, or cook the stuffing in a separate container outside the bird.

See also *Abdominal Pain/Stomachache.*

Fractures

See page 409.

Gastroesophageal Reflux

Infants often spit up small amounts of breast milk or formula after a feeding. This is quite normal in most babies. But spitting up or vomiting large amounts, as well as crying frequently after feedings, may be signs of reflux. Reflux is frequent regurgitation. Stomach acid in the regurgitated food can cause a baby so much pain that she cries most of the time and has trouble sleeping. In many infants, reflux goes away as the child grows and the muscles develop. In the meantime, you may be able to relieve your infant's reflux with some simple home remedies, like holding the baby upright after a feeding. If reflux is severe, the baby must see a doctor.

Signs and Symptoms

- *Vomiting* and/or spitting up regularly during or after feedings
- Choking, gagging, coughing during or after feedings
- Extreme fussiness, especially after feedings
- In babies, arching the back during or after feedings
- In older children, abdominal pain or "heartburn"

When severe:
- *Failure to gain weight* or grow normally, or trouble breathing

When to Call the Doctor
CALL THE DOCTOR IMMEDIATELY IF
- your child vomits blood.
- your child appears to be having trouble breathing.

CALL THE DOCTOR TODAY IF
- your baby vomits forcefully after every feeding, or the amount of vomit increases.

TALK WITH THE DOCTOR AT YOUR CHILD'S NEXT CHECKUP IF
- your baby spits up and/or vomits often and doesn't seem to be gaining weight.
- your baby consistently fusses after feedings, especially when lying on her back.

Essential Facts

Gastroesophageal reflux is the backward flow of the stomach contents into the esophagus, the tube that connects the throat to the stomach. In

Gastroesophageal reflux is the backward flow of the stomach contents into the esophagus, the tube that connects the throat to the stomach. Usually, a weakness or malfunctioning of the sphincter muscle between the esophagus and stomach is the cause of gastroesophageal reflux.

Esophagus

Diaphragm

Stomach

Small intestine

about 85 percent of affected babies, symptoms appear in the first week of life. The problem gradually diminishes over time, starting to improve at about 4 to 6 months of age, and is usually completely gone by 2 years of age.

Because the fluid that a baby spits up or vomits is highly acidic, it may irritate the esophagus, causing considerable pain. The pain makes the baby cry more than average and, unfortunately for household members, sleep less. In rare cases, a baby with reflux may also have apnea spells (see *Infantile Apnea*), when she stops breathing for several seconds. Apnea may be caused by the stomach contents' coming up and obstructing the airways.

When reflux is severe, babies vomit so much that they don't gain weight or grow properly (see *Failure to Gain Weight*). Other complications include increased risk of respiratory infections, especially middle ear infections (see *Earache/Ear Infection*) and aspiration pneumonia (see *Pneumonia*).

Causes

Usually, a weakness or malfunctioning of the sphincter muscle between the esophagus and stomach is the cause of gastroesophageal reflux. Normally, when children (as well as adults) eat or drink, this sphincter opens to let food pass into the stomach, then closes to keep the food down. With reflux, however, food and liquids flow back into the esophagus, throat, and often—when a baby is involved—out onto her bib or your shoulder.

The weakness of the sphincter is usually caused by an immaturity of the gastrointestinal tract, but a weak sphincter can be made even weaker by other factors, such as overfeeding, which puts undo pressure on it. Lying a baby down after a feeding, which most new parents do, can also increase the chance of reflux, because gravity can't help keep food down in this position. Reflux usually diminishes as the

upper intestinal tract develops and the baby spends more time upright.

What the Doctor May Do

Because most infants with reflux have no other symptoms of disease (such as irritability or growth problems), medical tests are usually unnecessary. But if a baby has severe symptoms or possible complications from reflux, the doctor may perform certain tests, such as X rays or blood tests, to detect physical abnormalities. To treat reflux, some doctors recommend feeding babies formula thickened with infant cereal, because thick food tends to stay down better. In addition, some medicines are used to treat reflux, including antacids and drugs that reduce the time it takes for food (including breast milk or formula) to leave the child's stomach. If reflux is severe, the doctor may suggest surgery to help the stomach stay closed after a feeding.

What You Can Do

Finding ways to alleviate reflux may take time, but these methods often help:

- *Avoid the slump.* Instead of placing your baby upright in an infant seat after feeding, ask your doctor about lying her on her stomach at a 20 to 30 percent incline with her head up. This position causes the stomach to fall forward, helping the sphincter to shut. You can keep your baby in this position by raising the head of her mattress. (One way to do this is by placing books or receiving blankets underneath it. Don't put your baby on a pillow, which can cause suffocation.) If your baby cries when lying on her stomach, try holding her upright. Don't allow your baby to sleep in this position, because it increases the risk of *sudden infant death syndrome.*

- *Try smaller, more frequent feedings.* Many children have an easier time keeping down small meals. But when you cut back on the size of the meals, you'll have to increase their frequency so that your baby gets enough to eat.

Prevention

Often, reflux cannot be prevented. But you may lessen or prevent mild cases by following the suggestions above.

See also *Abdominal Pain/Stomachache; Colic.*

German Measles

See *Rubella.*

Growing Pains

"Dad, my legs hurt. I can't sleep." Has your child awakened you in the middle of the night complaining of leg pain? You may even remember from your own childhood the achy feeling you experienced, mostly at night when you were just going to sleep. Your parents probably told you that they were just "growing pains." These are indeed normal, temporary pains in the limbs and joints of children mainly from 6 to 12 years of age. Often, the pains are not true growing pains but simply caused by overexertion after a busy day of physical activity.

Signs and Symptoms

- Aches and pains in thighs, calves, feet, or arms when the child is at rest
- Stiffness
- No sign of other illness

When to Call the Doctor
CALL THE DOCTOR TODAY IF
- the pain is constant, increasingly severe, or affects one leg only.
- your child recently experienced an injury.
- fever or swelling in the affected limb accompanies the pain.

Essential Facts

Most growing pains occur in a child's thighs, calves, and feet, but they can develop in any part of the body. Unlike other joint or muscle pains, your child may feel growing pains mostly when he is resting. Usually, growing pains aren't severe enough to interfere with your child's normal activities. Though they're not dangerous by themselves, growing pains can increase the risk of sports injuries. So be sure that your child stretches and warms up before playing organized sports to help prevent injuries.

Causes

True growing pains occur when your child is going through a growth spurt, and his muscles and bones are growing at slightly different rates, resulting in an achy soreness. Most of the time, however, the pains your child complains of are really the result of muscle fatigue caused by vigorous exercise. This fatigue occurs because your child's muscles have not yet completely developed and are vulnerable to strain.

What the Doctor May Do

In many cases, your child won't need to see the doctor. But if the pains persist, the doctor will probably examine your child to rule out potential causes of his pain, including influenza, sprains, fractures, or other injuries, as well as more serious conditions, such as arthritis or osteomyelitis (an uncommon bacterial bone infection). Sometimes, the doctor will order X rays to look for signs of injury or other causes of pain. Neither true growing pains nor the mild aches and pains caused by overexertion require medical treatment other than over-the-counter pain medications.

What You Can Do

Although growing pains are normal, they can be uncomfortable. Here are some tips to help your child feel better:

- *Relieve the pain.* Age- and weight-appropriate doses of acetaminophen or ibuprofen will ease muscle and joint discomfort.
- *Try home remedies.* Massaging the affected area can reduce the aching. Heat from a warm bath, a hot water bottle, or a heating pad can also provide relief. If using a heating pad, wrap it in a towel so that it doesn't burn your child's skin.
- *Encourage your child to stretch.* Gentle stretching exercises before exercise can help prevent muscle strain.

Prevention

Good physical health, regular exercise, and stretching before vigorous activity and sports can prevent muscle fatigue and the pains associated with it, but you cannot entirely prevent growing pains or the muscle aches and pains caused by physical activity.

See also **Back Pain; Joint Pain.**

▌ *Hand-Foot-and-Mouth Disease (Coxsackie)*

A child who complains of a sore mouth or throat or who has difficulty eating because of mouth pain may have the common childhood viral infection sometimes known as hand-foot and mouth disease. This usually mild but highly contagious virus, called the Coxsackie virus (after the town in upstate New York where doctors first identified it), usually affects children 6 months to 4 years of age. Its unusual name, "hand-foot-and-mouth disease," derives from the parts of the body where small blisters appear. Outbreaks are more common in the summer and fall.

Signs and Symptoms

- Small, painful ulcers in the mouth
- Small water blisters or red spots on the palms of the hands and soles of the feet, and between fingers and toes
- Low-grade *fever*

 When to Call the Doctor
CALL THE DOCTOR TODAY IF
- your child has the symptoms of hand-foot-and-mouth disease.
- the fever lasts for more than 3 days.
- the mouth pain becomes severe or it interferes with eating and drinking.

Essential Facts

This illness usually begins with a moderate fever followed by small, round blisters that develop inside the mouth and on the palms and the soles. The blisters may also appear between the fingers and toes. In about 1 to 2 days, the blisters begin to break, leaving shallow sores. These blisters and sores can make eating painful. Some children also develop a reddish rash of raised dots, usually on the buttocks. The red dots turn white briefly when you press them. The illness can last about 2 weeks.

What the Doctor May Do

Your doctor will probably be able to diagnose this common viral infection just by examining the blisters. But, as with most viruses, no cure or treatment for Coxsackie disease exists. The doctor will give you advice, however, on how to make your child more comfortable until the virus runs its course.

What You Can Do

Chances are, this mild disease won't hold your child back any more than the average cold would, which means she can attend day care or school once she feels well enough. However, if she is uncomfortable, follow these tips to help her feel better:

- *Offer soft, bland foods.* Tomato sauces and citrus, salty, and spicy foods are likely to irritate mouth sores. Since chewing may hurt your child, offer her soft foods—soups, pasta, mashed potatoes—and plenty of fluids. She'll probably enjoy cold drinks, sherbet, and ice pops, too.

- *Bring down the fever.* If a fever is running your child down, give her acetaminophen or ibuprofen and keep her home for a few days.

Prevention

The Coxsackie virus is common and hard to prevent, but you can reduce your child's chances of contracting this and other infections by encouraging frequent hand-washing and practicing the other good hygiene methods described on page 366.

See also *Canker Sores; Rashes; Sore Throat/Strep Throat.*

■ *Head Lice*

Oh no! Not another head lice warning. Any parent with a child in day care or school is likely to receive occasional written notification that head lice have been discovered on one or more of your child's peers. As unattractive and unlikely as it sounds, any child—including your own—can become infested with head lice. Fortunately, a lice infestation doesn't cause any harm and can be treated at home. Your child can return to school after the first treatment.

Signs and Symptoms
- Intense itching of the scalp
- Tiny, white eggs covering the hair roots

When to Call the Doctor
CALL THE DOCTOR TODAY IF
- home treatment doesn't work.
- your child has lice or nits in his eyebrows or lashes.

Essential Facts

Lice are tiny parasitic insects that attach themselves to human skin and hair, sucking the blood of their hosts for nourishment. As they feed, they inject their own salivary juices and digestive matter into the skin, which causes the intense itching that is the hallmark of a lice infestation. Head lice can become an epidemic in schools, camps, and other places where children congregate. Because they are so easy to acquire from even brief contact with children or their belongings, head lice can infest even the cleanest, well-groomed child with short hair!

Head lice have wingless, flat, translucent bodies that become dark brown when engorged with blood. They are visible to the naked eye, but are difficult to locate. Adult female lice have life spans of about 1 month, and each lays up to four or five eggs daily. The eggs, called nits, attach to the root of the hair until they hatch in about a week. At that point, the newly hatched lice bite the scalp to get blood.

Causes

Your child may get head lice through direct contact with an infested person: The insects cannot hop, jump, or fly. Children may unwittingly spread head lice by sharing hats, clothing, combs, and hairbrushes. Head lice may also be transmitted when children lie on infested sofas, carpeting, or bedding.

What You Can Do

First, if you find nits or lice in your child's hair, keep him home from school or day care until you have treated the infestation—and inform the school authorities, as well as other groups that your child may be involved with (such as Sunday school, scouts, and sports teams, as well as friends and their parents) of the infestation so that other children can be checked and treated. Ask the school nurse or day care director when your child can return. Then ask your doctor or pharmacist to recommend a shampoo for removing lice.

Follow the directions for use of the shampoo closely. Usually, head lice treatment is a two-step process: First use the louse-killing shampoo or lotion. Then remove the nits by combing the hair with a special fine-toothed comb made especially for nits. But because the nits are so close to the scalp, you may not be able to get all the nits out of your child's hair. Before combing, you can apply a special preparation that will help

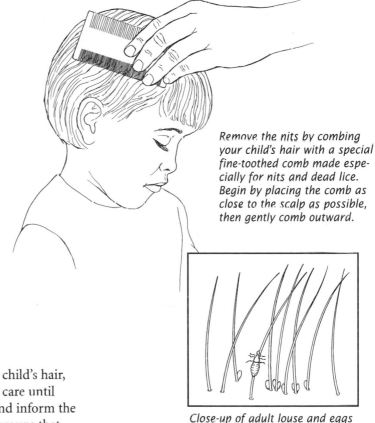

Remove the nits by combing your child's hair with a special fine-toothed comb made especially for nits and dead lice. Begin by placing the comb as close to the scalp as possible, then gently comb outward.

Close-up of adult louse and eggs (nits) on hair.

loosen the nits from the hair. If you follow the directions with care, these products are safe for both children and infants. In addition, you can also use cream rinses and/or a half-and-half solution of water and white vinegar to remove the dead lice from your child's hair strands. It is unnecessary to cut your child's hair.

Other alternatives recommended by some doctors and other health professionals are petroleum jelly or mayonnaise shampoo. Cover the hair thickly with petroleum jelly or mayonnaise, making sure every strand is coated, and cover the child's head with a shower cap. Leave it in place for several hours. If you leave it on overnight, remove the shower cap, which can be a suffocation hazard. Put a towel over the pillow case. The petroleum jelly or mayonnaise deprives the lice of oxygen, literally asphyxiating them. Shampoo your child's hair thoroughly. It may take several days of shampooing to remove all residues of petroleum jelly. Mayonnaise will shampoo out more easily.

In addition to applying treatment, always follow these tips to prevent other family members from becoming infested and your child from reinfestation:

- Soak combs and hairbrushes in louse shampoo for an hour or in water heated to 150°F (66°C) for 5 to 10 minutes.
- Launder clothing (particularly hats) and bed linen in hot, soapy water, or have them dry-cleaned.
- Vacuum rugs, upholstered furniture, and mattresses to dispose of any living lice or nits attached to fallen hairs.
- Examine other people who have had close physical contact with an infected person. Treat them if infested.

Do not . . .

- allow your child to share combs or head coverings, such as scarves or hats.
- leave any lice medication around where a child can reach and swallow it.
- use medications repeatedly without your doctor's advice. You can overdo it.
- get overanxious.
- stigmatize head lice. The condition is not at all caused by poor parenting or poor hygiene.

What the Doctor May Do

If home treatment fails, your doctor may prescribe another type or strength of shampoo. In some cases, the lice still do not go away. If they don't, your doctor may prescribe a stronger dose of permethrin than sold over-the-counter, to be used on the child's scalp overnight. There are reports that several strains of lice have developed resistance to permethrin, so if it doesn't work, your doctor may prescribe malathion or lindane, both of which have proved highly effective in killing lice and nits. There is some question surrounding the safety of chemical treatments, particularly that of malathion and lindane, which are potent insecticides that can be absorbed through the skin and mucous membranes. Malathion and lindane in particular may have long-term, as yet unknown neurotoxic effects. Talk to your doctor about the potential risks of any of these treatments, and if you decide to use one of them, be sure to follow your doctor's instructions for use precisely. Serious adverse effects of these products have been associated with misuses such as ingestion, excessive doses, or prolonged or repeated application.

If your child has nits in his eyelashes or eyebrows, the doctor will remove them with tweezers or a tiny comb, and show you how to do so at home if necessary.

Prevention

Do not use medicated shampoos to prevent head lice. The shampoos do not prevent head lice but only kill the lice that have already infested a child's hair. Even keeping hair clean does not protect against head lice. The only preventative measure you can take is to discourage your child from sharing hats, combs, and other objects or clothing that touch the head.

For more information, see the National Pediculosis Society, listed in Appendix: Parent Resources, Medical Conditions.

Headaches

"I've got a headache" is not an expression reserved for adults. Children also experience headaches. Usually, children have headaches related to mild infections like a cold or the flu, but some children experience severe headaches, most often due to migraines. Although most headaches are harmless, contact your doctor before attempting home remedies; some headaches are symptoms of serious conditions requiring medical attention.

Signs and Symptoms

- Aching or throbbing pains in the head, neck, or both
- Nausea and *vomiting* (occasionally)

When to Call the Doctor
CALL THE DOCTOR IMMEDIATELY IF

- a fever, vomiting, or a stiff neck accompanies the headache.
- a headache has occurred after a fall, a motor vehicle accident, or another trauma.
- the headache is so severe that your child cries, clutches her head, or has to lie down.
- the headache is rapidly progressing.
- your child has slurred speech or double vision.
- one eye pupil is larger than the other.
- your child is vomiting with considerable force (projectile vomiting).
- your child is confused or is not acting normally.
- your child is difficult to wake up.
- your child wakes up with a severe headache.
- the headache is accompanied by weakness in an arm or a leg.
- the headache is accompanied by your child's complaints of unusual smells, slurred speech, or visual difficulties (loss of vision, double vision).

CALL THE DOCTOR TODAY IF

- your child's headache is severe or prolonged.
- your child also has symptoms of infection, such as a fever or sore throat.
- your child frequently experiences headaches.
- the headache lasts more than 24 hours, even with acetaminophen or ibuprofen.

Essential Facts

Generally speaking, a headache is pain that occurs when certain nerves (pain fibers) located in the muscles, blood vessels, and other structures of the head become irritated. Tension headaches, for example, occur when stress causes neck and temple muscles to contract, which irritates the pain fibers.

Headaches usually affect children over 5 years old, but toddlers and infants may also experience them. About 40 percent of children get at least one headache by 7 years of age. Headaches in children usually result from mild, uncomplicated conditions.

Causes

Headaches may be classified into three categories according to their cause:

Disease- or Injury-Related

In infants and small children, a headache is usually a symptom related to a common condition, such as a cold, an ear infection, a sinus infection, or strep throat. Headaches also occur with fever, which causes blood vessels within the skull to enlarge temporarily. A headache will often accompany a blow to the head as the result of a fall or a sports injury.

Children with hemophilia or other clotting abnormalities may be at an increased risk for bleeding from blood vessels surrounding the brain under the tissues lining it (the dura). This subdural hemorrhage—which can pose a life-threatening emergency—may also accompany head injury following a trauma.

In rare cases, the headache is caused by a disease, such as encephalitis (an inflammation, usually an infection, of the brain) or a brain tumor (see *Cancer*).

Migraine

A migraine is another common type of headache. Migraines affect 4 to 10 percent of elementary school students. In most cases, migraines first occur in late childhood and early adolescence, but the condition has been diagnosed in children as young as 2 years old. No one knows what causes migraines, but they often run in families. Certain emotional and physical factors, including stress, missed meals, certain foods (especially chocolate and cheese), and head injuries, may trigger a migraine.

In childhood, a migraine is characterized by repeated attacks of a throbbing headache, loss of appetite, nausea, vomiting, and *dizziness.* Migraine attacks can occur anywhere from several times per week to several times per year, and the severity and duration of each may vary. Some attacks are accompanied by more severe symptoms, such as visual problems and vomiting, which can persist for a day or two. Children may be irritable, lethargic, pale, withdrawn, or dizzy during the attack. In some cases, children experience "auras," in which they feel different or strange, hear sounds, or have visual changes in one or both eyes, such as blind spots, brilliant flashes, or blurriness. These symptoms may precede the onset of a migraine.

For some children with migraines, a headache is not the most prominent symptom. Instead, these youngsters experience recurrent nausea and vomiting, abdominal pain, or vertigo, lasting minutes, hours, or even days. If a headache is a factor in these situations, it usually develops between attacks instead of during them.

Tension or Stress Headaches

Tension-related headaches due to nervous tension or stress (also known as psychogenic headaches) are uncommon in young children, who tend to develop stomachaches in response to anxiety instead.

What You Can Do

Most children's headaches pass within an hour or two and are no cause for alarm. If your child's headaches recur, follow these tips:

- *Try to determine the cause.* Did your child bump her head recently? Is she feverish? Look for uncommon triggers as well, such as sudden exposure to sunlight or allergic reactions to pets or other substances. If your child has recurrent headaches, the doctor may suggest that you maintain a calendar to track your child's diet, schedule, environmental exposures, and headaches to see if a particular food, mood, or activity precipitates headaches.

- *Keep track of what your child eats.* Caffeine, chocolate, cheese, the monosodium glutamate (MSG) in Chinese food, and peanuts are the most common food triggers of headaches. This is not a food allergy, but a chemical reaction in the blood vessels of the head that produces headaches. If your child's headaches occur after eating a particular food, help her avoid the food.

- *Make your child comfortable.* If fever and headache symptoms are present, reduce the fever and treat headache pain with acetaminophen or ibuprofen. If your child's nose is stuffed up, ask your doctor about using nasal spray or antihistamines. Have your child rest in a quiet room with the lights off and shades drawn, because noise and light can exacerbate headaches.

What the Doctor May Do

If your child's condition is severe or persistent enough to warrant a trip to the doctor, your doctor will examine your child, paying special attention to possible contributing factors, such as an ear infection or a cold. If the headache is severe and your child has a fever, the doctor will probably order special laboratory tests such as a blood culture or a lumbar (spinal puncture) to rule out a brain infection such as **meningitis** or encephalitis.

If a bacterial infection is involved, he may prescribe antibiotics. For simple headaches, the doctor will recommend bed rest and pain relievers such as acetaminophen or ibuprofen to reduce the pain.

If the doctor suspects a migraine headache, he will try to track down precipitating factors, such as certain foods, for your child to avoid. Most cases of migraine in children can be treated with acetaminophen or ibuprofen, given as early as possible when the headache develops. Occasionally, prescription drugs made specifically for migraine headaches may be necessary to alleviate the pain. If the headaches are frequent and severe, your child's doctor may prescribe daily use of preventative medication. For older children, behavioral modification methods, such as relaxation techniques including biofeedback, in which a child learns to control the pain with imaging techniques, are often helpful.

If a progressive headache follows a head injury, your doctor may order a computerized tomography (CT) or magnetic resonance imaging (MRI) scan of the brain to rule out bleeding and increased pressure. If this bleeding exists, a neurosurgical evaluation will determine whether pressure from the collection of blood needs to be relieved by a surgical evacuation of the blood.

Prevention

Often, headaches cannot be prevented, but most will go away when the underlying problem, such as a sinus infection or the flu, is resolved. Some

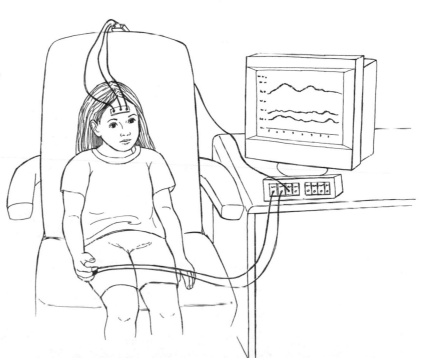

Biofeedback, in which an older child learns to control pain with imaging techniques, is often helpful for migraine headaches.

headaches that result from stress or lack of sleep or food may be prevented with early intervention. Protect your children from head injury by keeping them securely strapped into car seats, strollers, high chairs, or changing tables. Have older children wear appropriate protective headgear during sports.

Hearing Loss

Many children experience temporary hearing loss related to middle ear infections. In fact, 90 percent of temporary hearing loss involves inflammation of the middle ear. Normal hearing usually returns when the infection clears up. However, some children have permanent hearing loss unrelated to ear infections. The loss can be congenital (present at birth) or acquired. With care and attention, most children with permanent hearing loss can develop normal speech, language, learning, and social skills. Be alert to signs of hearing loss in your child so that any problems can be diagnosed and treated early.

Signs and Symptoms

For an infant under 6 months:
- Doesn't startle or turn head to noise
- Not responsive to parent's voice
- Doesn't turn toward sounds

For an infant over six months or an older child
- Doesn't turn to the sound of his name
- Speech and language delay in a toddler or an older child
- Frequent ear infections and draining ears
- Seems inattentive at day care or school
- Does not follow directions
- Has school problems
- Teacher describes child as "in his own world" or a "daydreamer"
- Withdraws socially from play with other children

When to Call the Doctor

CALL THE DOCTOR TODAY IF
- your infant seems inattentive to your voice or other sounds.
- you suspect that your child has a hearing problem.

TALK WITH THE DOCTOR AT YOUR CHILD'S NEXT CHECKUP IF
- your child has had one or more ear infections in the past year.

Essential Facts

A child's first hearing screening is often conducted before the age of 6 months, and in many states, it is a mandatory test given before a newborn leaves the hospital. For older children, hearing problems are sometimes discovered during a standard hearing test at school. (For ways to informally test your infant's hearing at home, see p. 98.)

Hearing loss results when the ear has deficits in hearing the range of pitches (high to low sounds), the range of intensities (loud to soft sounds), or both. Sounds travel in ripples (waves), much like the ripples created by dropping a stone in a body of water. These ripples have a pitch (frequency) and an intensity (loudness measured in decibels). When a ripple reaches a normal ear, the external ear captures it in much the way that a satellite antenna dish captures radio waves. The ripple then passes down the ear canal until it reaches the eardrum—a thin membrane separating the external ear from the middle ear—causing it to vibrate. In turn, the eardrum vibrations cause three tiny bones in the middle ear to vibrate. The inner ear membrane, which separates the middle ear from the inner ear, picks up these vibrations and passes them to the inner ear. Highly specialized structures in the inner ear convert the vibrations into electrical impulses that are sent via a special nerve to the brain, which completes the process by interpreting the impulses as sound. This entire process takes a fraction of a second.

Two main types of hearing problems exist:

- *Conductive hearing loss,* which refers to a condition in which a part of the external or middle ear malfunctions and interferes with a sound ripple's journey to the inner ear, is the most common type of hearing loss.

- *Sensorineural hearing loss* involves a malfunction of the inner ear, the nervous system, or the brain. In this case, the sound ripple may proceed normally, but something is wrong with the system that converts and interprets it. Sensorineural hearing loss is much less common, more severe, and more difficult to treat. Sensorineural hearing loss is generally not reversible.

Hearing loss of either type may be mild, moderate, severe, or profound. In four out of five cases of conductive hearing loss, the problem affects both ears. Most cases of hearing loss are conductive and are mild or moderate. A child with normal hearing can hear sounds in the 0 to 20 decibel hearing level (dBHL) range.

- *Mild hearing loss* (21 to 40 dBHL) affects a child's ability to hear soft sounds. If your child has already learned to speak, his speech is likely to be normal or nearly normal and his ability to converse is relatively unhindered. If the loss occurs before or while he's learning to speak, speech and language may be hindered, and he may need speech and language therapy.

- *Moderate hearing loss* (41 to 55 dBHL) significantly affects a child's ability to participate in conversations. Such children often do well with hearing aids and speech therapy and can usually attend a regular school with hearing children.

- *Severe hearing loss* (56 to 90 dBHL) makes normal conversation impossible and the learning of spoken language difficult. A child affected with severe hearing loss often can discern some words and detect some loud noises. These children can be helped by speech and language therapy and the use of hearing aids and may do well to attend a school for the deaf that has an emphasis on oral language.

- *Profound hearing loss* (90 or more dBHL) in both ears prevents a child from hearing most sounds, including normal speech. Retaining or acquiring useful spoken language is extremely difficult and often impossible. A child who learns to speak before becoming deaf may be able to retain his understanding of language, but speech is likely to be affected. A child who becomes deaf before learning to speak won't be able to acquire normal language or speech. Exposure to sign language at home or school or attendance at a school for the deaf that emphasizes sign language may be appropriate. The use of cochlear implants (see p. 588), developed recently, can increase the likelihood that children with profound hearing loss in both ears will develop spoken language.

Causes

Conductive hearing loss is common, and most often is caused by middle ear infection (see *Earache/Ear Infection*). Other causes of conductive hearing loss (including the accumulation of earwax in the ear canal or obstruction of the ear canal by an object, such as a piece of food or a button that the child has placed in his ear) are temporary, and the hearing will come back if the earwax or object is removed. Conductive hearing loss caused by a congenital structural abnormality is usually permanent.

Sensorineural hearing loss is often congenital, although it may occur after birth. It is caused by factors such as a specific malformation of the inner ear, diseases such as meningitis, a head injury, or inherited conditions. In up to half of the cases of sensorineural hearing loss, the cause is uncertain or unknown. In very rare cases, a viral infection during infancy can cause sensorineural hearing loss in a child, although many viral causes of such hearing loss are now prevented by vaccines (for mumps, measles, and rubella). The most commonly identified viral cause of sensorineural hearing loss in infants is cytomegalovirus (see p. 12), which causes hearing loss only if the fetus is exposed to the virus during pregnancy.

Permanent damage to the inner ear can also be caused by infections such as bacterial ***meningitis*** (inflammation of the protective covering of the brain and spinal cord) and German measles (see ***Rubella***). Exposure to extremely loud sounds—either once or over a prolonged period—can lead to temporary or even permanent sensorineural hearing problems.

What the Doctor May Do

The doctor will first examine your child's ears for signs of fluid, earwax, ear canal abnormalities, or an object that may have become lodged there. If the doctor suspects a hearing loss, she may send your child to an audiologist (who determines the extent and type of hearing impairment) or to an otolaryngologist (an ear, nose, and throat specialist) for a complete examination of the ears and upper respiratory tract. If the hearing loss is caused by a temporary medical problem, the specialist provides appropriate treatment, such as removing any earwax or the object that might be causing an obstruction or prescribing antibiotics for an ear infection.

If conductive hearing loss is due to fluid buildup in the middle ear, the doctor may prescribe antibiotics and recommend that you have your child's hearing retested in a few weeks to see if the condition improves. If your child's hearing shows no improvement within 3 months, the doctor may suggest inserting ventilating tubes surgically into the eardrum (see p. 550) to clear the middle ear fluid. If the conductive hearing loss is due to malformation of the outer or middle ear, a hearing aid may improve hearing to normal or near-normal levels. Your doctor may also suggest reconstructive surgery when your child is older.

Treatment for sensorineural hearing loss is more limited. Surgical treatment is not usually an option and won't restore normal hearing. But hearing aids and other assistive listening devices can help greatly and can be used in children of all ages—even newborns, depending upon the degree of hearing loss. A hearing aid will often "boost" hearing into the useful speech range. For children with profound hearing loss in both ears, a relatively new option is the implantation of an electronic device called a cochlear implant into the inner ear. The implant will provide a sensation of sound, which together with intensive speech and language therapy will provide increased environmental awareness (the ability to hear a doorbell, a telephone ring, or the child's name when called out). The combination of implants and therapy may also enable the child to develop spoken language.

A child with a significant hearing impairment—no matter what the cause—will probably require special help in learning to communicate, whether or not he uses a hearing aid or has an implant. Some, but not all, children with hearing impairments can learn to speak clearly with the help of appropriate speech therapy. Other communication techniques are also available and include lip-reading, sign language, and writing, which are often used in combination by children and adults with significant hearing loss.

What You Can Do

- *Treat all ear infections promptly.* By treating ear infections quickly, you may avoid or reduce the duration of the temporary hearing loss associated with middle ear inflammation. Be sure to treat ear infections in a child with a permanent hearing impairment, because inflammation and middle ear fluid accumulation can aggravate existing hearing problems.

- *Detect and treat hearing loss at an early age.* Report any suspicions of hearing problems you have to your child's doctor, and ask for a full hearing screening.

- *Learn to communicate with your child on his terms.* If your child learns sign language, make sure that you and your family learn this method as well so that you can communicate with him, teach him, and help him feel loved and accepted.

- *Be an advocate for your child's education.* By federal law, your school system must provide special education to hearing-impaired children. If you feel that your child needs extra help, speak to the director of special education or the principal, guidance counselor, or school administrator. Be persistent, and don't give up! You are your child's best advocate.

- *Encourage your hearing-impaired child to participate in his world.* There's no reason for children with hearing problems to isolate themselves from the hearing world around them. Make sure that your child uses his hearing aids or other assistive devices if recommended, gets speech therapy if needed, and is treated like the normal child—albeit with a hearing loss—that he is!

Prevention

While many cases of hearing loss cannot be prevented, you can help prevent some kinds of hearing loss.

- Help prevent hearing loss due to injury by teaching your child to never put anything in his ears—even cotton swabs—and to always wear seat belts in the car and proper headgear while playing sports or riding a bike.

- If you are pregnant, you can help prevent some forms of hearing loss by adhering to the healthy living guidelines in Chapter 1, including avoiding alcohol and drugs during pregnancy and protecting yourself from certain infections.

- Have your child vaccinated according to the current guidelines for immunizations (see p. 110).

- Avoid exposure to loud noises. Cumulative exposure to high-decibel noises, including lawn mowers, power tools, and amplified music, can gradually lead to hearing loss. Wear protective earphones. A single exposure to a very loud sound, such as a firecracker or a gunshot, can also cause permanent hearing loss.

■ *Heart Murmur*

Thanks to television medical shows and the experience of listening to our own heartbeats, most people know what a normal, regular heartbeat sounds like. When someone has a heart murmur, however, the heart has an extra sound. Most heart murmurs are normal and harmless (the medical term is "innocent"). They are simply extra sounds produced by the heart as blood is pumped through its chambers from the veins to the arteries.

Signs and Symptoms

- Usually none; murmurs are detected by physicians during routine exams

Essential Facts

Heart murmurs are common among children. More than half of newborns have a heart murmur sometime during their first 48 hours, and about 50 to 60 percent of children in the United States have a heart murmur at some point during their childhood. Most children who experience heart murmurs have structurally normal hearts, and the murmur has no adverse effects on health or the child's ability to participate in exercise. In a very small percentage of children with heart murmurs, however, extra heart sounds may signal structural heart disease.

Causes

Innocent heart murmurs are produced by vibrations caused by blood flowing normally through the heart chambers and blood vessels. Your doctor will usually be able to determine whether a murmur is innocent. Any conditions that increase normal heart rate, such as a fever and exercise, can increase the intensity of a heart murmur.

In some cases, the murmur may be related to a congenital heart defect, such as a narrowing of the blood vessels, defective or diseased heart valves, and abnormal openings in the heart wall or in a blood vessel near the heart. If a child has an infection that affects the heart (including infective endocarditis, rheumatic fever, or myocarditis), heart murmurs may develop. *Anemia* may also cause heart murmurs.

Different types of murmurs make different sounds (whistling, cooing, musical, high-pitched, rumbling). The murmur may occur between the "lub" and "dub" of the normal heartbeat, or it may occur before the "lub" or after the "dub." Where it occurs can offer the physician a clue as to the cause of the murmur.

What the Doctor May Do

Your doctor is most likely to detect your child's heart murmur during a routine examination.

Instead of hearing the heart make its normal "lub-dub" sound, he will hear other sounds, sometimes described as a buzzing, a rumbling, or a sound like the vibration of a tuning fork. If the abnormal sound indicates a potentially serious heart condition, the doctor will order other tests, such as electrocardiography (which electronically records the heart's actions) or echocardiography (which uses sound waves to form a picture of the internal structures of the heart and associated blood vessels). Rarely, cardiac catheterization (in which a thin, plastic sensor tube is guided through the veins to the heart) may be used to allow the cardiologist to make a precise diagnosis.

Children with innocent heart murmurs need no treatment. Treatment of other kinds of heart murmurs will depend on the underlying cause. Heart valve problems or congenital defects require evaluation by a cardiologist and possibly a surgical correction.

What You Can Do

Relax. If your child has an innocent heart murmur, she has a perfectly normal heart and requires no special treatment. You don't need to pamper her or restrict her diet or activities. When filling out health forms for schools, camp, or dentists, write "innocent heart murmur: no heart disease found," in the section under heart if your child has an innocent heart murmur. If your child has a structural heart defect, you will need to follow up according to your child's cardiologist. However, most children with cardiac problems can still lead full and active lives.

■ *Heat Rash (Prickly Heat)*

They don't call it heat rash for nothing. This faint red rash appears when your child gets overheated and sweats. It develops where his sweat glands are most numerous—around the face, neck, and shoulders, and in skin creases, such as the elbows, the groin, and behind the knees. It's a common and harmless rash that will clear up on its own or with a little help.

Signs and Symptoms

- Faint red rash over the face, neck, and shoulders or in the creases of the elbows, groin, and knees
- Small, pink or red bumps or water blisters
- Flushed, hot appearance

When to Call the Doctor
CALL THE DOCTOR TODAY IF
- the heat rash is very itchy.
- the heat rash appears infected.
- the heat rash gets worse or you have questions.

Essential Facts

A heat rash, also called prickly heat or a summer rash, consists of hundreds of tiny, pinhead-sized eruptions that may look like small, pink or red bumps or like tiny water blisters. Each bump extends from a skin pore and can be fairly itchy.

Causes

A heat rash is not due to exposure to sunlight but rather occurs when the body becomes overheated and the sweat glands become blocked. It often appears when children are sweating heavily, such as during hot, humid days or when the child has a fever. The skin may become further irritated by perspiration.

What the Doctor May Do

No medical treatment is necessary for heat rash, but call your doctor and describe the rash and its onset. That way she can rule out other possible causes of your child's condition. If the heat rash is very itchy, the doctor may recommend a mild

antihistamine to reduce the itchiness. If the rash is infected, a topical or an oral antibiotic may be necessary.

What You Can Do

Help your child feel better right away by cooling him down. Bathe him in lukewarm water, then pat him dry to remove most of the moisture. Allow the rest to evaporate, which will cool his skin. Dress him in comfortable, cool clothing.

Do not . . .

- use bubble baths, harsh detergents, or fabric softeners in your baby's laundry or oily lotions on your baby's skin while the rash persists: They tend to aggravate the condition.

Prevention

More than likely, your child will experience at least a couple of episodes of heat rash no matter how careful you are. Nevertheless, the following tips will reduce the chances:

- Keep the temperature in your child's room cool. Keep air flowing with a fan or by opening a window slightly.
- Don't overdress your child in hot weather.
- Make cotton the first layer. Don't put wool or synthetic fibers directly next to your child's skin.

See also **Rashes.**

Hemophilia

Hemophilia is a serious inherited bleeding disorder in which a child's blood doesn't have enough of a protein that helps blood to clot. Children and adults with this lifelong condition bleed longer than other people because their blood does not clot normally to stop the bleeding. The severity of the disease depends on whether the clotting factor deficiency is mild, moderate, or severe. There is no cure for hemophilia, but the condition can be managed and children with this condition can live a relatively normal life with some restrictions on physical activities that might cause injury or bleeding.

Signs and Symptoms

- In infants, unusual bleeding after circumcision
- Prolonged bleeding from a cut or wound
- Unusually large, dark bruises
- Bruises that swell and become painful
- Joint pain, tenderness, swelling
- Blood in the urine
- Prolonged nosebleeds
- Prolonged bleeding after dental work

When to Call the Doctor
CALL FOR EMERGENCY HELP IF

- your child has experienced a severe injury (such as a motor vehicle accident or fall).
- your child loses consciousness or shows signs of shock (dizziness, confusion, or rapid pulse—see p. 418).

For first aid information, see page 380 if your child is less than 1 year old and page 383 if your child is 1 year of age or older.

IF YOUR CHILD HAS HEMOPHILIA, CALL THE DOCTOR TODAY FOR ANY OF THE FOLLOWING:

- Pain, tenderness, swelling of the joints or extremities
- Paleness, weakness, or sudden sweating
- Irritability that lasts more than a few hours
- Unusually large, dark bruises
- A hard lump under the skin
- Complaints of a pulled muscle
- Numbness
- Inability or unwillingness to move a joint or limb
- Unusual headaches
- Abdominal pain
- Any accident involving the head, even if the child doesn't complain or cry

Causes and Essential Facts

Hemophilia runs in families and occurs in 1 in every 10,000 births. Hemophilia A (factor VIII deficiency) is the most common form of the disease and is inherited mainly by boys from the mother, who carries a gene for the disease on her X chromosome. It is called a sex-linked trait because the X chromosome is one of two sex chromosomes. Women have two X chromosomes, whereas men have one X and one Y. A woman who has one X chromosome with the hemophilia gene and one without will not have the disease but can pass it on to her children. Because boys have only one X chromosome, they can have the disease if they receive an X chromosome with the hemophilia gene. Girls can get the disease only rarely, such as in the unusual situation where the father has hemophilia and the mother carries the hemophilia gene on her X chromosomes. Occasionally, parents with no family history of the disease give birth to a child with hemophilia.

Two other kinds of blood factor deficiencies are hemophilia B and von Willebrand disease. Hemophilia B, also called Christmas disease or factor IX deficiency, accounts for about 15 percent of hemophilia cases and affects the body in much the same way as hemophilia A. Von Willebrand disease is about twice as common as hemophilia A and is caused by a deficiency of a different protein integral to factor VIII. It occurs in both boys and girls and is usually a relatively mild condition.

Minor cuts and scrapes on the skin of a person with hemophilia are not a significant problem. But internal bleeding, sometimes caused by a bump or a blow during physical activity or sometimes with no apparent cause, can lead to swelling in joints and organs, with resulting damage to those joints or organs or even death if not quickly treated with infusions of blood-clotting factor. Babies who have hemophilia usually experience no serious effects until they begin crawling, climbing, and walking, at which point they may develop large, swollen bruises. Before they reach toddlerhood, however, circumcision may also produce prolonged bleeding.

Other complications of hemophilia include abdominal bleeding, chronic arthritis and joint damage, brain hemorrhage, and blood-transmitted diseases acquired during transfusions, such as *hepatitis* or *HIV/AIDS infection.*

What the Doctor May Do

In addition to looking for the signs and symptoms of hemophilia (listed above), the doctor will inquire about a family history of the disease and order a blood test to see how well the blood clots. If the clot test is abnormal, the amounts of different clotting factors are measured to confirm the diagnosis and to identify the subtype of hemophilia. By identifying the subtype of hemophilia, the doctor will know which type of clotting factor to use as treatment if serious bleeding occurs.

Treatment for hemophilia involves caring for minor injuries, cuts, and scrapes at home as well as giving intravenous blood-clotting factor for more serious bleeding episodes. Your doctor can prescribe a blood-clotting factor that can be administered intravenously by health care professionals at the hospital or at home by a parent or an older child trained in the procedure. Early treatment of bleeding episodes is most effective. Deep muscle bleeding often requires follow-up treatment and observation by the doctor. Slings, splints, or crutches may help immobilize the joint for several days.

Children with hemophilia need to avoid aspirin, ibuprofen, and other drugs that tend to prevent blood from clotting. Acetaminophen is a good alternative for at-home pain relief.

What You Can Do

Parents of a child with hemophilia can help the child avoid serious bleeding episodes by encouraging him to avoid contact sports or other activities that might result in injury. To protect your child while he's playing, have him wear appropriate protective gear, such as a helmet or knee pads. Encourage low-impact exercise, such as swimming, to help joints and muscles stay healthy. The most important thing you can do is to stay alert for signs and symptoms of internal bleeding or joint bleeding, such as pain; tenderness; swelling; large, dark bruises; numbness; and headaches. Report any suspicious symptoms to your doctor quickly. Early treatment with blood-clotting factor is the most effective way to prevent the pain from becoming severe and to help speed recovery. Treat small cuts or scrapes with an ice pack, and apply pressure to the wound until bleeding stops.

Inform your child's caregivers, teachers, bus drivers, and friends that he has hemophilia. Give them a list of symptoms, and let them know that early treatment is important if symptoms appear. Make sure your child wears a medical alert bracelet.

Seek out support from other families who have a member with hemophilia. Join support groups and contact organizations that provide support and information for families with hemophilia. See Appendix: Parent Resources, Medical Conditions.

Prevention

Since hemophilia is an inherited disorder, preventative strategies are limited. For those with a family history of hemophilia, genetic counseling is an important step prior to pregnancy.

▌ *Hepatitis*

Don't assume that your child can't get hepatitis if she's been vaccinated against hepatitis B. While the vaccine protects against one of the most common forms of this potentially serious liver disease, it doesn't protect against the other strains. Hepatitis, an inflammation of the liver, can be contracted through eating contaminated foods or contact with infected people. It can even be caused by certain chemicals and drugs. It requires prompt medical attention.

Signs and Symptoms

- Flulike symptoms, including *fever*, aching joints, and *headache*
- Marked loss of appetite, often with nausea and *vomiting*
- Yellowish tinge to the skin and whites of the eyes (*jaundice*)
- Tea-colored urine
- Clay-colored stools

☎ *When to Call the Doctor*
CALL THE DOCTOR TODAY IF
- your child has hepatitis symptoms.
- your child has been exposed to someone with hepatitis.
- your child has eaten food, such as uncooked seafood, that might have been contaminated with a hepatitis virus.

TALK WITH THE DOCTOR AT YOUR CHILD'S NEXT CHECKUP IF
- you have any questions about the hepatitis vaccine or your child's vaccination status.
- you are planning foreign travel with your child.
- your child routinely requires transfusions of blood or blood products.

Essential Facts

Depending on the type of hepatitis, the symptoms and severity may vary widely. Five kinds exist, named with the first five letters of the alphabet. Hepatitis A, the most common type in children, is a relatively mild infection that often causes few symptoms and goes away completely. Symptoms may include fatigue, abdominal pain, *diarrhea*, vomiting, and jaundice.

Hepatitis B, the second leading type, accounts for about one-third of cases of hepatitis in children and is more serious. Symptoms develop slowly, about 2 to 3 months after infection. At first, they resemble those of the flu: nausea, vomiting, fatigue, and low-grade fever. Some children also develop jaundice. Within a few days, the symptoms may become worse and include abdominal and joint pain. The liver, spleen, and lymph nodes may become swollen and tender. About 10 percent of people infected with hepatitis B become chronic carriers of the disease, which means that even after the symptoms go away, they can still infect others. Carriers need regular checkups to monitor liver function and help prevent further liver damage. Hepatitis C, D, and E are uncommon or rare in children in the United States.

Causes

Hepatitis is usually caused by a virus. Hepatitis A is transmitted from person-to-person contact or from contaminated food or water. The virus, which lives in blood, saliva, and stools, can easily spread throughout a day care center, a school, or a house, especially if an infected person doesn't wash her hands carefully after having a bowel movement. In 1997, hepatitis A outbreaks occurred in several states when children ate imported strawberries that were contaminated.

Hepatitis B is spread through contact with an infected person's saliva, blood, semen, or breast milk. Infants born to infected mothers may therefore become infected before, during, or immediately after birth. Hepatitis B is especially prevalent among children with serious illnesses, such as AIDS (see *HIV/AIDS Infection*), or types of *cancer* associated with immune deficiency, as well as among adolescents and young adults, who become infected through intercourse or intravenous drug use.

Hepatitis C is less common in children and is caused by a virus transmitted through sexual contact, blood transfusion, or illicit, intravenous drug use. Also uncommon, hepatitis D is caused by a virus that occurs only in conjunction with the hepatitis B virus. Hepatitis E is rare in the United States and is caused by a virus found in water contaminated by sewage in some countries.

Children and adults can also get a noninfectious inflammation of the liver (chemical hepatitis) from swallowing substances that damage the liver. This damage occurs not from a virus, but from chemicals that harm the liver. Substances that can cause this damage include some prescription and over-the-counter drugs, such as acetaminophen, when taken in overdose amounts, and certain antimicrobial drugs, when taken as directed. Chemicals that can cause hepatitis when ingested include pennyroyal oil, alcohol, and carbon tetrachloride.

What the Doctor May Do

The doctor can diagnose hepatitis based on your child's symptoms; a review of her medical history and recent activities; and blood, urine, stool, and liver function test results. Many cases of viral hepatitis will clear up as long as the child gets enough rest and drinks enough fluids. The child may need to stay home and rest until the symptoms go away, which can take several weeks.

Severe and chronic cases may require hospitalization so that doctors can treat complications associated with hepatitis. For example, clotting factors such as vitamin K may be used to treat bleeding. Medications to treat kidney or brain complications may also be given. In addition, medical personnel will administer intravenous fluids to keep the child from becoming dehydrated. These fluids should be heavily monitored because, in severe cases of hepatitis where kidney function is affected, a child could slip into renal failure and thus not be able to eliminate the fluids easily.

Treatment also focuses on dietary restrictions to reduce the child's nitrogen levels (which rise because the damaged liver cannot process nitrogen) to prevent toxic effects to the brain. Nitrogen levels are lowered by reducing a child's protein intake. Hepatitis caused by acetaminophen and some other drugs can be treated with an antidote in the hospital if given early in the course of toxicity.

What You Can Do

If your child develops hepatitis, make sure that she drinks water throughout the day to prevent dehydration. Call the doctor immediately if you see signs of dehydration, such as loss of appetite or vomiting, or if your child appears lethargic, unresponsive, or delirious.

Don't give any medication unless the doctor tells you to do so. Most drugs must pass through the liver to be processed for use by the body. But as long as the liver is weakened by hepatitis, any medicine, even an over-the-counter painkiller, can harm the liver and impair its recovery.

Prevention

You can significantly reduce your child's risk of hepatitis by taking the following precautions:

- *Encourage proper hygiene.* Have children wash their hands after playing outside and using the bathroom and before eating. Make sure that you and other caregivers wash hands before and after handling dirty diapers. If someone in your household has hepatitis, be sure to wash food utensils with hot water and detergent, preferably in a dishwasher.

- *Travel with safety in mind.* When traveling abroad, drink only bottled, sterile water and eat only cooked foods. Avoid eating raw vegetables and fruits that may have been washed in contaminated water.

- *Take precautions if your child is exposed.* If you know that your child has been exposed to the hepatitis A or the hepatitis B virus, your doctor can give her a shot of gamma globulin, an immune system protein that combats infection. A gamma globulin injection can help prevent hepatitis A or hepatitis B.

- *Vaccinate your child.* The American Academy of Pediatrics recommends that all children be vaccinated for hepatitis B. Your child should have the hepatitis A vaccine if you live in a community with outbreaks of the disease or if you are planning to travel with your child to a developing country.

See also *Abdominal Pain/Stomachache.*

Hernia, Inguinal

A hernia is the protrusion of an organ—usually part of an intestine—into a space where it does not belong. The most common hernia in infancy and childhood is an inguinal hernia, which appears as a lump in the groin. It affects 1 in 20 children and is five times as common in boys as in girls, affecting approximately 5 to 10 percent of male infants. The condition is more common in premature infants. Fortunately, most of these hernias are easy to treat.

Signs and Symptoms

- A bulge in the skin near the groin

When to Call the Doctor

CALL THE DOCTOR IMMEDIATELY IF

- swelling, severe pain, vomiting, and/or extreme weakness related to hernia occur *(this is a medical emergency).*

CALL THE DOCTOR TODAY IF

- you suspect that your child has an inguinal hernia.

Essential Facts

An inguinal hernia appears as a lump in the groin that results when a portion of intestine pokes through a weakened area in the abdominal wall. The condition occurs more often on the right side than on the left in boys because the right testicle usually descends after the left, but it frequently affects both sides. The lump, which is usually painless, may move down into the scrotum in boys or toward the outer vaginal lips in girls. It may be visible continually or appear only when the abdominal muscles are under pressure, such as when a baby strains during a bowel movement or cries intensely. Once a child is old enough to walk, the lump may become progressively more noticeable during the day or "pop out" after an especially strenuous twist, stretch, or lunge while he is playing. Parents often first notice a hernia while bathing their child.

An inguinal hernia is usually minor, causing little or no pain. But if it isn't surgically repaired, the bulging intestine can, in rare cases, become trapped, causing cramping, vomiting, and abdominal bloating. Once trapped, the hernia may become strangulated, which means that its blood circulation is shut off by surrounding muscle and tissues. Without nutrients and oxygen from the blood, the bowel tissue can be injured or die, a serious complication.

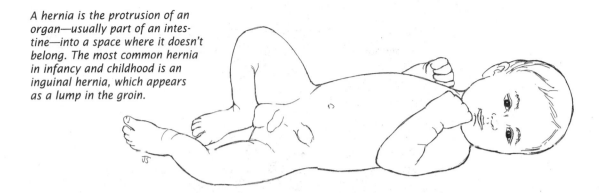

A hernia is the protrusion of an organ—usually part of an intestine—into a space where it doesn't belong. The most common hernia in infancy and childhood is an inguinal hernia, which appears as a lump in the groin.

Causes

Most hernias occur because of a slight abnormality in development that leaves the peritoneum (the membrane that lines the abdominal cavity) with a hole or a weak spot at birth. In the womb, the peritoneum has a sac-like projection that leads to the scrotum in boys and the labia in girls. Just before birth, this sac usually closes, sealing the peritoneum. If it doesn't seal, part of the intestine can bulge through the opening and into the groin area, resulting in an inguinal hernia. An inguinal hernia can appear at any age.

What the Doctor May Do

A doctor can usually diagnose a hernia based on the signs and symptoms and observation. If the doctor suspects that an infant has an inguinal hernia, she will press the abdomen while the baby is lying down; the pressure may cause the hernia to bulge out. With an older child, the doctor will firmly press the abdomen while the child stands and bears down with his abdominal muscles to see if an inguinal hernia appears.

Inguinal hernias must be repaired with surgery. In most cases, especially with infants, the

---

A FATHER'S STORY
The Bubble Gum Operation

When Nick was 9 years old, we noticed a painless bulge in his groin area while he was getting into his pajamas. Nick's doctor referred us to a pediatric surgeon, who confirmed that he had a hernia and scheduled him for surgery 3 weeks later, after we returned from a Thanksgiving trip.

When we arrived at the hospital at 8:30 in the morning, the nurses and anesthesiologist explained to Nick what was going to happen. They had him try out the mask they were going to use to put him to sleep and let him pick out which flavor of anes-

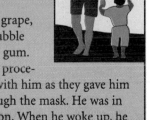

thesia he wanted: cherry, grape, strawberry, banana, or bubble gum. Nick picked bubble gum. When it was time for the procedure, his mother stayed with him as they gave him the bubble gum gas through the mask. He was in the recovery room by noon. When he woke up, he was a little tearful at first but was OK in a few minutes after he got his bearings. We were home by 1:30. Nick still remembers the experience as his "bubble gum operation."

surgeon will operate soon after diagnosis to prevent complications, such as strangulation of the hernia. The surgery involves removing the sac that protrudes from the peritoneum and strengthening the weakened abdominal muscles by stitching them together. When repairing an inguinal hernia on one side, the surgeon may use an endoscope (a slender instrument with a telescope and a light) to see if the abdominal wall on the other side has a similar opening or weakness. If so, the surgeon will repair it, too. Although it requires general anesthesia, the surgery is usually performed on an outpatient basis and doesn't require much recovery time. Your child can probably return to most of his normal activities almost immediately, although the surgeon usually advises that you notify your child's school and have him avoid gym class and strenuous activities for 3 or 4 weeks.

What You Can Do

Tell the doctor if you suspect an inguinal hernia. Call immediately if your child begins to vomit or experience abdominal pain and a bulge in the groin, signs that the hernia is trapped.

Prevention

To the extent that inguinal hernias are related to premature birth, you can prevent them by maintaining a healthy pregnancy to reduce the risk of premature birth (see A Healthy Pregnancy, p. 3). Otherwise, they cannot be prevented.

See also *Hernia, Umbilical; Hydrocele; Testes, Undescended.*

■ *Hernia, Umbilical*

An umbilical hernia is a soft lump beneath the navel. It may look like a handle or bulge where your child's navel should be. Alarming as it may seem, an umbilical hernia isn't serious and usu-

ally goes away without treatment. However, as with all hernias, consult your child's doctor for an accurate diagnosis, and watch it closely for signs of complications.

Signs and Symptoms

- Bulge in the skin of the navel

> ### *When to Call the Doctor*
> CALL THE DOCTOR IMMEDIATELY IF
> - swelling, severe pain, vomiting, and/or extreme weakness occur *(this is a rare medical emergency).*
>
> TALK TO THE DOCTOR AT YOUR CHILD'S NEXT CHECKUP IF
> - you suspect that your child has an umbilical hernia.

Essential Facts

An umbilical hernia is the second most common hernia in children, after an inguinal hernia. An umbilical hernia results when a portion of the intestine bulges through the abdominal wall. It is more common in girls, especially African Americans or premature babies. An umbilical hernia usually appears in the first few weeks or months of life and usually disappears without treatment by the fifth birthday.

Causes

An umbilical hernia is caused by either a weakness or an opening of the area around the navel called the abdominal ring. The weakness or opening occurs when the muscles in that area fail to close after the umbilical cord falls off.

What the Doctor May Do

The doctor can diagnose an umbilical hernia simply by examining your child. This type of hernia usually goes away by age five without

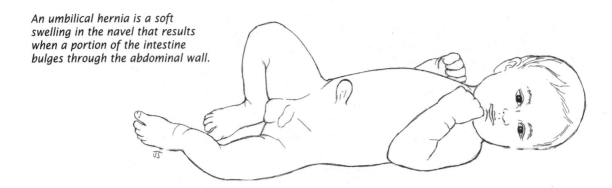

An umbilical hernia is a soft swelling in the navel that results when a portion of the intestine bulges through the abdominal wall.

treatment. But if it grows larger after a child's second birthday, or if at any age symptoms such as vomiting or sharp abdominal pain indicate that the hernia is trapped, surgery may be necessary. The surgery is a simple procedure that involves stitching the weak area of the umbilical ring.

What You Can Do

If the hernia causes no pain (which is usually the case), you needn't do anything except monitor it. The practice of binding the baby's abdomen is a folk remedy that does not work and can cause harm if the binding is too tight. Tell the doctor if the hernia is getting bigger. And call immediately if your child begins vomiting or experiences sharp abdominal pain. These are signs that the hernia has become trapped.

Prevention

To the extent that umbilical hernias are related to premature birth, you can prevent them by maintaining a healthy pregnancy to reduce the risk of premature birth (see A Healthy Pregnancy, p. 3). Otherwise, umbilical hernias cannot be prevented, because they appear to be hereditary.

See also ***Hernia, Inguinal.***

■ *High Blood Pressure (Hypertension)*

Although we usually think of high blood pressure as an "adult" disease, about 5 percent of children are diagnosed with this condition as well. Since high blood pressure, or hypertension, often has no symptoms, some cases go undetected. Hypertension is treatable and, at least in childhood, usually causes no serious health problems if treated appropriately. But it does require medical attention. If high blood pressure goes untreated for many years, it can lead to serious health problems later in life, including heart failure and stroke.

Signs and Symptoms

Often, there are no symptoms. Sometimes the following occur:

- *Dizziness*
- Shortness of breath
- *Headache*
- Visual disturbances
- Nosebleeds (rare)

When to Call the Doctor

CALL THE DOCTOR IMMEDIATELY IF

- your child with high blood pressure has headache, seizures, head trauma, vomiting, or blurred vision.

CALL THE DOCTOR TODAY IF

- your child has any symptoms of high blood pressure with no explanation.

Essential Facts

High blood pressure is a disease in which the force of blood circulating against blood vessel walls is too high. A health professional measures blood pressure with a sphygmomanometer—an inflatable cuff that goes around a child's arm and a meter that records two readings. Blood pressure is expressed as a two-part number.

- *Systolic pressure* is the first number, which measures the pressure in the arteries when the heart pumps blood out to the rest of the body.

- *Diastolic pressure* is the second number, which measures the pressure in the arteries when the heart relaxes between beats.

A child's blood pressure increases normally with age. To determine if your child's blood pressure is normal, a health professional will take three separate readings and determine whether they are within the normal range for your child's age group.

Causes

High blood pressure occurs under two general circumstances: when the heart must pump too large a volume of blood through normal blood vessels, or when the heart pumps a normal volume of blood through vessels, which, for many reasons, have grown inelastic or are too narrow and are resistant to blood flow.

Most children with hypertension, particularly infants, have what is called *secondary hyperten-*sion, which means that an underlying problem with the kidneys, heart, or blood vessels is causing the problem. In about 80 percent of young children who experience secondary hypertension, the condition is related to a congenital (present at birth) kidney irregularity. Other problems that may cause secondary hypertension include a narrowing of the aorta, the largest artery in the body; problems of the endocrine system (which produces and regulates hormones), especially thyroid or adrenal gland problems; or severe burns or serious injuries. Other problems include tumors, autoimmune diseases, and certain drugs, such as cocaine or amphetamines. Even over-the-counter cold and allergy medications containing ephedrine, pseudoephedrine, or phenylpropanolamine can cause dangerously high blood pressure.

Older children are more likely to develop *primary* (or *essential*) *hypertension,* a chronic, often progressive condition in which noticeable signs and symptoms are almost totally absent. Although the exact cause of primary hypertension is unknown, several factors increase the risk that a child will have the condition. In childhood, the primary risk factors are being overweight and inactive and having a family history of hypertension.

Uncontrolled hypertension can lead to serious kidney, central nervous system, eye, and heart damage. Termed *malignant hypertension,* this condition requires use of intravenous antihypertensive medications and hospitalization.

What the Doctor May Do

A health professional usually discovers hypertension in children by measuring blood pressure during a routine examination or, less often, during an investigation of another illness.

If hypertension is present, the doctor may decide to perform one or more of a series of increasingly specific tests, including blood and urine tests as well as kidney X rays or a renal

■ NORMAL BLOOD PRESSURE RANGES

Age	Systolic (First Number)	Diastolic (Second Number)
Birth	67–106	25–61
1 year	69–108	28–63
2 years	71–110	29–65
3 years	73–111	30–66
4 years	75–113	31–67
5 years	76–115	32–68
6 years	78–116	33–69
7 years	80–118	34–70
8 years	81–120	35–71
9 years	83–121	36–72
10 years	84–123	37–73

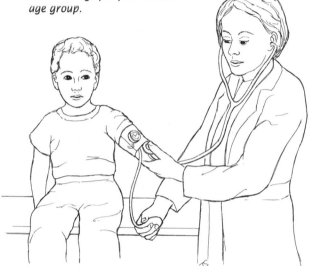

Doctors measure blood pressure by inflating a cuff around the upper arm and reading a dial, which is attached to the cuff by a rubber hose. To determine if your child's blood pressure is normal, a health professional will take three readings and determine whether they are within the normal range for your child's age group.

ultrasound, in order to diagnose an underlying cause of hypertension. If the tests identify a kidney problem, blood vessel abnormality, or endocrine system problem, the doctor will treat the condition as necessary with drug therapy, surgery, or both, depending on the cause and severity of hypertension and your child's general health.

Treatment for primary hypertension depends upon the severity of the condition. Some children with mild primary hypertension can control the problem with diet, weight reduction, and regular exercise. But if these measures don't bring blood pressure within the normal range, the doctor may prescribe one or a combination of special antihypertensive medications—sometimes a diuretic, which will cause your child to urinate more frequently and will reduce blood volume. Other medications include beta-blockers and calcium channel blockers, which lower the heart rate and reduce the force of the blood flow; hydralazine, a peripheral blood vessel dila-

tor; and ACE (angiotensin converting enzyme) inhibitors, which relax the blood vessels and allow the blood to flow more freely.

Any child diagnosed with high blood pressure needs to be checked regularly by a physician, who will monitor for possible development of serious related disorders, such as heart, nervous system, eye, or kidney problems. Even "borderline" hypertension during childhood may have serious consequences for health later on.

What You Can Do

If your child has secondary hypertension, work with your child's doctor in treating the underlying cause for the condition. If your child has primary hypertension, the condition will probably be lifelong. In that case, your doctor will help you devise a healthy diet and exercise plan to help manage the disease. Your first step will be to reduce the salt in your child's diet, which can help reverse mild hypertension. Consult a dietitian about what your child should and shouldn't eat. Next, your doctor may suggest that your child get regular exercise, which can help reduce mild hypertension. Find an activity your child likes, and sign her up. Or just encourage regular outdoor play with other children.

Prevention

Most cases of secondary high blood pressure can't be prevented. Only treating the condition causing the hypertension will help.

You may be able to prevent primary hypertension, or at least to prevent a mild case from becoming more severe, by helping your child maintain a normal weight; eat a healthy diet rich with fruits, grains, and vegetables; and get plenty of regular exercise.

For long-term prevention take these steps:

- Decrease your child's salt intake.
- Decrease your child's fat and cholesterol intake.
- Impart good dietary habits early in childhood.

■ HIV/AIDS Infection

Acquired immunodeficiency syndrome (AIDS) and the virus that causes it, human immunodeficiency virus (HIV), are rare in children. But some parents may worry that their children could be exposed to the life-threatening virus by coming in contact with someone who has the disease. Because the virus cannot be transmitted through casual contact or saliva—or through the air or via toilet seats and the like—no real risk of infection exists in routine contact, day care, or classroom activities. AIDS among children under age 13 years is rare. Most children with HIV or AIDS acquired the infection from their HIV-infected mothers in the womb or during birth.

Some of these children are infected with HIV but have not yet developed the clinical symptoms known as AIDS.

Essential Facts

HIV infection and AIDS are not the same thing. HIV is an infection caused by the human immunodeficiency virus. AIDS is the group of conditions that often develop as the result of the HIV infection. People infected with HIV, particularly if they are treated with medication, can live symptom-free for years before becoming ill with one or more of the infections that define AIDS. Nevertheless, even symptom-free people with HIV can infect others. As the disease progresses, life-threatening illnesses may develop.

Since the first AIDS cases appeared in the United States in 1981, doctors have learned much about AIDS and HIV, including what causes AIDS and how to protect people from the disease. Thanks to new drug therapy developments, both adults and children with HIV are now living longer. But doctors are still searching both for a cure and for a vaccine.

How the Disease Progresses

Once in the bloodstream, HIV attacks certain cells (lymphocytes) the body needs for protection against disease. When enough of these cells are destroyed, the body falls victim to various diseases, some life-threatening. This process of cell destruction, however, may take months or years.

Untreated infants with HIV infection may appear well at first, but gradually develop symptoms. They often don't gain weight (see *Failure to Gain Weight*) or grow at a normal rate and, as AIDS progresses, experience frequent bouts of diarrhea or skin infections. Other symptoms include enlarged lymph nodes and spleen and persistent fungal mouth infections known as candidiasis, or *thrush.* Neurological complications can include seizures and developmental delays in speech, motor skills, and cognitive abilities. As the disease progresses, life-threatening *pneumonia, cancer,* and other illnesses may develop. But some children are not as susceptible to infections as others, depending on various factors, including how these children respond to treatment.

Unless preventative treatment is started, about 20 percent of children born with HIV develop a profound immune system deficiency (AIDS) by their first birthday. This can lead to life-threatening infections. But some children with HIV develop few, if any, symptoms until about 4 years old, and some show no signs until 9 years old or even older.

How HIV Is Transmitted

HIV is present in blood, semen, and some other body fluids, including breast milk. It passes from person to person in the following ways:

- Through unprotected sexual contact with an infected person

- By sharing needles (typically for intravenous drug use) with an infected person

- Through transfusion or injection of contaminated blood or blood products

- From an infected mother to her child before birth or during delivery

- Through ingestion of breast milk from an infected mother

Since saliva is not considered a method of transmission for HIV, you and your child are not likely to contract the virus by coming in contact with an infected person's saliva. Studies of hundreds of families with HIV-positive members, including toddlers and infants, have found that HIV has not been transmitted through nonsexual contact unless blood was involved.

Some children were infected by transfusion of blood products in the 1970s and early 1980s. Blood is now carefully screened for HIV in the United States and in many other countries, and as a result, the transmission rate in these countries is low.

What the Doctor May Do

All women who are pregnant or considering a pregnancy should be offered screening for HIV infection, since effective drugs are available to prevent transmission of the disease to the fetus. After birth, children of HIV-infected mothers are often given medication at 4 to 6 weeks of age as a protective measure.

Determining whether an infant born to an HIV-positive mother has the virus can be complicated. The standard blood test for the virus antibody cannot confirm a diagnosis until around 18 months of age, when leftover maternal antibodies have cleared from the child's system. Other tests may need to be performed, including an HIV culture or an HIV-PCR (polymerase chain reaction), both of which test for virus in the blood. The HIV-PCR test gives a positive reading about 10 to 15 days after infection. These tests are recommended for the babies of HIV-infected mothers at birth, at 1 to 2 months of age, and again at 3 to 6 months of age. If all these tests are negative, there is a better-than-98-percent chance that the baby is not infected.

Treatment of a child with HIV/AIDS requires the attention of a multidisciplinary medical team. HIV treatment focuses on preventing AIDS symptoms from developing. AIDS treatment focuses on management of recurrent infections and proper nutrition. Treatment will depend on the age of the child, other conditions or illnesses, any symptoms that are present, reactions to the treatment, and the child's environment. Drugs such as zidovudine (AZT), didanosine (ddI), and protease inhibitors treat the virus itself, and can prolong HIV/AIDS patients' lives by reducing the amount of virus in their bodies. Such medications can sometimes be mixed with formula or food so that they are easier for a child to take. Since new treatments are constantly being developed, the family of a child with HIV infection should maintain regular contact with the child's doctors.

What You Can Do

- *During pregnancy:* If you are pregnant or planning a pregnancy, ask your doctor about testing. Practice safer sex during pregnancy by using condoms if your partner has not been tested recently for the HIV virus and if there is any risk that he has been exposed to the virus recently. If you are pregnant and you carry HIV, your doctor will discuss your options with you, including the medications that can prevent the disease from passing to your child.

- *Medication therapy:* If your child is diagnosed with HIV or AIDS, work closely with a medical team to keep him as healthy as possible. Make sure that your child takes any medication exactly as prescribed to ensure that the medication is most effective. Most children with HIV who receive modern treatments (especially those who start treatment before becoming immunodeficient) remain quite healthy, attend school, and lead relatively normal lives. But no one can predict the health of these children over the long term.

- *Protection from infections:* If your child has HIV or AIDS, keep him from coming into contact with children carrying infections such as chicken pox and measles, which can cause serious illness in children with HIV. HIV cannot be transmitted through casual contact or saliva, so infants and children with the disease can—and should—be held, stroked, touched, and loved exactly as healthy children are. Since the virus is not transmitted through the air or via toilet seats, no risk of HIV infection exists in routine day care or classroom activities. The Centers for Disease Control and Prevention recommend that HIV-infected children receive regular immunizations (except for the varicella/chicken pox vaccine) at the usual ages (see p. 110). The immunizations the child should get include the vaccines for polio; diphtheria, tetanus, and pertussis; measles, mumps, and rubella; hepatitis; pneumonia; and influenza. But be sure to ask your doctor about immunizations, because very immunodeficient children should not get certain vaccines.

- *Seek early medical attention:* If you notice signs of illness or infection, such as fever, listlessness, earache, or congestion, in your child, seek medical attention to avoid complications.

- *Provide a healthy diet:* Provide your child with a healthy, well-balanced diet that includes whole grains and plenty of fresh fruits and vegetables.

Prevention

Standard precautionary procedures ("universal precautions") for handling stool, blood, and body secretions protect others from infection with HIV. These precautions include immediately washing exposed skin with soap and water after any contact with stool, blood, and secretions of an HIV-positive person; cleaning soiled surfaces with bleach; and regular hand-washing.

If you are pregnant or planning a pregnancy and are unaware of your HIV status, you can help prevent your new baby from getting HIV by being tested and discussing your options with your doctor. If you do not have the virus, protect yourself and any future children by practicing safer sex (using condoms) and avoiding intravenous street drugs.

If you have a healthy child, there are ways to protect him from infection. When looking into child care, be sure the provider takes precautions against the spread of infection (see Is the Facility Clean? p. 326). Teach your child early about the dangers of intravenous drug use; contact with infected body fluids, such as blood; and (when he is older) the basics of safe sexual behavior. You can also encourage your school system to provide information about HIV and its prevention.

▌ *Hives*

"Mom, it itches!" is the all-too-frequent cry of a child with hives, a skin reaction usually triggered by allergies or certain medical conditions. Appearing as pink or white, itchy lumps or raised white lumps, hives can develop anywhere on a child's body and can last a few minutes to a few days. Hives are common; more than 20 percent of children have hives at least once.

Signs and Symptoms
- Itchy rash of raised pink or white spots
- Wheals (raised white lumps) that appear and disappear on various body parts
- Wheals that develop where your child scratches

When to Call the Doctor
CALL FOR EMERGENCY HELP IF
- hives are accompanied by difficulty breathing or swallowing. (This indicates allergic shock.)
- your child turns blue.

For first aid information, see page 380 if your child is less than 1 year old and page 383 if your child is 1 year of age or older.

CALL THE DOCTOR IMMEDIATELY IF
- hives develop immediately after your child takes medicine.
- abdominal pain occurs.

CALL THE DOCTOR TODAY IF
- your child has frequent bouts of hives that are not relieved by over-the-counter antihistamines.
- hives are accompanied by other symptoms such as vomiting and fever.

Essential Facts
Several categories of hives exist, classified by how long they last or how often they occur (acute, long-term, and recurrent) and their cause (allergic, physical, and stress-related).

- *Acute hives* are extremely itchy and develop anywhere on a child's body, including the face, sometimes causing the eyelids and lips to swell. These hives often appear suddenly and disappear without treatment within a few hours or days. Allergies to foods, medications, or substances that touch the skin usually cause acute hives.

- *Long-term hives* are often caused by an underlying illness, although the cause is frequently unknown. Long-term hives resemble acute hives in appearance, but develop more slowly and last until the underlying cause is resolved, and they disappear spontaneously.

- *Recurrent hives* appear repeatedly, usually in response to a repeated stimulus such as ongoing stress or repeat exposure to allergic triggers.

- *Physical hives* develop in reaction to physical stresses, specifically, sudden exposure to the sun or cold. Cold hives, for instance, result from exposure to cold air, cold drinks, or cold water. Solar hives appear within minutes of exposure to sunlight, often in children with systemic diseases that increase their sensitivity to the sun, such as lupus erythematosus, a chronic disease that causes inflammation of the connective tissues. Some medications also cause a similar reaction to the sun.

- *Allergic hives* may appear suddenly and may recur whenever the child is exposed to an allergic trigger. Food allergies or substances that touch the skin may produce allergic hives.

- *Stress-related hives* are uncommon in children but may appear in stressful situations.

Causes

Hives are usually caused by release of a chemical called histamine in response to allergies to medications (particularly aspirin, codeine, and penicillin) and foods (particularly shellfish, nuts, eggs, chocolate, strawberries, and food additives). Surface allergens, such as animal saliva, ointments, and plants, may also cause hives. In some instances, emotional stress or upset can trigger hives.

Less common causes of hives include viral infections such as **hepatitis** and **mononucleosis,** bacterial infections such as strep throat (see **Sore Throat/Strep Throat**) and **sinusitis,** and diseases such as **arthritis** and rheumatic fever (see **Fever**).

What the Doctor May Do

Once the doctor confirms that your child has hives, he will try to help you determine the cause. The doctor will ask what kinds of foods your child may have eaten that might have triggered the reaction or what kinds of substances your child may have been exposed to, including pet dander, detergents, or other triggers. The doctor may do a throat culture or a test for mono if he thinks an infection is causing the rash. Until the cause is determined, the doctor may recommend treatment for the symptoms, including home remedies (see below) and over-the-counter remedies such as antihistamines. Only the most severe cases require prescription medication.

What You Can Do

The most effective way to relieve the symptoms of hives is by administering an over-the-counter oral antihistamine such as diphenhydramine. Follow the dosing instructions carefully. Your doctor may instruct you to give an antihistamine every 4 to 6 hours for the next day or two or the hives will recur. Hives usually clear up an hour or two after your child is medicated.

Prevention

If you can identify the cause of your child's hives, you can help prevent future outbreaks by helping her avoid the offending substances or situations.

See also **Allergies; Rashes.**

▌ *Hoarseness*

See **Laryngitis.**

▌ *Hydrocele*

If you notice that your little boy's scrotum is swollen, don't be alarmed. Chances are, he's developed hydrocele, a relatively common and usually harmless condition in which fluid collects in the scrotum (generally on one side). In some cases, the surrounding area, including the penis, also swells. A hydrocele is not serious and usually subsides on its own without treatment.

Signs and Symptoms

- Scrotum swollen and pink or light blue
- Swelling in the scrotum that increases with crying or activity

When to Call the Doctor

CALL THE DOCTOR IMMEDIATELY IF

- your child feels tenderness or pain in the scrotal area.
- nausea or vomiting accompanies the discomfort (signs of a trapped hernia, which requires immediate surgery).

CALL THE DOCTOR TODAY IF

- you notice that your child's scrotum is swollen.

Causes

A hydrocele is usually caused by a minor problem. In infants, it may occur because the opening between the scrotal sac and the abdominal wall doesn't close completely, allowing fluid to collect in the scrotal area. This is called a communicating hydrocele. A hydrocele is noncommunicating if fluid is in the scrotal sac but no opening occurs between it and the abdominal wall. Sometimes a hydrocele is accompanied by an inguinal hernia (see **Hernia, Inguinal**), a piece of intestine bulging into the scrotal area. In older boys, a minor injury or even an insect sting can cause a hydrocele.

A similar congenital (present at birth) condition called a varicocele is an enlargement of veins in the scrotum that feels like a cluster of grapes. A varicocele can affect male fertility and usually needs surgical removal. Although present at birth, a varicocele may not become evident until later childhood or adolescence.

What the Doctor May Do

Your doctor will first determine by physical examination if it is a hydrocele and whether there is also a hernia present. She may also shine a bright light through the scrotum to see the fluid surrounding the testicle.

Hydroceles usually clear up on their own within the first year of life, though the doctor should check your child's hydrocele at each well-child visit. If the problem persists beyond 1 year, your doctor may recommend minor surgery to remove excess fluid and, if necessary, to close the opening in the abdominal cavity. A varicocele may effect fertility if left untreated into adulthood. Your doctor may refer your son for surgery to treat this condition and may also suggest surgery if your son has an inguinal hernia.

What You Can Do

If the swelling makes your child uncomfortable, have him lie down and elevate his legs to reduce the swelling. Otherwise, simply stay alert for signs of tenderness or illness, as these symptoms may indicate that an inguinal hernia has become trapped within the scrotal sac, a condition that requires surgery.

Prevention

Hydroceles cannot be prevented, but you can prevent complications by reporting signs of swelling, discomfort, fever, or vomiting to your child's doctor.

∎ Impetigo

Any time your child gets a cut, skinned knee, or open mosquito bite, she's at risk for an unwelcome side effect: impetigo. This contagious—but easily treated and benign—bacterial skin infection occurs after a minor injury becomes infected with either *Streptococcus* (strep) or *Staphylococcus* (staph) bacteria.

Signs and Symptoms

- A rash of tiny, fragile blisters that form honey-colored crusts

When to Call the Doctor
CALL THE DOCTOR IMMEDIATELY IF

- your child runs a fever, starts vomiting, or has tea-colored urine.

CALL THE DOCTOR TODAY IF

- your child has more than two sores distributed on more than one body area.
- the sores progress despite home treatment.
- after 4 or 5 days of home treatment, the rash has not cleared up.
- other family members get a similar rash.
- your newborn has the symptoms of impetigo described above.

Essential Facts

The rash of impetigo first appears as fragile blisters that begin to weep and eventually crust over to form yellow-brown scabs, often starting around the nose or mouth. Small children tend to get impetigo more often than adults because they play together, have more open cuts, and tend to get dirtier. The impetigo rash starts to form about 2 to 5 days after a child comes into contact with the bacteria and usually starts on the face, especially around the mouth and nose.

The infection sometimes occurs in epidemic outbreaks in camps, schools, and other places children gather. Although uncomfortable and unsightly, impetigo is not usually a serious medical problem.

Causes

This infection is caused by bacteria (*Streptococcus* or *Staphylococcus*) transmitted when a child touches an infected person or an object contaminated by the bacteria and then scratches one of her own open cuts, scrapes, or bites. Impetigo is usually spread by children who have visible signs of infection. Open cuts or sores offer a favorable environment for the bacteria to enter and multiply. Then, if a child scratches the first outbreak of sores, the bacteria spread to other body parts.

What You Can Do

Soak the sores and scabs with water to soften the crusts. Then, using soap and water, gently scrub off the scabs, under which bacteria can hide. A little bleeding is expected. You must completely remove the crusts. Pat the area dry. If your child has only one or two sores or a slightly infected cut or bite, an over-the-counter antibacterial ointment may be sufficient to clear it up. Otherwise, apply the antibiotic cream your doctor prescribes (see What the Doctor May Do). If possible, cover the area with gauze. Do this three to four times a day.

Encourage your child to touch the rash as little as possible. Scratching the rash can spread it to other body parts, and whatever your child touches may become contaminated with bacteria. Make sure she washes her hands and face often with soap and water. Keep her towels and washcloths separate from those of other family members. If the condition doesn't show signs of improvement within 4 to 5 days, visit your doctor.

What the Doctor May Do

If the condition does not clear with home treatment, your doctor may prescribe an antibiotic cream or oral antibiotics. Other skin rashes, such as herpes simplex infections or chicken pox, can resemble impetigo. Rare complications of certain strains of streptococcal impetigo, if left untreated, include inflammation of the kidney, kidney failure, and hypertension.

Prevention

While the lack of cleanliness doesn't cause impetigo, you can reduce your child's risk of developing the infection by encouraging her to wash her hands and face regularly with antibacterial soap to get rid of the bacteria that causes it. If the impetigo recurs or spreads to other family members, your child's doctor may recommend that everyone swab the area just inside the nose with an ointment containing bacitracin to prevent further spreading of the infection. Also, discourage sharing of combs, towels, and hairbrushes to further reduce the chance of contamination. Here are some other tips:

- Catch it early. At the first sign that a cut or scrape may be infected (redness, swelling, weeping), wash the area well and apply an over-the-counter antibiotic ointment.
- Keep children with impetigo away from other children until the infection is gone.

See also ***Diaper Rash; Rashes.***

Infantile Apnea

If you're like most new parents, you love standing and quietly watching your infant in his crib or bassinet. If so, you may notice that sometimes several seconds go by between breaths. Such a delay in respiration is perfectly normal. But if it lasts longer than 15 seconds or occurs regularly, your infant may be experiencing potentially serious apnea. Although this is unusual in full-term babies, it is more common in babies born prematurely. Most cases of apnea can be managed with medication and apnea monitors prescribed by the doctor. While apnea in infants generally resolves itself within a few months, the underlying causes need to be identified and treated.

Signs and Symptoms

- No breathing for periods exceeding 15 seconds
- Lack of movement
- Bluish color around lips and tongue (indicating lack of oxygen)

When to Call the Doctor

CALL FOR EMERGENCY HELP IF

- your child stops breathing for longer than 15 seconds, and you cannot rouse him.
- your child turns blue.

For first aid information, see page 380 if your child is less than 1 year old and page 383 if your child is 1 year of age or older.

CALL THE DOCTOR TODAY IF

- you have any concerns about your child's breathing or sleep patterns.

Essential Facts

The term "apnea" describes any period when breathing stops, particularly during sleep. Infant breathing patterns are often irregular, and pauses of a few seconds are normal, especially during dreams. When breathing stops for longer periods, apnea is considered potentially serious. In severe cases, reduced oxygen in the lungs can cause the blood and body tissues to accumulate acid and the small arterial lung branches to constrict, resulting in high blood pressure in the lungs. In rare cases, apnea can continue for more than a minute or so, and the lack of oxygen can cause brain damage or even death. Apnea is most likely to affect premature babies, whose central nervous systems aren't mature enough to regulate proper breathing patterns.

Causes

The cause of apnea is not fully understood. Apnea is extremely common in premature babies while they are in the hospital. Infantile apnea is most commonly due to central apnea, in which the airway remains open, but the brain is not sending signals to the body to breathe. Central apnea is caused by a disturbance in the brain's regulation of breathing in premature babies (called "apnea of prematurity"). Certain viruses and lung disease (in babies with immature lungs) can also cause apnea in premature babies.

Another type of apnea that occurs in premature infants and in full-term babies is obstructive apnea. In obstructive apnea, swollen or larger than normal tonsils or adenoids or other anatomical problems may cause apnea by blocking the airway. This type of apnea is often worse during sleep. Obstructive apnea may also occur in older children, and in this case is most often caused by large tonsils or adenoids.

Apnea is rare in full-term babies. Causes in full-term babies may include *gastroesophageal reflux* (the back flow of acidic fluid from the stomach into the esophageal tube to the throat and then into the mouth), *seizures,* significant infections (e.g., *meningitis*), and congenital heart disease (in extremely rare cases). Blood-borne bacterial infection (sepsis) as well as overdoses of some medicines, such as opiate narcotics, may also cause apnea in full-term babies as well as premature babies.

What the Doctor May Do

Most premature babies remain hospitalized long enough for the apnea to resolve itself as the baby develops and matures. Once home, if the premature infant gets sick (by catching a virus, for example), he is slightly more likely to develop apnea. A parent usually spots apnea in older infants, which is much less common, but sometimes the parent may notice it only after a severe apnea episode turns the baby's skin pale or blue. This can be life-threatening.

For a child who has had an apnea episode at home, the doctor will ask about the parent's observations, including what the baby looked like during the episode, what the circumstances of the episode were, and what other health problems the baby had then and previously. The doctor will take the child's medical history from the parent and thoroughly examine the child to try to figure out the cause of the apnea.

Treatment of apnea differs greatly depending on the affected infant's age, the duration and frequency of apnea, the underlying cause, and other possible conditions present. A baby with severe apnea may require observation in a hospital intensive care unit. Here, monitors will register breathing and heart rates and sound an alarm if the breathing or heart rate falls below normal.

Your doctor may prescribe medication, such as caffeine or theophylline, for premature infants with central apnea to stimulate more normal breathing rhythms. In rare instances, for severe apnea cases or cases that don't resolve themselves while the premature baby is still hospitalized, the doctor may send the baby home with an apnea monitor and instructions on whether to rouse your child or alert medical professionals if the alarm sounds. Such monitors have a sensor that

monitors heart rate and breathing and an alarm that rings if your baby stops breathing for a specific number of seconds or if the heart rate falls below normal. If your child is sent home with apnea, he will probably outgrow it within a few months.

What You Can Do

Know how to react. If your baby stops breathing for 15 seconds or more, follow these steps carefully:

1. Gently shake your baby's arm or leg and clap your hands loudly to rouse him. He should start breathing within a second or two.

2. If he still remains unresponsive, open his mouth and look inside to make sure nothing is obstructing his breathing. Loosen any tight-fitting clothing around his neck. If your baby is still not breathing, start CPR (see pp. 380 and 383) and call for help.

Prevention

Parents can prepare themselves for apnea spells by taking a CPR course in case of emergency and learning how to prevent choking and what to do if a child chokes (see pp. 380 and 383). Depending on the cause, the underlying condition may be treated to prevent apnea.

If your child was premature or has special health conditions, talk with your baby's doctor about precautions you can take at home. For example, most babies should be put to sleep on their back, but some premature babies benefit from the prone position (on the abdomen). Other precautions include keeping small objects that your child could choke on away from your child and providing a smoke-free home—particularly if you have a premature baby.

See also ***Sudden Infant Death Syndrome.***

Insect Bites and Stings

Most children love to be outdoors, but along with the fun of outdoor play come some risks, including that of stings from insects—mosquitoes, bees, wasps, spiders, and ticks, to name the most common. Insect stings can cause itching, soreness, and sometimes a more serious allergic reaction (see Allergic Shock, p. 389). But most insect stings are harmless, and most children and infants tolerate them well. Nevertheless, some insects carry disease and some children have allergies to certain insect bites, so be sure to identify the insect whenever possible and to carefully monitor your child's reaction to any sting or bite.

Signs and Symptoms

- Swollen, round wounds
- Redness, local area of warmth
- Itchiness or pain
- A small puncture mark, with or without a stinger

When to Call the Doctor
CALL FOR EMERGENCY HELP IF

- your child has a known severe bee sting allergy.
- your child has difficulty breathing or is turning blue.
- your child develops signs of allergic shock: rapid pulse; clammy, pale skin; shortness of breath; sweating; and faintness (see p. 390).
- your child is bitten by a known highly venomous insect, such as a black widow spider.

For first aid information, see page 380 if your child is less than 1 year old and page 383 if your child is 1 year of age or older.

CALL THE DOCTOR IMMEDIATELY IF

- your child vomits, becomes dizzy, or has a fever after being stung.

CALL THE DOCTOR TODAY IF

- your child has a large, local reaction to a bee or wasp sting (redness, warmth, and swelling that extend more than an inch or so beyond the sting).

Essential Facts

Bee and Wasp Stings Most bee and wasp stings are from yellow jackets, a type of small wasp. These stings may cause immediate, painful red bumps, which may swell and ache for up to 24 hours. Honeybees, hornets, and bumblebees may also sting. Although most kids experience only minor irritation from such stings, some are quite allergic to bee and wasp venom. Allergic reactions may be severe, ranging from swelling and pain to breathing difficulties and anaphylactic shock (also called allergic shock; see page 389), a life-threatening systemic reaction that can involve shortness of breath and loss of consciousness.

Mosquito, Mite, and Flea Bites These bites may cause itchy, red bumps, usually with minor swelling. However, a mosquito bite can swell up dramatically, although it remains a minor problem. Mosquito bites may itch for several days.

Horsefly, Sand Fly, Fire Ant, and Centipede Bites Bites from these animals can cause painful, red bumps that may ache for several hours, even a few days.

Spider Bites Although they are almost always harmless, spider bites may itch, ache, and/or swell for a day or so. Bites from poisonous spiders are rare in the United States, but they do occur. Two types of spiders can be particularly dangerous: Black widow (*Lactrodectus*) and brown recluse (*Loxosceles*) spiders both release poisons that often cause serious reactions. Both black widows and brown recluses are found throughout the United States. Glossy black with a characteristic red hourglass on its abdomen, a black widow is about $1/2$ inch long. Bites from a black widow may cause local pain, swelling, and muscle cramps. More serious symptoms include dizziness, muscle spasms, and seizures. The brown recluse is smaller than the black widow and has a violin-shaped marking on its body. Its bite can cause blistering and extensive skin damage that may require plastic surgery to heal. Both types of spiders tend to live in dark, secluded areas, such as basements and barns, and black widows also live in woodpiles. The brown recluse spider may hide in boxes of clothes and other items placed in storage.

Ticks A common biting insect, the tick lives in the woods and fields and often hides in the fur of animals (including house pets). Although its bite is usually painless, the tick attaches itself to the skin and can suck blood for up to 6 days if not removed. Most tick bites are harmless, but two types can cause disease. The wood tick may transmit Rocky Mountain spotted fever, and the deer tick may transmit *Lyme disease,* babesiosis, and ehrlichiosis. All these diseases are easily treated with antibiotics, but if left untreated, they can cause chronic symptoms.

What the Doctor May Do

Call your doctor if your child has difficulty breathing or exhibits signs of shock, or if symptoms get worse instead of better. If your child has an allergic reaction to an insect bite or sting, the doctor may prescribe antihistamines or steroids to inhibit the reaction, or prescribe the use of an epinephrine autoinjector. If he thinks the bite is infected (a condition called cellulitis), he may prescibe antibiotics.

If your child received a bite from a black widow, the doctor may administer an antivenin, which renders the poison harmless, and perhaps

prescribe steroids to reduce inflammation. Steroids are also the treatment of choice for brown recluse bites, although if the bite is severe and caught early, the doctor may recommend that he surgically remove the affected skin to limit the damage to surrounding tissue. Medication may be prescribed to control the infection.

If your doctor suspects Lyme disease, the treatment will include antibiotics.

What You Can Do

Most insect bites are harmless and resolve on their own. Follow the suggestions in the next paragraphs for home treatment if an insect bites or stings your child.

Bee and Wasp Stings First, check if the insect's stinger is still in your child's skin. If so, it will look like a little black dot in the middle of the bump. Remove it by scraping it off with the edge of scissors, a plastic credit card, or a fingernail or by plucking it out with tweezers. Once you've removed the stinger, apply an ice pack followed by a paste of baking soda and water to soothe the skin and relieve itching.

Mosquito, Mite, and Flea Bites These are less painful but itchier bites. The itch is often difficult to soothe. A paste of baking soda and water may help, as well as a dose of acetaminophen. If the itching is severe, ask your doctor if you should give your child an over-the-counter antihistamine to reduce the irritation.

Spider Bites If you have any reason to believe that a black widow or brown recluse spider bit your child, call your doctor immediately. Otherwise, clean the area around the bite and apply an ice pack to reduce swelling and soreness.

Tick Bites First remove the tick, using tweezers placed as close to the tick's head as possible. Pull with slow, steady pressure. Do not twist or jerk the tick, which may cause the body to break off, leaving the head and mouthparts embedded in the skin. If it doesn't come out easily, do not crush or tug at it. If the head remains in the skin, call your doctor. Once you've removed the tick, drown it in some water mixed with detergent. Some tiny ticks can be scraped off with the edge of a credit card or knife blade. Wash the wound and your hands thoroughly with soap and water. Methods such as touching the tick with a hot match head or covering it with petroleum jelly, alcohol, or fingernail polish are not effective in removing ticks.

Prevention

To reduce the likelihood of your child getting insect bites and stings, follow these precautions:

- *Repel insects.* If your child is over 2 years old, use insect repellents containing the chemical deet, but very sparingly. The chemical can be toxic. When choosing insect repellent containing deet, look on the label for a product containing less than 10 percent. Don't use insect repellents on skin that is cut, scratched, or wounded. For children under 2 years old do not use a repellent containing deet. Several safe, but somewhat less effective, repellents are available.

- *Perform an insect search.* You should check your child's skin for insects every time your child comes in from playing in the woods or in an area known to be infested with ticks or other insects. Do the same with your pets.

- *Cover your child up.* Protect your child from insect stings, or have him wear lightweight, long pants and long-sleeved shirts. Although some insects can sting right through some fabrics, you'll reduce the chances of a sting.

- *Bring your child indoors at dusk.* Dusk is the time of day when mosquitoes are most active.

Jaundice

The skin of most newborn babies has a soft, pink color. But some babies are born with jaundice, a yellowing of the skin and the whites of the eyes that occurs in approximately 60 percent of full-term newborns during the first week of life, and in an even greater percentage of premature infants. Older children can also develop jaundice as the result of underlying infection or other conditions that affect the liver.

Signs and Symptoms

- Yellow tinge to the skin and whites of the eyes
- Tea-colored urine and pale stools
- Nausea, loss of appetite (if liver infection is the culprit), or both

When to Call the Doctor
CALL THE DOCTOR TODAY IF
- your child has symptoms of jaundice.

Causes

Jaundice is caused by a buildup of bilirubin, a by-product of the body's normal, ongoing breakdown of old red blood cells. Normally, the liver rapidly removes bilirubin from the blood and excretes it in bile. But when the liver is immature, as in newborns, or not functioning properly for other reasons, bilirubin accumulates in the bloodstream. Because bilirubin is a yellow pigment, it turns the skin and the whites of the eyes yellow. The excess bilirubin may also enter the urine, turning it dark brown. The color of stools may become gray or chalky when a child is jaundiced, because of the lack of bilirubin in the intestines, where the stool forms. Very high bilirubin in the blood can lead to permanent neurological difficulties in newborns, including **developmental problems** and **hearing loss.**

The cause of jaundice varies with the child's age. In many babies, the liver isn't mature enough to process bilirubin. So, bilirubin builds up in the blood. Once the liver matures, after about 5 to 10 days, bilirubin levels tend to fall to within normal limits and jaundice goes away. Other, relatively rare causes of jaundice in infants include incompatibility with the mother's blood, blood disorders in the baby (such as *anemia*), severe infections (such as neonatal herpes simplex and salmonella), and structural problems of the liver or gallbladder. In older children, the most common cause of jaundice is *hepatitis,* a liver inflammation caused by infection or by drugs and other chemicals that can harm the liver.

What the Doctor May Do

If your child appears to have jaundice, the doctor will perform blood tests to check the bilirubin level. He also might take urine and stool samples to look for bacteria and viruses. Treatment of jaundice depends on its cause. For newborn jaundice, treatment is usually not necessary. But when jaundice is severe, the doctor might recommend light therapy (phototherapy), in which the baby is kept in the hospital and placed under ultraviolet lights, which help break down bilirubin. Light therapy prevents the complications associated with high bilirubin levels. If jaundice is very severe and light therapy fails, your child's doctor may recommend exchange transfusion (an exchange of the infant's blood with new blood by way of a transfusion) to reduce bilirubin levels in the blood.

What You Can Do

Keep an eye out for the signs of jaundice, and call the doctor as soon as you notice them. Be aware of any changes in your newborn's skin color or the coloring in the whites of the baby's eyes. Examine the baby in natural daylight or in a room with fluorescent lights. Press gently with your fingertip on the tip of your child's nose or forehead. If the skin looks white (this will happen with babies of all races), there's no jaundice. If you see a yellowish color, call the doctor.

Your doctor may recommend that you use light therapy at home: You can take your child outdoors to expose her to sunlight for a short time each day or use home phototherapy lights. Occasionally, a substance in mother's milk may cause a newborn's liver to work too hard. When this happens, a normal case of jaundice may be prolonged by breast-feeding. In this case, the doctor may recommend that you stop breast-feeding for several days until the baby's liver matures and can break down bilirubin more effectively. If this happens, use a breast pump to keep your milk supply flowing.

Prevention

Jaundice in newborn babies cannot be prevented. Prevention of jaundice in older children depends on the cause. For instance, there are ways to prevent hepatitis, which is a common cause of jaundice.

■ Jock Itch

See *Ringworm.*

■ Joint Pain

Aches and pains are normal side effects of an active childhood, and joints are particularly vulnerable. Joints are the hinges that allow bones to move. In most cases, joint pain is the result of either a minor injury that stretches the joint too far or a virus that causes an infection. Though it can be painful, joint pain in children is usually no cause for alarm.

Signs and Symptoms

- Pain, swelling, or both, in joints (knees, elbows, wrists, or hands)
- Other symptoms, including fever, rash, and inflammation of parts of the eyes (signs of juvenile rheumatoid arthritis)

When to Call the Doctor

CALL THE DOCTOR IMMEDIATELY IF

- severe pain occurs.
- a fever accompanies the pain.
- your child develops a persistent limp.
- your child cannot move a joint or limb, or has limited range of motion in one joint.
- your child has other symptoms, including a loss of appetite, a rash, or swollen glands.

CALL THE DOCTOR TODAY IF

- the pain persists for several days.
- the joints are swollen.
- your child experiences fatigue with the pain.

Causes

Children of all ages may experience joint pain, for various reasons. Joint pain may be caused by inflammation of the joint itself, the surrounding muscles, or other structures, or even inflammation of nearby bones from deep infection. Stretched ligaments or tendons, injury to muscles, *sprains and strains,* fractures (see p. 409), and *dislocations* all can cause joint pain, as can these conditions:

- *Growing pains:* These are the perfectly normal aches that sometimes occur during growth spurts. Unlike other types of joint pain, growing pains don't affect the child's ability to move the joint.
- *Injuries:* Sprains and strains, dislocations, fractures, and other injuries to muscles, tendons, or ligaments can cause joint pain.

- *Infections:* Both viruses and bacteria can cause joint pain and serious infection. Viruses that cause **chicken pox** or influenza (see *Colds/Flu*) can cause aches and pains. Bacterial arthritis can be caused by such bacteria as *Staphylococcus, Streptococcus, Gonococcus,* or *Haemophilus influenzae.*
- *Inflammatory conditions:* The inflammation of the kneecap, known as "jumper's knee" or Osgood-Schlatter disease, is a common cause of knee pain resulting from overexertion.
- *Chronic conditions:* Various conditions, such as **juvenile rheumatoid arthritis, sickle-cell disease,** and **hemophilia,** can cause joint pain.
- *Lyme disease:* This infectious disease is transmitted by deer ticks. If left untreated, it can result in chronic joint pain, swelling, and other symptoms (see *Lyme Disease*).
- *Infections or tumors:* In rare instances, a bacterial bone infection, which requires immediate medical intervention, can cause joint pain. The pain is usually severe and is accompanied by other symptoms, including fever. Also rare but serious is joint pain caused by bone cancer or leukemia (see *Cancer*).

What the Doctor May Do

Your child's doctor will attempt to identify the cause of the joint pain by performing a complete physical exam. The doctor will diagnose any growing pains or injuries by taking a history, performing a careful physical examination, and sometimes ordering an X ray or an MRI (magnetic resonance imaging, a detailed imaging test using a magnetic field). Usually, rest and perhaps treatment with an over-the-counter pain reliever, such as ibuprofen or acetaminophen, are recommended to treat growing pains or sprains and strains. Ice can provide additional relief for an injury (see *Sprains and Strains*). Depending on the injury, a brace might also help.

What You Can Do

If your child's joint pain is from a minor injury, you can promote healing by encouraging your child to rest. Elevate the affected area, and treat your child's pain with an over-the-counter pain reliever. For the first 3 days after an injury, apply cold compresses to the joint to decrease inflammation. After that, switch to warm compresses (from a hot water bottle or a heating pad). Heat encourages healing by increasing blood flow to the injury.

After a few days, be sure to get your child up and moving again in order to prevent the joint from stiffening. In addition, remain alert for other symptoms, such as fever, rash, severe or worsening pain, or extreme difficulty moving the joint, which could indicate a more serious condition. If any of these symptoms develop, consult your child's doctor.

Prevention

You can help prevent joint pain by taking precautions against injuries. Some precautions include having your child wear the appropriate protective equipment while playing sports and wear safety belts properly when riding in the car.

See also *Back Pain; Growing Pains.*

▌ *Juvenile Rheumatoid Arthritis (JRA)*

A strained knee from soccer practice or a sore elbow from baseball are the kinds of sports injuries that can cause *joint pain.* But if your child is experiencing chronic joint pain and it isn't the result of an injury, it may be caused by a more complicated disorder, such as juvenile rheumatoid arthritis (JRA), also known as juvenile chronic arthritis. Arthritis is inflammation

in one or more joints or in the tendons and ligaments that surround the affected joints. Typically, the pain and swelling associated with JRA waxes and wanes, becoming worse during "flares" of the disease. Though JRA can be disabling, most children fully recover with proper treatment and can lead normal, active lives.

Signs and Symptoms

- Pain and swelling of the joints lasting at least 6 weeks
- Some joints appear reddened and are warm to the touch
- Stiffness of the arms or legs, especially when the child gets up from sleep or a nap
- Child does not take part in normal play; prefers to watch others
- Child complains when activity is required; prefers to lie down in the middle of the day
- Fatigue and vague "unwell" feelings
- Eyes sensitive to light

Symptoms of the systemic form of JRA (see Essential Facts, on the next page) may also include the following:

- Generalized illness, including fever, rash, listlessness, loss of appetite
- Enlarged nodes and abdominal swelling

 When to Call the Doctor
CALL THE DOCTOR TODAY IF
- your child complains continually of joint pain and swelling.
- your child seems stiff or sore for many weeks.
- your child is not as active as other children.
- your child has a fever, a rash, and swelling of the abdomen or lymph nodes.

Essential Facts

JRA is one of the most common chronic joint diseases of childhood, affecting about 100,000 children in the United States. Three basic kinds of juvenile rheumatoid arthritis exist.

Pauciarticular

Pauciarticular juvenile rheumatoid arthritis is the most common type, affecting about 40 to 55 percent of children with JRA. It involves four or fewer joints, and the onset is usually gradual: A knee or an ankle swells initially, then causes the child to walk with a limp, although the child often feels no pain. This form of arthritis can also cause uveitis, a persistent inflammation of parts of the eye, including the uvea, iris, and surrounding tissue in the middle of the eye. If untreated, uveitis can cause permanent vision loss. Periodic examination by an ophthalmologist (eye doctor) is advisable, since uveitis can damage the eye with few warning signs.

Polyarticular

Polyarticular JRA involves many joints, including the small ones in the hands and feet. It usually strikes in a symmetrical fashion, so that if a joint on one side of the body is affected, the corresponding joint on the other side will also be affected. It is most common in girls and can also be complicated with uveitis. Often more severe than the pauciarticular form, polyarticular JRA causes more joint destruction. Other complications can include lung and heart disease.

Systemic

Affecting 10 percent to 20 percent of children with JRA, this form of the disease also affects many joints and often begins with a fever or a rash, as well as enlargement of the liver, spleen, and lymph nodes. In some cases, inflammation of the linings of the lungs (pleuritis) or heart (pericarditis) can cause cough, shortness of breath, and chest pain. It can take several months before the more classic symptoms of joint inflammation and pain occur. If left untreated, joint destruction can be extensive.

Causes

No one knows what causes JRA, but several theories exist. One is that it results from a viral infection. Another is that exposure to some unknown agent makes a child's immune system overreact and attack healthy joint tissue. Since some forms of arthritis run in families, genes may play a role.

What the Doctor May Do

The doctor may ask you to track your child's symptoms for several weeks or months before considering a diagnosis of arthritis. JRA must be diagnosed in part by excluding other causes of recurrent, chronic joint pain and swelling, such as systemic lupus erythematosus, a lifelong disorder characterized by inflammation of the body's connective tissues (tendons and ligaments); acute rheumatic fever; or Kawasaki's disease, characterized in part by fever, rash, and swelling of the hands and feet.

Often, he will order blood tests to look for signs of inflammation, anemia, and reactions to the immune system. One such test is for antinuclear antibodies (ANA test), which is positive in some children with JRA. Another is HLA (human leukocyte antigen) type B27, which may run in families.

To help diagnose JRA and treat any complications that may arise, your doctor may consult a pediatric rheumatologist, an ophthalmologist, physical and occupational therapists, and sometimes an orthopedic surgeon. If the diagnosis of JRA is made, children are typically seen periodically in a specialized rheumatology or immunology clinic so that their special needs can be coordinated. A counselor may be important to help your child adapt to her chronic illness and help her work through issues of self-esteem, school performance, and so forth.

Treatment for juvenile rheumatoid arthritis usually includes a combination of anti-inflammatory medication to help prevent damage to the joints and medications aimed at lessening the severity of the disease. Anti-inflammatory medications given include aspirin, ibuprofen, acetaminophen, and, in more severe cases, synthetic hormonelike medications called corticosteroids. Other treatments aimed at suppressing the immune system may include hydroxychloroquine, methotrexate, or sulfasalazine.

Your child should also take part in a regular physical-therapy program designed to maintain muscle strength and a full range of motion around the inflamed joints. Physical therapy is essential to avoid long-term side effects from joint inflammation. The therapist may recommend splinting during the day, at night, or both, to keep the joints loose and supple.

With proper management and medications, most cases of JRA will remit, with few long-term consequences to your child's health. In more severe, untreated cases, crippling joint destruction can occur. The joints can, in this case, become permanently stiff or frozen by scarring (known as contracture formation), which may require surgical repair. Most children do not outgrow JRA. Flares of symptoms may recur without warning for many years.

What You Can Do

If your child is diagnosed with JRA, your involvement is crucial to successful treatment. Here are a few ways you can help:

- *Ask lots of questions.* Make sure you understand the benefits and potential side effects of the medications you are using to treat your child. Keep appointments with specialists whom your doctor wants your child to see. They are your partners in dealing with this chronic illness.

- *Read all you can.* Check your local library and the Internet for resources on JRA. Your local chapter of the Arthritis Foundation is an excellent source for educational materials and support. See Appendix: Parent Resources, Medical Conditions.

- *Keep a diary.* Make note of good days and bad days, missed school, unusual symptoms, and so forth, to help you remember. You are the best observer of your child on a daily basis.

- *Encourage your child to be active.* Perform range-of-motion and muscle-strengthening exercises of the affected joints, under the guidance of a physical therapist. Only when in the midst of a "flare" should activities be restricted.

- *Join a parents' group in your community.* Ask your doctor about local support groups.

- *Be wary of unproven therapies.* Quick cures you can buy in a health food store or unconventional therapies usually offer only disappointment. Ask your doctor's opinion before trying a novel approach.

Prevention

Because no one knows what causes JRA, there is no way to prevent the illness. You can, however, help your child avoid the complications of the illness, such as joint deformity and poor joint function, by following the regimen of medicines, physical therapy, and other management strategies your child's doctor and consulting team of medical specialists recommend.

■ Ketoacidosis

See *Diabetes Mellitus.*

■ Lacerations

See *Cuts and Scrapes.*

Lacrimal Duct Problems

See *Tear Ducts, Blocked.*

Language Disorders

See *Learning Disorders.*

Laryngitis

Although many a parent of a talkative toddler might wish for a little silence, a case of laryngitis is often a source of worry. The good news is that laryngitis, an inflammation of the voice box (larynx), is usually harmless and resolves on its own.

Signs and Symptoms

- Hoarse cry in infants or a loss of voice in older children
- Dry *cough*
- Mild *fever*
- Sore throat

Inflammation of the larynx (laryngitis) is usually caused by respiratory viruses like those that cause colds and the flu.

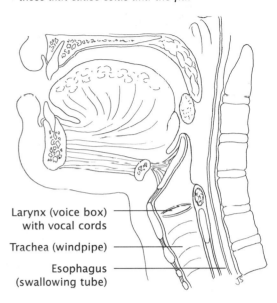

Larynx (voice box) with vocal cords

Trachea (windpipe)

Esophagus (swallowing tube)

When to Call the Doctor
CALL FOR **EMERGENCY** HELP IF

- your child has difficulty breathing and/or is turning blue.

  For first aid information, see page 380 if your child is less than 1 year old and page 383 if your child is 1 year of age or older.

  CALL THE DOCTOR IMMEDIATELY IF

- your child has difficulty swallowing or is drooling much more than usual.
- your child develops a sudden, high fever.

  CALL THE DOCTOR TODAY IF

- your child has been hoarse for days or weeks and is not getting better.

Essential Facts

Laryngitis often occurs as part of an upper respiratory infection. It can also be a symptom of *allergies,* such as hay fever, in the spring and fall. Children between 3 months and 5 years of age are most susceptible. The disease is usually accompanied by a mild cold or sore throat (see *Sore Throat/Strep Throat*).

Laryngitis is the most common cause of hoarseness—a rough and husky quality of voice—but it isn't the only cause. Hoarseness is also associated with *croup* or vocal strain that comes with excessive yelling and screaming. Hoarseness caused by consistent vocal abuse can lead to the development of vocal nodules, small thickened areas (calluses) of the vocal cords, which causes chronic hoarseness.

Less commonly, chronic hoarseness in children can be caused by papillomas, wartlike growths on the vocal cords that can cause respiratory distress. Hoarseness can also be a sign of *epiglottitis* or of a foreign body lodged in the larynx.

Causes

In most cases, laryngitis is caused by respiratory viruses such as those that cause colds and flu. For unknown reasons, some children are more vulnerable to laryngitis than others.

What the Doctor May Do

If your doctor suspects laryngitis, she probably won't prescribe medication. The condition should resolve within a few days, without treatment. Most cases of laryngitis don't require antibiotics, because they are caused by viruses that do not respond to antibiotic treatment. If your child is chronically hoarse, your doctor may refer you to an ear, nose, and throat specialist for further evaluation.

What You Can Do

- *Try the "silent treatment."* The less your child uses his voice, the faster the swelling and inflammation will heal. To make the enforced quiet more fun, devise a "code" of hand signals that your child can make when he needs something.
- *Discourage whispering.* Believe it or not, whispering strains vocal cords more than normal speech does. If your child can't completely rest his voice, have him speak in a low tone.
- *Use a vaporizer.* A vaporizer or humidifier in your child's room can help loosen the mucus that may be causing irritation. Also, dry air is much more irritating than moist air. If you use a vaporizer, clean it thoroughly and often to avoid recirculating viruses, bacteria, and fungi.

Prevention

You can reduce your child's chances of coming down with such infections by keeping him away from others who are coughing and sneezing, by protecting him from tobacco smoke, and by encouraging him to wash his hands often. If your child has laryngitis, encourage him to cover his mouth with a tissue when he coughs or sneezes to avoid spreading the infection to others.

Laryngotracheobronchitis (LTB)

See *Croup.*

Lazy Eye

See *Amblyopia and/or Strabismus.*

Lead Poisoning

Nothing is more natural than for small children to put things in their mouths. That makes babies and small children particularly susceptible to lead poisoning. Lead, a metal found in some paints, plasters, water pipes, house dust, and dirt and soil (in and around homes painted with lead paint), and some kinds of cookware and ceramics, poses health hazards when swallowed.

In young children, lead exposure poses the threat of impaired intellectual development. That's why it is important to protect your baby and young child from possible exposure to lead. A simple precaution such as washing your baby's hands frequently, as well as any toys she puts in her mouth, can help reduce the risk of lead poisoning. Be alert for signs of chipping, peeling paint, and never renovate an older home or sand or strip old woodwork in a home while a young child is living in it. Have your child's blood lead tested annually.

Signs and Symptoms

For mild cases of lead poisoning:

- Often, none until difficulties at school begin
- Fatigue
- Pallor
- Constipation
- Loss of appetite
- Irritability
- Behavioral changes
- Sleep disorders

For severe cases of lead poisoning:

- ***Vomiting*** and ***headaches***
- Abdominal pain (sometimes called "lead colic")
- Clumsiness (sometimes called "foot drop" or "wrist drop")
- Weakness
- Confusion, drowsiness, ***seizures***, or coma

When to Call the Doctor

CALL THE DOCTOR IMMEDIATELY IF

- your child has eaten paint chips or plaster or has otherwise been exposed to lead. Don't wait for symptoms to appear.

TALK WITH THE DOCTOR AT
YOUR CHILD'S NEXT CHECKUP IF

- you have questions about screening your child for lead poisoning.

Essential Facts

Lead poisoning is a common problem—about 1 million children in the United States had lead poisoning as of 1988, although it is less of a problem than it was 25 years ago, when lead-based paints and lead-containing car emissions were far more common. The total incidence of elevated blood lead levels dropped from 78.8 percent of people tested to just 4.4 percent in the past two decades, and average blood lead levels

in the United States have dropped more than 80 percent (probably due to the switch to unleaded gasoline) in the same period. If you suspect that your child may have swallowed lead or lead paint, have a doctor examine her immediately.

Also called plumbism, lead poisoning most often affects children 6 months to 6 years old who live in houses built before 1978 (the year that lead paint was banned) or in heavily industrialized and urban areas, where soil in yards and playgrounds may contain lead. Children under 2 years old are the most vulnerable to the neurotoxic (brain poisoning) effects, although older children can also suffer injury.

Lead poisoning occurs when a child ingests lead by swallowing contaminated paint chips or dust, plaster, water, or soil or, occasionally, by drinking or eating out of lead-contaminated vessels. About 10 percent of the lead swallowed is absorbed into the bloodstream, although in children with an iron deficiency, the bloodstream can absorb up to 50 percent, which is why lead poisoning tends to affect undernourished children. Lead tends to stay in the body for years, leaving slowly through urine, stool, sweat, saliva, and nails and hair.

How sick a child becomes from lead poisoning is determined by the amount of lead she is exposed to, how much her body absorbs, and the length of time over which absorption occurs. Lead poisoning interferes with body functions in many ways, including the following:

- *Brain growth and development:* Lead poisoning during fetal development or from infancy up to 5 years of age may permanently impair brain growth and development, leading to such problems as ***learning disorders, behavioral problems,*** or ***attention deficit disorder.*** Early signs include slow speech acquisition, impaired visual-spatial-motor skills, and hyperactivity.
- *Anemia:* Lead poisoning can cause severe ***anemia*** by inhibiting the production of the

iron-containing component of hemoglobin, a red pigment that carries oxygen to the tissues and removes waste.

- *Lead encephalopathy:* This rare, life-threatening complication of lead poisoning is caused by widespread toxic brain injury. Sudden, forceful vomiting and headache mark its onset, soon followed by seizures and coma. Children who survive lead encephalopathy may develop sensory impairments (*hearing loss* and blindness) and *mental retardation.*

Causes

Lead in Dust

The most common cause of lead poisoning in the United States is the consumption of lead-containing dust found in homes built before 1978. Windowsills and window wells often have high levels of lead dust, which can wind up on the floor or in other areas of the house. The lead in this dust comes from interior and exterior paint and from soil and airborne emissions, such as incinerators, smelters, and other machines. Millions of adult workers are exposed to lead on the job, and as a result, many children are poisoned by lead dust their parents bring home on their work clothes. Lead dust gets on children's hands and toys and then into their mouths through normal behavior, including thumb sucking.

Lead Paint or Plaster Chips

Children may chew on windowsills or other woodwork painted with lead-containing paint or put lead paint flakes or paint-laden plaster in their mouths. Furniture or toys with leaded paint are also contamination sources. Children who exhibit pica, an abnormal craving for substances that have no food value, are particularly at risk, as are babies and toddlers, who quite normally explore objects with their mouths.

Paint that contains lead tastes sweet, and therefore is appealing to toddlers.

Lead in Soil

Lead may contaminate the dirt in which your child plays at the playground or in your yard, the result of decades of peeling exterior building paint, air emissions from leaded car exhaust, and pollution from smelters and other factories.

Lead in Water

The Environmental Protection Agency (EPA) estimates that about 20 percent of lead exposure in the United States is through drinking water. The EPA's limit for lead in water is 15 parts per billion (15 ppb), and it may soon drop to zero tolerance. Lead leaches into the water from old lead pipes and service lines in city systems and from home plumbing. Even after lead pipes were banned in the 1960s, leaded solder was legal for use on drinking water lines until the 1980s and is still sold in hardware stores. Faucets and plumbing fittings may legally contain up to 8 percent lead. The greatest risk from lead-contaminated water is to infants who drink formula mixed with such water. If you are pregnant, be wary of lead in your drinking water. Be sure to have it tested.

Other Lead Sources

Lead can leach into food or beverages stored in imported ceramics or pottery and leaded crystal and china. Certain hobby items use products with lead (such as fishing sinkers, stained glass, and ceramics). Some indigenous or imported but unregulated health products can also be contaminated. For instance, lead can also be found in some cosmetics and natural folk remedies.

What the Doctor May Do

A simple blood test can measure lead levels. Doctors sometimes also take X rays to determine

the extent of lead deposits in bone tissue or to detect recently swallowed lead-containing objects or paint chips. In mild cases, treatment may involve simply preventing further lead intake and resolving nutritional problems, such as iron or calcium deficiencies.

More severe cases of lead poisoning require chelation therapy, or the administration of chemicals that latch onto the lead in blood (to *chelate* means to "hold onto tightly") and cause it to be eliminated in the urine. Most chelation therapy is now done with oral medications taken at home, after lead has been eliminated from the child's surroundings. Depending on the severity of the poisoning, this process may take weeks or months of daily medication. During this time, the doctor will monitor the child's blood lead levels and check for side effects every 2 to 4 weeks. The doctor may also prescribe vitamin supplements after chelation therapy to restore important metals, such as iron, lost during the therapy. Side effects of chelation therapy can include nausea, vomiting, diarrhea, rashes, bruising, and blood cells in the urine. Such symptoms may prompt the doctor to have the child discontinue the medication or switch to another medication.

A child with severe lead poisoning usually requires hospitalization, where strong chelating agents are given intravenously or intramuscu-

---

LEAD TEST RESULTS

In many areas, annual lead screening is required for preschool children. Lead levels in the blood are measured in micrograms per deciliter (mcg/dl). The federal Centers for Disease Control and Prevention have set the following guidelines:

- *Below 10 mcg/dl:* If your child's lead test results are below this level, you needn't be concerned: Lead poisoning is defined as a lead level of 10 mcg/dl and higher. Your child's doctor may recommend annual blood lead screening.

- *10–19 mcg/dl or higher:* If your child's lead level is at least 10 mcg/dl, your child's blood lead level should be monitored every 3 to 4 months. You'll need to identify the lead source that your child is exposed to and either remove it or help her avoid it.

- *20–44 mcg/dl:* In this range, your child will probably be treated for lead poisoning. Your doctor may recommend chelation therapy after the lead has been eliminated from the home environment. Blood lead levels should be screened every 3 to 4 weeks.

- *45–75 mcg/dl:* If the blood lead level is in this range, your child will probably be hospitalized and given medication to draw the lead out of her body. She will need to drink plenty of fluids in order to excrete the lead and medications in her urine. While your child is in the hospital, health professionals can inspect the home to try to find the source of the lead and help make arrangements for safe, alternative housing or recommend ways to eliminate the lead source. Your child's blood lead levels should be monitored every 24 to 48 hours.

- *75 mcg/dl or higher:* If blood lead levels are in this range, your child has a medical emergency and should be hospitalized for immediate treatment. Blood lead levels should be tested again within 24 hours.

larly. In severe cases, a child may require close observation and long-term care and medication.

Even after successful removal of lead from the body, affected children remain at high risk for recurrent lead poisoning. Therefore, any lead or lead products in the home must be completely removed before children return home. Symptoms of lead poisoning may remain apparent for some time.

What You Can Do

One important way to help avoid lead poisoning complications is to have your child's blood tested annually during the preschool years. Screening should start at 6 months for high-risk children—those who live near or in older houses or in heavily industrialized or urban areas. This is especially important when your child is between 1 and 5 years old, because lead poisoning occurs most frequently in this age range and the brain is most vulnerable to lead's toxic effects then. If any test shows an elevated lead level, plan to have your child screened more frequently. Even if you live in a low-risk area, bring your child in for a blood lead screening at least once before she turns 2 years old and once afterward.

Prevention

Act now to prevent your baby from being exposed to lead. Here are some ways to find lead sources and reduce lead levels:

- *Have your children tested annually for lead.*

- *Lead-test your home.* In some states, lead paint testing is required during the sale of the house. But if your house has not been tested, buy a lead-testing kit in a hardware store, and test surfaces that might contain lead, like painted walls, windowsills and trim, window frames, vinyl mini-blinds, and ceramic bowls. If you suspect that your home has lead paint, call your state health department, which will send an inspector who specializes in identifying lead contamination sources. Or hire a professional lead tester. Some independent contractors can both test for lead levels and remove lead paint.

- *Remove lead-based paint.* If you are renting your home, notify your landlord—most states require lead to be removed from rental properties where children live. If you own a house that has lead paint, hire a certified contractor who knows how to protect workers, the family, and the environment to remove the paint. Stripping the paint yourself or hiring someone inexperienced can worsen the problem by creating lead dust. You can poison yourself by breathing paint dust as you scrape and strip. To find a qualified contractor, call your state health department or the regional office of the EPA.

- *Don't allow young children to live in a house with lead paint during renovations.*

- *Discard mini-blinds and other items found to have lead.* For eating and serving food, don't use lead bowls, lead crystal, or cookware manufactured outside the United States.

- *Create barriers.* Keep contaminated windows closed. Windows with lead paint generate dust, which, when the windows are open, blows in and contaminates floors and other surfaces. Cover contaminated windowsills with duct tape. Use lead-encapsulating paint on exposed baseboards. Use paneling to cover walls painted with lead paint.

- *Consider replacing your home's windows.* Windows, where weathering and wear and tear cause paint to chip, flake, and peel more rapidly, are the biggest source of lead dust. Replacing your home's windows is one of the best investments you can make if you want to limit the amount of lead in your house.

- *Stress cleanliness.* If you're not sure whether your house contains lead or if you live in a high-risk area, keep home dust levels to a minimum. Clean up the dust with a damp mop and a solution of either trisodium phosphate (TSP) or other phosphate-containing detergents available at hardware stores, rather than vacuuming, which can scatter dust into the air. Phosphates in TSP and detergents can bind to the lead directly, thereby helping remove it from the floors and windowsills during cleaning. Wipe hard surfaces like floors and window frames in your home with TSP solution or automatic dishwasher soap.

- *Wash your younger children's hands and faces before eating,* and encourage older children to do so frequently. Also, regularly wash toys and pacifiers that your child puts in her mouth.

- *Provide healthy meals.* Since more lead is absorbed on an empty stomach and research suggests that calcium, iron, and protein help decrease the chance that children will absorb lead from dust in the environment, serving healthy meals with enough of these nutrients is crucial (see Feeding and Eating sections in age-by-age chapters for more information on nutrition).

- *Store and serve food safely.* Do not store food in open cans, especially imported cans, or in lead crystal or china, and do not serve or store food in pottery meant for decorative use only. Avoid using old cookware, family heirlooms, or yard sale cookware when heating baby formula.

- *Provide "clean" sand.* If the soil around your home may be contaminated with lead, build a sandbox with a solid bottom and a top that you can cover it with at night. Fill it with clean sand for your child to play in.

- *Test your drinking water.* If you are unsure whether your drinking water is safe, contact the EPA's Safe Water Hotline (see Appendix: Parent Resources, Safety). If the water pipes in your home or town contain lead solder, some of the toxic metal could be leaching into your drinking water. Have your water tested by an independent, state-certified laboratory. The lead level shouldn't exceed 15 parts per billion. If the lead content in your tap water is higher than the standard, let the water run for several minutes before using it, particularly in the morning after it has been sitting in the pipes all night. Use only cold water for drinking and cooking, because hot tap water sometimes leaches lead out more quickly. You can also reduce the lead in your water by installing a water purifier specifically designed to eliminate lead.

- *Leave contaminated clothing at work.* If you (or another family member) work in a high-risk industry (smelting, painting, or construction or remodeling), change your clothes and shower before going home.

Learning Disorders

Even children with average or above-average intelligence sometimes have difficulty learning. But some children have more difficulty than most. The most common form of learning disorder is in reading skills, but childhood learning disorders vary widely in degree, nature, and complexity. Teachers and parents can recognize a learning disorder by this red flag: A child is having learning difficulties in only one specific area, such as reading, writing, organizing information, or doing math—in all other areas, the child is keeping up with his peers.

It is important to understand that a child with a learning disorder can learn. The disorder usually affects a limited area of a child's development. A learning disorder is not **mental retardation.** And although learning disorders often persist, learning-disabled children who receive early instruction geared toward their specific problem can function well later in life.

Signs and Symptoms

In the preschooler:

- Late speech development
- Cannot learn or confuses the names of letters by 4 or 5 years of age
- Cannot understand rhyming by 5 years of age
- Trouble following simple commands or instructions
- Poor listener
- Frequently disturbs other children

In the early school-age child:

- Difficulty following instructions
- Inability to remember the alphabet sequence
- Inability to read words, sentences, and little stories by the end of first grade
- Rarely finishes things he starts
- Inattentive, easily distracted
- Frequently disturbs other children

In the older school-age child (third grade and beyond):

- Poor organizational skills
- Cannot make the transition from learning to read to reading to learn
- Frequently fails to finish the things he starts
- Easily frustrated
- Inattentive, easily distracted
- Teacher comments about poor achievement

 When to Call the Doctor
CALL THE DOCTOR TODAY IF

- you have questions or concerns about your child's intellectual or academic development.
- you suspect that your child may have a vision or hearing problem that is interfering with his ability to learn.

Essential Facts

People gain the intellectual tools necessary to learn about their surroundings and communicate during childhood. These tools include specific skills, such as speech, letter identification, and the more complex skill of reading. Children learn in different ways. Some have difficulty learning in a group setting, such as school, which isn't tailored to their individual needs, even though they may be able to learn at home.

Learning problems vary widely from child to child. Some children have problems distinguishing what they hear and what they see; others have difficulty in concentrating, writing, doing math, or remembering. Estimates of the prevalence of learning disorders range from 5 to 15 percent of school-age children. About 80 percent of children identified as learning disabled have— as their main problem—a difficulty in learning to read or, later, comprehending what they read. The term *dyslexia* describes children who have severe difficulties in reading and writing.

Children with learning disorders sometimes also have other problems, such as trouble paying attention (see **Attention Deficit Disorder**) or difficulty getting along with others. Sometimes learning problems can produce feelings of low self-esteem, a dislike of school, or a lack of motivation.

Learning problems don't necessarily limit future capabilities. For example, a National Institutes of Health study showed that 67 percent of young students at risk for reading difficulties achieved average or above-average reading ability when they received help by age 9. But the later a child's disability is identified, the later help can begin and the greater the chances the child will have continued learning problems. For this reason, identifying children with reading problems and providing appropriate treatment before third grade is extremely important. Diagnosis and treatment for children with learning disorders can begin as early as problems are identified—even in preschool, although most learning disorders aren't diagnosed until the child starts school. The following are among the more common issues associated with learning problems:

- *Speech and language disorders:* These disorders involve difficulty in producing speech sounds, using spoken language to communicate, or understanding what others say. Speech and language disorders are the basis of most reading disorders, and early diagnosis and treatment of speech and language problems is the first line of defense in treating learning problems.

- *Problems understanding the sounds of words:* Known as phonemes, the sounds that make up words are an important part of learning to read. Some children have trouble breaking words into sounds. For example, the word *ball* has two parts, "b" and "all."

- *Problems interpreting visual stimuli:* Some children have difficulty recognizing common letter patterns and may need to sound out slowly the words that other children spot quickly. Similar letters may be confused: The word *dog* may be perceived as *bog*, for instance.

- *Problems understanding time and other sequences; memory problems:* Some children have problems understanding the concept of time or learning to tell time. They may have trouble learning the days of the week, months,

and years. In addition, they may have difficulty manipulating numbers, especially multiplying. As children grow older, problems with understanding time and sequence may affect their organizational abilities.

- *Problems with complex thinking:* Some children have difficulty performing tasks that require complex thinking, such as reasoning, generalizing, or classifying information.

- *Problems producing schoolwork:* Some children have few problems learning, but have more difficulty producing their own work. When the emphasis in school shifts from learning skills to using the skills, these children start having trouble. They may have organizational problems, such as difficulty using time effectively, an inability or a reluctance to complete homework, a progressive loss of interest in school, or trouble with writing.

Causes

The cause of a learning disorder usually remains unknown. Learning disorders may result from a problem in the way the brain handles certain information, which impairs the ability to learn certain things. Such problems can begin before birth or may result from low birth weight, premature birth, or central nervous system infections at the time of birth. Other causes include the following:

- *Genetic causes:* Learning disorders can run in families. If a parent or sibling has a learning disorder, a child is more likely to have similar problems. The most clearly established inherited disorder is difficulty understanding phonemes. Even a child whose family members have no other obvious learning problems may have a genetic cause for this learning disorder.

- *Problems in the home or school:* New research shows that a home environment that doesn't support learning (due to a housing instability, a lack of books or reading at home, prolonged family stress, etc.) can contribute to or cause learning problems, as can inadequate teaching in the first few years of school.

- *Fetal exposure to pollutants, tobacco, alcohol, or drugs:* A pregnancy free from tobacco, alcohol, drugs, and exposure to environmental toxins such as pesticides and lead is more likely to produce a healthy child. For more about having a healthy pregnancy, see page 3.

- *School absence or adjustment problems:* Chronic illnesses or other problems that cause frequent or prolonged absences from school may contribute to learning problems.

- *Physical trauma:* Children who experience severe head injuries or who experience trauma before or during childbirth are also at increased risk for learning disorders.

What the Doctor May Do

Early identification is the key to helping a child with learning problems. If you or your child's teacher have concerns about your child's ability to learn, consult the doctor. The doctor may give your child a thorough physical and neurological examination to rule out underlying medical problems. If none are evident, your doctor may recommend that you visit a learning problem specialist, who will profile your child's learning abilities. If your child is school-age, a guidance counselor or other professional can administer the tests and procedures. Depending on the nature of your child's problem, he may see one or all of the following professionals:

- A psychologist, a psychiatrist, or another mental health professional, to assess psychological state

- A speech and language pathologist, to evaluate language and speech development

- A neurologist, to look for evidence of subtle brain abnormalities

- An ophthalmologist (eye doctor), to evaluate vision

- An otolaryngologist (ear, nose, and throat specialist), to evaluate hearing

- A reading specialist, to evaluate reading development

Your child may also benefit from counseling, in which he can discuss his frustrations, challenges, and successes in an atmosphere of privacy, support, and expertise. When a learning-disabled child has another problem, such as an **attention deficit disorder,** medication may be a useful supplement to other forms of therapy.

What School Professionals Do

Once you and your child's teacher have determined that your child needs to be evaluated, the program designed to meet your child's particular needs will be part of a process coordinated by the school, known as the individualized education program (IEP). The IEP is an evaluation and treatment plan that describes the type of support your child needs to learn and grow as efficiently as possible. Some plans focus on cultivating basic skills through intensive instruction. For example, if your child has difficulty learning the sounds of alphabet letters, a special reading teacher may spend time with him practicing his letter sounds. A parent can serve as a "coach," setting up practice sessions and helping to motivate your child with rewards. Your child can also get help from tutors and seek assistance from after-school programs and support groups.

In general, children identified as having a learning disorder are included in the regular classroom as much as possible. At times, they require extra help in a small group. Some children with severe learning issues may require an all-day special group.

What You Can Do

The best thing you can do for a child with a learning disorder is to stress his strengths. For instance, if you notice that your child is good at art, music, science, computers, or sports, help him pursue these talents.

Also, learn and understand the IEP you develop in cooperation with your child's educators. Help your child follow the plan, and encourage him by following these guidelines:

- *Work closely with the school system.* Federal law entitles children with learning disorders to special education, including special programs for infants and toddlers who have such problems or are at high risk for them. Ask the special education coordinator or the guidance counselor at your child's school about these programs in your school system.

- *Learn about your child's challenges.* The more you know about what types of learning are difficult for your child, what sources of aid are available, and what you can do to create a supportive environment for learning, the better. Keep a diary of your child's daily activities, including behavior, diet, study, and sleeping patterns. Consider joining a support group, which can provide information sources, practical suggestions, and mutual understanding.

- *Respect and challenge your child's abilities.* Most children with learning disorders have average or above-average intelligence that can be engaged in many ways by you and your child's teacher. Support your child for what he can do, rather than focusing on what he cannot do.

- *Provide structure and organization.* Help your child organize his study habits by providing a quiet, well-lit place to study and a regular time each day for homework.

Prevention

The recommended way to prevent long-term learning problems is to identify the problem early (before third grade) and follow through with effective instruction. Though some learning disorders can't be cured, early treatment and intensive training can strengthen the brain's learning pathways. Living a healthy lifestyle during your pregnancy and providing a safe, stimulating environment for your child may also reduce the risk of learning problems.

See also *Developmental Problems; Pervasive Developmental Disorder.*

Leukemia

See *Cancer.*

Lice

See *Head Lice.*

Limping

Limping, or walking with an uneven gait, is most often the result of a minor, easily treated injury. However, more serious underlying conditions sometimes cause limping. If your child is limping and you cannot discover the cause, or if the pain from an injury does not subside after a few minutes, be sure to call the doctor.

Signs and Symptoms
- Walking with an uneven gait
- Difficulty putting weight on one leg
- Pain

When to Call the Doctor

CALL THE DOCTOR IMMEDIATELY IF

- the pain is severe.
- your child cannot put any weight on her leg.
- swelling is present.
- bruising or redness is present.
- a fever accompanies the limp.

CALL THE DOCTOR TODAY IF

- your baby limps as soon as she starts to walk (symptom of developmental hip dislocation).
- your child suddenly develops a pronounced limp.
- your child has had a slight limp for several days.
- the pain is severe enough to wake your child up.

Causes

A limp develops if a child feels pain when she puts weight on her leg. Limping or refusal to walk can be caused by pain anywhere along the leg. Problems in the hip, leg muscles, knee, ankle, or foot can cause limping. Splinters, blisters, or tired muscles are common culprits, but sometimes a more serious cause exists, such as a sprain (see *Sprains and Strains*), fracture (see p. 409), hip dislocation (see *Dislocations*), viral or bacterial joint infection (see *Joint Pain*), or arthritis (see *Juvenile Rheumatoid Arthritis*). A limp caused by an injury tends to get worse throughout the day as the child walks, whereas a limp due to arthritis is most pronounced in the morning and improves with use as the day progresses.

What the Doctor May Do

Unless an injury or other minor problem (such as a splinter or blister) is clearly the cause of the limping, your child's doctor will perform a thorough examination of your child, paying special attention to the joints and muscle tissue of the affected leg. If he suspects an infection, the doctor will perform some blood tests. The doctor might also order X rays to help make the diagnosis.

Treatment of a limp depends on its cause. Minor injuries, sprains, and strains usually can be treated with simple first aid measures at home. Severe injuries such as joint dislocations, fractures, and joint infections must be treated by an orthopedic specialist. Arthritis or pain of unknown cause needs the attention of a pediatric rheumatologist (see *Joint Pain*).

Some inflammatory causes of limping are relatively common in early childhood. Hip inflammation in a toddler may cause a child to limp and complain bitterly of pain. She may run a mild fever and even refuse to walk or put weight on her leg. This condition, known as toxic synovitis of the hip, may be caused by a virus, an allergic reaction, or another problem. Although the symptoms can be quite upsetting to parents and children, the condition usually goes away on its own in a few days, but may recur. Your doctor will first try to make sure your child doesn't have a more serious condition, such as a bacterial infection of the hip, or inflammation of the spine (discitis), or, in school-age children, a hip inflammation called Legg-Calvé-Perthes disease. Perthes disease must be treated with physical therapy under the guidance of an orthopedic surgeon. In older children, Osgood-Schlatter disease (jumper's knee), an inflammation of the tendon attached to the knee, is a common cause of limping. Treatment includes anti-inflammatory medication, protection of the knee through the use of knee pads, and having the child avoid the sports that make it worse (such as basketball).

What You Can Do

Apply first aid at home if you know that the cause of limping is a minor condition such as *blisters, splinters,* or minor muscle strain (see *Sprains and Strains*). If further testing or treatment is necessary, comfort your child by explaining as much as she can understand about the tests and treatments while reassuring her that you will be there to help her feel safe.

Prevention

To help prevent limps related to muscle injuries, encourage your child to stretch out before playing sports or engaging in rigorous physical activity. Reduce the chance of blisters by making sure that your child wears shoes that fit properly, and reduce the chances of splinters by having her wear shoes when walking on any wooden surface, particularly play structures or wooden decking. You cannot prevent your child from developing a limp due to a developmental or congenital abnormality, a joint infection, or arthritis.

■ *Liver Disorders*

See *Jaundice.*

■ *Loose Tooth*

A rite of passage in every child's life, losing a first baby tooth is an occurrence that usually requires no medical care.

When to Call the Doctor or Dentist
CALL THE DOCTOR OR
DENTIST IMMEDIATELY IF

- a permanent tooth is loosened following a blow to the mouth or a fall.

CALL THE DOCTOR OR DENTIST TODAY IF

- a baby (primary) tooth is abnormally loose before your child is about 4 or 5 years old.
- a permanent tooth has become loose from an accident.
- you notice a permanent tooth coming in before the primary tooth it was to replace has fallen out.

Essential Facts

Most children start to lose their baby teeth between 5 and 7 years old, after permanent incisors (front teeth) are nearly finished forming beneath the gums. Usually (but not always) the first teeth to fall out are the lower front teeth, followed by the upper front teeth. By the time most children are 13 years old, all of their primary teeth will have been replaced by permanent teeth.

Causes

Most loose teeth are the result of the normal process by which primary teeth are replaced by permanent ones. But injury to the mouth can cause a tooth—primary or permanent—to come loose.

Normally children's primary teeth become loose (and eventually fall out) when permanent teeth are ready to erupt. The growth and maturation of a permanent tooth cause the root of a baby tooth to gradually dissolve (a process known as resorption). This process begins at the root tip and progresses until only the crown, the part of the tooth you see, remains attached to

Permanent teeth usually begin erupting around 6 to 7 years of age and follow a standard order that begins with the lower front teeth, known as the central incisors.

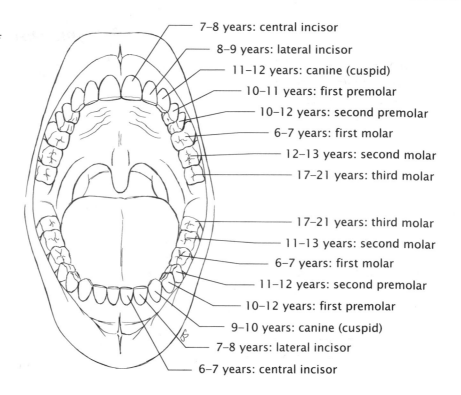

7–8 years: central incisor

8–9 years: lateral incisor

11–12 years: canine (cuspid)

10–11 years: first premolar

10–12 years: second premolar

6–7 years: first molar

12–13 years: second molar

17–21 years: third molar

17–21 years: third molar

11–13 years: second molar

6–7 years: first molar

11–12 years: second premolar

10–12 years: first premolar

9–10 years: canine (cuspid)

7–8 years: lateral incisor

6–7 years: central incisor

the gums. As the connection between the gum surface and the crown tears, the tooth loosens and falls out. The adult tooth emerges, usually within a few weeks or months.

What the Doctor or Dentist Might Do

A loose baby tooth usually requires no treatment; it will simply fall out by itself. But sometimes, permanent teeth will start to come in before primary teeth have had a chance to fall out. This usually occurs because the permanent teeth emerge slightly behind or in front of the primary teeth and don't trigger the normal resorption process. In that case, the dentist may decide to remove the primary teeth so that the permanent teeth can move into the proper location.

If, however, the loose tooth is a permanent one and has been loosened by injury, the doctor will stabilize it with a plastic splint or another device that secures the tooth to the adjacent teeth until the injury has healed. If a permanent tooth has been knocked out completely, the doctor will reinsert the tooth and secure it with a splint until it has healed. In some cases, a root canal procedure (a process by which damaged or infected pulp tissue within the tooth is removed) may be necessary within a few weeks.

A tooth that has been knocked out and reimplanted has a high likelihood of remaining permanently in place if reimplanted within an hour after the accident.

What You Can Do

If your child's tooth becomes loose as a result of an injury, bring him to the dentist as soon as possible, no matter what his age. If a tooth has been partially or totally knocked out, see What to Do on page 406.

When a baby tooth naturally becomes loose, the best thing you can do is simply reassure your child, who may be a little frightened or worried. If the area around the tooth is sore, you may give him acetaminophen or ibuprofen to reduce the pain. If the tooth is loose and really bothering him—particularly if it makes eating difficult—and doesn't seem to want to fall out on its own, you can try to twist it out the rest of the way by following these steps:

1. Rub the area around the tooth with an antiseptic mouthwash.
2. Take a clean tissue, and grip the tooth.
3. Quickly twist or turn the tooth both ways as if you are opening the cap to a bottle. It should come out in your hand.
4. Apply pressure to the wound with gauze or a clean, wet washcloth for a few minutes if any bleeding is occurring.
5. Have your child avoid vigorously sucking or chewing on anything in that area of his mouth for 24 hours so as not to disturb the healing process.

Prevention

You can protect your child's teeth by taking certain precautions. Active children in particular need proper mouth protection to prevent broken or knocked-out teeth. If your child participates in a contact sport, such as football, or simply rides his bike or enjoys in-line skating, ask your doctor or dentist for advice on choosing the proper mouth guard for your child. Also, discourage children from opening jars or bottle caps with their teeth.

▮ Loss of Consciousness

See *Fainting.*

▮ Lyme Disease

Nothing is more fun for a child than exploring the woods or playing in the fields in the summer. However, if you and your family live in certain areas of the United States—coastal areas of New England and the Middle Atlantic States, Minnesota, Wisconsin, or the Northwest Coast—examine your child carefully for tick bites at the end of the day. Some ticks found in these areas cause a potentially serious infection called Lyme disease, named after the town of Old Lyme, Connecticut, where the disease was first discovered. Fortunately, prompt treatment with antibiotics cures the infection before it causes any lasting damage. If left untreated, the disease can lead to a form of arthritis and neurological problems (which can, however, usually be treated effectively).

Signs and Symptoms

Early symptoms that appear within a few days of a deer tick bite:

- Red "bull's-eye" rash beginning at the site of a tick bite and growing larger for several days; lighter or whiter center with a pinkish and irregular border
- Similar rashes on other parts of the body appearing in the next few weeks
- *Headaches*
- *Fever*
- Fatigue
- Muscle pains
- Neck pain

Later symptoms that appear weeks or months after the tick bite:

- Symptoms of arthritis (joint pain and stiffness)
- Dizziness
- Encephalitis

- Pericarditis, dysrhythmias (see *Abnormal Heart Rhythm*)
- Facial palsy
- Chronic neurological problems

 When to Call the Doctor
CALL THE DOCTOR TODAY IF

- a red rash begins at the site of an insect bite and grows larger for several days.
- you notice other symptoms related to Lyme disease.

To locate ticks, perform a full body check, examining the armpits, ears, backs of knees, back of the neck, scalp, and groin area. The ticks are small, but they must remain attached to the skin for more than 24 hours in order to transmit Lyme disease.

The deer tick, one of the smallest ticks, which is the size of a sesame seed, causes Lyme disease.

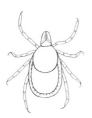
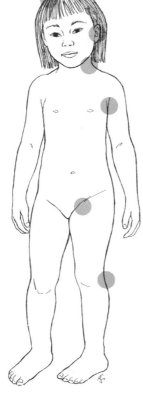

Essential Facts

After a child has been bitten by a tick that carries Lyme disease, the first sign of the disease is usually a large, doughnut-shaped or bull's-eye rash, sometimes up to 1½ inches across. Sometimes the child develops a red, raised bump that can expand into a 5-inch red ring. Only about half of children with Lyme disease develop this rash.

The earlier the condition is identified and treated, the more likely that the infection will be cured without complications. In some cases, especially if treatment is delayed, the joints may become swollen, sore, and difficult to move. Most commonly, one knee is involved. Severe cases of Lyme disease may also affect other organs, including the nervous system, heart, and kidneys. Usually, even these later complications of Lyme disease can be successfully treated.

Causes

The bite of a species of tick no bigger than a pinhead transmits this systemic disease. Called the black-legged or deer tick (*Ixodes scapularis* on the East Coast and in the Midwest, and a cousin, *Ixodes pacificus,* in the West), this tick often sucks the blood of white-tailed deer. The deer tick transmits a spirochete (a specialized spiral-form bacterium known as *Borrelia burgdorferi*), which first invades human skin, causing a distinctive rash. The organism later enters the bloodstream, causing other symptoms of infection.

What the Doctor May Do

Lyme disease can be difficult to diagnose, because the early signs and symptoms are variable and because the rash may not appear until 1 to 2 weeks after the bite occurs. Also, the blood test that detects antibodies to the infection is not accurate until between 3 to 6 weeks. If you suspect that your child has Lyme disease, ask to see a doctor experienced in diagnosing the condition. If a rash is present, your doctor will first examine your child's rash to see if it resembles the characteristic red pattern caused by Lyme disease infection. If the rash is typical, this confirms Lyme disease and he'll prescribe antibiotics. If the rash is gone before the doctor can examine it or if no rash ever developed, a blood test may be necessary.

As treatment, children 8 years of age and older usually receive oral amoxicillin or doxycycline (antibiotics). Children under age 8 usually receive amoxicillin. Only 1 percent of children treated with antibiotics develop more serious symptoms later. In those cases, the doctor may prescribe stronger antibiotic treatments for up to 30 days. If the disease progresses beyond its early stage, the doctor will prescribe treatment according to the symptoms that appear.

What You Can Do

Be alert for ticks on your child's skin, especially if your child has been outside in woods or areas of tall grass. If you notice a tick, remove it (see *Insect Bites and Stings*). If you suspect that it is a deer tick, save it by sticking it to a piece of transparent tape. Place the tape inside an airtight container like a zipper-seal plastic bag or a photo film container, and bring it to your doctor. Follow the instructions on page 613 for protecting your child from ticks and for performing a body search daily. Be alert for signs of a rash, particularly one that seems to grow larger from a central point over a few days. Watch for other signs and symptoms listed here, and report them to your doctor. Tell the doctor if your child has been playing in an area such as woods or tall grass where deer ticks may live.

Most children with mild cases of Lyme disease recover within a matter of days after beginning antibiotics. The period of convalescence for a very sick child, however, can last 2 to 3 weeks—or longer if the condition becomes chronic.

Prevention

A vaccine to prevent Lyme disease is available on a limited basis for people who live or work in high-risk areas. Also, protect your child against acquiring tick bites in brush or woodlands during tick season by making sure she wears protective clothing—lightweight but long-sleeved shirts, long pants, and hats—and using insect repellent, especially if you live an area where deer ticks are common. Consult your doctor or local health department if you have any questions.

Insect repellent containing deet (N, N-diethyl-meta-toluamide, no more than 10 percent strength) is effective when used sparingly on clothing and skin. (Do not use a repellent containing deet on a child less than 2 years old.) Wash it off later with soap and water. Because deer ticks are tiny, be sure to examine your child carefully before bathing each night. Perform a full body check, examining the armpits, the backs of knees, the back of the neck, the scalp, and the groin area. The ticks are small, but they must remain attached to the skin for more than 24 hours in order to transmit Lyme disease. If you find a tick on or in your child's skin, follow the tips provided in Insect Bites and Stings for removing it.

See also *Rashes.*

Lymph Nodes, Swollen

See *Swollen Glands.*

Lymphoma

See *Cancer.*

▮ *Measles*

Thanks to the combined measles, mumps, and rubella vaccine (MMR) that most children receive for the first time at about 12 to 15 months, the once-common childhood disease of measles is now rare. Outbreaks do occur, however, and because measles, also known as rubeola, is quite contagious, make sure your child is vaccinated against it.

Signs and Symptoms

- Eyes sensitive to the light (child prefers darkened room)
- Reddened eyelids with yellowish discharge
- Dry cough
- Fever as high as 104°F
- Bright red rash of small spots starting behind the ears and spreading to the rest of the body
- Pale, round spots inside the mouth

When to Call the Doctor
CALL THE DOCTOR IMMEDIATELY IF
- your child with measles acts confused or delirious.
- your child with measles has a cough and has difficult, congested breathing.

CALL THE DOCTOR TODAY IF
- you suspect that your child has measles.
- your unimmunized child has come in contact with someone who has measles.
- your child gets worse or complains of an earache while recovering from measles.

Essential Facts

Cough, runny nose, sore throat, and red and watery eyes are often the earliest signs of measles, also known as rubeola. A rash that eventually covers the whole body follows. The high fever that accompanies measles can be quite debilitating and may even cause a seizure (see *Seizures*). Often, a child with measles finds direct light annoying or painful to the eyes. Complications of measles, such as middle ear infections (see *Earache/Ear Infection)*, *pneumonia*, *croup*, and *diarrhea* may occur in younger children. In rare cases (about 1 in 1,000), measles can lead to brain damage or death. So be sure to alert your doctor if you suspect measles.

Measles usually lasts from 7 to 9 days or until the fever subsides and the rash begins to fade and peel in small flakes. A child with measles is contagious from 1 to 2 days before some symptoms appear and from 3 to 5 days before the rash appears. He remains contagious until 5 days after the rash has appeared. The average time between when a child is exposed and when the rash appears is 14 days.

Causes

Measles is caused by an RNA-containing paramyxovirus spread through direct contact with infected saliva, usually by coughing or sneezing. Highly contagious, measles affects 9 out of 10 unvaccinated people exposed to the disease.

What the Doctor May Do

The doctor diagnoses measles based on a child's symptoms, particularly by the characteristic rash and sensitivity to light. She may run special laboratory tests in order to confirm the diagnosis. No medication currently exists to treat the disease.

What You Can Do

- *Reduce the fever.* Use acetaminophen or ibuprofen to reduce your child's fever.
- *Quiet the cough.* Because measles is likely to cause a hacking cough, ask your doctor whether a cough medicine would be appropriate (see *Cough*).
- *Isolate your child.* Keep visitors away at this time to avoid spreading the disease.

- *Inform contacts.* Notify everyone your child comes into contact with, so that they can check their immunization status or receive appropriate care.

Prevention

The measles vaccine is part of the MMR (measles, mumps, and rubella) vaccine your child should receive at about 12 to 15 months of age. Your child should receive a second measles vaccine at around 4 to 6 years. Your doctor will assess whether your child needs another vaccine at 11 or 12 years old. Many measles outbreaks of the 1990s have involved teenagers and young adults who had previously been immunized but whose immunity had worn off. If your unvaccinated child is exposed to the virus, bring him to the doctor immediately. A vaccination within 3 days of exposure is about 70 percent effective in preventing the disease.

See also *Rashes.*

▌ *Meningitis*

A rare but serious condition, meningitis is an inflammation of the tissues that cover the brain and spinal cord. This uncommon illness usually affects infants and children under 5 years old. Although potentially life-threatening if untreated, children who receive prompt medical attention usually recover fully.

Signs and Symptoms

- Poor feeding
- Sudden vomiting
- *Fever* (101–106°F)
- Stiff neck
- Extreme lethargy or sleepiness
- Rash (occasionally)
- *Headaches*
- *Seizures*

When to Call the Doctor
CALL FOR EMERGENCY HELP IF

- your child has difficulty breathing and/or turns blue.
- your child is comatose.
- your child experiences a seizure (see *Seizures*).

For first aid information, see page 380 if your child is less than 1 year old and page 383 if your child is 1 year of age or older.

CALL THE DOCTOR IMMEDIATELY IF

- your child is under 6 months old and has a fever of 100.2°F or higher.
- your child is 6 months old or older and has a fever of 102°F or higher.
- your child has a fever and stiff neck and is vomiting.
- your child's headache is progressively worsening.
- your child is becoming more and more drowsy.
- your child has a fever and rash and is confused or lethargic.

Essential Facts

Meningitis occurs in two major forms: the more common viral form and the rarer, but more serious, bacterial form. Doctors still don't understand why some children get meningitis and others don't, but certain children are more susceptible than others, including

- babies under 2 months old, whose undeveloped immune systems cannot fight the infection.
- children with recent serious head injuries and skull fractures.

In children over 10 years old, symptoms usually appear suddenly. In children 2 to 10 years old, fever appears first, followed by lethargy or irritability. In infants, irritability, fever, vomiting, and poor feeding are accompanied by a tight or bulging fontanel (the soft spot on top of the head).

Causes

At least 20 viruses—including Coxsackie A and B (see *Hand-Foot-and-Mouth Disease*), the *mumps* virus, and the virus that causes polio—cause viral meningitis. Among the bacteria that cause meningitis are *Pneumococcus, Streptococcus, Meningococcus,* and *Haemophilus influenza.* All these organisms can pass from person to person through direct contact or by respiratory droplets.

Viral Meningitis

Also called aseptic meningitis, viral meningitis usually follows a previous viral infection that appears first as a nose and throat infection (like the common cold), a stomach or an intestinal problem, or some other usually minor viral illness. Viral meningitis usually lasts less than a week; in mild cases, recovery may begin as early as the third or fourth day. Children with viral meningitis almost always make a complete recovery.

Bacterial Meningitis

Especially dangerous in the child's first 6 months of life, bacterial meningitis is, fortunately, uncommon. The bacteria that cause meningitis can often be found in the mouths and throats of healthy children, but only a few children will develop meningitis after the bacteria invade the bloodstream. Although most children who receive prompt medical attention recover, complications can include seizures, learning difficulties, and permanent hearing loss.

What the Doctor May Do

The doctor can confirm the diagnosis of meningitis by performing a blood test to check for infection and a lumbar puncture (spinal tap) to obtain spinal fluid. A lumbar puncture involves inserting a needle into the child's lower back to draw out some spinal fluid after giving the child anesthesia. Signs of infection in this fluid suggest a diagnosis of meningitis.

If a child has bacterial meningitis, the doctor will admit her to the hospital for intravenous antibiotics and fluids and monitoring by the medical staff for complications. If an older child has viral (aseptic) meningitis, she may be treated at home with lots of rest, plenty of fluids, and acetaminophen for fever and discomfort. A child may be hospitalized for evaluation, however, until the doctors rule out the possibility of bacterial meningitis. No medication exists to treat viral meningitis; the illness simply must run its course.

What You Can Do

Stay alert to the signs of meningitis, and contact your doctor if its symptoms appear or if your child's playmate has been diagnosed with meningitis. In the latter scenario, your doctor can prescribe antibiotics for several days to protect your child from contracting the disease.

Prevention

Effective vaccines for poliomyelitis (the virus that causes polio), *measles, mumps,* the haemophilus influenza type B (Hib), and pneumococcal disease will help protect against meningitis. There is also a vaccine against certain types of meningococcus bacteria, which can cause meningitis. However, it is only recommended for children in certain high-risk groups. Consult your doctor about this, and ask him to make sure that your child's vaccination schedule is up-to-date (see p. 110)—the Hib vaccine, especially, is responsible for drastically reducing the number of bacterial meningitis cases. To date, you cannot protect your newborn from bacterial meningitis, but new vaccines are being developed. If someone in your family or circle of friends has bacterial meningitis, contact your doctor: You may be able to protect your child and other family members from the spread of the infection by taking prescribed antibiotics.

Mental Retardation

A child's intelligence and ability to adjust to his surroundings are highly individual. But when a child's intelligence is well below average, and he has difficulty acquiring the skills needed for everyday life, he may be diagnosed with mental retardation. About 2 percent of the population, or 4 million Americans, have mental retardation. Most have only mild impairment, however, and can learn many important skills, eventually achieving much independence.

Signs and Symptoms

- Inability to sit up unsupported by 10 months of age or walk unassisted by 18 months of age
- A significant delay in language, such as speaking no words at 2 years of age
- A significant delay in self-help skills, such as feeding, undressing, and dressing
- Trouble communicating and playing with peers

When to Call the Doctor
CALL THE DOCTOR TODAY IF

- you have concerns about your child's intellectual, physical, or social development.

Essential Facts

A child with mental retardation moves through the same developmental stages as a child who is not intellectually impaired, only more slowly. The final level of development may be lower,

however, limiting the child's ability to adapt and become self-sufficient. Like children of normal intelligence, those with mental retardation develop faster in some areas than in others. A child who has intellectual impairment may develop gross motor skills—the ability to walk and play ball, for example—yet be severely delayed in language development. A child with intellectual impairment frequently has other developmental impairments as well, such as in physical motor skills or coordination.

Parents usually become aware if a young infant is not developing normally. The two most common parental concerns are a child's slowness in talking and walking. Early delays in these types of skills (see the developmental milestone charts in the age-by-age chapters of this book) are sometimes accompanied by mental disabilities, as well. Many children experience slight delays in certain development areas, but children with mental retardation show a pattern of general delay within one or more areas. In some instances, however, children with mild mental retardation show no signs of early physical impairment. Their intellectual disability appears later as a delay in language development or still later, in preschool or elementary school, as difficulty performing academic skills at grade level.

No solid dividing line exists between mental retardation and normal development. IQ scores are sometimes used to differentiate between levels of intellectual ability. Although IQ scores are a limited and imperfect method of assessing a child's level of functioning, they continue to be used as one test of a child's intellect. About 95 percent of the population fall between 80 and 120 on the IQ scale. Because of cultural or language variations, however, IQ scores may not be fully accurate and further evaluation may be necessary. The following IQ ranges may give a rough estimate of a child's present abilities:

- *Normal intelligence:* An IQ score around 100 on standardized tests is generally considered average, and a score near 70 is regarded as the lower limit of normal intelligence.

- *Mild retardation:* A score between 50 and 70 corresponds to mild retardation, a category that includes about 85 percent of children with cognitive impairment. These children generally achieve considerable independence.

- *Moderate retardation:* About 10 percent of people with mental retardation score between 35 and 49 on standardized IQ tests. These people have more difficulty adapting than their more mildly affected counterparts and require skilled teaching to enhance self-help skills.

- *Severe and profound retardation:* These children have an IQ score of 35 or lower. Their language skills and their ability to learn and care for themselves are limited. They need considerable personal care and, often, medical supervision.

Causes

Often, no cause can be pinpointed for mental retardation. But the condition may result from factors including genetic causes, problems that arise during pregnancy or childbirth, and environmental exposures during pregnancy or later.

Genetic Conditions

Rare genetic diseases, such as phenylketonuria (PKU, which can be successfully treated if detected early, see p. 44), Tay-Sachs disease, neurofibromatosis, and some other neurological syndromes, may cause mental retardation. Down syndrome, one of the most common causes of mental retardation, results from the presence of an extra chromosome 21. Another chromosomal abnormality, fragile X syndrome, is a cause of mental retardation.

Problems During Pregnancy

Alcohol consumption during pregnancy may cause fetal alcohol syndrome, which is marked by mental retardation, heart disease, and altered facial characteristics. Since experts don't know what level of alcohol consumption is safe for the fetus during pregnancy, the best advice is for pregnant women to abstain from drinking alcohol. Infection with toxoplasmosis (see p. 12) or cytomegalovirus (see p. 12) during pregnancy raises a woman's risk of having a child with mental retardation. Premature birth and its complications may also result in developmental delays, including mental impairments.

Problems During Delivery

Birth injuries or difficulties may contribute to developmental delays. Internal bleeding in the brain, caused by a difficult delivery or a lack of oxygen to the brain, may also be a cause.

Other Causes

During childhood, mental retardation is occasionally caused by brain injury, illness, or environmental exposure to toxic substances, such as lead (see **Lead Poisoning**). In addition, severe neglect of infants and small children can cause a variety of developmental impairments, including mental retardation. Severe neglect of children has emerged as a problem for adoptive parents, considering the increasing number of adoptions from countries in which conditions in some orphanages have been seriously deficient.

Rarely, a brain tumor is a cause of mental retardation. Some children develop retardation as a complication of severe childhood infections, such as **meningitis** (inflammation of the protective membranes covering the brain and spinal cord) and encephalitis (inflammation of the brain).

What the Doctor May Do

Today, much can be done to help the intellectual and social development of a person with mental retardation. If you or your doctor suspect developmental delays in your child, a careful diagnostic approach is necessary. Diagnosing mental retardation is complex and involves a team of health professionals who evaluate a child's physical condition, gross and fine motor skills, language and cognitive skill development, and social adaptation. Parents often wonder about the future for their children, but predicting how well a child with early developmental delays may function later in life is difficult.

To evaluate a child, a doctor will begin by performing a thorough examination and taking a careful prenatal, postnatal, developmental, and family history. Tests may include a chromosomal study to detect abnormalities, and vision and hearing tests. A physical therapist will measure muscle strength and control, a speech and language pathologist will test language and speech development, and an audiologist will test hearing ability. A psychologist will use tests to measure intellectual and emotional development, while a special educator will test for specific learning abilities. You may also decide to consult a neurologist or a developmental pediatrician. Start early: A child's disability can be dramatically reduced if the diagnosis is made early and an educational and developmental plan is established promptly.

What You Can Do
Your job as a parent is mainly to give your child love, support, and informed assistance. First, follow the health and educational program that you, your doctor, and other health team members develop for your child.

During the first few years of life, a baby with special needs may take part in early intervention programs. The federal government requires that these programs be made available locally to your child at no cost. Your child's doctor can tell you how to get in touch with these programs. Once your child reaches school age, federal law guarantees educational opportunities for all children, regardless of how complex their needs are. An individualized education program (IEP) designed to encourage optimal growth in all

development areas requires participation by educators and health professionals, including child development workers; physical, occupational, and speech therapists; nurses; and special education and preschool teachers. An IEP includes academic goals; training in self-help skills and socialization; and, eventually, vocational training.

Children with intellectual impairment have emotional needs like those of any other child. In fact, your child may need extra love and attention to deal with the frustration of his disability. He needs to feel like a valued member of the family and community, and he depends on you to help him develop a good self-image. Like other children, those with mental retardation need to know that their parents are proud of them.

Prevention
Often, mental retardation cannot be prevented. But parents can take steps to lower the risk. Living a healthy lifestyle during pregnancy (see p. 3) and protecting your child from exposure to environmental toxins, such as lead, both during pregnancy and after birth are important steps to take.

See also *Developmental Problems; Learning Disorders.*

Middle Ear Infection

See *Earache/Ear Infection.*

Migraine

See *Dizziness; Headaches.*

Mites

See *Scabies.*

Molluscum Contagiosum

Molluscum contagiosum is a common and benign viral infection that appears on the skin as pearl-like clusters of pimples that can each grow to ¼ inch or an inch or more in size. This infection is most common among young children, but also affects adolescents and adults. In most cases, molluscum contagiosum is a mild condition that disappears by itself within 18 months. However, in children with **HIV/AIDS infection** or other diseases that compromise the immune system, the infection can be chronic and quite disfiguring.

Signs and Symptoms

- Firm, waxy, flesh-colored pimples with sunken centers, most often appearing on the face, eyelids, neck, thighs, and genital area

When to Call the Doctor
CALL THE DOCTOR TODAY IF
- your child develops symptoms of molluscum contagiosum.

Causes

A mildly contagious virus (poxvirus) causes molluscum contagiosum. It passes from person to person or child to child when your child touches an infected person's lesions.

What the Doctor May Do

Your doctor usually can diagnose molluscum contagiosum on the basis of the appearance of the pimplelike eruptions, with the dimple or indentation in the center of each pimple being the most important clue. Usually, no medical treatment is necessary, especially in infants and toddlers. In older children or in severe cases, the doctor may use the same techniques to remove the lesions as he does to remove warts—applying a topical irritant solution, such as phenol, salicylic acid, or cantharidin, to destroy them, or freezing them with liquid nitrogen (cryosurgery).

What You Can Do

In most cases, you need only ignore the skin eruptions until they pass on their own, which may take up to 18 months. Or, if your doctor decides to treat the condition, follow your doctor's instructions about caring for your child's skin after treatment. Don't attempt to treat the condition without your doctor's advice, but over-the-counter wart removal products may be effective.

Prevention

The best thing you can do to prevent your child from developing this infection is to encourage frequent hand-washing and help your child avoid skin-to-skin contact with anyone who has the condition.

Mononucleosis

Often known as the "kissing disease" because of the way it is sometimes transmitted between dating teenagers, infectious mononucleosis is common in younger children, too. When it strikes preadolescents, however, the disease is often mild—so mild that you might not be aware that your child has it. Some children, however, experience more severe symptoms of fever, sore throat, and fatigue. Mononucleosis is spread easily by contact with an infected person. It usually is not a prolonged illness, but occasionally can be severe enough to warrant hospitalization. Because the symptoms tend to be mild in small children, it frequently goes undiagnosed.

Signs and Symptoms

In infants and young children:

- *Fever*
- Sore throat or enlarged tonsils or adenoids
- Fatigue
- Swollen lymph glands, especially in the neck

In adolescents:

- Swollen lymph glands, especially in the neck
- Severe sore throat
- *Fever*
- Lethargy and exhaustion
- Runny nose
- Aches and pains
- Abdominal pain and tenderness

When to Call the Doctor

CALL FOR EMERGENCY HELP IF

- your child has trouble breathing and/or is turning blue.

  For first aid information, see page 380 if your child is less than 1 year old and page 383 if your child is 1 year of age or older.

  CALL THE DOCTOR IMMEDIATELY IF

- your child has difficult, congested breathing.
- your child seems lethargic or dehydrated.
- your child can't drink fluids at all.

  CALL THE DOCTOR TODAY IF

- your child has a severe sore throat.
- your child has trouble swallowing.
- lymph nodes in the neck area are very swollen and painful.
- your child has abdominal tenderness.

Causes

The Epstein-Barr virus (EBV), a herpesvirus, causes mononucleosis. Children contract the virus by contact with infected saliva, such as through coughing, sneezing, or sharing cups, toys, or utensils that go in the mouth. Epstein-Barr is not highly contagious compared to other viruses, and not everyone who comes into contact with the virus will become ill. It may take 30 to 50 days for symptoms to appear after your child is exposed to this virus. The virus can cause severe complications and even become life-threatening in children with *HIV/AIDS infection* or other illnesses that compromise the immune system.

What the Doctor May Do

Often the doctor can diagnose mononucleosis on the basis of your child's symptoms, such as weakness and extreme fatigue, swollen lymph nodes in the neck, and a red throat with pus on the tonsils. These symptoms, however, are difficult to distinguish from strep throat and other causes of throat infection. As a result, your doctor may also examine your child's abdomen for signs of a swollen, tender liver and spleen, which is typical of EBV infection. She may use a blood test to confirm EBV infection. The tests are less accurate in children under 4 years old but more accurate in older children. The test for mononucleosis, known as a monospot, or heterophile test, identifies the virus in about 90 percent of older children and adults and a lower proportion of younger children who carry it. Your doctor may also test for the presence of certain types of lymphocytes (infection-fighting white blood cells) in the blood, which are almost always present with mononucleosis. Other blood tests measure antibodies to specific parts of the EBV protein structure in the blood.

As with most viruses, the disease must run its course. The doctor may prescribe corticosteroid medication to reduce inflammation in children and adolescents with markedly enlarged tonsils and adenoids that are causing breathing trouble. Some children who are dehydrated may need a short course of intravenous fluids.

What You Can Do

Although mononucleosis in children may be mild, it remains contagious. Follow these tips until your doctor says the infection has passed:

- *Keep your child home from school.* Keep children and adolescents home from day care and school until they feel well enough to return. This period varies considerably: Younger children may experience mild—even unnoticeable—symptoms and can thus return to school or day care sooner. Older children and adolescents may not feel well enough to return to their normal activities for several weeks.

- *Encourage your child to rest.* Although complete bed rest is not necessary, mononucleosis can be debilitating to older children and adolescents, especially while fever is present.

- *Ease your child's sore throat.* Give acetaminophen or ibuprofen to bring down the fever and lessen the pain of a sore throat. Provide milkshakes and cold drinks. Avoid orange and grapefruit juices, whose acidity may irritate the throat.

- *Monitor your child's hydration.* A child with mononucleosis has difficulty swallowing. Give him plenty of fluids and notify the doctor if you think he is getting dehydrated (see *Dehydration*).

- *Have your child avoid contact sports if his spleen is swollen and his abdomen is tender.* For the next 3 to 6 months, have your child avoid participating in contact sports or other activities that might result in injury to the spleen, which can become enlarged during mononucleosis.

Prevention

Preventing mononucleosis is difficult, but you can reduce your child's chances of contracting it by avoiding contact with children who have it, and by encouraging frequent hand-washing and following the good hygiene methods described on page 366.

■ *Motion Sickness*

"Mommy, I think I'm going to be sick!" is a refrain most parents dread while traveling. For many families, motion sickness is a common but disruptive side effect of travel. Never serious and always temporary, motion sickness can often be prevented with behavioral techniques or medication.

Signs and Symptoms

- Nausea
- *Dizziness*
- Fatigue
- *Vomiting*
- Sweating
- Crying

> **When to Call the Doctor**
> CALL THE DOCTOR TODAY IF
> - you need advice about treating your child's motion sickness.

Essential Facts

The symptoms of motion sickness usually develop slowly, starting with a vague feeling of nausea and queasiness. Your child's palms and forehead may become clammy, and she may feel nauseous and finally vomit. Often, motion sickness occurs only on a first boat or plane ride or when the motion is intense, such as that caused by rough water or turbulent air. But some children are so sensitive to movement that even short car rides trigger symptoms. Older children sometimes experience motion sickness if they try to read in the car.

Causes

Certain movements, such as the rolling of a boat or the bouncing of a car, cause a disturbance of the body's inner ear, where the balance center is located. Trying to focus on rapidly moving objects, such as passing cars or scenery, aggravates the condition. Nerves affected by this imbalance send a message to the brain and to the stomach, resulting in nausea or vomiting.

Children may be more susceptible to motion sickness than adults for two reasons: Their nervous systems are not completely developed, and they haven't learned the tricks that adults unconsciously use to keep their sense of balance. Why some children don't outgrow the condition or some adults develop it later, however, remains a mystery.

What You Can Do

If your child feels sick in the car, park in a safe place and allow her to get out, breathe deeply, and regain her balance. If the event occurs in a plane or boat over which you have no control, have her lie down and keep her eyes open and focused on a stationary object, which may alleviate the nausea. This technique can also be used in a car if you cannot pull off the road immediately. Or, in a boat or car, have your child stare at the horizon, which does not move. Here are some other tips to reduce the incidence and severity of the problem:

- *Keep your child occupied.* Focusing on games or puzzles or looking at pictures may distract your child from her symptoms and from looking at objects the car or boat travels past. But don't let your child read in the car. This will probably only cause her worse discomfort.

- *Have your child lie down and breath fresh air.* If you're traveling in a car or boat, put your child near an open window. Reclining as much as possible, even lying down in the back seat, may also help her (unless she is vomiting).

- *Offer bland snacks.* Crackers, flat carbonated beverages, and gum may settle a queasy stomach. Make sure that your child eats only a small snack before your trip begins and that she doesn't travel on either a full or a completely empty stomach. Some parents also find

that giving a child ginger ale or ginger candy (if she's over 3 years old) helps prevent motion sickness.

- *Use medication wisely.* If you choose to use an antihistamine or antinausea medication, be sure to give the right medication, in the right dose. Many medications are not appropriate for small children, so consult your doctor or pharmacist first. Give the medication to your child about an hour before you travel and about every 4 hours during the trip (or as often as directed).

What the Doctor May Do

Apart from making sure your child isn't experiencing an illness (such as the flu) that causes similar symptoms, your doctor will probably suggest some of the tips we have just discussed to comfort your child while traveling. He may suggest over-the-counter remedies appropriate for children, such as antihistamines (which block nerve signals between the inner ear and the part of the brain that triggers vomiting) or other antinausea medications. Follow your doctor's instructions about choosing the right medication and dose—some drugs aren't appropriate for young children. If your child has severe motion sickness, consult a neurologist: Some motion-sick children may also have trouble with migraines (see **Headaches**).

Prevention

You may be able to reduce your child's chances of experiencing motion sickness by following the tips discussed earlier in this section.

▌ *Mouth Sores*

See *Canker Sores.*

Mumps

Many of today's parents remember having the puffy, swollen neck and cheeks of mumps. Luckily, if you keep your child's vaccinations current (see Childhood Immunization Schedule, p. 110), he probably will never have mumps. Although mumps may be uncomfortable, it is rarely serious.

Signs and Symptoms

- Swollen, sore salivary glands
- Facial swelling on one or both sides
- Mouth pain when eating citrus fruits (oranges, grapefruits)
- *Fever*
- Weakness and fatigue
- *Headaches*
- Swollen, painful testes (in boys) and ovaries/abdomen (in girls)

When to Call the Doctor

CALL THE DOCTOR IMMEDIATELY IF

- your child with mumps develops a stiff neck, extreme sleepiness, or vomiting.

CALL THE DOCTOR TODAY IF

- your child has the symptoms of mumps.

TALK WITH THE DOCTOR AT
YOUR CHILD'S NEXT CHECKUP IF

- you have any doubts that your child's vaccinations are current.

Essential Facts

The virus that causes mumps attacks the parotid salivary glands found in front of the ears, causing them to swell and become tender and sore. The swelling may be so severe as actually to change the shape of the child's face until the infection clears. In about one-third of cases, though, no swelling or tenderness occurs. Mumps can also lead to a mild viral *meningitis* if the virus enters the cerebrospinal fluid (liquid surrounding the brain and spinal cord). Fortunately this viral meningitis clears up within a few days.

Fever often accompanies mumps. In older children, the virus attacks the ovaries in girls or testes in boys, causing swelling and pain. In rare cases, it can cause sterility in boys. In other cases, however, mumps may be so mild as to go unnoticed. It can also cause permanent hearing loss in either boys or girls, and before the vaccine became available, it was the most common cause of acquired sensorineural (i.e., due to malfunction of the inner ear) *hearing loss.*

Mumps usually appears from 16 to 18 days after exposure. The disease tends to run its course in about 7 to 10 days. During this period, chewing and swallowing may be difficult. An accompanying fever may make your child tired and cranky. In extremely rare cases, the mumps virus can cause meningitis or encephalitis, diseases of the central nervous system.

Cause

A paramyxovirus causes mumps. Mumps is transmitted by person-to-person contact or by airborne droplets produced by sneezing and coughing. Household objects and personal possessions may be contaminated by a sick child's saliva.

What the Doctor May Do

If your unvaccinated child has been exposed to mumps, be sure to tell your doctor, who will examine your child for signs of swelling. Because mumps is now rare, the American Academy of Pediatrics recommends that the diagnosis be confirmed by sampling the throat or urine. A blood test may also be used.

If mumps is confirmed, the doctor will instruct you on how to make your child more comfortable until the infection clears. Your doctor or school nurse may advise you that your child must be excluded from school or day care for 9 days after the swelling starts. As with most viral infections, the disease must run its course naturally; no medication can cure it.

What You Can Do

Encourage your child to rest until the infection runs its course. In the meantime, you can help him feel better by following these tips:

- *Relieve the fever.* Give your child acetaminophen or ibuprofen to relieve any accompanying fever. Check the package directions for the correct dosage for your child's age and weight.

- *Offer moist, soft foods.* With mumps, the parotid glands fail to produce saliva to moisten food. If your child finds eating difficult, offer him food with a high liquid content, such as soups, yogurt, pudding, or oatmeal.

- *Avoid acids.* Acidic foods, like citrus fruit, tomato sauce, or salad dressing with vinegar, can stimulate saliva production, which is a painful process during a mumps infection.

Prevention

Making sure that your child receives all his vaccinations on schedule is the best way to prevent mumps. The mumps vaccine is not effective in preventing mumps after exposure to the virus.
See also *Swollen Glands.*

Myopia

See *Vision Problems.*

Nearsightedness

See *Vision Problems.*

Neck Pain

If your child is old enough, she'll tell you if her neck hurts. But in a younger child, you may notice that your child has difficulty tilting her head to one side or turning her head (stiff neck). Most neck pain is the result of minor infection or muscle strain, but neck pain can be a symptom of a more serious central nervous system infection, such as *meningitis* or encephalitis (inflammation of the brain), or another disorder that requires immediate professional medical treatment.

Signs and Symptoms

- Difficulty holding the head straight
- Neck pain, stiffness, or tenderness
- Neck swelling, bruising, or redness

When to Call the Doctor
CALL FOR **EMERGENCY** HELP IF

- neck pain occurs after a trauma, such as a fall, motor vehicle accident, or sports injury.
- your child is listless, unusually sleepy, and unable to respond to your questions or commands.

CALL THE DOCTOR IMMEDIATELY IF

- a fever accompanies the pain or stiffness.
- your child's eyes seem sensitive to light.
- your child is vomiting.

CALL THE DOCTOR TODAY IF

- the neck pain is constant.
- your child keeps tilting her head to one side.
- your child cannot touch her chin to her chest or shoulders.
- your child's neck is swollen or very red.
- pain or discomfort makes it difficult for your child to hold her neck straight.

Causes

A young child's neck pain or stiffness is most likely a temporary symptom related to the aches and pains that accompany an illness, an uncomfortable night's sleep, or a minor injury due to strenuous activity. The following conditions can cause neck pain in children.

Infections

Neck pain is often a symptom of a relatively minor viral infection, such as a cold or the flu. With an infection, the lymph nodes in the neck may become enlarged and tender. When accompanied by fever, sensitivity to light, listlessness, and vomiting, neck pain may be the result of several serious infections, including meningitis and encephalitis.

Injuries

A stiff or painful neck may also result from an injury, such as a muscle strain from strenuous activity, or even sleeping in an unusual position. In a more serious trauma, neck pain can be caused by dislocations or fractures of the cervical vertebrae. High-energy trauma can cause compression of the disks situated between vertebrae and can also cause other life-threatening neck injuries. If neck pain begins after a fall or another injury, call for emergency help and don't try to move your child. Emergency personnel may need to stabilize the head and neck with sandbags and a cervical collar in the neutral position (eyes forward) before your child is moved.

Torticollis (Wryneck)

A painful condition called torticollis causes a child's head to tilt to one side. Straightening the neck for more than a few seconds at a time is difficult or impossible because of the pain. In older children, torticollis is more often caused by an inflammation of the throat and lymph nodes as a result of an upper respiratory infection, an injury, or an unknown factor. The inflammation may cause asymmetrical spasms in the neck muscles, causing the head to tilt to one side. If untreated, the asymmetry will become more pronounced, making the child's face look lopsided. But prompt treatment can prevent this problem.

Infantile (Congenital) Torticollis

Sometimes newborns suffer from congenital neck stiffness and may not have full motion of the head. They hold it to one side, and the neck muscles seem swollen and hard. The most common cause of torticollis in infants is an injury to the muscles connecting the head, neck, and breastbone that most likely occurs either during delivery or during pregnancy. Fortunately, infantile torticollis usually clears up in a few days to weeks with treatment.

What the Doctor May Do

A complete physical exam, including a careful neurological exam and sometimes X rays, computed tomography (CT), magnetic resonance imaging (MRI), or some combination of these tests, will help the doctor determine the cause of your baby's discomfort. If the doctor diagnoses torticollis, he may recommend that you exercise your baby's neck to increase muscle flexibility. This treatment works in more than 90 percent of infants with torticollis within weeks. If a baby doesn't show significant improvement, surgery may eventually be recommended.

If your doctor suspects that the neck pain is the result of an illness, he may order blood tests, X rays, or both. If a bacterial infection is present, the doctor will prescribe antibiotics. If an injury is the cause, your child may need a neck brace and bed rest while the injury heals.

What You Can Do

To treat neck pain due to an injury or a strain, give your child over-the-counter pain relievers. If your child wakes up with a stiff neck and can't turn her head, help relieve her discomfort by applying a hot water bottle or a heating pad to her neck, encouraging her to rest and, if necessary, giving her pain-relieving medicine. If your baby has wryneck, gently exercise her neck as directed by the doctor, probably twice a day while she lies on her back. You can also use warm (not hot) washcloths as directed by your baby's doctor.

Prevention

You cannot prevent most cases of neck pain, but you can reduce your child's risk of head and neck injuries by encouraging the use of seat belts in cars and helmets while riding bicycles. In addition, you can prevent some forms of meningitis by making sure that your child is immunized with the Haemophilus influenza type b (Hib) vaccine.

See also *Back Pain; Sprains and Strains.*

▌ *Nosebleed*

A nosebleed can be frightening to both parent and child, producing alarming amounts of blood in a short amount of time. But nosebleeds are extremely common, are almost always harmless, and usually last no more than 10 or 15 minutes. You can usually treat a nosebleed at home.

Signs and Symptoms

- Sudden bleeding from one nostril or both nostrils

When to Call the Doctor

CALL THE DOCTOR IMMEDIATELY IF

- your child starts bleeding from the nose after a severe blow to the head or nose.
- you cannot get the bleeding to stop after about 20 minutes.
- the bleeding results from a blow that may have broken the nose.

CALL THE DOCTOR TODAY IF

- your child has a medical condition (such as *hemophilia*) or is taking medications that inhibit blood clotting.
- the bleeding is caused by an object your child has put in his nose.
- your child regularly has several nosebleeds a month.

Essential Facts

A nosebleed occurs when a small blood vessel in the lining of the nose breaks. This lining is extremely thin and contains many fragile blood vessels, especially on the septum (the wall dividing the two sides of the nose) near the opening of the nose. Nosebleeds occur more frequently in childhood because nasal infections that inflame the tissue are more common at this time. They also occur more in the winter, when the air is dry and can irritate the lining of the nose. Children also tend to pick and scratch the inside of their noses. But many nosebleeds occur at night, even when a child is not touching or picking his nose. Nosebleeds can recur if a child picks at, or otherwise disturbs, the scab that heals over the original scratch; indeed, one nosebleed often leads to several more in the following weeks.

Causes

Any condition that causes the nasal passages to become inflamed or dried out might lead to a nosebleed. Among the most common culprits are upper respiratory tract infections, *allergies,* overly dry air, inserting an object into the nose, and picking or hitting the nose. Rarely, bleeding or blood vessel disorders such as hemophilia, thrombocytopenia, or hypertension (see ***High Blood Pressure***) cause nosebleeds. Abnormal growths in the nose (such as polyps) or overly prominent blood vessels may cause nosebleeds as well.

What You Can Do

First of all, stay calm, and try to calm your child. In most cases, the bleeding will last only a few minutes. Follow these steps to stop the bleeding

1. Keep your child in a sitting or standing position, and have him lean slightly forward, as if sniffing a flower, so the blood drips out, not down the back of the throat.

2. Firmly pinch your child's nose closed at the front of the nose with your thumb and index finger. Have your child breathe through his mouth.

If your child is having a nosebleed, keep him in a sitting or standing position and have him lean slightly forward, as if sniffing a flower, so that the blood drips out, not down the back of the throat. Pinch the soft parts of his nose between your thumb and two fingers, and hold this position for 10 minutes.

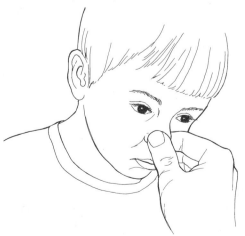

3. Hold this position for 10 minutes. Don't release the nose during this time, even to see if the bleeding has stopped.

4. After 10 minutes, if the bleeding resumes, apply pressure for another 10 minutes. If the bleeding persists, call your child's doctor.

5. If a blow to the nose caused your child's nosebleed, place an ice pack on his nose for an hour or so to reduce the swelling.

6. Keep your child quiet and calm while trying to stop the bleeding. Encourage him to remain quiet; restrict physical activity for a few hours to prevent the bleeding from resuming.

7. Offer an over-the-counter nasal decongestant spray for children, such as oxymetazoline (Afrin), to help slow the bleeding. Try this only once: Don't repeat the dose.

8. Teach your older child how to stop a nosebleed himself by following the previous instructions, if he has recurrent nosebleeds.

Do not . . .

- lay your child down, which will only increase pressure in the blood vessels.

- let your child put his head back. With the head in this position, blood will run down his throat and into his stomach, which may irritate the stomach lining and cause him to vomit.

- pack the nose with cotton, tissue, or gauze without your doctor's guidance. Removing the impacted material may only reopen the broken vessel.

- let your child blow his nose, no matter how stuffed up he feels; doing so could dislodge the forming clot, resulting in another nosebleed.

What the Doctor May Do

In most cases, your child need not see a doctor. If you have trouble getting the bleeding to stop or if your child has nosebleeds regularly, take him in for an evaluation.

To find the cause of a nosebleed, your doctor will probably examine the inside of your child's nose with a lighted otoscope (often also used to examine ears) or a lighted fiber-optic scope and use gentle suction to remove all blood clots. If the bleeding hasn't stopped, the doctor may pack the nose with gauze, sometimes coated with petroleum jelly or antibiotic ointment, to be left in place for 24 to 48 hours. The doctor may also use other types of packing, such as gel foam, which is easier to remove than gauze. If the bleeding persists, the doctor may cauterize the bleeding blood vessels with a chemical (silver nitrate) to close them off. The doctor may also apply topical antibiotics to prevent infection.

If your doctor suspects that anything more serious than local inflammation or irritation is causing the nosebleeds, she'll conduct a complete physical examination and occasionally order blood tests (e.g., complete blood count and blood clotting studies). When a nosebleed is caused by an underlying disease (such as a bleeding disorder), the doctor will treat that problem.

Prevention

Nosebleeds cannot be prevented altogether, but you can take steps to reduce the chances that your child will experience a nosebleed:

- Teach your child not to pick or scratch the lining of the nose.

- Keep indoor air moist with a vaporizer or humidifier, especially in the winter.

- If your child's nose is irritated or inflamed, keep it coated by applying a bit of petroleum jelly or antibiotic ointment with a cotton swab, just inside the nostril on the septum.

∎ *Nose Injury*

In most cases, the only result of a blow to the nose is some swelling, bruising (see *Bruises*), and occasionally a *nosebleed.* Occasionally, however, a blow to the face can cause a fracture of the bony upper part of the bridge of the nose or displace the septum (the inside wall dividing the two sides of the nose).

Signs and Symptoms

- Swelling
- Bleeding
- Redness and bruising around the nose and under the eyes
- Breathing difficulties
- Disfigured nose

When to Call the Doctor
CALL THE DOCTOR IMMEDIATELY

- your child's nose is disfigured by a blow or an injury.
- the pain is severe.
- the bleeding cannot be stopped.

CALL THE DOCTOR TODAY IF

- pain and swelling develop and last more than 3 days.
- the nose appears crooked or off-center as the swelling decreases.

What You Can Do

If your child's nose is injured by a blow, apply an ice pack immediately to reduce the swelling and to minimize the bleeding. (Never apply ice directly to the skin. Instead, use a cold pack or wrap ice in a towel.) Take your child to the doctor if you notice swelling, black eyes, lots of bleeding, or a crooked nose or if your child is having trouble breathing.

What the Doctor May Do

The doctor will examine your child's nose and ask how the injury occurred, to assess the extent of the damage. The doctor will also examine the inside of the nose to check for bleeding, septal deviation, or a hematoma (blood clot) within the septum. If the doctor suspects that your child's nose is broken or if the injury displaced the cartilage, he may take an X ray to confirm the diagnosis. In most cases, the injury will heal on its own, although the doctor may decide to reposition and tape the nose to protect it from further injury and help it heal properly, or he may need to drain a hematoma of the septum. These procedures often require general anesthesia.

Over the long term, many nasal fractures heal with no permanent disfigurement. But sometimes, even if the nose is "set" by the doctor, it may heal in a somewhat misshapen fashion. The more often a nose is broken, the more likely this is to occur. If the child's nasal septum is severely deviated (crooked) or cannot be straightened, she might continue to have breathing problems and corrective surgery might be necessary.

Prevention

Although you can't prevent all nose injuries, you can encourage your child to use protective head-gear with face guards while playing contact sports or those involving the use of a stick (baseball, hockey), to reduce the risk of fractures and bruising. Encourage children to use soft, not hard, balls when playing sports such as baseball or football.

■ Nose (Object Lodged in Nose)

Children under 5 years old are most likely to insert objects into their noses, including small pieces of food, crayon pieces, toys or parts of toys, paper wads, beans, and pebbles. If a foreign object remains in the nasal passages, it can cause breathing difficulty and infection. Usually, these problems easily resolve themselves once you or a doctor removes the object. The only real danger is if the object travels from the nasal passages into the back of the throat and causes your child to choke. To make sure this doesn't happen, get your child to a doctor quickly if you can't easily remove the object yourself.

Signs and Symptoms

- Nasal discomfort
- Foul-smelling yellow or green discharge from one side of the nose
- Sneezing
- *Nosebleed*
- Breathing difficulties
- Swelling and pain if the object remains in place

When to Call the Doctor
CALL FOR EMERGENCY HELP IF
- your child has difficulty breathing and/or is turning blue.

  For first aid information, see page 380 if your child is less than 1 year old and page 383 if your child is 1 year of age or older.

CALL THE DOCTOR IMMEDIATELY IF
- your child has an object lodged in his nose.
- your child has a foul-smelling discharge coming from his nose.
- your child has swelling and pain in his nose.

What the Doctor May Do

The doctor will examine the inside of the nose and try to remove the object. X rays cannot usually detect small, nonmetallic objects, such as food, paper, or sponges. If the object cannot be easily removed, your doctor may refer you to an ear, nose, and throat specialist for treatment. The specialist may need to anesthetize the area or place your child under general anesthesia to keep him completely still while removing the object using suction or an appropriate grasping instrument. She may then prescribe antibiotics if any sign of infection exists.

What You Can Do

If a foreign object protrudes from a nostril and you can easily remove it, do so. Otherwise, bring your child to a doctor right away.

Do not ...

- try to remove an object from your child's nose unless it's protruding from the nostril.
- instruct your child to blow his nose. It might cause him to suck the object in further.
- stick a cotton swab or another probe into the nose in an attempt to remove the object.

Prevention

Watch your toddler carefully to make sure that he doesn't put any small objects into his nose, and as soon as he's old enough, teach him the dangers of doing so. Examine your toddler's toys for small parts from under 3/4 to 1 inch in diameter; items this small may be hazardous. Eliminate any small objects, such as marbles, beads, button eyes on stuffed animals, small building block pieces, and any other small objects, from your child's reach.

▌ Obesity

See *Overweight.*

▌ Obsessive-Compulsive Disorder

See *Anxiety Disorders.*

▌ Otitis Externa

See *Earache/Ear Infection.*

▌ Otitis Media

See *Earache/Ear Infection.*

▌ Overanxious Disorder

See *Anxiety Disorders.*

▌ Overweight

Nothing is cuter than a chubby baby. Indeed, during your baby's first few years, fat cheeks, body, and limbs are considered normal unless your doctor says your child is significantly overweight, meaning that her body weight is consistently 20 percent or more above that considered normal for her height. But helping your child establish healthy eating and exercise patterns from the start is a good idea. Overweight and obesity patterns can be set at a very young age, and childhood obesity rates keep climbing. During the 1980s and 1990s, the prevalence of obesity in children nearly doubled to almost 20 percent.

Signs and Symptoms

- Weight consistently 20 percent or more above that considered normal for the child's height (see Appendix: Growth Charts)

> **When to Call the Doctor**
> CALL THE DOCTOR TODAY IF
> - weight gain develops unexpectedly and is associated with poor growth or other general medical problems, such as poor energy or problems sleeping.
>
> TALK WITH THE DOCTOR AT YOUR CHILD'S NEXT CHECKUP IF
> - you are concerned about your child's weight.

Essential Facts

The struggle with excess weight is widespread in the United States. The prevalence of high-calorie, refined foods and the lack of physical activity, compounded by sedentary pastimes like television, computers, and video games, has led to a general lack of fitness in today's youth. Young children are particularly vulnerable to this combination. These activities not only keep children sedentary but also encourage unhealthy snacking.

For children under 2 years old, the greatest risk factor for being overweight as adults is having overweight parents. For other children, the greatest risk factor for becoming obese as an adult is being overweight as a child. Obesity places children at a much greater risk of developing numerous serious medical problems in adulthood, including heart disease, stroke, *diabetes mellitus,* and *cancer.* In addition, childhood obesity can cause many immediate health problems, including **high blood pressure,** high cholesterol, **asthma,** sleep apnea (see *Infantile Apnea*), musculoskeletal problems, exercise intolerance, digestive problems, and emotional difficulties.

Causes

Scientists continue to search for the cause of obesity. They have discovered that many factors influence a child's weight and metabolism,

including genetics, diet and exercise habits, and general health.

Genetics

A tendency to become overweight can be inherited. Some obese children may have inherited both an increased number of fat cells and an increased ability to store fats, which means that they gain weight more easily than their peers (even if they eat the same amount) and have extra fat cells even after losing weight. Having overweight parents doesn't predetermine a child's weight, but it does make it more important to set healthy eating and exercise patterns.

Poor Diet and Exercise Habits

Children and adults gain weight because they consume more calories (especially from high-calorie, refined foods and fast foods) than they burn.

Medical Problems

Several medical conditions—including hypopituitarism (in which the pituitary doesn't produce certain hormones), Cushing's syndrome (too much cortisol, a steroid hormone), or hypothyroidism—may cause excess fat accumulation. However, since such conditions generally interfere with growth, an overweight child who is growing well probably doesn't have a hormone problem. Abnormal weight gain can also result from certain genetic syndromes or prolonged inactivity (caused by paralysis, for example).

Psychological Factors

Children may overeat because of **depression,** stress, poor self-esteem, or poor self-image, as a means of comforting themselves.

What the Doctor May Do

Your doctor will diagnose a weight problem by assessing your child's weight compared to height, amount of body fat, eating habits, medical history, and family history of weight problems. Body mass index (BMI) is another, more precise measurement of fat distribution than weight alone. (See Appendix: Growth Charts for more information on BMI.) The doctor will also perform a complete physical exam and may order blood and urine tests. Overweight children should have their cholesterol and triglyceride levels checked (see p. 234). If your doctor rules out underlying medical conditions, he will work with you and your family to develop a healthy eating and exercise plan or refer you to a program specializing in treatment of childhood obesity.

Your doctor may recommend a behavior modification program to teach your child new eating patterns. He may also recommend a nutritionist to help create an appropriate diet. If your child is having related emotional, social, or psychological problems, your doctor may suggest bringing your child to a mental health professional for counseling. In rare cases, the doctor may hospitalize your child for specialized medical care, such as a very low calorie diet.

What You Can Do

Obesity may require consistent, lifelong treatment. As a parent, you can keep your child on track by teaching her about proper nutrition, encouraging her to stay active, and setting a good example by eating healthy, unprocessed, high-fiber foods (such as fruits, vegetables, and whole grains) and exercising daily. These tips may help you work with your overweight child:

- *Reassure your child.* Before you tackle your child's weight problem, try to bolster her self-esteem. If she's in school or preschool, she's probably already received negative messages about her weight. Remind her that people come in various shapes and sizes and that she is a good, smart, capable child, no matter how much she weighs.

- *Never nag or tease.* Any negative attention you give your child's eating habits or weight gain is likely to decrease her self-esteem, which may trigger overeating.

- *Choose low-calorie foods.* Trimming excessive calories from your family's diet may be easier than you think. Ice cream, milk, yogurt, and other dairy products are now available in reduced-fat varieties. Fruits and vegetables are low in calories and high in fiber (which creates a feeling of fullness and helps maintain a healthy digestive tract). Make such foods readily available, and limit access to high-fat foods, such as those found in fast-food restaurants and in prepared, prepackaged foods. Choose whole grains (bran cereals, whole-wheat bread, brown rice) instead of refined grain products (white bread, many breakfast cereals, and cookies). Dessert, other than fruit, should be an occasional treat only, not a regular reward for eating.

- *Low fat does not equal low caloric.* Remember that many low-fat foods, especially juices, sodas, and punch, are high in sugar and add unneeded calories. Water, diet soda, and other drinks with artificial sweeteners are good substitutes. Your child will gain weight if she eats more calories than she burns, even if most of those calories are from low-fat snacks and desserts. Limit the portion size of starchy foods (a large, fat-free bagel can have over 500 calories).

- *Never deny your child food.* If your child is hungry, feed her low-calorie, healthy food. Withholding food will only lead to overeating later, so offer healthy snacks or mini-meals (e.g., plain tuna on a few crackers or an apple with a slice of reduced-fat cheese or sugar-free, low-fat yogurt).

- *Limit television and video games; increase activity.* Because sitting in front of a television screen is a primary risk factor for obesity, especially in children, enroll your child in an afternoon activity, such as soccer or scouting. Encourage her to walk or ride her bike to school instead of getting a ride.

- *Make healthy living a family affair.* Modeling a healthy lifestyle is the best thing parents and siblings can do for an overweight child. Assess the whole family's diet and exercise habits. Adopt family-wide changes rather than focusing solely on your overweight child's needs. Try television "blackouts" or scheduling family-oriented exercise (bike riding, walking, hiking). Have the whole family take a short walk after dinner.

- *Seek help.* Be sure to keep follow-up appointments with your child's doctor and nutritionist. Encourage your child to join a community exercise group or a peer support group.

Prevention

In some cases, establishing a healthy eating and exercise routine early in life will prevent your child from developing a weight problem. However, obesity is a complex disease, and some children may have difficulties with weight control despite their best efforts. Support, encouragement, good nutrition, and physical activity will help your child maintain balance and give her lifelong healthy habits and a positive attitude toward weight control.

When children reach school age, parents should check out school lunches for nutritional value and caloric content. Some school lunch programs offer food from fast-food franchises that is high in fat, sodium, and calories. If this is the case, consider packing a lunch for your child and advocating for better school lunches.

▌ Palpitations

See *Abnormal Heart Rhythm; Heart Murmur.*

▌ Panic Attacks

See *Anxiety Disorders.*

▌ Parasites

See *Worms: Pinworm and Other Parasitic Worms.*

▌ Pervasive Developmental Disorder (Autism)

The term *pervasive developmental disorder* (PDD) is used to describe a group of developmental disorders related to and including autism. The disorders are characterized by impaired social interaction, problems with communication, severely restricted ranges of play and interest, and various types of unusual, repetitive behavior. While PDD may vary greatly in terms of severity—with autism generally being the most severe—all forms of it are a result of abnormalities in brain function. There is no treatment known to cure autism or other forms of PDD, yet tremendous strides in education and behavioral interventions have enabled children with these disorders to learn to function productively and, in less severe cases, live virtually normal lives.

Signs and Symptoms

Symptoms usually become apparent sometime during toddlerhood. Yet, in many cases, after a toddler is diagnosed with a PDD, parents recall certain behavioral or developmental quirks that baffled or concerned them when the child was an infant.

In infants:

- Resists being touched or cuddled
- Routinely goes limp or stiffens up when cuddled

- Appears unresponsive most of the time

In toddlers and preschoolers:
- Limited language or pointing before 15 months
- Communication skills regress
- Few attempts to communicate
- Little eye contact
- Resists cuddling with parents
- Appears extraordinarily sensitive to noises at times and deaf at other times
- Repeats words or sounds over and over
- Engages in repetitive movements, such as hand flapping, rocking, or head banging
- Ignores other children and prefers solitary play
- Does not engage in imaginative play
- Exhibits an intense need to stick to the routine

When to Call the Doctor
CALL THE DOCTOR TODAY IF
- your child exhibits some of the symptoms above.

Essential Facts

Pervasive developmental disorders are not rare, but rather strike 10 to 20 out of 10,000, according to some estimates. Others are even higher. Several states are reporting apparently significant increases in the number of children diagnosed with an autism-related disorder, but it is unclear whether this reflects a true increase or better understanding of these conditions. Three to four times more males than females are afflicted.

Differentiating between conditions that fall under the umbrella of PDD is often difficult, given that autism alone has a wide range of symptoms and characteristics that can present themselves in a variety of combinations, from mild to severe. The following are general descriptions of some forms of PDD. The common thread among all of them is a lack of social and interaction skills. PDD is often accompanied by *mental retardation.*

Autism

On the most severe end of the PDD spectrum, autism is characterized by much of the stereotypical behavior mentioned in the symptoms list. An autistic child may display a profound lack of responsiveness to others. Many do not talk, but may instead engage in repetitive movement rituals, such as echoing dialogue or phrases, arm flapping or hand rocking. They resist change of any sort. Other stereotypical behavior centers on dulled or heightened sensory responses. A child may seem deaf and then may suddenly tune in to a noise in the distance. He may have a high tolerance for pain, yet scream when his shirt tag touches his back.

Asperger Syndrome

Children with this disorder exhibit some deficit in areas of communication, social interaction, and play. They tend to have much better verbal expression than autistic children and sometimes a greater interest in interpersonal social activity.

Rett Syndrome

This is a progressive disorder that occurs only in girls and is characterized by normal development up to about a year, followed by regression in language, social function, head circumference growth, and loss of previously acquired hand function that's replaced with repetitive hand-wringing movements.

Childhood Disintegrative Disorder

Childhood disintegrative disorder (CDD) is typified by normal development for at least the first 2 years, often up to 5 years, followed by significant loss of previously acquired skills. Children with CDD often speak in full phrases or sentences before losing their language skills.

Pervasive Developmental Disorder— Not Otherwise Specified

If a child does not meet the criteria for a specific diagnosis, yet there is a severe and pervasive impairment in specified behavior, he may be given a diagnosis of PDD-NOS. This is sometimes referred to as atypical autism.

Causes

The causes of autism and other forms of PDD remain largely a mystery. Researchers believe that several genes may play a significant role, along with environmental toxins, such as viruses or pollutants, that have yet to be identified.

Scientists have found abnormalities in several regions of the brain in people with autism. For example, smaller-than-usual neurons and faulty brain circuit wiring indicate that PDD may result from interference in normal brain development during early fetal stages. This finding, however, requires further study.

The theory that vaccines, particularly the MMR (measles, mumps, rubella) vaccine, can cause autism has been disproved. Because PDD manifests itself in the first 3 years of life, during the same period that children are being vaccinated, some people had pointed to a possible connection between vaccination and the onset of autism. Several studies have found that the timing is only a coincidence. In those studies, researchers found similar PDD rates among children who received the MMR vaccine and those who had not.

What the Doctor May Do

A diagnosis of a pervasive developmental disorder can be made only after a thorough and complete evaluation that involves much more than a brief observation in a single setting. When you visit your pediatrician or family doctor, you may first be asked to give a complete, detailed history of your child's development. The doctor may order some tests to rule out other conditions, but no medical test can confirm the existence of autism or related conditions.

To get a true picture of an individual's abilities and behavior, your doctor may refer you to a multidisciplinary team of specialists that may include a neurologist, psychologist, developmental pediatrician, speech/language therapist, and learning consultant. If your child is diagnosed with a PDD, he will be referred to the appropriate specialists and will begin intense, one-on-one behavioral therapy. He will also participate in a specialized educational program. If your child is under 3, a special early intervention education program will be offered to him. If he is 3 or older, a team of specialists along with school professionals will coordinate an individualized education program (IEP). The IEP is an evaluation and treatment plan that describes your child's individual educational needs. These interventions are highly structured and offer intense skills training aimed at correcting specific behavioral symptoms that your child displays. These strategies are usually most effective when started at an early age and although they do not cure a PDD, they can result in substantial improvements.

If your child shows more troublesome behavior, such as self-injurious conduct, your doctor may prescribe medication to help ease these symptoms. Your doctor may also prescribe a drug to treat *seizures,* which may accompany your child's condition, but no medicine will cure the disorder itself.

What You Can Do

Parenting a child with autism or a related disorder can be daunting and isolating. The best thing you can do is learn all that you can about your child's condition and the behavioral and educational programs available to you in your community. Keep in mind that a good intervention program will also incorporate training for parents and support systems to help alleviate the stress that you are likely experiencing. Seek out a local support group for parents of children with autism and PDD; see Appendix: Parent Resources, Disabilities/Special Needs.

Prevention

There is no known way to prevent pervasive developmental disorders. Early, intense, one-on-one behavioral treatment, however, may reverse some symptoms or prevent them from emerging.

See also *Developmental Disorders.*

Phobias

See *Anxiety Disorders.*

Piercing

See *Ear and Body Piercing Infections.*

Pigeon Toes

See *Toeing-In.*

Pimples

See *Acne.*

Pinkeye (Conjunctivitis)

Your child wakes up with bloodshot eyes and a gooey discharge sticking to her eyelids. Chances are, she has conjunctivitis, which is cause for immediate attention. Conjunctivitis, also known as pinkeye, is the most common eye problem of young children and, if treated promptly, will quickly subside.

Signs and Symptoms

- Redness of the white part of the eye
- Undersides of the eyelids are beefy red and inflamed
- Watery eyes, tearing
- Eye discharge, especially at night, that causes eyelashes to stick together
- "Sandy" or burning sensation in the affected eyes

When to Call the Doctor
CALL THE DOCTOR IMMEDIATELY IF

- your child's eye is swollen shut.
- your child has a fever along with eye symptoms.
- the inflamed eyelid seems dark red or violet and the other eyelid is swelling, as well.
- your child complains of blurred or double vision.
- the eyelid and surrounding skin are beginning to swell.

CALL THE DOCTOR TODAY IF

- you suspect that your child has early signs of conjunctivitis.

Essential Facts

Highly contagious, conjunctivitis is an inflammation of the filmy membrane (the conjunctiva) covering the white of the eye and the inner eyelids. This condition usually signals infection, but it may also be caused by irritation or an allergic reaction. In rare cases, a more serious illness may be causing it. Conjunctivitis usually causes no long-term harm if treated promptly.

If your child has conjunctivitis, her eyes may be sensitive to light. Viral conjunctivitis often causes a more watery discharge than do bacterial infections and may be accompanied by other viral infection symptoms, including fever, sore throat, and diarrhea.

Causes

Bacterial Infections

Various bacteria, including *Streptococcus pneumoniae, Moraxella catarrhalis,* and *Staphylococcus aureus,* may cause this infection. Your child can spread the infection from one eye to the other by rubbing. Infections of the nose and sinuses can travel up the tear ducts to cause conjunctivitis as well. A child with bacterial conjunctivitis can transmit the condition to others by sharing tissues, towels, or anything else that houses the bacteria. A much more serious form of conjunctivitis is caused by gonorrhea, a common sexually transmitted disease, carried by the mother and transferred to the infant during birth. Your child could also contract bacterial conjunctivitis by swimming in polluted water or a poorly sanitized pool.

Viral Infections

Some viruses directly cause conjunctivitis. Other cases of conjunctivitis occur when another viral disease, such as measles, affects the entire body.

Noninfectious Causes

Various *allergies*—to materials such as grasses, tree pollen, and animal dander—can cause a watery conjunctivitis, which is often seasonal and associated with other symptoms, such as a runny nose and respiratory problems. Chemical irritants, such as household cleaning substances, smog, smoke, and industrial pollutants, can irritate the eye membranes and are all potential causes of conjunctivitis. Chlorine or bromine used to sanitize swimming pools can also cause chemical conjunctivitis. Finally, injuries to the eye may scratch the surface and cause inflammation of the conjunctiva.

What the Doctor May Do

The doctor will examine your child's eyes carefully. He will look for redness or discharge, and he may also take a sample of any discharge for a culture. A thorough examination is necessary to help the doctor distinguish the infection from a more serious infection—periorbital cellulitis, an inflammation of the tissues lining the eye socket. Periorbital cellulitis can cause complications such as sepsis (infection of the blood) and meningitis and requires hospitalization and treatment with intravenous antibiotics. The doctor must rule out other more serious illnesses that can lead to a loss of vision. These include iritis (an inflammation of the pigmented part of the eye, which can be caused by infection) and *juvenile rheumatoid arthritis.* If he suspects trauma, he may touch a paper strip with fluorescein (a type of temporary, fluorescent dye) to the film of tears on top of the eye, to help detect injuries or scratches on the eye's surface.

For more common cases of conjunctivitis caused by bacterial infection, the doctor will prescribe antibiotic eyedrops or ointment. Because conjunctivitis tends to be contagious, the doctor will treat both eyes even if pinkeye affects only one. Anti-inflammatory eyedrops (usually hydrocortisone) and antihistamines can help relieve the itchiness of allergic conjunctivitis. For children with allergic conjunctivitis, cool compresses relieve discomfort.

The condition should clear up—or at least significantly improve—within 24 hours after treatment begins. If the eyelid appears violet or red or the eyelid swells so much that your child cannot open it, call the doctor immediately. If several days pass and you see no improvement or if your child develops other symptoms (such as an **earache** or a **fever**), call your doctor.

What You Can Do

Follow your doctor's treatment instructions, including applying medication according to the schedule prescribed. If the treatment involves eyedrops or ointment, your child is likely to struggle and resist. If so, try these techniques to make it a bit easier:

- Make the treatment into a game, or promise a reward.

- Get someone to help you hold and soothe your child while you apply the drops.

- If your child is extremely resistant, ask your doctor about the possibility of using oral antibiotics, especially if your child has an infection that extends beyond her eye.

To avoid infecting other children, keep a child with infectious conjunctivitis out of child care or school while she has a pink or red eye with a white or yellow eye discharge. A physician can decide when she can safely return, usually 48 hours after starting an antibiotic. You can also soothe discomfort by these methods:

- *Clean it up.* Cover the affected eye with a clean, moistened washcloth, holding it gently against your child's eye to soften the discharge. Wipe the discharge off your child's eyelids and eyelashes with the washcloth.

- *Encourage a "no-itch" policy.* Discourage eye-rubbing; this may only aggravate the irritation and spread infection.

- *Protect your family.* The bacteria and viruses that cause conjunctivitis are easily spread among family members. Separate the towels, washcloths, sheets, and pillowcases your infected child uses from those that others use. Launder them separately in hot water, and wash your own hands to avoiding spreading the infection yourself. Clean anything that touches your child's eyes.

- *Eliminate allergens.* If you can determine that certain substances, such as tobacco smoke or other allergens, are causing your child's eye irritation, try to eliminate those substances from her environment. See **Allergies.**

Do not . . .

- put previously opened medication or someone else's medication into your child's eye. It could cause serious damage.

Prevention

Not all cases of this common infection can be prevented, but there are a few steps you can take to help protect your child:

- Swimming goggles may prevent conjunctivitis caused by chemical irritation. Avoid swimming where there are unsanitary water conditions.

- Help your child avoid, if possible, any allergens—including cigarette smoke—that may be linked to past conjunctivitis outbreaks.

- Don't put any chemicals or medicines in your child's eye unless directed by the doctor.

- Encourage frequent hand-washing, and use other good hygiene methods to prevent the spread of infection, as described on page 366.

- At birth, the use of antibacterial ointment or silver nitrate drops can help prevent gonorrhea infection of the newborn.

See also **Eye Injuries; Sty.**

Pinworm

See *Worms: Pinworm and Other Parasitic Worms.*

Pneumonia

Despite its alarming reputation, pneumonia is actually a common lung infection that can be treated effectively, usually leaving no lasting health effects. Pneumonia, an infection of the lung tissues, causes a cough, shortness of breath, fever, an increased breathing rate, or some or all of these symptoms. People with *asthma* and other chronic lung diseases are more susceptible to recurrent bouts of pneumonia. Severe *gastroesophageal reflux* (the backup of fluid from the stomach into the esophagus and throat) can also cause recurrent pneumonia. Pneumonia is not uncommon in childhood but requires prompt medical attention if complications are to be prevented.

Signs and Symptoms

- Fast, labored, sometimes painful breathing
- Flaring of the nostrils (indicating difficulty breathing)
- *Fever* or chills
- *Chest pain* that is worsened by breathing
- Abdominal pain
- Loss of appetite
- Persistent *cough*
- Wheezing

When to Call the Doctor
CALL FOR EMERGENCY HELP IF
- your child has difficulty breathing and/or is turning blue.

  For first aid information, see page 380 if your child is less than 1 year old and page 383 if your child is 1 year of age or older.

CALL THE DOCTOR IMMEDIATELY IF
- your child's lips or nails become bluish.
- your child makes grunting sounds when breathing.

CALL THE DOCTOR TODAY IF
- your child continues to seem run-down after having a cold or croup.
- your child cannot sleep, because he is coughing and wheezing.
- your child is not drinking enough fluids or has persistent vomiting.
- your child has a fever and abdominal pain.
- your child's symptoms are worsening.
- your child is coughing up mucus that is yellow or green or streaked with blood.
- your child has a lingering cough.

Essential Facts

The term *pneumonia* describes an infection that causes fluid to collect in the air sacs of the lungs. In infants and children, pneumonia usually develops from an upper respiratory tract infection—usually viral—which then spreads to the chest. In some cases, this virus weakens the lungs' natural defenses and a bacterial infection sets in. In contrast, a healthy child may suddenly develop pneumonia without evidence of prior infection. Children whose immune defenses or lungs are weakened by other illnesses, such as *asthma, cystic fibrosis,* or immune deficiency (see *HIV/AIDS Infection*), are more likely to develop pneumonia than other children.

Viral pneumonia symptoms usually develop over a couple of days. You may even be unaware that your child has developed pneumonia. Instead, you may think that your child's cold or bronchial infection is getting worse, or that he's having trouble recuperating from a typical respiratory illness.

In some cases, however, your child will become quite ill. His skin may be hot and dry, and he may be weak and drowsy. He will develop a fever, may cough, and may be short of breath. As the disease progresses, he may cough up thick, yellow mucus. Less common symptoms include nausea, *vomiting, diarrhea*, and *headaches.* Sometimes, whole segments of the lung (called lobules) may become filled with fluid and collapse. In other instances infected fluid can collect around the lungs, a condition commonly called a pleural effusion or an empyema. If pneumonia symptoms appear, or if you suspect that your child has developed the infection, call your doctor immediately.

Causes

Pneumonia can be caused by either viruses or bacteria. Each type has different symptoms.

Viral Pneumonia

Viral pneumonia usually starts as an upper respiratory tract infection. The bronchial tubes—the two main branches of the windpipe and the tubes branching from them—often become inflamed. Viral pneumonia can be mild or severe, and localized or spread throughout one or both lungs. A child with a mild case may seem to have a prolonged cold and cough and feel tired. Viral pneumonia can sometimes involve wheezing, most commonly in young infants with *bronchiolitis.* Common viruses include respiratory syncytial virus (RSV), influenza A or B, parainfluenza virus, Epstein-Barr virus (which also causes *mononucleosis*), and varicella *(chicken pox).* Uncommon viruses, such as the measles virus, can cause pneumonia.

Bacterial Pneumonia

Bacterial pneumonia is sometimes more severe than viral pneumonia. In some cases, a viral infection comes first and disturbs the lungs' natural defenses, allowing the bacteria to settle in the air sacs of the lungs. Inflammation occurs, causing coughing, fever, and rapid breathing. White blood cells are drawn into the lungs to fight the bacteria and combine with dead bacteria to form pus, which may be coughed up as mucus. Bacteria that cause pneumonia include *Streptococcus pneumoniae* (which causes one type of strep throat—see **Sore Throat/Strep Throat**), and *Staphylococcus aureus.*

Other Causes

Other causes include organisms such as yeasts, fungi, mycoplasmas, *Pneumocystis carinii, Chlamydia trachomatis,* and rickettsia. Pneumonia can also be a complication of **tuberculosis.** Mycoplasma pneumonia is common in children and can linger for days or even weeks. Since mycoplasma is contagious, other family members may also develop the harsh, persistent cough, fever, and run-down feeling typical of mycoplasma pneumonia. The condition can be treated with antibiotic medications.

Aspiration pneumonia may result when a child inhales substances such as food, small objects, or even vomit. Inhalation of some solvents, gasoline, kerosene, or other volatile substances can cause chemical pneumonia.

Pneumonia is a common complication of some chronic illnesses in childhood, such as cystic fibrosis and bronchopulmonary dysplasia, and immune deficiencies such as AIDS.

What the Doctor May Do

Your doctor can diagnose pneumonia by listening to your child's breathing with a stethoscope and by taking chest X rays. She may perform a blood test to measure your child's white blood cell count, which may be high.

The doctor will assess whether your child has a bacterial infection in the lungs or elsewhere (e.g., the throat or ears). If the doctor suspects a bacterial infection, she may take blood and tracheal or bronchial mucus cultures to help identify the infection-causing bacteria, and she will prescribe antibiotics. Pneumonia caused by tuberculosis is treated with antituberculosis medications for months. Viral pneumonia usually requires no treatment with medication. The doctor may treat other symptoms, such as wheezing, with inhaled bronchodilator medications to help reduce airway inflammation and make breathing easier for your child.

Depending on the cause of the pneumonia, your doctor may suggest that you isolate your child from other children until after the most contagious stage of the illness. Occasionally, if your child is exhausted from coughing and a lack of sleep, your doctor may prescribe a nighttime cough suppressant. But this is not routinely done, because coughing is the body's natural way of clearing mucus from the airways, and suppressants may actually worsen the infection. Proper physical therapy can also help treat the pneumonia by facilitating the drainage of mucus and pus from the affected parts of the lungs.

In more severe cases, the doctor may give your child an antibiotic injection, which is sometimes more effective than oral antibiotics. If your child is an infant, is dehydrated, or is very ill with pneumonia, the doctor may hospitalize him for treatment. Rarely, a child with pneumonia may develop respiratory failure, requiring intravenous fluids, antibiotics, and breathing assistance. Other reasons for hospitalization include evidence of a blood infection or a severe abnormality on the chest X ray, such as an abscess (a collection of pus); the need for oxygen; rupture of the breathing sacs; inflammation of the lining of the lung; or collapse of the lung, leading to respiratory failure. A child with cystic fibrosis will often require special antibiotics and hospitalization when pneumonia complicates his chronic illness.

What You Can Do

Most cases of pneumonia can be treated at home after diagnosis by a doctor. To comfort a child with pneumonia, use the following steps:

- *Bring down the fever.* Use acetaminophen or ibuprofen to lower your child's fever, which can be a debilitating part of any illness. Placing lukewarm cloths on his forehead (unless it makes him shiver) may also soothe him. For more suggestions on treating fevers, see *Fever.*

- *Monitor fluid levels.* Encourage your child to drink plenty of fluids to prevent dehydration. Fluids also loosen secretions and mucus, making it easier to cough them up.

- *Prop your child up.* If your child is having trouble breathing, you can also prop extra pillows behind his head and shoulders while he is awake or asleep.

- *Use physical therapy.* You can help your child's lungs drain by "clapping" on his chest and back (chest percussion) after proper positioning in bed. This procedure loosens secretions and helps re-expand the lungs. It helps your child's cough. Ask your doctor or a physical therapist about how to do this at home.

Prevention

To protect your child from the viruses and bacteria that cause pneumonia, encourage frequent hand-washing and practice the other good hygiene methods described on page 366. A vaccine is now available for children at high risk of contracting pneumococcal pneumonia (see p. 112). Discuss this vaccine, as well as the flu vaccine, with your doctor if your child has a chronic illness or is at higher risk for some other reason. Protect your child from exposure to secondhand tobacco smoke, and don't allow anyone to smoke around a child who has pneumonia.

■ *Poison Ivy, Poison Oak, Poison Sumac*

"Leaves of three, let them be" is a familiar adage and one that remains as true for children today as it was when you were a child exploring the woods and fields. Certain plants, specifically poison ivy (*Toxicodendron radicans,* a three-leaved plant), poison oak (*Toxicodendron quercisolium,* another three-leaved plant), and poison sumac *(Toxicodendron vernix)* can produce similar allergic skin reactions when they touch the skin.

Signs and Symptoms

- Intense itching
- Swollen, red skin spots
- Pin-sized, clear blisters
- Rash that appears in straight lines (showing where the leaf rubbed the skin)

When to Call the Doctor
CALL THE DOCTOR TODAY IF

- the rash hasn't cleared up in a week or two, is particularly severe, or appears infected.
- the rash is on the face, eyes, mouth, or genital area.

Essential Facts

Once your child comes in contact with the plant, the first signs of redness and itching usually appear within 24 to 72 hours, although the rash may appear a few days later. Most often, the rash erupts on exposed areas of the arms, legs, and face, but it can appear on other parts of the body that have touched the leaves. It may appear in surprising places as the result of the plant's having come in contact with clothing or shoes, which your child touches later.

The worst stage of the eruption occurs 4 to 7 days after contact. Even with prompt treatment, an outbreak may take up to 2 weeks to clear. Unless the rash becomes infected (usually due to constant scratching), the rash will disappear on its own.

Causes

Sensitivity to a chemical contained in the oils of the plants causes the symptoms. The degree of sensitivity varies: Some children react only slightly or not at all to the oil, whereas others remain highly allergic throughout their lives. Contact with the leaves and stems of these plants—or even smoke from their burning—exposes a child to the oils. Shoes and pets may also carry the oils, which can be transferred to a child's skin. Poison ivy is not contagious and doesn't spread unless the oil is transferred from the source (the plant) to parts of the body.

What the Doctor May Do

If the rash is particularly stubborn or severe, the doctor may prescribe a topical or an oral steroid. The topical steroid cream can be rubbed on the skin to reduce swelling and itching.

What You Can Do

First, carefully wash the clothes your child was wearing, so that you don't risk exposing her to the offending substances again. If you think a pet has been exposed, bathe it, too. Then, try these steps to relieve the itching:

- *Coat the rash with calamine lotion.* This over-the-counter preparation remains the recommended method for soothing the itch and drying up the blisters.
- *Give your child a soothing bath.* Soak her in a warm—but not hot—tub of water mixed with baking soda, oatmeal, or commercially available oatmeal (colloidal) preparations.

- *Use a topical steroid cream, such as hydrocortisone.*
- *Give your child an antihistamine.* If the itching is severe, consider giving an over-the-counter antihistamine. Do not give antihistamines to children under 2 years old without a doctor's supervision.

Do not . . .

- use a topical antihistamine lotion or topical antiseptic containing benzocaine. Your child could become sensitized to these medications and end up with a different rash.

Prevention

If your child likes the outdoors, she'll probably end up in a patch of poison ivy, poison oak, or poison sumac at some point. To reduce the risk, follow these tips:

- *Identify the enemy.* As soon as your child is old enough to play outside by herself, teach her how to identify potentially irritating plants (see illustration).

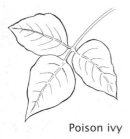

Poison ivy, poison oak, and poison sumac can be identified by their distinctive shapes. The best defense against these rash-causing plants is to recognize and avoid them.

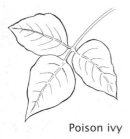
Poison ivy

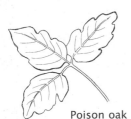
Poison oak

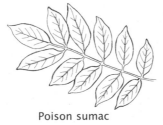
Poison sumac

- *Avoid burning poison ivy.* The smoke contains the toxin. Also, if you know that you have poison ivy, oak, or sumac in your yard, dig it up and cart it away while wearing gloves and long sleeves and pants. Wash yourself and your clothes with strong soap and water.
- *Cover up.* When you know that your child may be exposed to poison plants, make sure she wears long-sleeved shirts, socks, and long pants. This will help her avoid direct contact with the plants. Wash her clothes and shoes thoroughly.

See also *Rashes.*

Port-Wine Stain

See *Birthmarks.*

Prematurity (Preterm Birth)

Tiny and very pink, a baby born more than 3 weeks early is said to be premature or preterm. A preterm infant is any child born before the 37th week of pregnancy. Full-term infants are born from 37 to 43 weeks of pregnancy. Medical care for preterm infants has improved significantly in recent decades with the result that infants born as early as 23 to 24 weeks of pregnancy have a chance at survival. Infants born after 30 weeks are nearly certain to survive. Along with this good news, however, remains the fact that premature infants are more likely than full-term infants to experience medical complications and delays in development. The earlier a baby is born, the more likely the baby will have medical complications that require care in the neonatal intensive-care unit (NICU) of a hospital. The NICU is specially equipped and staffed to care for the typical needs of a preterm infant.

Essential Facts

Your "preemie," as preterm infants are often called, is a new little person who is different from the fetus developing quietly in your womb just a short time ago and also from the larger, full-term infants whom you've probably seen. Until the time of birth, most preterm infants develop normally, but because they are born early, their development is not as far along. For example, if your baby was born 2 months early, by the time he is 2 months old, he will likely resemble a full-term newborn. Prematurity is common, occurring in 6 to 8 percent of all births in the United States.

Preterm infants look different from full-term babies. A preterm infant's skin is thin and reddish and may be covered with fine body hair. The muscle tone and reflexes are, as yet, poorly developed. Bones are soft and flexible, and in a boy, testicles may still be undescended.

Because of their small size and low birth weight, preterm infants are susceptible to a variety of medical problems. Very young babies will have poorly developed lungs and trouble with the respiratory control center in the brain. As a result, these babies often experience episodes of apnea (failure to breathe). These infants also have difficulty maintaining their body temperature, and their heart rates may be variable, sometimes going too low to maintain good blood pressure and blood flow. The more underdeveloped the baby, the greater the danger of serious or life-threatening complications caused by underdeveloped parts of the body such as lungs, brain, liver, kidneys, gastrointestinal tract, and muscles. Your infant may require intensive care for such disorders as *jaundice,* respiratory distress syndrome (a disease of the premature lungs), apnea (periodic pauses in breathing—see *Infantile Apnea*), feeding problems, *anemia,* low blood pressure, low blood sugar, and others.

What the Doctor May Do

A preterm infant will have a multidisciplinary team in the NICU working to improve his chances for a healthy life. The health professionals may include a neonatologist (doctor specializing in newborn intensive care), clinical nurse specialist, primary nurse, social worker, respiratory therapist (trained in the management of oxygen and breathing machines), physical therapist, and other doctors and health care professionals.

Treatment depends on your infant's medical condition. Most infants will be placed in a warm incubator and be fed by intravenous tubes that provide nutrients, vitamins, and mineral supplements. The health professionals in the NICU will monitor your child's blood for the proper levels of oxygen, sugar, acid, and other chemicals. If your baby has jaundice, they may use special lights or, occasionally, blood transfusions to treat the condition. Your child may need a breathing tube and breathing assistance with a machine and supplemental oxygen until his lungs and brain respiratory center are mature enough to take over. Your child may also need help eating, either through intravenous lines or by way of tubes inserted into the mouth or nose. Many premature infants will need to have antibiotic medications to help prevent bacterial infections.

What You Can Do

If you have a preterm baby in the NICU, here are some things you can do to get involved:

- Learn all you can about your baby's physical and developmental condition.

- Ask your doctor and nurses questions, and write everything down so you'll remember it later.

- Take one day at a time—your baby's condition may change from day to day.

- Touch and love your baby as much as possible.

The health professionals in the NICU encourage parents to spend as much time as possible with their infants. Babies are calmer, their blood pressure lowers, and their breathing improves when parents hold their hands, stroke them, and cuddle them.

Because your infant may be able to breast-feed once his digestive system develops, it's a good idea to express your breast milk several times a day in order to keep your milk flowing and ready for your baby (see p. 68 for information on expressing breast milk). Some preterm babies who have not yet developed a strong sucking reflex begin with gavage feeding, a way of delivering a mother's breast milk to the infant's stomach with tubes. Freeze your breast milk to be used if needed.

Once you are home with your preterm infant, you may discover that sleep is not easy to get. Preterm infants sleep for shorter periods at

Touching or holding your premature baby as often as medically allowed will foster his comfort, his sense of security, and the bond that you share.

a time and cry more than full-term babies, the result of having a less mature nervous system. In addition, you will need to protect your infant from infection by keeping him away from crowds and other members of the family or friends who have colds, the flu, or other illnesses. Many very premature babies develop complications, such as chronic breathing difficulties (known as bronchopulmonary dysplasia), growth disturbances, and vision or hearing impairments. Parents of preterm babies with medical conditions will have many extra responsibilities, including these:

- Learning how to administer their baby's medications
- Bringing the baby in for frequent medical examinations
- Learning about and dealing with developmental issues
- Getting extra help at home
- Obtaining financial coverage for medical and related costs

Rely on doctors, nurses, local support groups, and parents of children who have the same or similar medical conditions for guidance in these matters. A visiting nurse or home health aide can really make a difference. Ask your child's doctor about the possibility of getting help in your home.

Investigate community services, especially respite care—a specialized in-home nursing program that allows parents to have some time off from the stress and challenges of caring for a medically complex child.

Keep an eye out for developmental delays such as lateness in achieving developmental milestones such as sitting up, rolling over, walking, and talking. The milestones are described in the age-by-age chapters in the front of this book. Early diagnosis and treatment of *developmental problems* can help a child develop skills that may otherwise lag.

Prevention

It is not possible to prevent every case of preterm birth. But there are some steps you can take during pregnancy to reduce your risk of premature labor. Make sure to attend your regular prenatal checkups. Do not smoke or drink alcohol. Avoid exposure to drugs not prescribed by a doctor who knows you are pregnant. Talk with your obstetrician about any risks in your workplace, such as exposure to industrial solvents, lead, pesticides, or other substances that may harm a developing fetus. Also discuss any hobbies you may have that may expose you and your fetus to these substances. Avoid sports that may result in any high-impact blow to your abdominal area—sports such as horseback riding or high-speed skiing. Avoid infection by washing hands frequently and avoiding contact with raw meats and cat feces. Report symptoms of vaginal discharge (watery or bloody) or abdominal pain or discomfort to your doctor immediately.

■ Prickly Heat

See *Heat Rash.*

■ Punctures

See *Cuts and Scrapes.*

■ Rabies

See *Bites, Animal and Human.*

■ Rashes

It's a rare child who doesn't develop a rash at one time or another during infancy or childhood. Although most rashes are minor and easily treated at home, a rash can be caused by an infectious disease (e.g., fifth disease, chicken pox), an allergy, an insect infestation, or—very rarely—a potentially serious disease.

Signs and Symptoms

- Red, rough, itchy, and/or blistering skin over small or large areas of the body

When to Call the Doctor

CALL THE DOCTOR IMMEDIATELY IF

- your child suddenly develops a purple or blood-colored rash.
- your child develops a fever and otherwise appears unwell.

CALL THE DOCTOR TODAY IF

- your child has any rash you cannot easily identify.

What the Doctor May Do

Treatment depends on the cause of the rash. The doctor will first determine whether the cause of the rash is a systemic infection, such as *fifth disease* or *chicken pox,* or an allergy, such as a local reaction to laundry detergent. To treat *hives* or other allergic rashes (see *Allergies*), the doctor may prescribe antihistamines and show you ways to help your child avoid the offending substances. For rashes caused by infectious diseases, the doctor will treat either the disease or the symptoms, depending on the nature of the infection. If your child has a rash caused by an irritating substance, the doctor will work with you to discover what substance may be irritating your child's skin and then recommend ways to avoid

COMMON SKIN RASHES

Skin Problem	Fever	Description	Location	Duration
Acne	No	Elevated, red pimples; sometimes blackheads	Face, back, chest	Until treated
Athlete's foot	No	Colorless or red rash; mild to intense itching; cracking; scaling; oozing blisters	Between toes	Until treated
Chicken pox	Yes	Flat, red spots become raised bumps, then blisters, then crusts; intense itching during blister stage; irritability; headache; fatigue; loss of appetite	May begin anywhere, appearing in new crops every 1 to 2 days; highest concentration on torso and face	5 to 14 days
Cradle cap (seborrhea)	No	Rash changing from white to yellow to red; some crusting and occasional itching; fine, oily scales	Scalp, eyebrows, eyelids, behind ears, groin	Until treated
Diaper rash	No	Red rash; no itching	Under diaper	Until treated
Eczema	No	Red rash; moderate to intense itching; moist or oozing	Elbows, wrists, knees, cheeks	May get better or worse for months or years despite treatment
Fifth disease	Yes	Bright red "slapped cheeks" rash with flat, lacy appearance; rash comes and goes	Starts on face; spreads to arms and legs; then entire body	7 to 10 days
German measles	Yes	Swollen glands; flat, or slightly raised, red rash; headache; inflamed eyes; runny nose; sore throat; loss of appetite	Starts on face; spreads to torso; then extremities	2 to 4 days
Hives	No	Pale, raised lesions with flat tops, surrounded by red; intense itching	May appear anywhere	Minutes to days
Impetigo	Maybe	Red sores with golden crusts; occasionally itchy	First appears on arms, legs, face; then most of body	Until treated
Measles	Yes	Cough; red eyes; eyes sensitive to light; runny nose; flat, pink spots changing to red	Starts on face; spreads to chest, abdomen, arms, legs	4 to 7 days

█ COMMON SKIN RASHES (continued)

Skin Problem	Fever	Description	Location	Duration
Pityriasis rosea	No	Oval pink or beige flat spots in a "fir tree" pattern over back and extremities; often preceded by larger "herald patch"; can be very itchy	Starts on back or upper extremities	6 to 8 weeks
Poison ivy	No	Red, linear, elevated blisters; intense itching; oozing; swelling	Exposed areas	7 to 14 days
Prickly heat	No	Slightly raised, white or red dots; surrounding skin may be red, itchy	Torso, neck, skin folds on arms, legs	A few days
Ringworm	No	Slightly raised, red rings; occasionally itchy, flaky, or scaly	Anywhere, including nails and scalp	Until treated
Roseola	Yes	Itchy, flat, pink rash, occasionally with some bumps; high fever sometimes with convulsions; runny nose; sore throat	Starts on torso; spreads to arms, neck, face, legs	1 to 2 days (rash); 3 to 7 days (fever)
Scabies	No	Red, crusting, slightly elevated rash; intense itching	Arms, legs, torso, wrists, armpits, between fingers and toes (older children); head, neck, hands, feet (infants)	Until treated
Scarlet fever	Yes	Flat, pink rash resembling a sunburn, rough to touch; sore throat; red tongue	Starts on face, elbows; rapidly	5 to 7 days

it. If your doctor suspects purpura—purplish (or sometimes red, brownish-yellow) bruiselike areas that can indicate various underlying conditions—he'll probably perform blood tests and other laboratory tests to identify the source of the problem. For most other common rashes, the doctor will recommend a soothing lotion or methods for reducing itching or perhaps prescribe a stronger steroid cream for particularly severe cases.

What You Can Do

Try to determine what's causing the rash. Call your doctor if the rash looks like bruises or if you suspect chicken pox, **measles**, or another infectious disease. Otherwise, you can probably treat the rash yourself.

If the rash is localized in the diaper area, **diaper rash, impetigo,** or a yeast infection (see **Thrush**) may be the cause. If a rash develops after your child plays in the woods, it might be a reaction to a toxic plant (see **Poison Ivy, Poison Oak, Poison Sumac**). If she's eaten something new, like chocolate or berries, or started a new medication, then an allergic reaction might be causing the problem. If you are unsure what's causing the rash, call your doctor and describe the rash. To comfort your child, give her a lukewarm baking soda or oatmeal (colloidal) bath, pat her rash dry, and cover it with calamine lotion. Discourage her from scratching, and keep her hands clean and nails short to prevent her from aggravating the rash or causing an infection.

Red Eye

See *Pinkeye.*

Reflux

See *Gastroesophageal Reflux.*

Rett Syndrome

See *Pervasive Developmental Disorder.*

Rheumatoid Arthritis

See *Juvenile Rheumatoid Arthritis.*

Rheumatic Fever

See *Fever; Sore Throat/Strep Throat.*

Ringworm

Ringworm has nothing to do with worms. Identified by its characteristic red ring of rash—and not by a worm, as its name implies—the fungal infection ringworm is a common childhood rash. It causes both athlete's foot and jock itch. In children, it appears most commonly on the scalp or the trunk, although ringworm can develop on any body part.

Signs and Symptoms

- Small, red spots that form sores that heal from the center, leaving a characteristic ring
- White, blistered skin between and underneath the toes (athlete's foot)
- Yellow, cracked toenails (athlete's foot)
- Rash around the groin area (jock itch)

When to Call the Doctor
CALL THE DOCTOR TODAY IF
- the rash appears on the underside of your child's foot.
- the toenails are distorted or yellowing.
- self-help measures fail to improve the condition within 3 or 4 weeks.
- your child's scalp is infected.

Essential Facts

This fungal infection begins as small, round red spots that grow to the size of a dime or larger. They begin to heal from the center outward, creating a ring of scaly, red skin around a smooth center. The affected area is usually itchy and inflamed, but easily treated and not serious. Ringworm can invade the hair shafts; the skin of the arms, legs, trunk, or face; or the fingernails.

Feet

One of the more common types of ringworm is athlete's foot (tinea pedis), which is caused by the fungus *Trichophyton rubrum*. Swimming pools, locker rooms, and shower rooms—places where children congregate—are the perfect breeding ground for the fungi that cause athlete's foot. Athlete's foot causes the skin above and between the toes to scale and crack, and the infection can easily spread to the soles. Blisters may also develop.

Hair and Scalp

If your child has a chronically itchy, flaky scalp with hair loss, consider the possibility of head ringworm (tinea capitis), which is caused by the fungus *Trichophyton tonsurans*. (If your child is under 1 year old, however, he may have cradle cap.) Two types of infection involve the hair and scalp. In both, the fungus directly invades the hair shaft, causing it to become brittle and then break. In the milder form of the infection, the fungus doesn't invade the scalp. The more severe form causes the scalp to become inflamed and pus to form at the base of the hair shafts. In many cases, the infection causes the hair to fall out, sometimes in clumps.

Trunk or Upper Extremities

Ringworm appearing on the chest, abdomen, or back (the trunk of the body) is known as tinea corporis and is caused by *Trichophyton tonsurans* or *Microsporum canis*. Its symptoms are round, scaly patches. Tinea corporis is one of the most common forms of ringworm in young children. Ringworm noted for small, teardrop-shaped and reddish, white, or tan spots is known as tinea versicolor. It appears in clusters on the chest, back, or upper extremities. Tinea versicolor, appearing as white or tan flat spots on the trunk or upper extremities, is caused by *Pityrosporum orbiculare*.

Causes

Yeasts and other fungi cause various types of fungal skin diseases. Even the healthiest children can develop the infection if exposed. Inadequate nutrition, poor hygiene, and illness increase the likelihood of infection. People living in a humid climate are more likely to get ringworm. Contact with contaminated combs, brushes, hats, or seat backs spreads hair and scalp infections. Cats and dogs infected with the fungus may transmit the infection. A child can get a fungal infection from walking barefoot on damp, contaminated surfaces or walking in infested soil. Constantly wearing rubber and nylon shoes makes fungal infections more likely because they trap heat and moisture close to the feet, creating an environment where the fungus can thrive.

What the Doctor May Do

Your doctor will identify ringworm by examining scales or the roots of your child's hair under a microscope. The doctor may also need to culture (grow the cells of) the flaky skin, pus, or

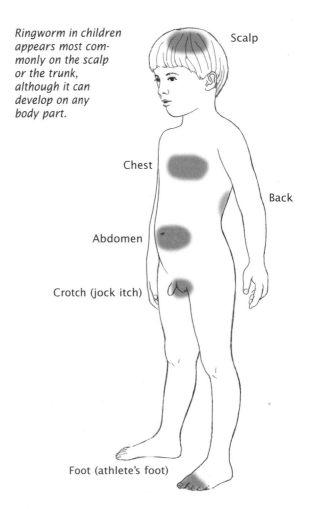

Ringworm in children appears most commonly on the scalp or the trunk, although it can develop on any body part.

Scalp

Chest

Back

Abdomen

Crotch (jock itch)

Foot (athlete's foot)

hair roots. In most cases, you should be able to treat ringworm at home. If the scalp is affected, your doctor will prescribe 2 or 3 months of an oral antifungal medication called griseofulvin. A 2 percent selenium sulfide shampoo may be recommended for tinea capitis or tinea versicolor. Your child's doctor may recommend a 1 percent tolfanate powder or topical miconazole or fluconazole for tinea corporis or tinea pedis. For most other cases, topical prescription antifungal ointments used for 3 to 6 weeks are effective.

What You Can Do

Antifungal creams or solutions, available over the counter, are sometimes effective for infections of the trunk, groin, legs, arms, neck, and face. After washing and drying the area, apply the treatment according to the manufacturer's instructions. The infection should start fading in several weeks, but you should continue treatment for another week or two to make sure that all the fungi are gone. In addition, follow these tips until the infection clears up:

- Keep your child's towel, bath mat, and hairbrushes separate from the rest of the family's (to avoid spreading the infection), and wash them every day (to avoid reinfection).

- Check your pets for signs of ringworm infection, and treat them accordingly.

- For athlete's foot, use clean cotton socks. Wash them thoroughly in hot water.

Do not . . .

- allow your child to go barefoot.

- use creams or ointments containing cortisone.

Prevention

Because the fungi that cause ringworm are so common, preventing infections may be difficult. Nevertheless, you can reduce the chances of his contracting ringworm by having your child avoid sharing hats, combs, and hair ornaments and by keeping his feet as dry as possible to discourage the growth of microorganisms. Have your child wear shoes or sandals in locker rooms.

See also **Rashes.**

▌ *Roseola*

Although you may be alarmed if your baby develops a high fever that persists for several days and a rash that appears on her body and arms after the fever breaks, chances are good that she has roseola, also known as exanthem subitum, a relatively harmless viral infection that is most common in children under 2 years old. You'll know for sure in about 3 days, when the fever passes and a rash—pink and itchy, with flat or raised spots on the chest, abdomen, or back—appears and then, within 24 hours, clears up without treatment. During the course of the infection, your child may be irritable or more tired than usual, but probably will pass through the illness easily.

Signs and Symptoms

- Fever, often high, lasting 3 to 7 days
- Rash on upper body that appears after temperature returns to normal
- Slightly swollen eyelids
- Reduced appetite
- Mild *diarrhea*
- *Cough*
- Irritability
- Fatigue
- Febrile seizure

When to Call the Doctor
CALL FOR EMERGENCY HELP IF

- your baby has a seizure (see *Seizures*).

CALL THE DOCTOR TODAY IF

- your child has the symptoms of roseola.
- your infant under age 6 months has a fever.
- your older baby or child has a fever over 102°F.

Causes

A virus of the herpes family called human herpesvirus 6 (HHD-6) causes 80 percent of roseola cases. Other viruses (HH7, enterovirus, parainfluenza virus, adenovirus) cause the remaining 20 percent of cases. How the virus is transmitted remains unknown, but doctors suspect that the virus is present in oral secretions. That means that sharing objects that children put in their mouths can transmit roseola.

What the Doctor May Do

Your doctor may not know what's causing the fever—at least not until the characteristic rash appears, and by then the illness is nearing its end. Your doctor will suggest ways to control the temperature and advise you to call again if the fever increases or lasts for more than 4 days. If your child has a febrile seizure (see *Fever*), the doctor will examine her and advise you on how to handle future seizures.

What You Can Do

Apart from lowering your child's fever according to your doctor's instructions, you can't do much but wait out the infection. It should clear up completely within 5 to 7 days. Keep your child out of day care or school until the rash is gone.

Prevention

Roseola is a highly contagious childhood viral infection and is difficult to prevent once your child has been exposed.

■ *Rubella (German Measles)*

Thanks to the now routine vaccination (MMR—measles, mumps, and rubella), this once common childhood disease is rare. Rubella is a viral disease usually accompanied by a rash of tiny and flat or slightly raised, pinkish red spots that may appear behind the ears, on the forehead, around the mouth, or elsewhere on the face. The potential danger with rubella is usually not to the child with rubella, but rather to the fetus of a pregnant woman who may contract rubella during her pregnancy. Rubella during pregnancy can cause a variety of birth defects.

Signs and Symptoms

- Slight fever
- Tiny pink spots starting behind the ears, then spreading to the forehead and the rest of body
- Enlarged, swollen glands at the back of the neck
- Occasional joint pain

When to Call the Doctor
CALL THE DOCTOR TODAY IF

- your child is exposed to rubella and has not received his vaccinations.
- your child has the symptoms of rubella.
- you are pregnant and your child has rubella.

Causes

Rubella is caused by a virus in saliva or nasal secretions transmitted by coughing, sneezing, or sharing drinking or eating utensils. It takes about 14 to 21 days to develop symptoms after exposure.

What the Doctor May Do

The doctor may first confirm a rubella diagnosis by performing blood tests or examining throat cultures. She may then advise you to keep your child home from school or child care during the contagious phase of the illness and give suggestions for helping your child feel more comfortable. Rubella is contagious from 7 days before the rash erupts until 4 to 7 days afterward.

What You Can Do

Fortunately, the rash that accompanies rubella does not usually itch. So, unless your child's fever runs him down, the illness should be mild. Give your child acetaminophen or ibuprofen to reduce the fever, and isolate him from playmates and—especially—pregnant women until your doctor gives you the OK, usually about 7 days after the rash begins.

Prevention

You can prevent rubella by making sure your child receives all his vaccinations. Also see page 11 of the pregnancy chapter of this book for ways to avoid infection while pregnant.

Salmon Patch

See *Birthmarks.*

Salmonella

See *Food Poisoning.*

Scabies (Mites)

One of the itchiest rashes around is scabies—a common insect infestation in young children. This rash, caused by tiny mites that burrow under the skin's surface, is highly contagious and spreads from child to child and family member to family member if not treated promptly.

Signs and Symptoms

- Red bumps often seen around the wrists, ankles, armpits, and genitalia
- Small, curved lines on skin's surface, resulting from insect's burrowing under the skin
- Small blisters

When to Call the Doctor
CALL THE DOCTOR TODAY IF
- your child scratches constantly, or if you suspect scabies.

Essential Facts

Scabies appears as itchy, red, swollen bumps, usually at the wrist and armpit, in the webbing between the fingers and toes, and on the genitals and buttocks. Infants commonly become infested on the face, scalp, palms of the hands, and soles of the feet.

Causes

A mite causes scabies. This mite spreads most easily through contact with people who are infested, although clothing and bedding can also be a source of infestation. Mites burrow under the skin and lay eggs, producing a rash. Once the mite gets into the skin, the rash may take 2 to 4 weeks to appear. The rash is caused by an allergic reaction to the mite.

What the Doctor May Do

Your doctor can identify scabies by examining skin scrapings taken from around the rash. In addition, he'll ask about your child's recent activities and recent scabies outbreaks in the community to see if your child might have been exposed. If he confirms that scabies is the cause of the rash, he'll prescribe an anti-mite lotion containing 5 percent permethrin. No over-the-counter preparations treat scabies effectively. Your doctor may also recommend that the entire family use the lotion, applied over the entire body from the ears down, to prevent reinfestation. In infants, the scalp, forehead, and temples should be treated. A second treatment may need to be applied a week later. Your doctor may also prescribe an oral antihistamine or steroid cream to reduce itching and inflammation and to help prevent infection.

What You Can Do

Apply the anti-mite preparation as instructed by your doctor. Thoroughly massage the cream into your child's skin from her head to the soles of her feet. About 8 to 12 hours after you apply the treatment, wash the medication off your child, and dress her in clean, mite-free clothes. Wash all bedding and clothing in hot water, or place clothing in a hot dryer for 10 minutes. Unfortunately, even after the mites and eggs die—usually within 72 hours after the treatment—your child is likely to be itchy and uncomfortable, sometimes for a week or two, because although the mites are gone, the allergic reaction may recede slowly. Try the following home remedies to help your child feel more comfortable:

- Ask your doctor about giving your child an antihistamine to relieve severe itching.

- Soak your child in an oatmeal bath or over-the-counter bath designed to relieve itching.

Prevention

Keeping your child away from people or clothing known to be infested will help prevent scabies infestation.
See also *Rashes*.

Scarlet Fever

See *Sore Throat/Strep Throat*.

School Phobia

See *Anxiety Disorders*.

Scoliosis

Thanks to increased awareness and public health campaigns, doctors and school nurses now routinely screen children for this once chronic and debilitating curvature of the spine. Although scoliosis still occurs (about 2 percent of the population have it), early treatment successfully prevents the development of serious complications.

Signs and Symptoms

- Poor posture and spinal curve to one side
- Hump on the upper back, with the body bending forward
- Unequal hip position or shoulder level

When to Call the Doctor
CALL THE DOCTOR TODAY IF
- you are concerned about your child's posture.
- your child's hips or shoulders look uneven.
- your child's school nurse recommends an evaluation.

Essential Facts

Everyone's spine has a natural curve that makes the shoulders slightly rounded and the lower back somewhat arched. With scoliosis, however, the spine also curves from side to side, causing an abnormal bending of the back and a mis-alignment of the entire body. Scoliosis may be accompanied by another condition called kyphosis, in which the normal curve of the spine is accentuated, creating a hump on the top of the spine. Scoliosis often develops after about 10 to 12 years of age, and is most common in girls, possibly because sex hormones play a role.

If your child has scoliosis, your first hint that a problem exists will probably be that her clothes no longer fit properly: A hem or waistband becomes uneven, for example, or one pant leg appears longer than the other. If left untreated, scoliosis can cause profound deformity and disability. With treatment, however, most children with the condition grow and develop normally.

Causes

Four types of scoliosis exist:

- *Idiopathic:* The most common type of scoliosis, it affects healthy children. Though the cause is unknown, another family member often has this same type of scoliosis, indicating a genetic predisposition. It is more common and significantly more likely to require treatment in girls. Idiopathic scoliosis often begins late in childhood or in early adolescence, when hormonal changes and rapid growth occur.

- *Congenital:* In rare cases, scoliosis is present at birth and is therefore considered a congenital abnormality. As with idiopathic scoliosis, the cause is unknown. This form of scoliosis often accompanies other congenital abnormalities.

- *Neuromuscular:* Children who have neuromuscular conditions such as *cerebral palsy* often develop scoliosis and other skeletal abnormalities as they grow.

- *Disease-related:* In rare instances, scoliosis can be caused by various disorders, such as Marfan's disease (which affects the connective

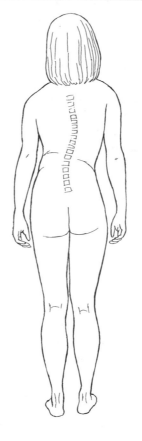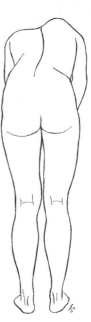

With scoliosis, the spine curves from side to side, causing an abnormal bending of the back and a misalignment of the body.

tissue), spinal cord tumors, or muscular dystrophy.

What the Doctor May Do

The doctor will first examine your child's back. If he thinks that a pronounced curve exists, he will take X rays to measure the degree of curvature. If the curvature of the spine is mild, the doctor may monitor your child with X rays periodically to see if it gets worse as your child's bones grow. More than half of scoliosis cases correct themselves and require no treatment except periodic examination and measurement observation by an orthopedic specialist.

If the condition gets worse, however, the doctor may recommend the use of an orthopedic back brace, such as a Boston brace, to reduce the curve. This brace usually must be worn for at least 18 hours a day for 1 to 3 years. An orthopedic specialist will monitor your child to determine whether the brace may need to be refitted or replaced periodically.

In some moderate to severe cases, surgery is necessary to correct the curvature. Surgery is best done during adolescence or young adulthood, when the bones heal more quickly and the risk of complications is lower than when done later. Surgery involves fusing some of the vertebrae in the curve and inserting a rod to tighten the spine. After the operation, a child may need to wear a back cast for up to 6 months.

What You Can Do

Take your child to the doctor if you notice any symptoms of scoliosis. Early diagnosis and treatment provide the best chance for a complete recovery. You can further increase the odds of recovery by encouraging your child to strengthen her back muscles with good posture, sports, and exercise. A physical therapist can suggest appropriate exercises. Follow the doctor's treatment plan, and reassure your child that she, you, and her doctor will work together to improve her posture, and that in all likelihood, she'll be a healthy, active, normal adult.

Prevention

Scoliosis cannot be prevented, but early diagnosis and treatment can correct the problem.

■ Scrotal Swelling and Pain

Boys commonly experience swelling and pain of the scrotum at some point, usually because of an injury. A blow to the groin can produce intense, lingering pain and swelling of the scrotum, the thick-skinned pouch that contains the testicles. The symptoms usually clear up without treatment, but occasionally these symptoms indicate serious problems of the genital tract. Therefore, have a boy with scrotal swelling or pain checked by a doctor immediately.

Signs and Symptoms

- Persistent or lingering pain in the groin or genitals
- Swelling or redness in the groin or genitals
- Discomfort or tenderness in the groin or genitals after an injury or a blow
- Nausea and vomiting along with genital pain

 When to Call the Doctor
CALL THE DOCTOR IMMEDIATELY IF
- your son has any pain, swelling, or discoloration in his groin or genitals.
- your son feels a mass in his scrotum.

Causes

At one time, ***mumps*** was a significant cause of scrotal swelling and pain, but immunization has virtually eliminated that disease in the United States. Today, the condition is usually caused by the factors described in the following paragraphs.

Injury to the Testicles A blow to the groin forces the testicles against the body, causing excruciating pain. The pain usually decreases within minutes, although a boy's groin may feel sore for a day or two. The more severe the injury, the more severe and long-lasting the pain. In rare cases, an extremely sharp blow to the groin (from being hit by a car, for example) can cause a testicle to rupture or move into the abdomen or upper thigh. Surgery may be needed to repair the damage.

Hydrocele A *hydrocele* (swelling and accumulation of fluid in the scrotum) is a common condition in boys of all ages. It usually affects only one side of the scrotum, causing it to become swollen, firm, and pink, but not painful.

Varicocele Varicocele is an uncommon condition in which the veins surrounding one or both testicles become enlarged (see *Testes, Undescended*). It tends to appear during puberty. Though a varicocele is painless, it can interfere with the testicles' growth and possibly with sperm production and fertility if left untreated.

Torsion of the Testicle With this condition, the torsion, or twisting, doesn't involve a testicle but rather a spermatic cord, the structure that connects a testicle to the internal reproductive organs. The spermatic cord contains blood vessels, nerves, muscles, and the tube that carries semen. Any twist to the cord could pinch off the blood supply to the testicle, killing cells in the testicle. Torsion of the spermatic cord can destroy a testicle in as little as 6 to 12 hours. Though rare, this condition requires immediate emergency treatment.

Torsion of the Testicular Appendix Boys frequently have small attachments or growths on their testicles that are remnants of testicular development. They are called appendix testes, and they sometimes become twisted. The symptoms are virtually identical to those of torsion of the spermatic cord, but the problem is far less serious. Because no vital blood vessels connect the appendage to the rest of the testicle, it does not put the child at risk of losing a testicle.

Testicular Tumor Though rare, a painless mass in the testicle can be caused by either a benign or a malignant tumor. Tumors are more common in adolescence, but can occur at any age.

What the Doctor May Do

In addition to performing a physical exam, the doctor may order a sonogram to observe blood flow in the testicle in order to identify the cause of the swelling or pain. Abnormal blood volume—either too great or too little—can help the doctor make a diagnosis. Treatment for the problem depends on its underlying cause.

- *Injury:* Most injuries heal by themselves within a few days. But if a boy experiences a ruptured or dislocated testicle, he may need surgery to repair the damage. Otherwise, your doctor will probably tell you how to ease your son's pain until the condition heals.

- *Hydrocele:* This condition often subsides without complications or treatment in young boys. But have a doctor examine your son to rule out an inguinal hernia, an associated condition that might require surgical treatment (see *Hernia, Inguinal*).

- *Varicocele:* If testicular growth is delayed, surgery is needed to tie off the affected vein, forcing the blood to find a different pathway to the heart.

- *Torsion of the spermatic cord:* Usually, the boy must undergo immediate surgery in the groin area so that the doctor can see if a cord is twisted. If necessary, the surgeon will untwist the cord and fix the testicle into place. She may also put the other testicle in its proper place to prevent torsion from occurring on that side. If the testicle is dead or dying, the doctor may remove it. This step is necessary only when the spermatic cord has been twisted for more than 12 hours. Loss of one testicle will not interfere with a boy's fertility or sexual function, because the remaining testicle can compensate fully. The boy's scrotum will look normal except that it contains only one testicle.

- *Testicular tumor:* If a tumor is felt or suspected, the child needs to see a surgeon. The doctor might first order a sonogram or a CT (computed tomography) scan, then take a biopsy of the mass by making an incision in the groin. If the biopsy reveals **cancer,** the testicle will probably have to be removed and further treatment may be needed.

What You Can Do

If your son's scrotum is injured, call the doctor and apply an ice pack wrapped in a towel as soon as possible to reduce the swelling and pain. Never put ice directly on the scrotum: Wrap the ice in a towel to avoid injury to the delicate skin. Acetaminophen or ibuprofen may ease the pain. Several hours after the injury, a warm bath may relieve the soreness. For other causes of scrotal swelling or pain, follow your doctor's instructions.

Prevention

You can reduce your son's risk of injury by encouraging him to wear protective equipment such as a cup, an athletic supporter, or both when playing sports. As your son gets older, ask his doctor to explain to him how to examine himself for scrotal masses.

■ *Seizures (Convulsions)*

If your child loses consciousness and twitches and shakes for several seconds or minutes, don't panic. Seizures—sudden, temporary changes in physical movement, behavior, or consciousness—are fairly common in childhood and are usually short-lived. More than 50 percent of seizures affect children.

Signs and Symptoms

- Convulsions or rhythmic jerking of the limbs

- Loss of consciousness
- Involuntary urination and/or defecation
- Drooping of the eyelids or blinking
- Loss of awareness (child appears to be in a trance or daydreaming)
- Déjà vu (a sense of having been in the exact same situation before)
- Child complains of strange smells
- Infant has unexplained repetitive movements, decreased alertness, weakness, or irritability

 When to Call the Doctor
CALL FOR EMERGENCY HELP IF

- your child has difficulty breathing and/or is turning blue.

  For first aid information, see page 380 if your child is less than 1 year old and page 383 if your child is 1 year of age or older.

  CALL THE DOCTOR IMMEDIATELY IF

- your child has a seizure for the first time.
- your child with seizure disorder controlled by medication has a seizure that lasts for longer than 10 minutes.
- your child shows signs of meningitis (e.g., fever, neck stiffness, or drowsiness).

Causes and Essential Facts

A seizure, also known as a convulsion, is an uncontrolled spasm of the body's muscles caused by a temporary disruption of the brain's normal electrical patterns. Seizures are sometimes accompanied by a loss of consciousness, which may be quite brief or more prolonged. A seizure can affect any function controlled by the brain—thoughts, sensations, or movements. Seizure symptoms can vary in intensity, from a split-second reaction to a violent shaking of the entire body for several minutes or longer. Fever is the most common trigger of seizures in infants and children.

Fever One common form of seizure that occurs in infants and young children with a high fever is called a febrile seizure (see *Fever*). The faster a fever rises, the more likely a febrile seizure is to develop. About 2 to 4 percent of children experience these usually harmless seizures with a very high temperature that rises rapidly. They occur most between 6 months and 3 years of age.

Infections Seizures may also accompany certain infections, such as that caused by *Shigella,* bacteria that are found in contaminated water or food and that cause diarrhea. If your child experiences a seizure, ask your doctor for an evaluation—especially on the first occasion—so that he can exclude the possibility of infection.

Poisoning Poisoning by specific drugs and chemicals, such as cocaine, nicotine, pesticides, tricyclic antidepressants, and certain mushrooms of *Gyromitra* species, may also cause seizures. Other causes include brain injury from lack of oxygen or trauma, lack of glucose, or other metabolic problems.

Epilepsy Sometimes, seizures recur over a long period, even throughout a person's life. This condition, called epilepsy, requires medical attention and ongoing care. In about 50 percent of cases, children "outgrow" epilepsy by adolescence if it is treated and controlled during childhood. Even if the condition persists, however, epilepsy does not affect intelligence or, in most cases, normal development.

There are four types of seizures, which are discussed in the following sections.

Grand Mal Seizures Also known as convulsions or generalized tonic/clonic seizures, grand mal seizures are the most dramatic. During a classic grand mal seizure, a child may fall to the floor, unconscious, with all muscles tense. Her eyes roll back in her head, and excess salivation begins. Within seconds after falling, the child's entire body begins to shake, or convulse, violently and rhythmically. The child has trouble breathing and may lose control of her bladder or bowels. These seizures are generally not dangerous unless the seizure lasts more than 20 or 30 minutes or is repeated without the child's regaining consciousness between seizures (so-called status epilepticus).

Petit Mal Seizures Far less obvious than grand mal seizures, a petit mal seizure (also called an absence seizure) typically involves a momentary loss of consciousness, which observers may not notice. During a petit mal seizure, a child's face may fall blank for a few seconds or she may appear to be staring into space. Sometimes her eyelids droop and blink or her muscles twitch. In other cases, the child's arms and legs twitch slightly, and she may drop what she is holding. Whatever the symptoms, the entire episode lasts only a few seconds, after which the child resumes what she was doing as though nothing happened. Petit mal seizures are often misidentified—a teacher may think a child is ignoring him, for example, or not paying attention in class.

Complex Partial Seizures Because complex partial seizures (also known as psychomotor or limbic seizures) originate in one part of the brain, their symptoms vary according to which part of the brain is involved. These seizures are quite common in children and are relatively benign, but need to be treated if they continue. A common type of partial seizure arises in the temporal lobe, which is responsible for language, perceiving smells, and storing feelings and memories. When a partial seizure occurs, a child may "smell" an unpleasant odor, become exceedingly anxious, or have other strange feelings. When a partial seizure affects memory, a child may have a vivid memory or she may experience déjà vu (a sense of having been in the exact same situation before), although such feelings do not always indicate a seizure. If the seizure affects another part of the brain, a child may jerk her arm and leg on one side or turn her head to one side (sometimes called a myoclonic seizure). Often, the child doesn't remember having the seizure and the diagnosis is made by the symptoms that a parent, another relative, or a teacher observes. Sometimes, a complex partial seizure is the first sign that a grand mal seizure is about to begin.

Infantile Seizures Also called infantile spasms, infantile seizures usually occur in the first year of life and consist of flexion or extension of the body lasting several minutes and occurring in clusters.

What the Doctor May Do

Although many seizures don't require medical treatment, contact your doctor whenever your child has a seizure. If your child has a fever, the doctor will try to determine if your child has an infection and, if necessary, will treat the underlying illness. He may explain how to reduce a high fever and how to cope with a febrile seizure in case another occurs.

If no fever is present, your child's doctor will probably try to determine the cause of the seizure by first taking a thorough history of the symptoms and the circumstances under which the seizure occurred. He will then conduct a physical examination, paying special attention to neurological functions such as reflexes and coordination. The doctor may recommend that you visit a pediatric neurologist, who may conduct tests including blood tests, X rays, an EEG (electroencephalogram), or brain-imaging techniques such as a CT scan (computed tomography) or an MRI (magnetic resonance imaging).

If the doctor finds that a metabolic disorder or another disorder caused the seizure, he will treat that problem. If the neurologist diagnoses epilepsy, he will probably prescribe one of several medications to help control the seizures. These medications, called anticonvulsants, work to prevent nerve cells from abnormally firing. Common anticonvulsants include phenobarbital, phenytoin, carbamazepine, valproic acid, primidone, ethosuximide, benzodiazepines, ACTH (for infantile spasms), gabapentin, and trileptal. The type and dosage of medication varies for each child and must be carefully regulated because of the danger of side effects. No matter how seldom a child's seizures occur, anticonvulsants are effective only when taken regularly. A doctor will monitor the child's condition carefully and, if appropriate, wean a child off the medication to see if the condition has resolved.

In some cases of brain injury or scarring, surgery may be needed to restore more normal brain function. Sometimes seizures cannot be controlled by medication or surgery. Another option is a strict seizure-control (ketogenic) diet. Ask your doctor about your child's options.

What You Can Do

If your child has a seizure, stay calm, ease your child onto the floor, and move away any furniture or other nearby objects that might cause injury. Unless your child previously has had a seizure and you are experienced in caring for her through such an episode, call your doctor or call for emergency help. If your child experiences frequent febrile seizures, see *Fever* for more information about fevers and how to reduce them.

If your child is diagnosed with epilepsy, you'll work closely with a health care team to provide medication or other measures to reduce the number and severity of the seizures she experiences. Your most important job, however, will be to support, love, and encourage your child. Here are some other tips you can use to cope with epilepsy:

■ *Get support* Contact your local chapter of the epilepsy advocacy agency (AEA) and a parental support group (see Appendix: Parent Resources, Medical Conditions).

■ *Help family and friends understand the disorder.* Many people have misconceptions about epilepsy's effects. After educating yourself (with help from your doctor and support groups), explain to people that epilepsy is not contagious, nor does it affect intelligence or development. Also, make sure your child's caregivers know what to do if a seizure occurs.

■ *Treat your child naturally.* That means establishing rules you expect her to follow. A child with epilepsy—like any child—benefits from consistent, loving rules and expectations.

■ *Advocate at school.* Meet with your child's teacher before each school year to discuss how epilepsy affects your child and what to do if a seizure occurs. If medication slows her level of functioning (an occasional side effect), tell the teacher and ask that your child be given extra time to finish her work. Also consult your child's doctor, who may adjust her medication. Remember, too, that your child has a legal right to be in school and to receive extra help.

■ *Protect your child.* Children with very frequent seizures may require special precautions, such as constant supervision around water and the use of protective head gear.

During a seizure, do not . . .

■ rub the child with alcohol. Rubbing alcohol can be absorbed through the skin and is toxic.

■ place your child in a tub of cold water. This might injure your child or reduce the fever too rapidly.

■ bundle up your child. This could cause a fever to rise.

■ give your child medicine or anything to drink until your child is fully awake.

■ force anything between the teeth.

■ restrain your child. You cannot stop a seizure once it has started. Do, however, protect her from injuring herself.

Prevention

Proper medication can prevent seizures from recurring. You can help prevent febrile seizures by treating the fever with acetaminophen or ibuprofen before it gets too high. Avoiding environmental toxins such as lead will prevent some seizures. If your child has a seizure, you can protect your child during the episode, to prevent injury.

Separation Anxiety

See *Anxiety Disorders.*

Sexually Transmitted Diseases

See *Vaginal Infections, Irritations.*

Shingles

See *Chicken Pox.*

Short Stature

Your 8-year-old child gets frustrated shooting baskets with neighboring children. He still climbs on the counter to open kitchen cabinets, because he can't even reach them on tiptoe. He is shorter than all his classmates, and he sometimes comes home crying because they tease him about being short. You wonder if he's ever going to catch up to his peers. Your child may have what doctors call short stature.

Signs and Symptoms
- Your child doesn't gain height appropriate for his age.
- Your child is shorter than 95 percent of his peers.

When to Call the Doctor
TALK WITH THE DOCTOR AT YOUR CHILD'S NEXT CHECKUP IF
- you have concerns about your child's height.
- your child seems to have stopped growing.
- your child has deviated significantly from his previous growth pattern.

Essential Facts
Your child's growth rate—and the size he ultimately attains—depends on heredity, the quality and quantity of nutrients he eats, and his overall health. Heredity plays a large role. If a child's parents are short, he will probably be short no matter how well he eats or how healthy he is—short is healthy for him. But various health conditions, including chronic illnesses, poor nutrition, and hormone deficiencies, may also cause short stature. So be sure to consult your child's doctor about any concerns you have about his height.

Causes
The most common causes of short stature in an otherwise healthy, well-nourished child are genetic short stature or a constitutional delay in growth. Growth hormone (GH) deficiency is rare.

- *Genetic short stature* is an inherited, normal condition. If a child's parents or grandparents are short, the child is likely to be short as well.

- *Constitutional growth delay* is a pattern of slow growth during childhood and a late onset of puberty. A child with constitutional growth delay eventually achieves a normal height. Constitutional growth delays often run in families and are more common in boys. In some parts of the world, malnutrition is a common cause.

- *GH-deficiency syndrome* occurs when the pituitary gland secretes too little growth hormone. It occurs in about 12,000 to 15,000 children every year in the United States.

- *Hypopituitarism* is a condition that includes GH deficiency and other pituitary hormone deficiencies, in which the pituitary is damaged and doesn't release its hormones. Most cases of hypopituitarism occur after surgery or because of a tumor. In hypopituitarism, thyroid function and sexual development may be

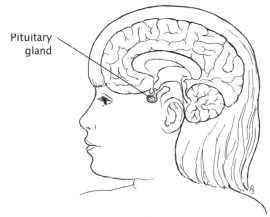

Your child's pituitary gland regulates and controls her body processes, such as growth and reproduction, by secreting hormones that stimulate other glands to produce hormones.

affected, since the damaged pituitary releases neither the hormones regulating these activities nor GH.

- *Genetic disorders,* such as Turner's syndrome, which is caused by a genetic defect (and affects only females), can also cause short stature. In addition, the condition causes ovarian failure; girls with ovarian failure do not undergo puberty without treatment.

- *Chronic illnesses,* such as chronic renal insufficiency, a kidney disorder that causes both kidney- and growth-related problems, can also be at the heart of short stature. Most untreated or inadequately treated chronic childhood diseases cause short stature. Other chronic illnesses that cause growth problems include **cystic fibrosis;** malabsorption, a gastrointestinal disorder that interferes with food absorption; and Crohn's disease, a chronic inflammation of the gastrointestinal tract (esophagus, stomach, and intestines). Still other causes of short stature include malnutrition, bone disorders, hypothyroidism, and emotional deprivation.

What the Doctor May Do

If you are concerned about your child's height, consult your child's doctor. She'll look at your child's growth history on a growth chart and compare your child's weight, height, and head circumference with normal standards. She'll also examine your child physically, emotionally, and developmentally. In most situations, your doctor will advise you that your child's short stature is simply the result of family genetics and that all you need to do is help your child eat a nutritious diet and get plenty of exercise to ensure normal growth.

In some cases, your child's doctor may take an X ray to determine your child's bone age (one measure of growth) and conduct blood tests to check blood chemistry, organ functioning, hor-

mone levels, and the like. If necessary, your doctor will consult nutrition, child development, and psychology specialists to help diagnose your child. Children who grow poorly are often referred to an endocrinologist for a parent-doctor consultation.

If your child is diagnosed with GH deficiency, chronic kidney problems, or, in rare cases, Turner's syndrome, an endocrinologist may prescribe GH injections to improve growth. GH injections are not recommended unless the child has a deficiency of this hormone. Researchers are still trying to determine if children with constitutional or genetic short stature will benefit from treatment by achieving a greater final height than that predicted from the target height. Turner's syndrome and chronic renal failure are the only non-GH-deficiency disorders for which growth hormone treatment is approved.

What You Can Do

Most importantly, maintain a positive attitude and help your child accept his size. Try to promote self-esteem; point out his advantages and good qualities; and suggest activities appropriate to his height. Soccer, swimming, gymnastics, and ice skating, for example, may be better choices than basketball. Try not to convey the message that something is wrong. Instead, point out that many short people have achieved great things! Next, try to relax. As long as you follow the doctor's advice, you can probably keep your child's growth on track.

Prevention

Although you cannot change genetic short stature, good nutrition and treatment of diseases that can affect growth can prevent abnormal short stature. Avoid cigarettes and ethanol (ethyl alcohol) during pregnancy, since these can cause fetal growth retardation and lasting effects on both height and weight.

How Tall Will My Child Be?

If you're like most parents, you imagine how your child will appear as he grows up. If he is your biological child, you can get as accurate a picture as possible by looking in a mirror. Your child's height and even his basic body type are largely determined by his genes.

To determine your biological child's approximate adult height, use the following formula developed by pediatricians. (To convert inches to centimeters, multiply the number of inches by 2.54. To convert back to inches, multiply the final number of centimeters by 0.394.)

▮ Add the mother's and father's heights in centimeters.

▮ If your child is a boy, add 13 centimeters to that figure and divide by 2.

▮ If your child is a girl, subtract 13 centimeters from your combined height and divide by 2.

Most children, when they become adults, fall within 10 centimeters (about 4 inches) of the resulting measurement, called the target height. Of course, this is just an estimate, and other variables may influence your child's ultimate height.

▮ Sickle-Cell Disease

Sickle-cell disease is an inherited blood disorder that causes the red blood cells to change into a sickle, or curved, shape. Because of this shape, the red blood cells are fragile and tend to become stuck in the blood vessels, causing blockages that can damage organs and result in a shortage of red blood cells, a condition known as **anemia.** A child born with sickle-cell disease will develop normally but will need regular treatment with antibiotics to prevent infection, and

may require oxygen, blood transfusions, pain relief, and other medications during times of sickle-cell crisis.

Signs and Symptoms

- Symptoms vary widely depending on which organs are affected.

When to Call the Doctor

IF YOUR CHILD HAS SICKLE-CELL DISEASE, CALL THE DOCTOR TODAY IF

- your child has a fever.
- your child is breathing rapidly or has difficulty breathing.
- your child is experiencing pain.
- your child is irritable or is crying more than usual.
- your child has a severe headache.
- your child suffers from fatigue and lack of energy.
- your child is pale.
- your child has a poor appetite.
- your child is vomiting.
- your child has diarrhea.

Essential Facts

Every red blood cell contains hemoglobin, a protein that carries oxygen from the lungs to every part of the body. But people with sickle-cell disease have hemoglobin that is different from normal hemoglobin and causes blood cells to take on a sickle shape rather than the normal, round, doughnut shape.

Cells in the sickle shape tend to become trapped and be destroyed in the liver and spleen, resulting in anemia, a shortage of red blood cells. Anemia, if severe, may cause shortness of breath and fatigue, although most children with sickle-cell disease do not experience these symptoms on a regular basis. Blood cells trapped in certain organs can block the delivery of oxygen, causing swelling and pain. Blood cells trapped in the lungs can cause life-threatening breathing difficulties. Children with sickle-cell disease may also develop serious bacterial infection in the blood. Other complications may include slow growth, blindness, gallstones, kidney failure, and stroke (blockage of blood flow to the brain).

Causes

Sickle cell is an inherited disorder. To inherit this disease, a child must receive two sickle-cell genes, one from each parent, or one sickle-cell gene plus a gene for any one of several other abnormal hemoglobin disorders. If a child inherits only one sickle-cell gene, she is said to have the sickle-cell trait and will not have the disease but can pass it on to her children. Sickle-cell disease occurs most commonly in children of African descent. Among this population, 1 in every 10 people carry the gene and 1 in every 600 people have the disease.

What the Doctor May Do

Doctors can diagnose sickle-cell disease in newborn babies by way of a routine blood test. Most states now require that all newborn babies be tested for sickle cell. If your baby tests positive for sickle-cell disease, the doctor will test again to make sure. The doctor may also ask one or both parents to have a similar blood test.

A baby who has this disease will be placed on oral antibiotics (usually penicillin) beginning by age 2 months to prevent dangerous infections. Children with sickle-cell disease should continue on antibiotics indefinitely or until the doctor decides that the medication is no longer necessary. Because of the risk of infection, it is important to call the doctor if a child with sickle cell develops a fever.

Children with sickle-cell disease need to receive all the normal childhood vaccines as well as an annual flu shot and vaccines for pneumococcal bacteria. The doctor will also prescribe folic acid (folate), a vitamin that helps promote the production of new red blood cells and prevent severe anemia. Routine eye exams are also recommended because sickle-cell disease can sometimes lead to vision problems.

A pain episode, sometimes referred to as a sickle-cell crisis, results when the blood cells pile up and block the blood vessels. This cuts off the blood supply to nearby tissues so that no cells can get through to bring oxygen to them. Without oxygen, the tissues or organs begin to swell, causing pain. In mild cases, the pain episode can be treated at home with pain relief medications. For very severe symptoms, including breathing problems, strokes, and severe anemia, hospitalization, oxygen by mask, and blood transfusion of red blood cells are sometimes necessary.

What You Can Do

If your baby has sickle-cell disease, work with your child's doctor to provide the best medical care for your child. Your child may be treated by a pediatrician or a pediatric hematologist (children's blood specialist) or at a special sickle-cell clinic. You may need to administer daily doses of antibiotics to your child to protect her from severe infection.

Make sure to give your child all the antibiotics and vitamins (folate) prescribed by your child's doctor. You will need to provide your child with a healthy diet that includes a balance of nutrients. Since dehydration can bring on painful episodes, give your child plenty of liquids. Your doctor may also advise you to keep your child warm. Cold air or cold baths can slow the blood flow and cause blood circulation problems.

If you are considering having more children, seek advice from a genetic counselor who can explain your future chances of giving birth to a baby with sickle-cell disease. You may also want to seek help from a social service agency or a social worker who can help your family cope with the emotional, social, and financial burdens of caring for a child with sickle-cell disease. For information on organizations that can provide information and support for families with sickle cell disease, see Appendix: Parent Resources, Medical Conditions.

Prevention

Because sickle-cell disease is inherited, prevention strategies are limited. For those with a family history of the disease, genetic counseling is an important step prior to pregnancy.

▌ *Sinusitis (Sinus Infection)*

If your child has a cold that seems to linger longer than usual or if he cries and fusses or complains of a headache along with the cold, his sinuses could have become inflamed—a condition called sinusitis.

Signs and Symptoms

- Upper respiratory tract infection that lingers longer than usual
- *Headaches*
- *Fever*
- Nasal congestion and discharge
- Bad breath
- Tiredness
- Sore throat persistent for several days

When to Call the Doctor

CALL THE DOCTOR IMMEDIATELY IF
- your child has difficult, congested breathing.

CALL THE DOCTOR TODAY IF
- the symptoms don't improve more than 7 days after the start of a cold or the flu.
- your child has a fever above 102°F.
- your child has a thick, yellowish or greenish nasal discharge.

Essential Facts

Sinusitis is a common condition that occurs in up to 10 percent of children with colds or the flu. It involves inflammation and infection of the mucous membrane that lines the sinuses, a group of air-filled hollows within the bones of the face and skull. During infancy and early childhood, most cases of sinusitis are acute, self-limited, and uncomplicated. Acute sinusitis occurs more often after 2 years of age, when the sinuses are more fully developed. An acute episode typically lasts 7 to 10 days.

In addition to a chronically runny nose, many children with sinusitis also experience headaches, a fever, nasal congestion, bad breath, and a *cough*—and most cases of sinusitis occur when your child has a cold. As uncomfortable as the condition may be, sinusitis is usually easy to treat with medication.

In rare cases, the infection spreads beyond the sinuses, causing other problems. The areas around the eyes and the brain are the most likely sites of secondary infection. If your child has a severe headache, becomes sensitive to light, or is increasingly irritable, contact your doctor immediately.

Causes

Most cases of sinusitis are caused by bacteria that become trapped when the sinus passages

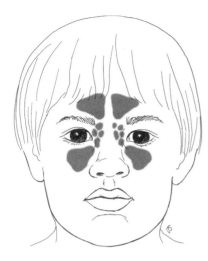

The sinuses are hollow cavities within the facial bones. They are not fully developed until after 12 years of age. Most cases of sinus infection are caused by bacteria that become trapped when the sinus passages swell or become blocked with fluid, or both.

swell or become blocked with fluid, or when both conditions occur. The primary cause of sinus blockage in children is the common cold, but several other culprits exist, including allergies, chronic respiratory illnesses, injury to the nose, nasal growths, and inhaled water or chlorine during swimming.

What the Doctor May Do

If your child's symptoms indicate a sinus infection, your doctor will examine his nose to detect inflammation and the presence of yellow, greenish, or milky discharge. If your child has an underlying problem causing chronic sinus blockage, such as allergies, your doctor will treat the sinus infection with antibiotics first and then try to treat the underlying condition for the long term. For sinusitis caused by nasal congestion due to an upper respiratory infection, your doctor will usually prescribe a combination of decongestants (to clear the sinuses by reducing

nasal passage swelling) and antibiotics (to combat the bacterial infection and prevent complications). Although your child may need to take antibiotics for 10 days to—in some cases— as long as 3 to 4 weeks, the acute symptoms should diminish within a few days. For chronic sinusitis that doesn't respond to antibiotics, the doctor may recommend that an otolaryngologist surgically enlarge the sinus openings to encourage better fluid drainage.

What You Can Do

Your child is apt to be uncomfortable until the blockage clears and the inflammation dies down. Here are some tips to help him feel more comfortable:

- Offer acetaminophen or ibuprofen to reduce the pain and fever.
- Place a vaporizer or humidifier in your child's room.
- Have your child breathe warm, moist air in the shower or tub.

Prevention

Depending on the cause of the sinusitis, you may be able to prevent recurrences by treating the underlying problem with your doctor's help. Talk to your doctor about a vaccine now available for sinusitis caused by pneumococcal bacteria (see p. 112). Your doctor may also prescribe occasional preventative treatment using antibiotics or other medications such as decongestants or antihistamines, especially if your child's condition seems to be caused by allergies.

▌ *Sleep Apnea*

See *Infantile Apnea.*

Sneezing

See *Colds/Flu.*

Snoring

"I never thought a four-year-old could make so much noise sleeping!" says one parent of a child who snores. Snoring in small children can be disruptive—to the child and other family members. Most cases of childhood snoring are caused by a cold or the flu and will disappear as the underlying condition subsides.

When to Call the Doctor

CALL THE DOCTOR TODAY IF
- your child snores loudly and regularly, interrupted by several seconds of silence.
- your child pauses or gasps for breath while snoring.

TALK WITH THE DOCTOR AT YOUR CHILD'S NEXT CHECKUP IF
- you have concerns about your child's snoring.

Causes

Snoring occurs whenever an obstruction of the nasal passages and upper airways is present. Children tend to snore when their noses are congested from a cold, the flu (see *Colds/Flu*), or *allergies* or when their adenoids or tonsils swell as the result of colds, the flu, tonsillitis, or other upper respiratory infections. Some children who snore were born with larger-than-normal tonsils or adenoids. Some children's adenoids or tonsils swell during an infection and don't return to their original size after the infection is gone. As a result, the children continue to snore over the long term.

What the Doctor May Do

In most cases, no treatment for snoring is necessary; the snoring will stop after the allergy attack, cold, or tonsillitis clears up. If a permanent obstruction—such as large adenoids or tonsils—causes the problem, the doctor may recommend surgery to remove it.

What You Can Do

If your child's snoring is triggered by an allergy or upper respiratory tract infection, try these ways to relieve her congestion before bedtime:

- *Avoid antihistamines.* Unless your doctor recommends an antihistamine to treat an allergy, avoid giving your child these medications, which can dry and thicken nasal secretions, possibly causing snoring.

- *Use decongestants.* If the snoring is related to a cold, a decongestant before bedtime can open up your child's air passages.

- *Try a different sleep position.* Propping up your child's head with an extra pillow may help her breathe more freely and easily. Or try turning her on her side or stomach. Don't, however, place an infant on her stomach to sleep.

Prevention

Encouraging frequent hand-washing and practicing the other good hygiene methods described on page 366 will help protect your child from many common infections that cause snoring.

Sore Throat/Strep Throat

Sore throats are almost as common as stomachaches, and usually as easy to treat. A sore throat is a symptom accompanying more than one-third of acute childhood respiratory illnesses. Peak ages for sore throats are from 5 to

10 years, although a child of any age can be affected.

Sore throats occur whenever the throat becomes irritated or infected, which causes the tonsils (if present) and surrounding tissues to become inflamed (swollen, red, tender). Even a child who has had his tonsils or adenoids removed can still get a sore throat or strep throat. Although most sore throats are not serious, make sure that you identify the cause of any sore throat accompanied by *fever* or lasting more than 24 hours. Certain throat infections, if left untreated, can lead to rheumatic fever, an acute disease characterized by fever, inflammation, pain in muscles or joints, and possible heart damage.

Signs and Symptoms

- Complaints of pain and swallowing difficulty
- Fussiness, persistent crying, and difficulty feeding in infants
- Red, raw-looking throat
- Enlarged or tender lymph nodes in the neck
- Pus appearing at the back of the throat or on the tonsils

When to Call the Doctor
CALL THE DOCTOR IMMEDIATELY IF
- your child cannot swallow or fully open his mouth.
- your child cannot breathe normally.
- your child sounds as if he has marbles in his mouth.

CALL THE DOCTOR TODAY IF
- the sore throat is severe and not getting better, despite home remedies after a day or two.
- a fever accompanies the sore throat.
- your child has an accompanying rash on his body.

Causes

Viral Infections Viruses that infect the throat and upper respiratory tract cause most sore throats and usually resolve on their own. These infections include the common cold, the flu, and *mononucleosis.* Your child may or may not exhibit other symptoms, such as *fever* and *cough.* Children with mononucleosis, however, are often quite ill, with severe sore throats, fever, swollen lymph nodes in the neck, and occasionally trouble breathing because of enlarged tonsils and adenoids.

Bacterial Infections Only about 10 percent of sore throats are triggered by infection with *Streptococcus* (strep) or other bacterial infections. Strep infections, also known as strep throat, can cause infection and inflammation of throat tissues, including the tonsils. In addition to a sore throat, a strep infection may cause a high fever, *headaches, abdominal pain/stomachache, vomiting, swollen glands,* and the rash known as scarlet fever. Bacterial infections of the throat are potentially serious conditions that require treatment with antibiotics. Untreated strep throat can lead to rheumatic fever (a disease that can cause joint pain and heart damage) or to a kidney inflammation known as poststreptococcal glomerulonephritis (an illness noted for swelling of the extremities, cola-colored urine, and high blood pressure).

Inhaling Irritants Breathing in dust, smoke, chemicals, pollen—even dry air—can irritate the mucous membranes of the throat.

Vocal Abuse Shouting and prolonged talking or singing can also irritate the throat.

What the Doctor May Do

After performing a physical exam, the doctor may take a throat culture by swiping the back of your child's throat and tonsils with a cotton-tipped applicator and placing it into a special growth medium that allows bacteria to grow. Although some doctors perform a "quick" strep test that can show the presence of strep bacteria within 5 minutes, this test isn't 100 percent accurate. If the result is negative, a standard culture may be needed for definite diagnosis.

Treatment of a sore throat depends on its cause. If a virus is responsible, your doctor will advise you on comforting your child while the infection runs its course. If strep or other bacteria are present, your doctor will treat the sore throat with antibiotics such as amoxicillin or penicillin. In cases of recurrent and severe sore throat, the doctor may recommend a visit to an ear, nose, and throat specialist, who would evaluate the possibility of surgically removing your child's tonsils. Removing a child's tonsils, although done less frequently than in the past, is still performed about 500,000 times a year in the United States.

What You Can Do

If a bacterial infection is causing the sore throat, make sure your child takes all the medication your doctor prescribes. If an allergy is responsible for throat irritation, you, your child, and the doctor will cooperate to determine what might be causing the allergic reaction and to minimize exposure to the offending substance. Your doctor may recommend an allergy medication that helps relieve your child's symptoms.

In most cases, however, the sore throat is the result of a virus and will run its course, usually within a week. By following these tips, you can help your child feel better in the meantime:

- *Offer lozenges.* Sucking on throat lozenges (for children over age 4 years) can soothe the throat and help reduce pain but does not shorten the course of infection.
- *Use painkillers.* Give over-the-counter pain medication such as acetaminophen or ibupro-

fen. If your child is under 2 years old, consult your doctor for the proper dosage.

- *Moisten the air.* A cool-mist vaporizer or humidifier in your child's bedroom adds moisture to the air and may soothe the throat.
- *Make your home smoke-free.* Inhaling cigarette and cigar smoke—even secondhand—can irritate an already sore throat and cause many other health problems. The best thing you can do for your child—and for yourself—is to limit exposure to these toxic chemicals.
- *Keep your child home.* If your child's doctor diagnoses strep throat, your child is mildly contagious and should stay home from school or day care for at least the first 48 to 72 hours after starting treatment with antibiotics.

See also *Bronchiolitis, Colds/Flu.*

Speech Disorders

See *Learning Disorders;* sections on Communicating in the age-by-age chapters of this book.

Spina Bifida

Spina bifida is one of the most common and most disabling birth defects. It is a type of neural tube defect—a condition that results when the fetus's spine fails to close properly during the first month of pregnancy. Spina bifida is present in about 1 in every 1,000 births and is usually, but not always, detected during prenatal testing. The symptoms range from minor to severe. Children born with severe spina bifida will need to undergo immediate (within the first 24 hours after birth) spinal surgery and will likely need long-term care by a multidisciplinary team of medical professionals. Spina bifida may be accompanied by a number of physical, mental, and emotional impairments. Children with this condition can attend school, however, and the majority will be of normal intelligence. Some may have learning disabilities and will benefit from appropriate testing and special education at school age.

Signs and Symptoms

- An opening in the spinal column sometimes covered by skin or a thin membrane
- Neurological impairments, including weakness or paralysis of limbs and lack of bladder and bowel control
- Possible swelling of the head and brain with excess fluid (hydrocephalus)
- Difficulty breathing or swallowing

Essential Facts

The degree of impairment and the complications that accompany spina bifida vary with the severity of the spinal defect (see illustration). In very mild cases (occulta) the defect is so minor that it is not visible and causes little or no impairment. In more severe cases (meningocele) part of the spinal sac is defective and can lead to more motor and sensory impairments. In severe cases (meningomyelocele) nerve circuits may remain incomplete, leaving the child unable to walk or control bladder and bowel function.

A large percentage of children born with spina bifida also have hydrocephalus, the accumulation of spinal fluid in the brain. Other complications are the result of neurological damage and include muscle weakness or paralysis. Some children with spina bifida will have problems caused by Arnold-Chiari type II malformation. This condition occurs when the brain stem, the lower part of the brain that controls involuntary functions such as breathing and heartbeat, is compressed downward toward the spinal column. The symptoms can be difficulty swallowing and breathing, and weakness in the arms and hands.

Causes

The spinal cord normally closes during the first 3 to 4 weeks of pregnancy. The reasons this

The only symptom of the mildest form of spina bifida (occulta) may be a birthmark or dimple on the skin of the lower back. In more severe forms (meningocele), the gray and white matter of the spinal cord is exposed and appears as a skin defect. In the condition's most severe form (meningomyelocele), the spinal sac and nerves are exposed.

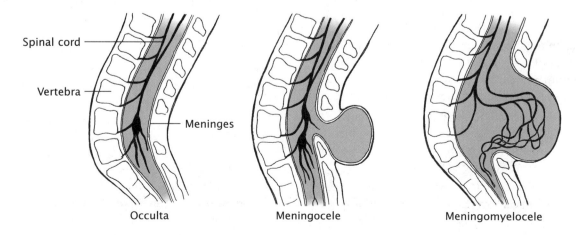

Spinal cord

Vertebra

Meninges

Occulta   Meningocele   Meningomyelocele

sometimes fails to happen (causing spina bifida and other neural tube defects) are not fully understood but are thought to be a combination of genetic and environmental factors. When the spinal cord and nerves are exposed by this defect, further development of spinal nerves is impaired and the nerve circuits needed for functions such as walking or bladder control never completely form.

Parents who have spina bifida in their family are more likely than others to have a child with this condition. However, some environmental factors may also play a role. In particular, a lack of sufficient folic acid (folate) in the diet early in pregnancy, or even before pregnancy, and exposure to certain drugs, such as methotrexate, used to treat rheumatoid arthritis and cancer, increase the risk of neural tube defects. Other environmental factors that may contribute to the development of neural tube defects include exposure to radiation (X rays), drugs, and toxic chemicals, and malnutrition.

What the Doctor May Do

During pregnancy, your doctor or health care professional will keep a careful watch for signs of neural tube defects during ultrasound exams. At about 16 weeks of pregnancy, your doctor will perform a blood test called the maternal alpha-fetoprotein (MAFP) test. Elevated levels of alpha-fetoprotein in the blood can indicate a neural tube defect and will prompt the doctor to perform an ultrasound exam to look for visible signs of the defect. Women who have the amniocentesis test (the insertion of a needle through the abdomen to take a sample of amniotic fluid) can also be screened for elevated levels of alpha-fetoprotein. Most but not all instances of spina bifida are detected before birth.

An infant born with spina bifida may appear normal at first, except for a small bulge of fluid-filled tissue along the spine. A surgeon will assess the extent of the neurological problem and perform a procedure to close the spinal defect, usually within the first 24 hours after birth. The surgery protects the spine from infection and further damage but does not repair any neurological damage that may already have occurred. A child born with fluid on the brain (hydrocephalus) will have a shunt surgically implanted to drain the fluid. Because hydrocephalus may occur later in some children, the child's doctor will watch carefully over the ensuing months to determine whether the child's head is growing at a normal rate. If the doctor suspects hydrocephalus, the condition can be confirmed by X rays, and an internal shunt can be surgically inserted to help drain the fluid. The doctor will also assess whether Arnold-Chiari type II malformation is present and will initiate treatment for the symptoms. A multidisciplinary team of health professionals (often including a neurologist, neurosurgeon, child development specialist, physical therapist, nurse specialist, and pediatrician) will be necessary to help you and your child cope with impairments such as muscle weakness, paralysis, or bowel and bladder incontinence.

What You Can Do

Early intervention can help a child with spina bifida to develop physically, socially, and academically. You can assist your child by providing a supportive, caring home and family life and by advocating for her to receive as much in the way of medical, physical, and educational support as she needs. Along the way, you will assist your child with a variety of needs, including helping her cope with her physical disabilities. Most children can become independent in managing their bowel and bladder problem with the help of new medical technologies.

During infancy and toddlerhood, watch your child's developmental progress, and have your child assessed by the doctor if you think one or more developmental skills (e.g., talking, walking, using hands) is lagging. Your child may be a candidate for early developmental enrichment programs in your area (see *Developmental Problems*).

Once your child reaches school age, have her learning skills assessed by way of neuropsychological testing to help define areas of academic strength and weakness. If she requires special education, you can participate in developing her individualized education program (see *Learning Disorders*). Physical disabilities such as those that accompany spina bifida can affect a child's emotional and social development. Make sure that your child's teachers understand your child's physical and intellectual capabilities, and encourage them to help provide the necessary assistance in a positive and supportive manner.

For further information and support for families of a child with spina bifida, see Appendix: Parent Resources, Disabilities/Special Needs.

Prevention

As many as 75 percent of cases of neural tube defects, including spina bifida, could be prevented if all women of childbearing age took 400 micrograms of folic acid each day. Neural tube defects occur in the first 3 to 4 weeks of pregnancy, often before a woman knows she is pregnant. For this reason, all women of childbearing age should take this vitamin. For those with a family history of spina bifida or other neural tube defects, genetic counseling is an important step prior to pregnancy.

▌ Splinters

A barefoot race across the deck or a climb up a wooden play structure may end suddenly in tears when your child gets a splinter. Many parents dread the chore of trying to extract a splinter from a squirming child's foot or finger, but most splinters are harmless and can be handled at

home unless the splinter is particularly deep or shows signs of infection.

The skin, the largest and most resilient organ, forms a remarkably effective protective sheath around our muscles, blood vessels, and internal organs. Nevertheless, as soon as your child is old enough and curious enough to explore, he's bound to get a splinter or two—usually on the hands or feet.

Signs and Symptoms

- A piece of material, usually a sliver of wood, embedded under the skin
- Pain, soreness in an area when touched
- Redness, swelling of the skin

When to Call the Doctor
CALL THE DOCTOR IMMEDIATELY IF
- the splinter is very large and deeply embedded.
- the skin around the splinter is red, hot, and painful, with red streaks going away from it.
- metal shards, glass, or other material is embedded deeply.

CALL THE DOCTOR TODAY IF
- you can't remove the splinter and your child is in pain.
- the wound shows signs of infection (redness, swelling).

Causes

Almost any small, sharp object can become embedded in the skin. Wood, metal, glass, or plant material (such as a thorn or nettle) are the most likely culprits.

What You Can Do

First, determine what the splinter is made of and where it came from. Unless it's glass, metal, or covered with a germ-ridden material such as animal feces, you can try to remove it yourself. If the end of the splinter sticks out of the skin, take a pair of tweezers and pluck it out slowly but firmly. Try not to break off the tip, which would leave the body of the splinter embedded in the skin. Sometimes soaking the affected area in warm water will soften the skin and make it easier to push the splinter up and out.

If this fails, sterilize a needle by holding it over an open flame. When it cools, use the needle to gently probe the area, lifting the splinter's tip until you can grasp it with your fingers or tweezers and remove it.

Clean the area thoroughly, dab on some antibiotic cream, and cover the wound lightly with a bandage. Encourage your child not to pick at it or press against it.

What the Doctor May Do

Take your child to the doctor if the splinter looks as if it might or has become infected, or if you can't remove the splinter and it's causing pain. The doctor may remove the splinter using a local anesthetic to numb the area, then evaluate the wound for infection. If there is a chance that glass, metal, or other material remains deep in the wound, the doctor may gently probe the wound under local anesthesia. In some cases, an X ray can reveal the location of the embedded material. Depending on your child's age and the date of his last tetanus shot, the doctor may give him a booster.

Prevention

No matter how careful you and your child are, splinters are bound to occur. You can reduce the risks, however, by encouraging your child always to wear shoes (even inside, if you have wooden floors). Also, regularly sand and paint or stain play structures, decks, and other wooden surfaces where your child may be playing. Dispose of old timbers with rough surfaces and other debris that might cause splinters.

■ Sports Injuries

See *Back Pain.*

■ Sprains and Strains

Once your child starts to walk, it won't be long before she starts to run, skip, jump—and fall down. Besides getting many cuts, bruises, and scratches, she also may eventually sustain sprains (injuries to the ligaments) or strains (injuries to the muscles). Sprains and strains are most common among schoolchildren, especially those who play sports. These injuries rarely occur among younger children, because their ligaments and muscles are stronger than their bones. (As a result, they're more likely to experience fractures than sprains.) While not serious, sprains and strains can cause much discomfort and may require medical care.

Signs and Symptoms
- Throbbing pain
- Swelling of the joint
- Difficulty moving or putting weight on the joint

Note: These symptoms can indicate fractures (see p. 409), as well as sprains or strains.

When to Call the Doctor
CALL THE DOCTOR IMMEDIATELY IF
- the pain is severe.
- the joint is swollen and discolored (evidence of bleeding into the joint).
- your child can't bend the joint.
- your child can't walk or bear weight on her feet or legs, or can't move her hands and fingers normally.

CALL THE DOCTOR TODAY IF
- the pain or swelling persists or worsens after 1 to 2 days.

Causes

Strains and sprains are usually caused when a child falls, lands forcefully on a joint, and stretches or tears the tissues. A strain is an overstretched muscle. Though they can be uncomfortable, muscle strains are minor injuries that usually heal relatively quickly. A sprain is more serious; it is a tearing of the ligaments, the tough tissue that connects the bones and provides strength and stability to the joints. Though any joint can be sprained, including a finger, a shoulder, an elbow, or a knee, the ankle is the most common site of a sprain.

RICE *RULE FOR SOFT TISSUE INJURIES*

When your child comes home with a strain or sprain, remember the RICE rule:

R*est:* Don't allow your child to continue using her injured joint. Have her sit or lie down as you continue first aid treatment.

I*ce:* Wrap ice or an ice pack in a towel, and apply it to the area immediately for 10 to 15 minutes. If the swelling doesn't decrease, apply the ice for 10 minutes at a time at 30-minute intervals until the swelling decreases. Cold reduces the pain, bleeding, and swelling that accompanies a soft-tissue injury.

C*ompression:* Compressing the joint helps reduce the swelling. Wrap the joint in an elastic bandage made especially for this purpose. Make the bandage firm but not so tight that it turns the skin blue or causes tingling or numbness. Such bandages are available in drugstores. Do not use a tourniquet.

E*levation:* Elevate the injured limb to control the local internal bleeding, swelling, and pain. One way to do this is to prop the arm or leg on several pillows.

What the Doctor May Do

First, the doctor will make sure that your child has no injury more serious than a sprain or a strain. If your child has a strain or sprain, the doctor will tell you how to keep her comfortable until the injury heals. Strains and mild sprains usually heal within a few weeks without treatment. For a severe sprain, the doctor may recommend the use of a sling for arm injuries and braces for knees and ankles in order to allow the muscles and ligaments to rest. The doctor might also refer your child to a physical therapist for special exercises.

What You Can Do

The most important treatment is rest—the more your child uses the injured ligament or muscle, the more slowly it will heal. Strains and mild to moderate sprains can usually be treated at home with the RICE rule (see box). If necessary, give your child an over-the-counter anti-inflammatory medicine, like ibuprofen, to reduce pain and swelling. When your child is no longer in pain, she can resume normal—but not vigorous—activity, taking care not to reinjure the joint. Your child can engage in vigorous activity again when she regains full range of motion and strength in the affected joint.

The pain and swelling should diminish within 1 to 2 days for mild strains and from 4 to 6 weeks for severe sprains. If they don't, or if the pain is severe, see a doctor; otherwise, complications and permanent damage, such as poor flexibility and a loss of the joint's full range of motion, may result.

Prevention

You can reduce the risk of sprains and strains by encouraging your child to warm up and stretch before and after vigorous activity and by providing safe and fairly level playing areas. Make sure that your child wears well-fitting shoes and protective gear (see Playing It Safe, p. 274).

Stiff Neck

See *Neck Pain.*

Stitch in the Side

See *Chest Pain.*

Stomachache

See *Abdominal Pain/Stomachache.*

Stork Bite

See *Birthmarks.*

Strabismus

See *Amblyopia and/or Strabismus.*

Strawberry Hemangioma

See *Birthmarks.*

Strep Throat

See *Sore Throat/Strep Throat.*

Sty

Your toddler wakes up rubbing his eye and complaining that it itches and hurts. When you look at his eye, you see a red, pimple-like bump on the edge of his eyelid. Called sties, these bacterial infections are unsightly and uncomfortable and cause painful swelling. Sties most frequently occur on the sweat glands and hair follicles of the eyelids. Most sties are not serious and disappear within a few days without complications.

Signs and Symptoms

- Stinging, itchy eyes
- Painful, red pimple on the eyelid edge
- Puffy, swollen eyelid

When to Call the Doctor

CALL THE DOCTOR TODAY IF

- your child's symptoms remain longer than a few days.
- your child is in pain.
- the sty is caused by an infection that is spreading.
- the eyelid becomes so swollen or red that your child can't open his eye.

TALK WITH THE DOCTOR AT YOUR CHILD'S NEXT CHECKUP IF

- your child frequently gets sties.

Essential Facts

Children often have more than one sty at a time, for unknown reasons. Within a few days, the sty usually forms a tiny, pus-filled head on the edge of the eyelid, near the base of the lash. Once a child has had a sty, he's likely to get sties again. Although most sties heal without a problem, in rare cases a persistent sty may need surgical drainage by an ophthalmologist.

Causes

Most sties are caused by blocked ducts of the glands in the lid, causing a backup of secretions. We do not know what causes most of these obstructions. But infection by staphylococcal bacteria can sometimes cause sties. Unlike conjunctivitis (see *Pinkeye*), a common eye infection, most sties are not contagious.

What You Can Do

Cleansing and warm compresses can often soothe a sty and help it heal. Wash your child's face daily with a dilute solution of baby shampoo and water, which is less irritating than normal soap, but be careful to keep it out of your child's eyes. To bring the sty to a head quickly, apply warm compresses to the eyelid using cotton balls or a clean washcloth.

Do not . . .

- try to burst a sty. Doing so may damage the tissue, spread the infection (if there is one), and cause unnecessary pain.

- use alcohol or any other substance to clean the eye.

What the Doctor May Do

If a sty lasts for more than a few days after you start home treatment, call your doctor for advice. If the sty is caused by a bacterial infection, she may prescribe antibiotic ointment or drops to heal the sty quickly. If this treatment doesn't heal the sty, the doctor may open and drain the sty surgically. This procedure usually requires general anesthesia and hospitalization. A deeper infection, called chalazions (infected collections of cheesy cellular material), may take several months to disappear.

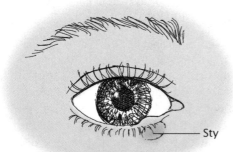

A sty is a small, pus-filled bump caused by blockage of the ducts of glands in the lid, causing a backup of secretions. If the sty is uncomfortable for your child, you can place warm compresses against his closed eye.

Prevention

To reduce the frequency of sties, encourage hand-washing with an antiseptic soap and the use of good hygiene methods, as described on page 366.

■ Sudden Infant Death Syndrome (Crib Death)

As its name implies, sudden infant death syndrome (SIDS) is the unexpected and unexplained sudden death of an infant under 1 year old. Although this condition accounts for one-third of U.S. infant deaths, and more than 95 percent of SIDS cases occur between the ages of 1 month and 6 months of age, the syndrome is uncommon and occurs at a rate of less than 1 per 1,000 births.

When to Call the Doctor
CALL FOR EMERGENCY HELP IF

- your baby appears to stop breathing for longer than 15 seconds.

   For first aid information, see page 380 if your child is less than 1 year old and page 383 if your child is 1 year of age or older.

   TALK WITH THE DOCTOR AT YOUR CHILD'S NEXT CHECKUP IF

- you have any questions or concerns about SIDS.

Essential Facts

In a typical SIDS case, an apparently healthy baby goes to bed in the evening and is discovered dead during the night or the next morning. The death occurs rapidly, and the baby does not struggle or cry out. In some instances, another person sleeping in the same room hears nothing. In some cases, infants have died silently in car seats or in a parent's arms. For unknown reasons, more SIDS deaths are reported in the fall and winter, and more boys than girls tend to die of SIDS.

Causes

Despite decades of research, we do not know what causes SIDS. According to the National SIDS Resource Center, babies who die of SIDS are probably born with one or more unknown conditions that make them especially vulnerable to stresses occurring in an infant's normal life. Other influences may include the following:

- *Exposure to cigarette smoke:* Smoking during pregnancy and around new infants significantly increases the risk of SIDS.

- *Sleep position:* Because sleeping on the stomach (the prone position) increases the risk of SIDS, the American Academy of Pediatrics recommends that healthy infants be placed on their back for sleep.

What the Doctor May Do

To provide a healthy environment for your child, your obstetrician-gynecologist and your child's doctor will probably encourage you to stop smoking before, during, and after you give birth. They will also recommend certain sleep positions for your infant.

What You Can Do

Parents of a baby who dies of SIDS can seek support—from their doctors, family and friends, counselors, and SIDS support groups—to help cope with the loss. Professionals and other parents whose babies have died of SIDS can help parents identify and deal with the grieving process and the side effects of grief, including interpersonal problems among family members and feelings of guilt and blame.

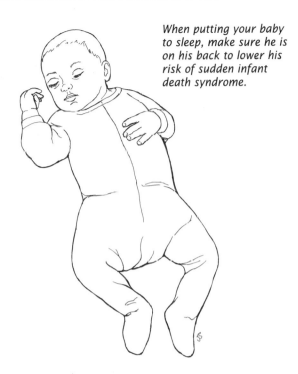

When putting your baby to sleep, make sure he is on his back to lower his risk of sudden infant death syndrome.

Prevention

Although you cannot prevent SIDS, you can protect a baby by protecting her from exposure to cigarette smoke. Above all, don't smoke during pregnancy. Additional preventative steps include placing her on her back to sleep, keeping the room at a moderate temperature, using a firm mattress with a tight-fitting sheet, and placing no pillows, toys, or loose blankets in the crib. For more information, see Appendix: Parent Resources, Safety.

See also *Infantile Apnea.*

▌ Suicide

See *Depression.*

▌ Summer Rash

See *Heat Rash.*

Sunburn

No one is immune—not the tiniest infant or the most careful preteen—to sunburn, the inflammation of the skin by overexposure to the sun's ultraviolet rays. Fortunately, most sunburns are minor, first-degree burns that turn the skin pink or red. But long-term sun exposure does raise the risk of skin cancer later in life. And most people get more than half their lifetime exposure to the sun's damaging ultraviolet rays before 18 years of age. So be sure to protect your child routinely from sun exposure using hats, clothing, and sunscreens.

Signs and Symptoms

- Red, hot skin that feels tender
- *Blisters*
- Itchy skin

When to Call the Doctor

CALL THE DOCTOR IMMEDIATELY IF

- the burn is extensive and extremely painful.
- a fever over 102°F accompanies the burn.
- your child feels dizzy, confused, and drowsy (signs of heatstroke).

CALL THE DOCTOR TODAY IF

- your child has widespread blistering.

Essential Facts

When mild sunburn occurs, the skin may feel hot, tender, itchy, and sore, making a child quite uncomfortable. This type of burn will resolve itself, perhaps with a little peeling of the top skin layer, within a few days or a week. More severe burns cause blistering. If your child has widespread, painful blisters on his sunburned skin, take him to a doctor for an evaluation. See Burns, page 394, for more on burns of all kinds.

Although sunburn usually heals within a few days, exposure to the sun over the years can cause skin cancer later in life, particularly in fair-skinned people. Even one or more severe sunburns in childhood increase the risk of skin cancer in adulthood.

What the Doctor May Do

Your doctor will treat your child's burn as she would any other burn (see p. 395). If the sunburn has become infected, she may suggest treatment with antibiotics.

What You Can Do

If your child experiences a minor sunburn, you can help ease his discomfort by giving him a lukewarm bath with baking soda or oatmeal or applying cool compresses. Aloe vera gel helps soothe the burn. Dress him in loose, lightweight clothing, and give him plenty of water to drink.

Do not . . .

- apply petroleum jelly or other oily ointments or lotions. They may feel good at first, but they actually may prevent the skin from healing.
- break any blisters. If they break on their own, keep the area clean and covered. (Consider applying an over-the-counter antibacterial cream to prevent infection.)
- apply lotions or creams containing benzocaine or diphenhydramine. They can sting and cause an allergic reaction.

Prevention

Prevention is the best cure when it comes to sunburn. Every child needs protection from potentially damaging ultraviolet rays. Make sure to apply sunscreen with an SPF (sun protection factor) rating of 15 or above to all exposed areas about 30 minutes before your child goes outside, to allow the lotion or cream to penetrate the skin. Hats, long-sleeved shirts, and long pants provide even better protection. Zinc oxide on highly exposed areas like the ears and nose provides maximal protection against sunburn.

▌ *Swimmer's Ear*

See *Earache/Ear Infection.*

▌ *Swollen Glands*

Swollen glands, the small lumps and bumps that may appear in several places on your child's body—but particularly around the neck—are inflammations of the lymph nodes. Although they may be alarming, they are simply the body's response to infection and are not, of themselves, usually a cause for concern.

Signs and Symptoms

- A swollen lump of tissue under the skin usually in front of or behind the ears, at the base of the skull, under the chin, down the sides of the neck, or in the armpit or groin
- Tenderness in the armpit or groin

When to Call the Doctor
CALL THE DOCTOR TODAY IF
- lymph glands are swollen for more than 2 or 3 days.
- a fever accompanies the swollen glands.
- the glands appear to be swollen throughout the body.
- the glands enlarge rapidly or the skin near them turns purple.

Essential Facts

Also called lymphadenopathy, swollen lymph glands commonly occur when the body is fighting an infection or healing an injury. The glands that swell are lymph nodes, small collections of infection-fighting tissue. Since swollen lymph nodes can, in rare cases, be a sign of a more serious disorder, be sure to pay attention to any swollen glands your child experiences.

Lymph nodes are part of the body's immune system: They filter lymph, a watery fluid composed of different kinds of white blood cells and plasma cells. These cells help destroy bacteria and viruses and aid the body in healing. When an infection or injury occurs and causes inflammation, it causes the nodes to swell as they filter bacteria or viruses from the inflamed area.

Causes

Any infection—serious or mild, generalized or localized—can cause the lymph nodes to swell. The most common causes of swollen glands are mild viral or bacterial infections of the upper respiratory tract. A mouth or tooth infection can also cause lymph nodes—especially those of the head and neck—to swell. When nodes swell in one arm or leg, that limb is probably infected or injured. *Mononucleosis* is a common cause of severely swollen lymph glands in the neck. *Tuberculosis* is a less common cause of lymph node enlargement. An allergic reaction to the anticonvulsant drug phenytoin can also cause enlarged nodes.

In rare cases, swollen lymph nodes indicate a more serious problem. AIDS (see *HIV/AIDS Infection*) can cause lymph nodes to swell, as can certain types of *cancer,* including Hodgkin's disease, leukemia, and lymphoma.

What the Doctor May Do

If your child's lymph nodes are swollen and painful, the doctor will perform a careful physi-

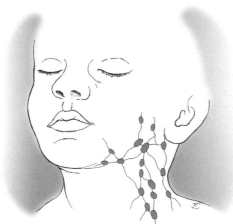

Lymph nodes, small collections of infection-fighting tissue, are part of the body's immune system that may swell when cells in the lymph glands are fighting an infection in the body.

cal examination and take a history of all signs and symptoms. He'll pay special attention to any recent infections, skin wounds, or rashes that might have triggered the swelling. If the doctor identifies an underlying infection, he'll treat it accordingly. For example, if a bacterial infection is the cause, he may prescribe antibiotics. If he can't identify a specific cause of the swollen lymph nodes and they persist or are very large, he may recommend other tests, such as a CT (computed tomography) scan or blood tests. In uncommon cases of a persistent, swollen node that doesn't respond to treatment, your doctor may suggest that it be surgically removed and examined by a laboratory. Once the doctor identifies the cause, the doctor will treat it accordingly.

What You Can Do

If you notice that your child has swollen glands, touch the nodes gently. In most cases, a swollen lymph node will feel relatively soft and mobile and, although tender, not particularly sore or hot to the touch. If it's hard, immobile, or very painful, consult your doctor.

A warm washcloth applied to the red, swollen area can often be soothing to your child. Give your child ibuprofen or acetaminophen for a fever and to relieve pain.

Prevention

Swollen lymph nodes are a sign that the immune system is fighting an infection. Consequently, the only way to prevent them is to protect your child from infection with frequent hand-washing and other good hygiene techniques described on page 366.

▌ Swollen Scrotum

See *Hydrocele; Scrotal Swelling and Pain.*

▌ Tattooing

See *Ear and Body Piercing Infections.*

▌ Tear Ducts, Blocked

Although babies cry frequently, excessive or constant tears from your baby's eyes may mean that the tear ducts of one or both eyes are blocked. Blocked tear ducts (sometimes called congenital dacryostenosis) are very common among newborns and young babies. Fortunately, more than 90 percent of cases of congenitally blocked tear ducts clear up without medical treatment, and even the cases requiring surgery usually result in no permanent damage. However, blocked tear ducts may make your baby more likely to contract *pinkeye.*

Signs and Symptoms

- Tears
- Mucus or pus formation
- Swelling of the eyelid

When to Call the Doctor

CALL THE DOCTOR TODAY IF

- your infant's eyes are inflamed or are leaking pus.

TALK WITH THE DOCTOR AT YOUR CHILD'S NEXT CHECKUP IF

- your infant's eyes drain small amounts of whitish water.
- your infant's eyes tear when she's not crying.

Essential Facts

Glands located under the upper eyelids produce tears to keep the eyes clean, lubricated, and free of foreign matter. These tears wash over the eyes' surface and then drain into the nasal passages through ducts near the nose, where the upper and lower eyelids meet.

Should the tear ducts become blocked, tears leak out of the inner corners of the eyes. Sometimes, a bacterial infection accompanies the blockage, causing a sticky discharge.

Causes

In cases of blocked tear ducts, a child is born with a thin, invisible membrane covering the nasal end of the duct. Your baby's excess tears could also be caused by one of several conditions, including these:

- *Infection:* viral or bacterial infections (colds, pinkeye)
- *Irritation:* chemicals, dust, air pollution
- *Allergy:* pollen, dust, animal dander, soaps, or cosmetics

- *Blocked tear ducts:* congenital (present at birth) condition accompanied by swelling and pus formation
- *Dacryocystitis:* infection of tear duct resulting from blockage
- *Glaucoma:* abnormal pressure inside the eyeball
- *Dendritic keratitis:* eye infection caused by virus
- *Uveitis/iritis:* inflammation of blood vessels in the iris, caused by infection, toxic substances, drugs, or autoimmune disease such as rheumatoid arthritis
- *Corneal ulcers:* caused by viral or bacterial infections that may lead to blindness

What the Doctor May Do

In most cases, your doctor will simply show you how to massage your child's tear ducts gently to open them, and how to carefully clean the eyelid

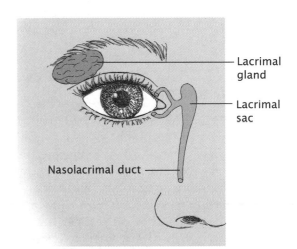

Glands located under the upper eyelids produce tears to keep the eyes clean, wet, and free of foreign matter. These tears wash over the eye's surface, then drain into the nasal passages through ducts near the nose, where the upper and lower eyelids meet.

with moistened cloths or pads. If an infection exists, the doctor may prescribe an antibiotic ointment. Occasionally, a surgeon may need to open blocked ducts by inserting a small probe into the tear duct opening. This procedure is fairly common (although most cases clear up on their own), usually requires general anesthesia, and is performed on an outpatient basis.

What You Can Do

First, don't worry. Your baby will probably outgrow his blocked tear duct soon. Just follow your doctor's instructions about massaging the tear duct—usually with downward strokes—using a warm washcloth to clean your baby's eyes of discharge and applying antibiotics in case of infection.

Prevention

Congenitally blocked tear ducts can't be prevented. Nevertheless, you can reduce the chances of your infant's developing an infection by keeping his eyes and hands and your hands as clean as possible.

Testes, Undescended

Before birth, a male fetus's testicles develop in the abdominal cavity next to the kidneys. During the final weeks of pregnancy, they're supposed to descend into the scrotum. But in about 3 percent of full-term newborn boys, at least one testicle fails to descend. In most cases, it moves into the scrotum by the time the boy is 1 year old. But if it doesn't, surgery is usually necessary to correct the problem.

Signs and Symptoms

- One or both testicles cannot be seen or felt in the scrotum.

When to Call the Doctor
CALL THE DOCTOR TODAY IF
- you think that your son has undescended testicles.

Essential Facts

Undescended testicles are most prevalent among premature infants because of their overall delay in physical maturity. In some babies, the testicles remain high in the abdominal cavity. In others, they progress downward but stop short of the scrotum. If both testicles are undescended, his scrotum will appear small. If only one testicle is undescended, the scrotum may look lopsided. If the testicles seem to be present at some times and absent at others—such as when your son is cold or excited—they are said to be retractile, a normal condition that requires no treatment.

Undescended testicles are painless and often eventually descend into their proper position without treatment. Undescended testicles increase the chance of male infertility. Normally, by lying outside the abdominal cavity in the scrotum, the testicles stay about 6 degrees cooler than the core body temperature. Undescended testicles are exposed to warmer temperatures inside the body, which can impair the development of the testicles and the production of fertile sperm. In addition, undescended testicles are more prone to testicular cancer, possibly because they are abnormal to begin with.

Causes

Why testicles sometimes do not descend normally is not fully understood. But it may be because the testicle is abnormal and therefore may not respond to hormones. Another possibility is that the hormone levels are abnormal.

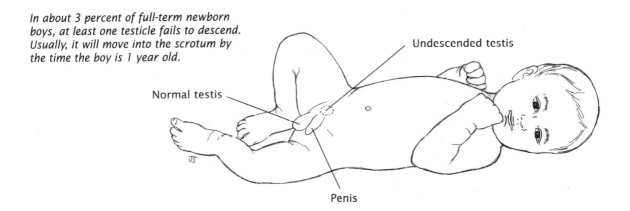

In about 3 percent of full-term newborn boys, at least one testicle fails to descend. Usually, it will move into the scrotum by the time the boy is 1 year old.

Undescended testis

Normal testis

Penis

What the Doctor May Do

The doctor will examine your child's scrotal area and feel for one or both testes, trying to move them into the scrotum (indicating retractile testes). If she can move the testes into the scrotum, she will likely suggest watching the situation for a while, because retractile testes require no treatment. She will reexamine your child's scrotum again in 3 to 4 months.

If your child has undescended testicles, the doctor will probably suggest scheduling treatment to correct the problem when your son is about 1 to 1½ years old. Treatment is a form of surgery called orchiopexy, in which the testicle is moved into the scrotum. If the testicle can be felt in the groin, orchiopexy will probably be done through a small incision in the groin. But if the testicle can't be felt in the groin, the doctor will try to find it in the abdomen either with ultrasound imaging or laparoscopy, a surgical procedure that involves looking into the abdomen with a minute telescope. Sometimes, it takes two operations to bring the testicle into the scrotum.

Your son may feel some discomfort after the surgery, but most boys feel better after about a day. Your doctor will probably recommend that your child avoid riding toys for about 6 weeks in order to prevent injury to the testicle and avoid inadvertently pushing the testicle back into the groin.

Prevention

To the extent that undescended testicles are related to premature birth, you can prevent the problem by maintaining a healthy pregnancy to reduce the chance of premature delivery (see p. 3). Otherwise, you cannot prevent this congenital abnormality. But early detection prevents later problems. The earlier the condition is treated, the better the results. If your son has an undescended testicle, it will probably be diagnosed during a routine newborn checkup.

See also *Scrotal Swelling and Pain.*

Thalassemia

See *Anemia.*

Thrush

Just as you and your new baby are settling into your new life together, this stubborn infection may appear. Thrush is an extremely common yeast infection that occurs mostly in infants under 6 months old, but can affect older babies and even toddlers. It must be treated by a doctor and may take several weeks to cure.

Signs and Symptoms

- A layer of milky matter in the mouth—over the tongue, palate, or inner cheek—sometimes in streaks, sometimes in patches
- *Diaper rash*
- Irritability, due to mouth pain when feeding

When to Call the Doctor

CALL THE DOCTOR TODAY IF

- your child has the symptoms of thrush.

TALK WITH THE DOCTOR AT YOUR CHILD'S NEXT CHECKUP IF

- your child gets thrush or yeast diaper rash frequently.

Essential Facts

Thrush most often affects a baby's mouth, appearing as a white coating (that persists long after feeding) on the tongue, inside the cheeks, or on the roof of the mouth. It can also spread through the digestive tract to the diaper area, where it appears as an angry-looking red rash. The nipples of breast-feeding mothers may also become infected.

Thrush may make your baby's mouth sore, making feeding painful. If your baby suddenly refuses to nurse or eat, check her mouth for signs of yeast infection. If you see any white patches on her tongue or inside her cheeks, gently try to wipe them away with a clean handkerchief. If they don't come away easily or if the skin looks raw once you've removed the coating, bring your baby to the doctor for an evaluation.

Cause

A yeast called *Candida albicans* causes thrush. Yeast is a type of fungus that normally lives in the intestines and mouth and on the skin. Most of the time, the body naturally keeps the amount of yeast in the body in check. In infants, though, the yeast often grows out of control. Sometimes, a yeast infection occurs because a baby is taking antibiotics, which kill the bacteria that normally control the yeast. Most of the time, however, thrush occurs for no apparent reason.

What the Doctor May Do

To confirm a diagnosis, the doctor may take a sample of the white patches to be tested in the lab for signs of the fungus. Most often, however, he'll be able to diagnose the infection just by looking at the telltale rash. Once he confirms a thrush infection, he'll prescribe an antifungal medication (usually nystatin) and a cream for any associated diaper rash. You give the medication by dropper in the front and on the sides of your baby's mouth to coat the affected areas several times a day. If your nipples are infected (red, cracked, or sore), your doctor may prescribe an antifungal cream that is safe for use by breast-feeding mothers. Ketoconazole, fluconazole, or itraconazole are sometimes prescribed for more severe or stubborn infections.

What You Can Do

Your infant may find sucking on a bottle or pacifier, or even your breast, uncomfortable and irritating. To make your baby more comfortable, try the following suggestions:

- Reduce sucking time by limiting or avoiding pacifier use.
- Soak all bottle nipples and pacifiers in water at 130°F (hot tap water is about this temperature), to help eliminate the yeast.

See also **Rashes.**

■ *Toeing-In (Pigeon Toes)*

A baby or young child often has toes that tend to point toward each other. Parents who notice this condition may be concerned that it will interfere with their child's ability to develop a natural walking and running gait. But about 70 percent of babies are born with a condition in which the bone of the thigh, lower leg, ankle, or foot turns in. In most cases, toeing-in is caused by the baby's position in the uterus, such as an excessive inward rotation of the hip, shinbone, or foot.

In older children, toeing-in can be caused by conditions as diverse as knock-knees and *cerebral palsy.* Regardless of the cause, the position of the toes usually improves after a child starts walking and often disappears entirely by the time he is 3 years old. In the meantime, the condition usually doesn't interfere with a child's ability to walk, run, or engage in other physical activities.

Signs and Symptoms
- Both feet turn in
- Both legs turn in

When to Call the Doctor
TALK WITH THE DOCTOR AT
YOUR CHILD'S NEXT CHECKUP IF
- the condition interferes with your child's ability to stand or walk.
- the condition persists past 4 years of age.
- your child complains of leg or foot pain after physical activities.

Causes
Most babies are born with their toes turned in, usually as a result of the normal position of the feet in the womb. Most babies outgrow the condition within a few years. In rare cases, a bone malformation may cause the toes to turn in. In children older than 2 years of age, toeing-in or pigeon toes may be caused by one or more of the following conditions, whose cause is unknown:
- internal tibial torsion, in which the shinbone turns in
- medial femoral torsion, in which the thighbone turns in
- forefoot adduction, in which the foot turns in

What the Doctor May Do
The doctor will examine your child, noting the position of his feet, knees, and hips while your child stands, walks, sits, and is lying down. The doctor might also order X rays to rule out bone malformations or diseases.

Usually, the doctor will send you home with instructions to observe your child's feet and monitor any changes. She may suggest some exercises you can do with your child at home. For older children, activities that help improve positioning are skating or ballet, because they develop the muscles that turn the leg out. In severe cases, usually in children who have reached adolescence or whose condition interferes with the ability to walk or run properly, your doctor may refer your child to an orthope-

Most babies are born with their toes turned in and outgrow the condition within a few years. But in rare cases, a bone malformation may cause persistent toeing-in that requires medical attention.

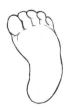
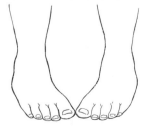

dic specialist. If toeing-in is severe in an infant, the doctor may prescribe braces to be worn at night for several months to encourage the child's feet to turn outward. Very few children require surgery to correct the problem.

What You Can Do

Monitor your child's progress, and report any changes to the doctor. If recommended, gently massage your baby's feet by turning them outward while he sleeps. For a preschooler, a common remedy is to encourage him to sit cross-legged whenever possible to help turn the feet out naturally as the bones, ligaments, and muscles develop. Be wary of expensive corrective shoes (called reverse last shoes) or shoe inserts that are promoted for children with pigeon toes. They are usually unnecessary or unhelpful. Ask your doctor before buying them.

Prevention

You cannot prevent toeing-in, but you can monitor your child's development to avoid future problems.

Tonsillitis

See *Sore Throat/Strep Throat.*

Toothache

You notice your child holding the side of her face or having difficulty chewing her food. Chances are, she has a toothache, which is cause for immediate attention.

Signs and Symptoms

- Pain
- Redness or swelling of gums

When to Call the Doctor or Dentist
CALL THE DOCTOR OR DENTIST TODAY IF

- your child complains of continuing pain or sensitivity to hot, cold, or sweet foods.
- your child complains of throbbing or stabbing pain in the jaw or in the teeth.
- your child has swelling or marked redness around a tooth or the face or jaw.

Causes

Most toothaches are caused by the decaying process. This causes pain when the decay reaches the soft center of the tooth, which contains blood vessels and nerve cells (see *Cavities*). Other causes of toothaches include a crack in a tooth, eruption of a new tooth, irritation of the gums caused by a piece of impacted food, abscess (infection) of the tooth, *canker sores,* and infection of the gums or other oral tissues. Sinus infections may cause tooth pain because the roots of many of the top teeth are anatomically close to the sinuses. In infants and small children, ear pain may be difficult to distinguish from tooth pain (which in small children is usually related to teething).

What the Doctor or Dentist May Do

The dentist will examine and X ray the tooth to determine what's causing the pain. If he finds a cavity, he will remove the decay and fill the tooth, or if severe decay exists, he may perform a root canal or even remove the tooth. If the tooth is cracked, he'll probably use specialized bonding materials to repair it. If the source of the pain is a particle of food caught in the gums, the dentist will remove it.

What You Can Do

Your child may complain of a toothache when it is sometimes an ear infection or other problem in the head or neck region that is causing the pain. To decide whether a dental problem is responsible, examine the affected area for discoloration of the tooth or gums around it. Also, tap her teeth gently one at a time to locate the tooth causing her discomfort.

In the meantime, make your child feel more comfortable by following these tips:

- *Ease the pain.* Offer acetaminophen or ibuprofen to reduce the pain and inflammation.
- *Add some heat.* Place a hot water bottle covered with a cloth against her cheek.
- *Offer soft, bland foods.* Avoid giving excessively hot or cold foods.
- *Apply over-the-counter pain relief products to the tooth or gum.* Use products recommended by your doctor or dentist for children. Don't exceed the recommended dosage.

Prevention

The best way to prevent toothaches is to prevent decay. See *Cavities.*

▌ Tooth Decay

See *Cavities.*

▌ Tooth-Grinding (Bruxism)

Worse than nails against a chalkboard, the sound of a child grinding his teeth during sleep can be disturbing to parents and siblings alike. Also known as bruxism, tooth-grinding is a habitual grinding together of the top and bottom teeth. The result is an audible sound and visible wearing of the teeth. It is quite common in infants and toddlers and is usually no cause for alarm. Most children outgrow the habit by the time their permanent teeth grow in. However, severe and chronic bruxism can cause excessive wear of tooth enamel, which can lead to sensitivity and periodontal (gum) problems.

Signs and Symptoms

- Loud, grating noise made by the grinding of teeth
- Headache or jaw pain, if tooth-grinding is severe

When to Call the Doctor or Dentist
TALK WITH THE DOCTOR OR DENTIST AT YOUR CHILD'S NEXT CHECKUP IF

- tooth-grinding is severe, bothering other family members.
- you have questions or concerns about tooth-grinding.

Causes

The causes of tooth-grinding are not fully understood. Tooth-grinding is a subconscious neurological reaction that can be exacerbated or triggered by a misaligned bite (malocclusion).

What the Doctor or Dentist May Do

In most cases, the dentist will do nothing but reassure you and your child that the tendency will most likely pass. Tooth-grinding tends to decrease with age for unknown reasons. The improvement may be caused by better alignment (bite) of the teeth. If tooth-grinding continues, it could affect the permanent teeth by excessive wear or muscle and joint problems. For older children or adolescents, the dentist may prescribe a thin, plastic splint or mouthpiece that fits over the teeth during sleep to keep the upper and lower teeth from making contact, to decrease grinding and prevent further wear of the teeth.

Prevention

While you can't do anything to prevent your child from grinding his teeth, bringing him to the dentist for regular exams can help identify treatable malocclusions that may contribute to bruxism.

Torsion of the Testicle

See *Testes, Undescended.*

Torticollis

See *Neck Pain.*

Tuberculosis

Once the scourge of civilization, tuberculosis (TB) was known in historical times as "consumption" and accounted for one-third of all deaths at autopsy. In the 1940s, the first of several drugs to treat TB was discovered. That, along with public health measures, such as less crowded living conditions, improved community-wide sanitation, improved hygiene, and better nutrition, virtually eliminated TB in the United States.

As recently as the 1980s, however, tuberculosis has made a resurgence among indigent and other vulnerable groups of people. Some new strains of the bacteria that cause TB are resistant to many drugs that have been effective against the disease in the past. In 1993 alone, more than 25,000 cases of TB were reported, according to the Centers for Disease Control and Prevention.

Signs and Symptoms

- Persistent, chronic cough, sometimes producing thick, yellowish or blood-tinged sputum
- Chest pain
- Weight loss
- Low-grade fever
- Night sweats and chills
- Fatigue, weakness, loss of energy
- Poor appetite
- Painless swelling of lymph nodes
- In infants, poor feeding, lethargy, irritability

When to Call the Doctor
CALL THE DOCTOR TODAY IF
- your child has come into contact with a person known or suspected to have untreated TB.
- your child has a chronic cough.
- your newly adopted baby is from a developing country and has not been tested for TB.
- your child has had a chronic cough, enlarged lymph nodes, unexplained weight loss, night sweats, or other symptoms.
- you are planning a trip overseas with your children.

Essential Facts

TB usually begins as an infection in the lungs. However, the bacteria can be transported through the blood to infect almost any organ. Besides pneumonia, TB can cause meningitis, hepatitis, kidney disease, eye or skin infections, infections of the lymph glands, or even bone disease.

Indigent populations; those who are malnourished (drug abusers, chronic alcoholics, the homeless, impoverished people from developing countries); health care workers; the immunocompromised; and those living in unsanitary, crowded conditions are particularly prone to infection. People immigrating from developing countries and infants adopted from impoverished circumstances in other countries may bring TB infections with them to the United States.

TB is highly contagious and is spread by the inhalation of droplets in the coughs and sneezes of those with active lung infections.

Causes

TB is caused by a type of bacterium, *Mycobacterium tuberculosis*, also known as acid-fast bacilli. Other types of mycobacteria, such as *Mycobacterium avium intracellulare*, may cause illness in healthy children or those with compromised immune systems, such as those with HIV infection and AIDS (see *HIV/AIDS Infection*). Some types of mycobacteria, such as *Mycobacterium bovis*, also infect animals and may be transmitted through food to humans. One notable source of *Mycobacterium tuberculosis* is raw, unpasteurized milk.

What the Doctor May Do

Children carrying the TB bacillus may not have any symptoms of illness. The American Academy of Pediatrics no longer recommends that all children receive a TB skin test at 1 year of age. Children who may have been exposed to TB, however, should have a skin test. To do the TB skin test, also known as a PPD (purified protein derivative) test, a small amount of TB-reactive protein is injected under the skin of the arm. The injection site is read 2 to 3 days later; an itchy, red bump greater than 1 centimeter in diameter indicates exposure to the bacteria. This does not, however, necessarily mean that your child has the disease.

If the skin test is positive, your doctor will take an X ray of your child's chest. If the X ray is negative, he will start your child on daily therapy with isoniazid medication for 6 to 12 months to prevent the TB germs from starting an active infection.

A positive chest X ray indicates an active infection. Having the lung or other organ systems infected with TB calls for the use of several anti-tuberculous medications (isoniazid, rifampin, rifapentine, pyrazinamide, ethambutol, streptomycin, and others) and regular monitoring of your child's progress to prevent complications. Some newer strains of mycobacteria are difficult to kill with some of the drugs; people infected with these strains are said to have multi-drug-resistant TB. Your doctor may, in that case, have to try several drugs before finding one that works.

What You Can Do

Take all the medicine. If your child or other members of your family are placed on anti-tuberculous medications, make sure they take all the daily doses as prescribed. Even missing just a few doses can lead to the development of multi-drug-resistant TB, resulting in the complications of TB or another long-term, chronic disease.

Prevention

There are many things you can do to ensure that your children don't become infected with TB:

- *Good nutrition:* Include plenty of fresh fruits, vegetables, and adequate protein in your child's diet.

- *Good health habits:* Make sure that your child gets enough sunshine, fresh air, sleep, and exercise.

- *Sanitary living conditions*

- *Testing members of your household:* Encourage TB testing of grandparents or other adults in the household who may be susceptible to TB or who have a chronic cough.

- *TB testing of yourself and partner:* Especially if you work in an institution, a nursing home, a health care facility, a prison, a homeless shelter, or another social services facility, where you are at a higher risk of contracting TB, you should routinely be tested for TB. Your spouse or partner should be tested as well.

Tumor

See *Cancer.*

Tumor, Vaginal

See *Vaginal Bleeding.*

Umbilical Cord Bleeding/Infection

During the 2 or 3 weeks after birth, the stump that remains from your baby's umbilical cord is supposed to dry up and fall off. But for a few babies, it ends up bleeding and becoming infected. If this happens, call the doctor, because an umbilical cord infection requires prompt medical treatment.

Signs and Symptoms

- Redness and swelling of the umbilical stump and the surrounding area
- Bleeding or a thick, yellowish discharge from the stump
- Foul odor from the stump

When to Call the Doctor
CALL THE DOCTOR IMMEDIATELY IF
- you see bleeding or other symptoms of an umbilical cord infection.

CALL THE DOCTOR TODAY IF
- you have any questions about the care or condition of the umbilical cord.

Essential Facts

A newborn baby's umbilical cord stump requires simple care to remain free of infection and irri-

tation. With each diaper change, wipe the stump gently with a cotton ball wet with rubbing alcohol to help prevent infection from germs in the dirty diaper. It's normal to see a drop of blood or a bit of clear fluid leaking from the stump in the first day or two after birth. But if bleeding or discharge occurs more frequently or in greater volume, looks yellowish, smells foul, or persists longer than a day or so, or if there is redness around the cord, call the doctor.

Causes

Most umbilical cord infections are caused by bacteria from stool that leaks from an infant's diapers to the navel. The main symptom is bleeding that lasts longer than the second day after birth in amounts larger than a few drops.

What the Doctor May Do

If your baby's umbilical area is infected, the doctor will probably prescribe an oral antibiotic. If the infection is severe, the doctor may hospitalize your baby.

What You Can Do

Keep the area clean and dry. Don't try to pull or twist the cord off, even if it seems to be hanging by just a thread of tissue. Let it fall off by itself.

Prevention

Cleaning the umbilical cord stump with rubbing alcohol after each diaper change can reduce the chance of infection. Make sure that the cord is not covered by the diaper when diapering your baby.

Umbilical Hernia

See *Hernia, Umbilical.*

Underweight

See *Failure to Gain Weight.*

Undescended Testicles

See *Testes, Undescended.*

Urinary Tract Infection

If your baby is irritable, feverish, or fussy during feedings or if your older child has the urge to urinate more often than usual or tells you she feels pain when she urinates, she might have a urinary tract infection. This infection occurs when excessive amounts of bacteria enter the bladder, kidneys, or other parts of the urinary tract. The condition is readily treated with antibiotics that your child's doctor can prescribe.

Signs and Symptoms

In infants:
- Feeding difficulties
- **Fever**
- **Vomiting**
- **Diarrhea**
- Bloody urine
- Strong-smelling urine
- Lethargy
- Crankiness

In older children:
- Pain while urinating
- Frequent urge to urinate
- Waking up at night to urinate
- **Bed-wetting** when previously toilet trained
- Dribbling urine
- Strong-smelling or cloudy urine
- Bloody urine
- **Back pain**
- **Fever**

When to Call the Doctor
CALL THE DOCTOR TODAY IF
- your child has some of the symptoms of a urinary tract infection.

Essential Facts

Urinary tract infections occur mainly in children 5 years and older. They are more common in girls than in boys, because the female urethra, which drains urine from the bladder, is shorter than the male's, making it easier for bacteria to enter the bladder. If a young girl wipes herself from back to front, she may bring stool (which contains bacteria) close to the urethra, further increasing the chance of infection. Some people are more prone to urinary tract infections than others. Susceptibility runs in families.

Urinary tract infections tend to recur. About one-third of girls who have one will have at least one more within a year. Urinary tract infections mean more than just discomfort; if left untreated, they can lead to a kidney infection, such as nephritis, which is characterized by inflammation of the kidney, and other long-term kidney problems. So be sure to get prompt treatment for urinary tract infections. Symptoms of nephritis include decreased urine output in addition to one of the following: coffee-colored urine, puffiness around the eyes, blurred vision, fever, weakness, vomiting, headache, convulsions (see *Seizures*), or severe **chest pain.**

Causes

Most urinary tract infections are caused by bacteria from the rectum—such as *E. coli*, the most common bacterium causing urinary tract infections—that enter the urinary tract through the urethra. But bacteria can also reach the urinary tract through the blood if a child has a bacterial infection such as strep (see *Sore Throat/Strep Throat*) or sepsis. Bacteria are usually washed out of the urinary tract by urination, but certain problems can prevent this from happening. One is a blockage in the urinary tract, and another is vesicoureteral reflux, a condition in which urine backs up from the bladder into one or both ureters (the channels that carry urine from the kidneys to the bladder) and sometimes into the kidneys, instead of passing out of the body.

What the Doctor May Do

To diagnose a urinary tract infection, the doctor will ask for a urine sample. Be sure to get a sample that is uncontaminated by the assorted bacteria that normally live on the skin in the groin area. To get a clean sample, wash your child's genitals with mild soap and water, then have her urinate into the container provided. The test will help identify which bacteria are

Urinary tract infections are more common in girls than in boys, because the female urethra, which drains urine from the bladder, is shorter than the male's, making it easier for bacteria to enter the bladder.

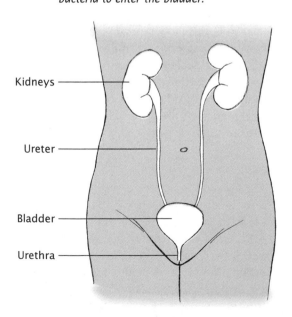

Kidneys

Ureter

Bladder

Urethra

present in the urinary tract. The doctor will also examine your child, paying close attention to any abdominal tenderness that might indicate a urinary tract infection.

If your child has a urinary tract infection, the doctor will probably prescribe antibiotic medication. After your child has been on the medication for a week, the doctor may test another urine sample to see if the medicine is working. If it is not, he will prescribe a different antibiotic. For repeated infections, the doctor might recommend that a child take antibiotics daily for several months to see if they prevent recurrences.

If the doctor thinks that your child might have vesicoureteral reflux, he will order an X ray or a sonogram to make the diagnosis. Treatment of reflux depends on a child's age, how long she has had the problem, and the number and severity of her urinary tract infections. Children with mild cases are usually treated with low doses of antibiotics daily until the reflux resolves, which can take years. Most children with reflux recover fully without complications, but doctors usually suggest frequent follow-up appointments to be sure that the condition is not getting worse. Surgery may be necessary if urinary tract infections recur, if the kidneys aren't growing normally, or if urinary tract infections persist despite repeated courses of antibiotics.

What You Can Do

If your child has a urinary tract infection, make sure that she takes all her medication. Call the doctor if your child still has a fever 48 hours after starting antibiotics. Even if symptoms disappear after a few days, your child must take the full course of antibiotics, or else the bacteria may grow again, causing further infection and possibly serious damage to the urinary tract. Also, make sure that your child gets adequate amounts of vitamin C. This keeps the urine mildly acidic, and an acid environment restricts bacterial growth. Drinking cranberry juice, an acidic beverage, is helpful for the same reason.

Prevention

You can reduce your child's risk of contracting urinary infections by following these suggestions:

- *Choose cotton.* When dressing your daughter, choose cotton underpants and avoid tight or nylon underpants, which can trap bacteria and moisture in and around the urethra.

- *Teach proper hygiene.* Encourage your daughter to wipe her bottom from front to back to avoid bringing fecal matter near her urethra.

- *Give your child water.* Drinking plenty of water every day will help flush harmful bacteria from the urinary tract.

Vaginal Bleeding

The last thing you expect to see when changing your new daughter's diaper is blood. Though it is disturbing, in newborns vaginal bleeding is common and normal and has a hormonal cause: It is a result of withdrawal from the large amount of estrogen in the mother's bloodstream that the infant was exposed to before birth and during delivery. Vaginal bleeding in babies over 3 weeks old and in prepubescent girls is not normal and requires a doctor's attention.

When to Call the Doctor
CALL THE DOCTOR IMMEDIATELY IF
- your daughter bleeds from the vagina after 3 weeks of age but before puberty (usually between 10 and 15 years of age).

Causes

Vaginal bleeding in newborns is usually the result of estrogen withdrawal after the baby is born. After 3 weeks of age, vaginal bleeding is uncommon and may be caused by one of the following:

- *Vulvovaginitis:* This infection of the vulva and vagina causes a yellowish or white discharge that is often blood-tinged.

- *Pinworms:* These are parasites that infect the gastrointestinal tract and produce an intense itching in the anal area. Pinworms (see **Worms: Pinworm and Other Parasitic Worms**) can also enter the vagina, causing a vaginal infection. They can cause vaginal bleeding indirectly when a girl scratches the itchy area and causes minor injury.

- *Foreign objects in the vagina:* Pieces of toilet paper can get stuck in the vagina, irritating the tissue to the point that it bleeds. Some girls have been known to put toys and other objects, including buttons, crayons, small toys, even wads of paper, in their vaginas.

- *Injuries:* The vulva and vagina can be injured during a fall—for example, if a girl slips from the seat of her bicycle and her groin hits the front bar. Injury to the vagina can also be caused by sexual molestation or rape, a factor doctors consider when diagnosing the cause of vaginal bleeding at a young age.

- *Precocious puberty:* Some girls experience an exceptionally early (before 8 years of age) onset of menstruation.

Other Causes of Vaginal Bleeding

Less common causes of vaginal bleeding in young girls include abnormal blood clotting, as well as polyps (growths on the cervix), and cancerous or noncancerous tumors. Urethral prolapse, a protrusion of the end of the urethra (the tube that carries urine from the bladder) through the urethral opening, may also cause a bloody discharge.

What the Doctor May Do

The first step in diagnosing the cause of vaginal bleeding is a complete physical, including a general checkup and gynecological exam. The doctor will probably first look for signs of infection or injury. The treatment of vaginal bleeding depends on the cause.

Vulvovaginitis is usually treated with oral antibiotics. For pinworms, the doctor will prescribe oral antiparasitic medication both for the affected child and for the entire family to prevent the infection from spreading.

If your daughter's bleeding is caused by a foreign object in the vagina, the doctor will first remove it, and then try to determine how the object got there. If your child has a history of putting objects in her vagina, the doctor may suggest counseling. This behavior is sometimes a child's reaction to sexual abuse. Counseling is especially important if the child has been raped or sexually molested. Most injuries to the vulva and vagina, whether caused by abuse or accident, heal by themselves. But injuries that cause extensive damage must be repaired with surgery.

Some causes of vaginal bleeding require special treatment. If your child experiences precocious puberty, your doctor may recommend hormone therapy in order to delay further development (see Girls and Early Puberty, p. 251). In the rare cases of tumors and polyps, surgery may be necessary both to evaluate and to treat the problem.

Mild cases of urethral prolapse can sometimes be treated at home with warm baths to reduce inflammation. If this doesn't work after about 2 weeks, a prescription cream containing a female hormone (estrogen) can usually cure the problem. But if the estrogen cream isn't effective

or if the prolapse is severe, surgery might be necessary.

What You Can Do

Follow your doctor's directions for treatment, and comfort and reassure your daughter. Depending on her age, she may be frightened or confused by the sight of blood.

Prevention

You may prevent some causes of vaginal bleeding by telling your daughter that putting foreign objects into her vagina is dangerous and giving her age-appropriate information to help her protect herself from sexual abuse. By doing so, you can reduce her risk of vaginal bleeding from injury or trauma. For information about preventing vaginal infections and pinworms, see the entries devoted to these topics.

See also *Vaginal Infections, Irritations.*

■ *Vaginal Infections, Irritations*

Various factors can cause a girl's vaginal area to become irritated or infected. Although vaginal infections are most prevalent in girls after puberty and the onset of sexual activity, they can also occur in girls who haven't yet reached puberty. Most vaginal infections and irritations are easily treated and, if treated, pose no danger to a girl's health or reproductive future.

Signs and Symptoms

- Itchiness and/or tenderness of the vaginal area
- Thick, white or yellow vaginal discharge
- *Vaginal bleeding*
- Foul-smelling discharge
- Irritation or redness of the vulva
- *Bed-wetting* after a child has been dry at night

When to Call the Doctor
CALL THE DOCTOR TODAY IF

- an abnormal discharge (thick, white or yellow, or foul-smelling) is in your child's diaper or underpants.
- your daughter complains of itching or soreness in her vaginal area.

Essential Facts

Girls normally have a slight vaginal discharge that consists of mucus secreted by glands in the cervix (the neck of the uterus), the vaginal cells, and harmless bacteria from the vagina. This mixture, called leukorrhea, is clear or whitish and odorless. The amount, consistency, and color of vaginal discharge changes depending on many factors, including a girl's age. Newborn girls have heavy mucus secretions caused by their exposure to high levels of estrogen before birth. But from 3 weeks of age until puberty, girls produce a relatively small amount of leukorrhea.

One reason girls are susceptible to vaginal infections is because the mucous membranes of their vaginas are thin and therefore easily penetrated by bacteria. When a girl has a vaginal infection, she has more discharge than usual. It becomes thicker, turns white or yellow, and may have an unpleasant odor. It also irritates the vaginal area, causing itching, redness, or tenderness.

Causes

The most common cause is poor hygiene, particularly wiping from back to front after a bowel movement and spreading bacteria and other organisms from the rectal area to the vagina. Another cause is pinworms (see *Worms: Pinworm and Other Parasitic Worms*), a type of parasite that tends to infect the rectum, but also can spread to the vagina when a child scratches the anus to relieve the itching. Fungi (yeasts) can also infect the vagina. Fungus infections are most common in girls who have been taking antibiotics, because these drugs tend to kill the beneficial organisms that keep fungi in check. *Diabetes mellitus* can also predispose a girl to vaginal infections. Other organisms that cause vaginal infections are transmitted through sexual intercourse or abuse. These include gonorrhea, *Trichomonas,* herpes, and chlamydia.

Not all cases of vaginal irritation, itching, and abnormal discharge are caused by vaginal infections. In young girls other factors can lead to vaginal irritation or bleeding and include chemical irritation from detergents and shampoos, foreign objects such as paper or beach sand, masturbation, skin conditions, and early puberty.

What the Doctor May Do

Your doctor will begin by asking about your child's symptoms and general health, including any recent infections she has had. Expect the doctor to ask how your child wipes herself, whether she uses bubble baths, and if she is taking any medications. The doctor will also examine your child's vagina. If the discharge appears to contain pus—a sign of infection—he will take a specimen for laboratory analysis to identify the organisms that are there.

Even if your child has a bacterial infection, the doctor might not prescribe antibiotics right away. He may simply recommend that she improve her hygiene by wiping herself from front to back to avoid infecting the vagina. Bacterial infections sometimes clear up by themselves once a girl practices proper hygiene. If after several days the infection has not cleared up, or if it is severe, the doctor may prescribe an antibiotic cream or oral antibiotics to cure it. If your child experiences recurrent vaginal infections, the doctor may also prescribe an estrogen-containing cream in order to thicken the vaginal walls and make the vagina more resistant to germs.

To cure a yeast infection, the doctor will probably recommend that your daughter use a prescription antifungal ointment or cream, usually containing nystatin or an azole drug (e.g., clotrimazole or miconazole), to be applied to the vaginal area. If the vaginal infection is caused by a sexually transmitted disease, your child may need oral antibiotics.

What You Can Do

Vaginal infections and irritations will usually clear up by themselves or with treatment within a few weeks. In the meantime, you can make your daughter more comfortable by giving her a warm bath. Sitting in a tub of warm water for 10 minutes several times a day will relieve the pain and irritation. After your child takes a bath, pat her dry and dress her in clean, cotton underpants to reduce irritation further.

Prevention

You can help your daughter avoid infections by following these tips:

- *Teach proper hygiene.* Show your older daughter how to wipe herself from front to back to avoid bringing germs from the anal area into the vagina. Make sure she knows to wash the external area of her vagina gently with water and mild soap when she bathes.

- *Use proper hygiene when changing diapers.* Wash your hands before and afterward.

- *Choose loose-fitting, cotton underpants.* Cotton underpants absorb moisture, helping the area stay dry and discouraging the growth of bacteria.

■ Varicella-Zoster

See *Chicken Pox.*

■ Varicocele

See *Testes, Undescended.*

■ Vertigo

See *Dizziness.*

■ Vision Problems (Myopia, Hyperopia, Astigmatism)

Vision is a precious gift—a gift your child uses from the earliest moments of life to learn about people and places. So be sure to have the doctor check his vision early and often so that any vision problems can be detected and treated promptly.

Signs and Symptoms

- Inability to make steady eye contact by 3 to 4 months of age
- Difficulty tracking close, moving objects by 3 to 4 months of age
- Squinting and frowning
- Frequent head tilting
- *Headaches* in an older child
- Eye soreness or discomfort
- Covering one eye while reading or viewing a picture book; cross-eyed look
- Complaints of double or blurry vision in an older child

When to Call the Doctor

CALL THE DOCTOR TODAY IF

- your child has any of the above symptoms of vision problems.

TALK WITH THE DOCTOR AT YOUR CHILD'S NEXT CHECKUP IF

- you are concerned about a vision problem.

Essential Facts

In normal vision, the circular eye opening (the pupil) brings light to the lens, which focuses the image onto the retina (the rear portion of the eye that receives light rays). The image is focused first by the cornea, the transparent membrane covering the eye, which bends light rays before they strike the lens, which performs the final focusing. The picture is projected on the retina and transmitted to the brain.

When something goes wrong with this normal process, a vision problem may result. Vision problems are common in children. Three different focusing problems may develop in children: myopia (nearsightedness), hyperopia (farsightedness), and astigmatism (blurred vision). Children who were born prematurely are more likely to develop myopia and astigmatism, as well as a condition called strabismus (see *Amblyopia and/or Strabismus*), than other children. An uncorrected vision problem may lead to eyestrain (fatigue, discomfort, teariness, and headaches from eye use), which does not permanently affect vision.

Myopia (Nearsightedness)

The most common visual problem in children is myopia, the inability to see distant objects clearly. A nearsighted, or myopic, child can't see distant objects clearly, because the image is focused in front of, instead of on, the retina. The problem usually results from having a longer-than-average eyeball. Myopia tends to gradually develop in children between 6 years of age and adolescence and often runs in families. While it occurs occasionally in preschoolers, it is uncommon in this age group.

Hyperopia (Farsightedness)

When a child is farsighted, or hyperopic, he has difficulty seeing objects at close range because light rays focus behind the retina. His eyeball is usually shorter than average. Most children are born farsighted. Newborns can focus on things about 12 to 15 inches away. But as they grow, their eyeballs get longer and farsightedness diminishes. Long-term farsightedness, however, tends to run in families.

Astigmatism (Blurred Vision)

A child with astigmatism tends to see objects at any distance as blurred. Light rays entering the eye are refracted (bent) irregularly because of an uneven cornea or lens curvature, distorting vision. Astigmatism may occur alone or with myopia or hyperopia. A mild degree of astigmatism is common among children and may not require treatment.

Causes

Any deviation in the eye's normal size, shape, and dimensions, including those in the cornea or lens shape or in the eyeball dimensions (especially the distance between the lens and the retina), can cause vision problems. These traits are usually inherited, although eye injuries or foreign objects in the eye can also cause vision problems (see *Eye Injuries*).

Preterm children are at greater risk for developing vision problems, as well as a condition called retinopathy of prematurity (a problem with the blood vessels of the retina). So it is doubly important to have a child who was born prematurely screened for vision problems throughout childhood.

Some parents wonder whether too much time in front of a television or computer screen will damage a child's vision. While a child's eyes may tire after a few hours in front of a screen, and he may develop eyestrain (aching or discomfort), he won't permanently damage them, no matter how long he uses them. Sitting close to a television will not damage your child's vision. But make sure he takes frequent breaks and wears corrective lenses (if necessary) to avoid eyestrain. If he sits particularly close to the television, it may be a sign that he is nearsighted. In that case, have his vision checked.

What the Doctor May Do

Depending on your child's age and vocabulary, your physician or ophthalmologist may use different tests to evaluate your child's vision. She may test an infant or a toddler's vision by watching how he follows brightly colored, moving objects. Once a child has a sufficient vocabulary, the doctor may have him identify and name small pictures held at increasing distances. This is part of a standard vision screening for preschoolers.

If the doctor suspects that a young child has vision problems, she may perform a test in which your child chooses between looking at a black and white, striped image or a plain, gray one. A child with normal vision will instinctively choose the striped image. In addition, the tester may show smaller and smaller striped patterns until the child can't tell the difference between the patterns and the gray. Older children can be checked for color blindness, an inherited condition occurring more commonly in boys, with a

simple screening test.

Once the ophthalmologist has made a diagnosis, she may prescribe corrective lenses. Until your child is old enough to accept responsibility for thoroughly cleaning and caring for contact lenses, eyeglasses are recommended. Children with focusing problems occasionally begin wearing eyeglasses before 12 months of age.

What You Can Do

Make sure to have your child's vision screened annually by his doctor beginning at 2 years of age. This is usually part of a regular checkup. If your child has a vision problem, bring him in for regular eye exams, as your doctor suggests. If he needs eyeglasses, follow these tips:

- *Help choose the right eyeglasses.* Choose a store with a certified optician experienced in fitting children and with a broad selection of children's frames, which have special hinged temples that make them more flexible. Make sure the glasses seem to fit well. Always buy shatter-resistant lenses (preferably polycarbonate) to avoid eye injuries and unnecessary expense.

The eye's view: In myopia, or nearsightedness, light rays from a distance focus sharply in front of the retina. In hyperopia, or farsightedness, light rays from close objects focus sharply behind the retina.

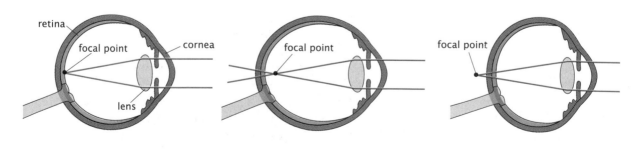

Normal eye   Myopic (nearsighted) eye   Hyperopic (farsighted) eye

■ *Visit the eye doctor regularly.* As your child grows, his eyesight will continue developing until around 14 years of age. Be sure that his eye doctor reevaluates his vision at least once a year, or more if recommended by the ophthalmologist.

Prevention

You can't prevent vision problems in your child, but early detection and correction will maximize his eyesight. To protect your child's eyes from injuries, see *Eye Injuries.*

■ *Vomiting*

Vomiting can start slowly: Your baby becomes fussy or gets the hiccups, or your older child first complains of a stomachache. Or it can happen in a flash: Your child suddenly bends over and vomits. Vomiting is one way the body expels germs and other irritants, such as bacteria, viruses, poisons, and foods that provoke an allergic reaction. Often, the cause is stomach flu, but vomiting can also be induced by allergies, overeating, food poisoning, and motion sickness.

Signs and Symptoms

■ Throwing up or heaving often accompanied by clammy skin, sweating, rapid heartbeat, weakness, or sore throat

When to Call the Doctor
CALL FOR EMERGENCY HELP IF
■ your child has difficulty breathing and/or is turning blue.

For first aid information, see page 380 if your child is less than 1 year old and page 383 if your child is 1 year of age or older.

CALL THE DOCTOR
IMMEDIATELY IF
■ your baby is under 1 year old and vomits (not just spits up milk).
■ your child has abdominal pain that is not relieved by vomiting.
■ your child also has diarrhea or signs of dehydration (dry mouth, dry skin, deep yellow urine).
■ the vomit is red or looks like coffee grounds (possible signs of bleeding).
■ your child vomits after a head injury, seizure, or headache.
■ your child has a fever, a headache, or a stiff neck.
■ your child is confused or lethargic after vomiting.
■ you suspect poisoning (call your local poison control center).

Essential Facts

Vomiting usually occurs when a part of the brain called the vomiting center is stimulated by such things as stomach or intestinal tract irritation, chemicals in the blood such as alcohol or medication, unpleasant sights or smells, or inner ear disturbances (from *motion sickness,* for example). Most episodes of vomiting end on their own and require no treatment apart from replacing lost fluids with regular sips of water or other liquids.

Causes

Vomiting has a wide range of causes. Here are the most common ones in children:

■ *Infection:* In toddlers and older children, the most common culprit is gastroenteritis, otherwise known as the stomach flu (see *Colds/Flu*). Viruses are the usual causes. Fever often accompanies the stomach flu, as does diarrhea and abdominal pain. Food-borne bacteria and viruses (see *Food Poisoning*) also cause vomiting. Infections of other parts of the body may also cause a child to vomit. Many of these infections require medical attention. Infections to watch out for include strep throat (see *Sore Throat/Strep Throat*), ear infections (see *Earache/Ear Infection), pneumonia, meningitis, appendicitis,* and Reye's syndrome—a severe illness characterized by brain disease and deterioration of liver function that is linked to aspirin use.

- *Overeating:* Filling the stomach with too much food can trigger the vomiting reflex by stretching the stomach. When your baby turns away from the bottle or breast or your older child says that she's full, don't try to make her finish the meal.

- *Gastroesophageal reflux:* Infants frequently have reflux, a condition in which the gastrointestinal tract fails to keep all of the food down (see *Gastroesophageal Reflux*).

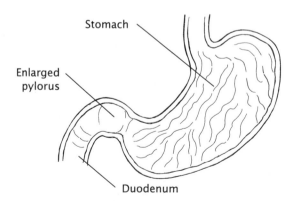

With pyloric stenosis, the pylorus (a strong muscle at the lower end of the stomach) is larger than normal, making it difficult for food to pass into the small intestine. Because the food can't go down, it is pushed out of the stomach and into the throat. The main symptom is projectile vomiting—forcefully throwing up.

- *Food allergy and intolerance:* Vomiting is sometimes a symptom of an allergy or intolerance to a particular food (including shellfish, milk, and wheat) or intolerance of certain medications (see *Allergies*).

- *Poisoning:* Swallowing poisonous substances such as mushrooms or overdosing on common medications such as aspirin or iron can sometimes induce vomiting.

- *Ipecac:* A medicine used to induce vomiting in instances of childhood poisoning, ipecac will cause vomiting in more than 90 percent of children within 15 to 20 minutes.

- *Motion sickness:* The dizziness associated with motion sickness stimulates the brain's vomiting center.

- *Pyloric stenosis:* This physical abnormality usually begins around the third week of life and requires immediate medical attention. With this condition the pylorus (a strong muscle at the lower end of the stomach) is larger than normal, making it difficult for food to pass into the small intestine. Because the food can't go down, it is forced out of the stomach and into the throat. The main symptom is projectile vomiting—forcefully throwing up. Pyloric stenosis usually requires surgical correction.

What the Doctor May Do

You needn't call the doctor right away unless your child has any of the signs listed in When to Call the Doctor, page 723. If your child needs medical care, the doctor will examine her, take a thorough history of her symptoms, especially those related to the vomiting, and perhaps order laboratory tests and X rays to look for signs of infections or other possible causes of vomiting. If the doctor thinks that your child has a severe illness, such as meningitis or pneumonia, he may hospitalize her.

The treatment will depend on the cause of the vomiting. If your child has strep throat, for example, she'll need antibiotics. Often the cause is an intestinal flu, which goes away by itself. Meanwhile, the doctor can tell you how to make your child more comfortable at home.

What You Can Do
Vomiting can be an upsetting—and exhausting—ordeal, so simply being there with your child, holding her hand, stroking her forehead, and offering words of reassurance will comfort her. Here are some other ways to help:

- *Watch for signs of dehydration.* All children, but especially infants, risk becoming dehydrated if their fluids are not replenished following bouts of vomiting (see **Dehydration**).

- *Reintroduce food.* If your child wants solid foods to nibble on and she can hold them down, let her eat. You needn't restrict her diet, except to have her avoid foods that are high in fat and sugar, which can upset the stomach.

- *Avoid over-the-counter antinausea medicines.* These medications can have dangerous side effects. Only use them under the guidance of a physician.

Prevention
You can reduce your child's risk of contracting infections that cause vomiting by encouraging frequent hand-washing and following the other good hygiene methods described on page 366.

■ Warts

Unsightly and sometimes uncomfortable, warts are a very common, harmless—though sometimes difficult to treat—skin condition.

Signs and Symptoms
- Small, hard lumps of dried skin, sometimes forming in clusters on any part of the body
- A hard, rough-surfaced, sometimes painful area on the sole of the foot

When to Call the Doctor
CALL THE DOCTOR TODAY IF
- your child is uncomfortable, or if the wart interferes with his ability to walk or otherwise participate in day-to-day activities.

Essential Facts
Warts occur more often in children but also affect adults. Caused by a human papilloma virus, which stimulates the rapid multiplication of skin cells that clump together on the surface, warts spread from person to person and from one part of the body to another by direct contact. Warts often recur. They most commonly occur on the hands and feet (on the feet, they're called plantar warts), but they may sprout anywhere on the body. Warts often appear at the site of an injury, because broken skin is highly susceptible to infection.

Types of Warts
Four varieties of warts may affect children and are described in the following sections.

Plantar Warts Occurring on the soles of the feet, plantar warts *(Verruca plantaris)* are usually small, but may spread to 1/4 inch or more in diameter. Plantar warts usually become embedded in the foot, making walking painful and treatment difficult.

Flat Warts Flat, flesh-colored, and occurring in great numbers, flat warts *(Verruca plana)* are small—about 1/16 to 1/4 inch in diameter. They tend to grow together into a large, flat mass. Plane warts often appear on the face.

Common Warts Ranging in size from $1/8$ to 1 inch across, common warts *(Verruca vulgaris)* have a rough surface and a tan, yellow, or even dark brown color. They may occur anywhere on the body, but concentrate in areas where the skin is constantly being injured, such as around bitten fingernails and cuticles.

Genital Warts Genital warts *(Condylomata acuminata* or *Condylomata lata)* arise on the skin of the mucous membranes of the genital and rectal areas, ranging in frequency from small and isolated to masses of hundreds. They are usually transmitted through sexual contact with a person infected with the virus. An infant can contract genital warts through contact with warts in the mother's genital areas during birth.

Causes

A human papilloma virus causes most warts, although one form of genital warts *(Condylomata lata)* is caused by the syphilis infection. Your child can develop warts by coming into direct contact with the virus or by scratching warts on one part of his body and then touching another area of skin. He can be exposed to plantar warts by walking barefoot on surfaces contaminated by the virus.

What the Doctor May Do

In most cases of warts on the hands or feet, the doctor may advise waiting to see if the warts disappear on their own (usually within a year or two). Genital warts, however, require immediate treatment. Genital warts may be a sign of sexual abuse in children. (See pp. 211 and 334 for other signs of sexual abuse in children.) Otherwise, the doctor may recommend an over-the-counter

remedy for you to apply at home. She may also suggest consulting a dermatologist.

The doctor or dermatologist can remove warts in several ways. The most common method involves freezing the wart with a liquid nitrogen solution, which causes it to fall off or disintegrate shortly after treatment. Laser surgery is another possible treatment, or your doctor may recommend using an over-the-counter remedy. If your doctor freezes the wart or uses laser surgery, she may first give your child an injected local anesthetic so that the procedure isn't painful.

What You Can Do

If you have any doubt that the growths on your child's skin are warts, visit your doctor to confirm the diagnosis. If you decide to treat the wart with an over-the-counter remedy, read the manufacturer's instructions carefully and follow them exactly. Usually, you will cover the wart with a bandage containing a salicylic acid solution every day to cause the wart to gradually peel away after several weeks or months of treatment.

Do not . . .
- attempt to remove warts that appear on the genitals or face.
- continue treatment on raw or bleeding skin.
- attempt to cut the warts off.

Prevention

Wearing shoes to prevent cuts and scrapes on the feet and to protect the soles from exposure to the virus may reduce your child's risk of getting plantar warts. There is not much you can do to prevent other types of common warts, except to have your child avoid touching other people's warts, particularly if your child has cuts or scrapes that could easily become infected with the virus.

Weight Problems

See *Failure to Gain Weight; Overweight.*

Worms: Pinworm and Other Parasitic Worms

Parasites are organisms, in this case worms, that live in and feed off other organisms or hosts to survive. They can cause infection in people of all ages and are very common among children, who tend to put their unwashed fingers and hands in or near their mouths.

The most common parasitic infection in the Unites States is pinworm—a small, round worm that inhabits the large intestine of humans. Several other parasitic worms not as common as pinworm—including hookworm, ascaris, and tapeworm—will also be briefly discussed in this section.

Signs and Symptoms

Pinworm
- Rectal itching, particularly at night
- Vaginal itching
- Restlessness, irritability, or insomnia

Hookworm
- Itching and rash near the point of entry
- Fever
- Diarrhea
- Abdominal pain

Ascaris
- Slight fever
- Vomiting
- Mild abdominal pain

Tapeworm
- Often no symptoms in mild cases
- Increased appetite
- Weight loss
- Weakness

Trichinosis:
- Often no symptoms in mild cases
- Fever
- Headache
- Muscle pain
- Abdominal swelling
- Loss of appetite
- Nausea and vomiting

When to Call the Doctor
CALL THE DOCTOR TODAY IF
- your child has any of the above symptoms that are unexplained by other causes.

Essential Facts

Pinworm

Approximately 10 to 30 percent of children and many adults experience at least one bout of pinworm *(Enterobius vermicularis),* which, fortunately, is easily treated. Children can contract pinworm from playing in dirt and dust, but pinworm infestation does not necessarily indicate poor hygiene.

A pinworm is a type of round worm so hardy that its eggs can survive for weeks in dirt, house dust, furniture, bed sheets, clothing, toys, and pets' fur. To become infected, a child must ingest pinworm eggs. This can easily happen if she touches something with pinworms on it, then puts her fingers in her mouth.

Once in the body, pinworms live in the large intestine. Female pinworms deposit their eggs in the skin of the anus—it is this activity that causes the hallmark symptom of intense itching. The parasites can quickly spread through a household when an infected child touches doorknobs, towels, cups, and other objects, or shares food with a family member. Some children with pinworms have no symptoms. In such cases, a parent's first clue that a child is infected may be the sight of the adult worms—which look like whitish gray threads about $^1/_4$ to $^1/_2$ inch long—around the child's anus.

In girls, pinworms sometimes infect the vagina, where they can cause pain and a slight discharge. The pinworms can crawl there by themselves from the anus or spread there when a girl scratches a pinworm-related itch or wipes herself from back to front.

Hookworm

Hookworm *(Ancylostoma duodenale* and *Necator americanus)* is so named because of the small, hooklike appendages it uses to attach itself to the inside of the small intestine. The worm can enter the body through the skin of a person who walks on soil contaminated with the worm. It can then pass from person to person through close contact or shared food. Hookworm is rare in the United States but more common in developing countries, especially in areas where soil is contaminated with human feces. **Anemia** may result in severe cases. An oral antiparasitic drug is effective.

Ascariasis

Ascariasis *(Ascaris lumbricoides)* is a parasitic infection common in preschool children or early-school-age children, especially in the tropics and in areas of poor sanitation where human feces are used as fertilizer. The parasite is a long, pinkish white worm resembling an earthworm. Its eggs are spread by contact with contaminated soil or human or animal excrement where the worms have laid eggs. Complications include intestinal obstruction and allergic pneumonia.

Tapeworm

A long, white, flat worm, tapeworm *(Taenia)* may be found in contaminated fish, beef, or pork. For this reason, you should make sure to fully cook these foods before they are consumed. Once the worm reaches the intestines, it may compete with the child's body for nutrients. For more on food-borne illness, see **Food Poisoning**.

Trichinosis

Trichinosis is caused by a worm *(Trichinella spiralis)* found in infested, undercooked meats, especially wild game. Because of improvements in meat inspection regulation, trichinosis is rarely seen in the United States. Wild game not subjected to government inspection is more likely to carry this parasite. People become infected when they eat meat containing the encysted larvae (juvenile stage) of the worm. The larvae eventually mature into adult worms, which mate and produce more larvae in the intestines. From there, the larvae are carried in the bloodstream to other parts of the body. Here, the larvae grow and bury into muscle fibers. For more on food-borne illness, see **Food Poisoning**.

What the Doctor May Do

To diagnose pinworm, your doctor may ask you to apply a strip of ordinary transparent adhesive tape to your child's anal area at night, when the worms are active, then bring the tape in for laboratory examination. Other parasitic worms may be diagnosed by laboratory examination of stool samples, body fluids, or body tissue. If muscle pain is present, a muscle biopsy (removal of a tiny tissue sample for microscopic examination) may be performed to determine whether trichinosis is present. If worms are present, the doctor will then prescribe the appropriate oral antiworm medicine for your child and perhaps for your whole family. These include pyrantel pamoate or mebendazole to treat pinworm, hookworm, or ascariasis; praziquantel to treat tapeworm; and mebendazole or thiabendazole to treat trichinosis.

What You Can Do

Here are some tips to make your child feel better and to prevent pinworms or other parasites from spreading to the rest of the family:

- *Practice good hygiene.* Have all members of the family wash hands frequently, particularly before eating. Do not allow your children to put toys, pacifiers, or other items that have been on the ground or in other children's mouths into their own mouths. Cook all meats, poultry, and fish completely.

- *Reassure your child.* The thought of having worms may be upsetting, especially to a young child. Let your child know that having this infection doesn't mean she's "dirty." Also assure her that the worms can't hurt her and that the medicine will make them go away.

- *Draw soothing baths.* Giving your child a warm bath can provide temporary relief from itching. Wash and store your child's washcloths and towels separately.

- *Give your child a manicure.* Help prevent reinfestation by clipping and cleaning your child's nails. Long fingernails provide convenient hiding places for pinworm eggs.

- *Clean sheets, underwear, and pajamas daily.* Use hot water. And don't let your child share bed linens or pajamas.

Prevention

It is impossible to completely prevent worm infestation among children, but taking the following precautions will reduce the chances your child will get worms:

- Teach your child to wash her hands after playing outside, before meals, and after using the bathroom—and to avoid putting her fingers in or near her mouth.

- Be sure your child wears shoes at all times when walking in areas where there is even the slightest possibility of contamination by untreated sewage.

- Cook meats and fish completely before eating. The temperature at the center of the meat should reach at least 150°F (66°C).

▋ *Yeast Infection*

See *Thrush; Vaginal Infections, Irritations.*

Growth Charts

Babies and children are bigger today, on average, than ever before. That is one of the reasons the Centers for Disease Control and Prevention (CDC) has revised growth charts for the first time in more than two decades. The new charts, presented in this section, were revised and released by the CDC in 2000. They more accurately represent today's population in the United States, with its cultural and racial diversity, than the charts they replace. These charts reflect a heavier population of children—with the number of overweight children doubling since the late seventies. Height averages have remained unchanged over the years.

Growth charts can be used to track your child's physical growth over time. Pediatricians and other health professionals rely on them to help identify any problems in a child's growth and development. For instance, a new BMI (body mass index) chart is meant to assist health professionals in recognizing a child's propensity to be overweight, as early as age 2. BMI is a single number that evaluates an individual's weight status in relation to height. (See the formula below to calculate body mass index.)

All of the charts are based on a series of curves, called *percentiles* (see p. 57) that are meant to illustrate how your baby or child's measurements (height and weight) compare to those of others in the same age group.

If you have any concerns about your child's growth, talk to his or her doctor.

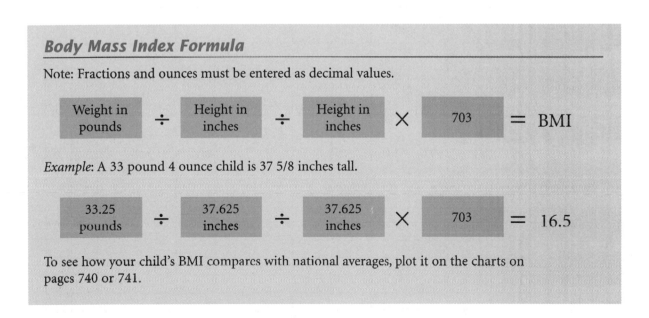

Example: A 33 pound 4 ounce child is 37 5/8 inches tall.

To see how your child's BMI compares with national averages, plot it on the charts on pages 740 or 741.

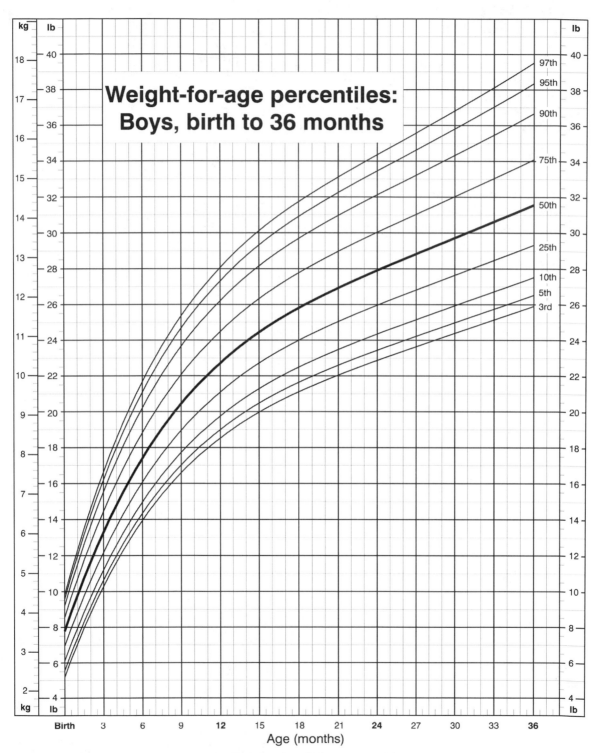

Weight-for-age percentiles: Boys, birth to 36 months

SOURCE: Developed by the National Center for Health Statistics in collaboration with the National Center for Chronic Disease Prevention and Health Promotion (2000).

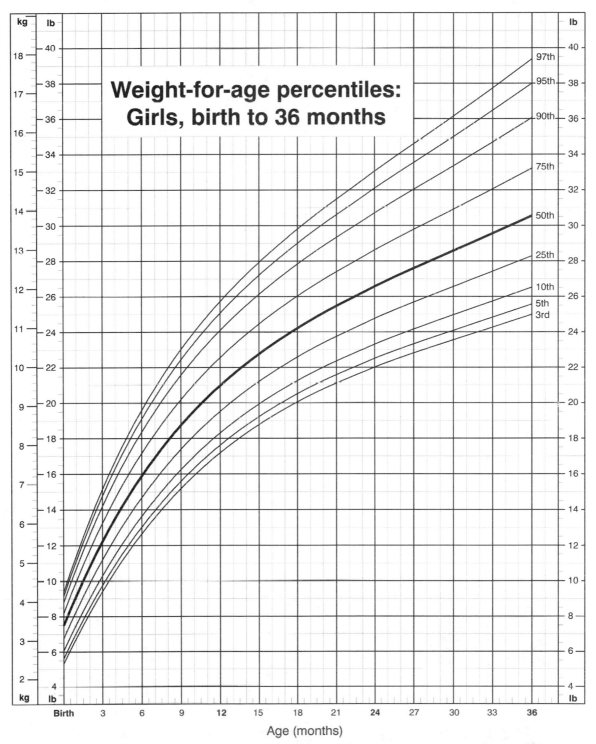

Weight-for-age percentiles: Girls, birth to 36 months

Age (months)

SOURCE: Developed by the National Center for Health Statistics in collaboration with the National Center for Chronic Disease Prevention and Health Promotion (2000).

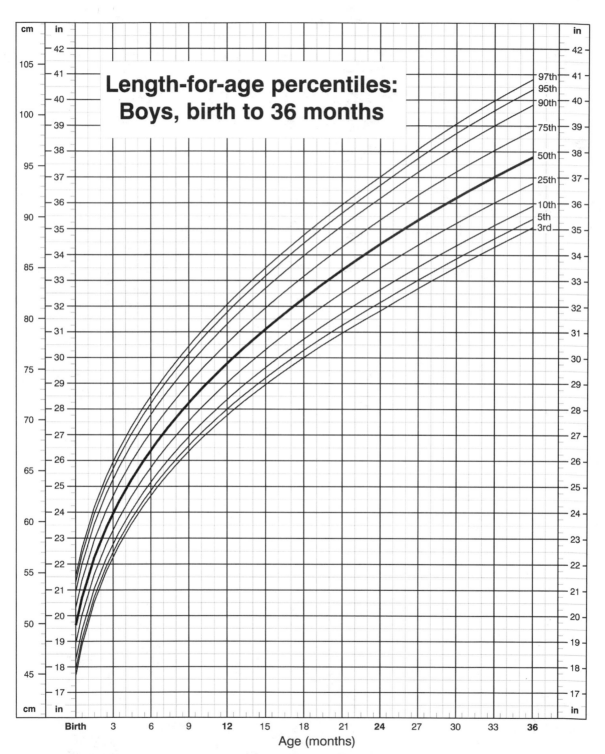

**Length-for-age percentiles:
Boys, birth to 36 months**

SOURCE: Developed by the National Center for Health Statistics in collaboration with
the National Center for Chronic Disease Prevention and Health Promotion (2000).

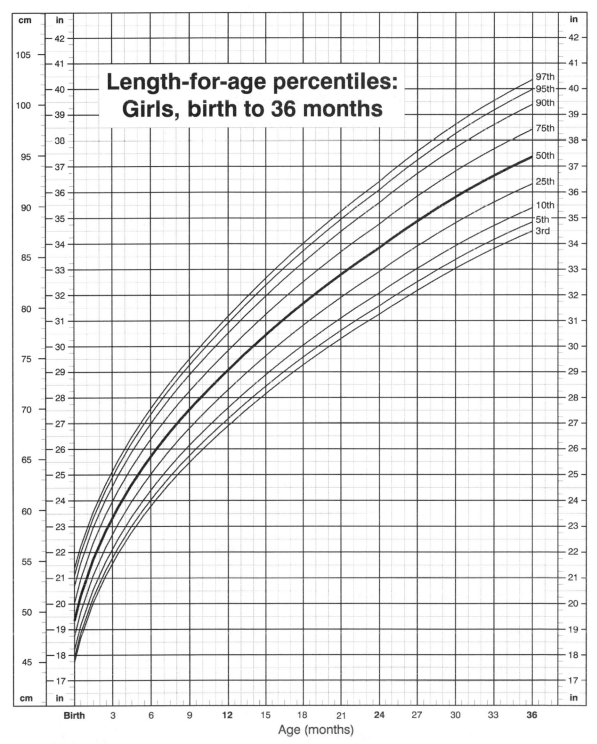

Length-for-age percentiles: Girls, birth to 36 months

SOURCE: Developed by the National Center for Health Statistics in collaboration with the National Center for Chronic Disease Prevention and Health Promotion (2000).

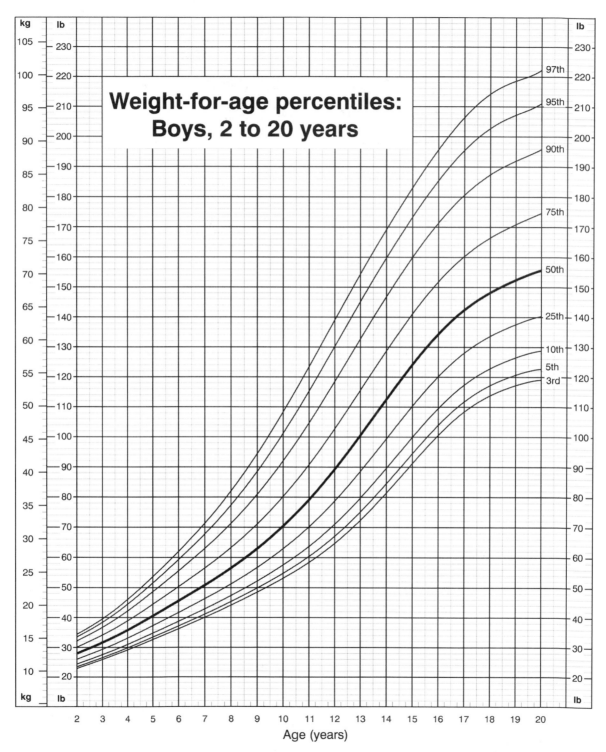

Weight-for-age percentiles: Boys, 2 to 20 years

SOURCE: Developed by the National Center for Health Statistics in collaboration with
the National Center for Chronic Disease Prevention and Health Promotion (2000).

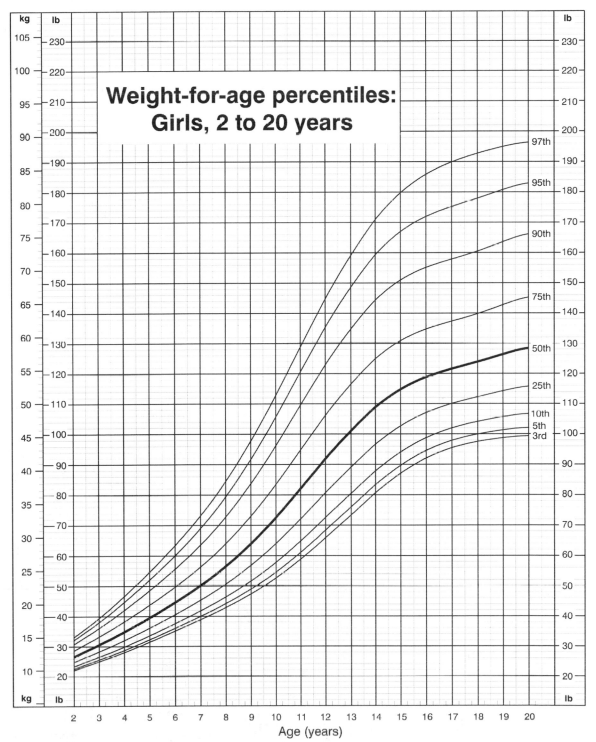

Weight-for-age percentiles: Girls, 2 to 20 years

SOURCE: Developed by the National Center for Health Statistics in collaboration with
the National Center for Chronic Disease Prevention and Health Promotion (2000).

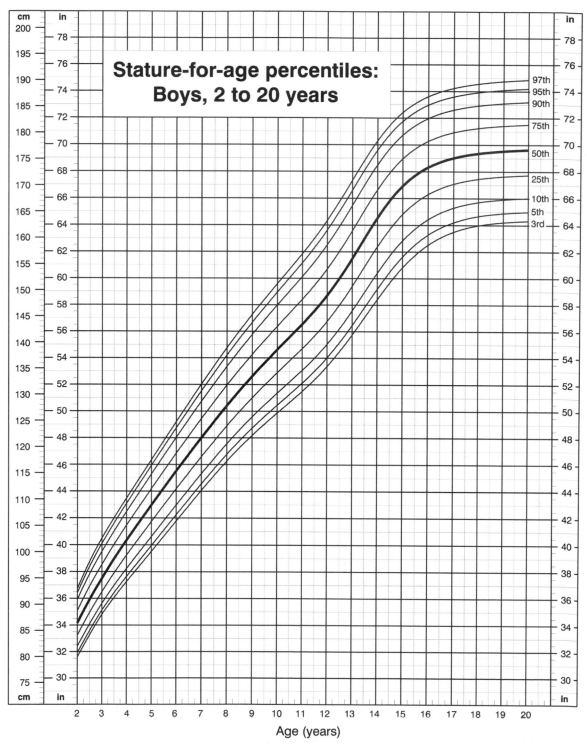

Stature-for-age percentiles:
Boys, 2 to 20 years

Age (years)

SOURCE: Developed by the National Center for Health Statistics in collaboration with
          the National Center for Chronic Disease Prevention and Health Promotion (2000).

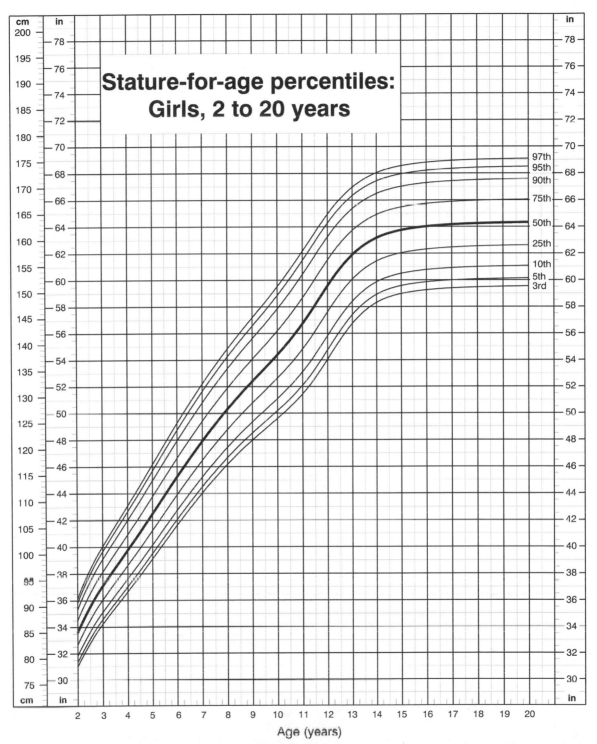

**Stature-for-age percentiles:
Girls, 2 to 20 years**

Age (years)

SOURCE: Developed by the National Center for Health Statistics in collaboration with
the National Center for Chronic Disease Prevention and Health Promotion (2000).

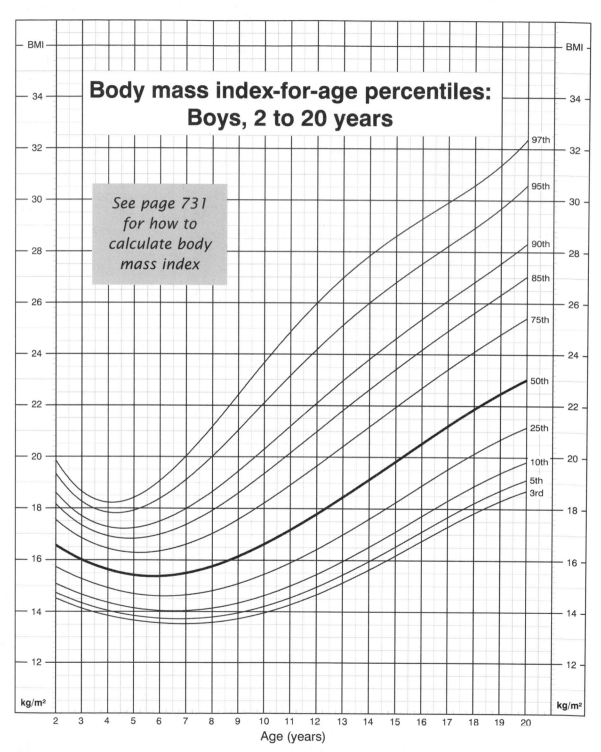

Body mass index-for-age percentiles: Boys, 2 to 20 years

See page 731 for how to calculate body mass index

97th
95th
90th
85th
75th
50th
25th
10th
5th
3rd

Age (years)

kg/m²

BMI

SOURCE: Developed by the National Center for Health Statistics in collaboration with the National Center for Chronic Disease Prevention and Health Promotion (2000).

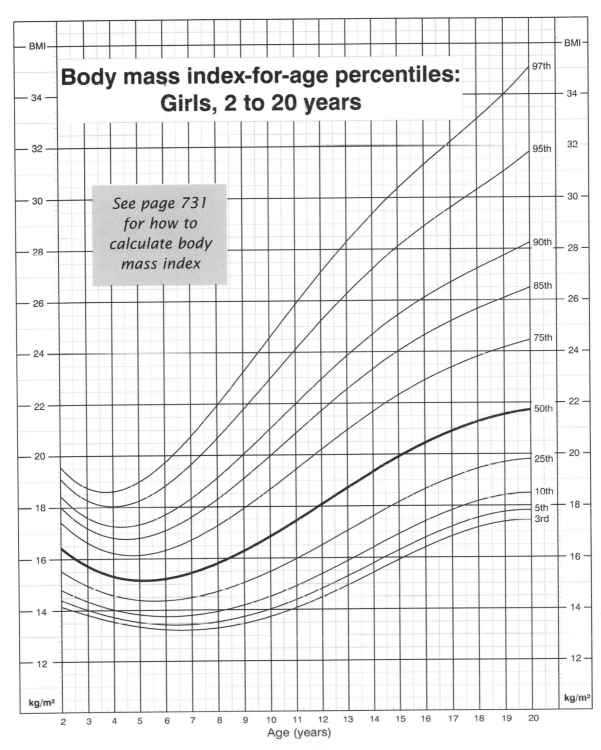

Body mass index-for-age percentiles: Girls, 2 to 20 years

See page 731 for how to calculate body mass index

97th
95th
90th
85th
75th
50th
25th
10th
5th
3rd

Age (years)

kg/m²

SOURCE: Developed by the National Center for Health Statistics in collaboration with the National Center for Chronic Disease Prevention and Health Promotion (2000).

Parent Resources

Adoptions

Allergies

Alternative Medicine

Breast-Feeding/Lactation

Child Care

Child Development

Child Health (General Resources)

Dental Health

Disabilities/Special Needs

Hearing Problems

Medical/Financial Assistance

Medical Conditions

Mental Health

Parenting

Poison Control

Pregnancy/Childbirth

Safety

Vision Problems

You and Your Child's Doctor

The following listings are for the information of our readers and do not represent an endorsement of any organization by Children's Hospital Boston. The contact information in the listings was accurate at the time of publication but may be subject to change.

Children's Hospital Boston
300 Longwood Ave.
Boston, MA 02115

(617) 355-6000
www.childrenshospital.org

Adoptions

Adoptive Families of America
2309 Como Ave.
St. Paul, MN 55108
(800) 372-3300 or (612) 645-9955
Fax: (612) 645-0055

Children Awaiting Parents, Inc.
700 Exchange St.
Rochester, NY 14608
(716) 232-5110
Fax: (716) 232-2634
www.ggw.org/cap
Adoption service for special-needs children

Deaf Adoption News Service
www.erols.com/berke/deafchild
    ren.html

National Adoption Center
National Adoption Exchange
1500 Walnut St., Suite 701
Philadelphia, PA 19102
(800) TO-ADOPT
(215) 735-9988
www.adopt.org

*National Adoption Information
    Clearinghouse*
330 C St., SW
Washington, DC 20447
(888) 251-0075 or (703) 352-3488
Fax: (703) 385-3206
www.calib.com/naic

National Council for Adoption
1930 17th St., NW
Washington, DC 20009-6207
(202) 328-1200
Fax: (202) 332-0935
www.ncfa-usa.org

*National Council for Single
    Adoptive Parents*
PO Box 15084
Chevy Chase, MD 20825
(202) 966-6367
www.adopting.org/ncsap.html

*National Resource Center for
    Special Needs Adoption*
Spaulding for Children
16250 Northland Dr., Suite 120
Southfield, MI 48075
(248) 443-7080
Fax: (248) 443-7099
www.spaulding.org

*North American Council on
    Adoptable Children*
970 Raymond Ave., Suite 106
St. Paul, MN 55114-1149
(651) 644-3036
Fax: (651) 644-9848
www.cyfc.umn.edu/adoptinfo
Includes local support groups

Allergies

*American Academy of Allergy,
    Asthma, and Immunology*
611 E. Wells St.
Milwaukee, WI 53202
(800) 822-2762 or (414) 272-6071
Fax: (414) 272-6070
www.aaaai.org

*Asthma and Allergy Foundation of
    America*
1125 15th St., NW; Suite 502
Washington, DC 20005
(800) 7-ASTHMA, (800) 727-8462,
or (202) 466-7643
www.aafa.org

Food Allergy Network
10400 Eaton Pl., Suite 107
Fairfax, VA 22030-2208
(800) 929-4040 or (703) 691-3179
Fax: (703) 691-2713
www.foodallergy.org

*Medic Alert Foundation
    International*
2323 Colorado Ave.
Turlock, CA 95382
(888) 633-4298 or (800) 432-5378
www.medicalert.org
*Information on allergies; identifica-
tion bracelets or necklaces*

*National Institute of Allergy and
    Infectious Diseases*
National Institutes of Health
31 Center Dr., MSC 2520
Building 31, Room 7A50
Bethesda, MD 20892-2520
(301) 496-5717
Fax: (301) 402-0120
www.niaid.nih.gov

Alternative Medicine

*American Academy of Medical
    Acupuncture*
5820 Wilshire Blvd., Suite 500
Los Angeles, CA 90036
(213) 937-5514
www.medicalacupuncture.org

*American Association of
    Naturopathic Physicians
    (AANP)*
8201 Greensboro Dr.
McLean, VA 22102
(703) 610-9037
Fax: (703) 610-9005
www.naturopathic.org

*The Center for Holistic Pediatric
    Education and Research*
Children's Hospital
300 Longwood Ave.
Boston, MA 02115
(617) 355-2576
Fax: (617) 355-4924
www.childrenshospital.org/holistic

*Federation of Chiropractic
    Licensing Boards*
901 54th Ave., Suite 101
Greeley, CO 80634
(970) 356-3500
www.fclb.org

Herb Research Foundation
1007 Pearl St., Suite 200
Boulder, CO 80302
(303) 449-2265 or (800) 748-2617
Fax: (303) 449-7849
www.herbs.org

Longwood Herbal Task Force
Children's Hospital
300 Longwood Ave.
Boston, MA 02115
(617) 355-2576
Fax: (617) 355-4924
www.mcp.edu/herbal

*National Center for
    Complementary and
    Alternative Medicine
    Clearinghouse*
National Institutes of Health
PO Box 8218
Silver Spring, MD 20907-8218
(888) 644-6226
Fax: (301) 495-4957
www.nccam.nih.gov

National Center for Homeopathy
801 North Fairfax St., Suite 306
Alexandria, VA 22314
(703) 548-7790
Fax: (703) 548-7792
www.homeopathic.org

Breast-Feeding/ Lactation

International Lactation Consultants Association (ILCA)

4101 Lake Boone Trail, Suite 201
Raleigh, NC 27607
(919) 787-5181
Fax: (919) 787-4916
www.ilca.org

La Leche League International

1400 N. Meacham Rd.
Schaumburg, IL 60173
(800) LALECHE *(Breast-feeding questions)*
(847) 519-7730
Fax: (847) 519-0035
www.lalecheleague.org

National Alliance for Breastfeeding Advocacy (NABA)

http://hometown.aol.com/marsha
lact/Naba/home.html

Child Care

Child Care Aware

1319 F St., NW; Suite 810
Washington, DC 20004
(800) 424-2246 *(Parent information)*
www.childcareaware.org
Local referrals for sick-child care and quality child care programs; child care tips page

International Nanny Association

900 Haddon Ave., Suite 438
Collingswood, NJ 08108
(856) 858-0808
Fax: (856) 858-2519
www.nanny.org

National Association of Child Care Resource and Referral Agencies

1319 F St., NW; Suite 500
Washington, DC 20004-1106
(800) 570-4543 or (202) 393-5501
Fax: (202) 393-2533
www.naccrra.net

National Association for the Education of Young Children (NAEYC)

1509 16th St., NW
Washington, DC 20036-1426
(800) 424-2460 or (202) 232-8777
Fax: (202) 328-1846
www.naeyc.org
Names of accredited child care centers and preschools in your area

National Association for Family Child Care

PO Box 10373
Des Moines, IA 50306
(800) 359-3817 or (515) 282-8192
Fax: (515) 282-9117
www.nafcc.org

Child Development

Touchpoints Project

Children's Hospital Boston
1295 Boylston St., Suite 320
Boston, MA 02215
(617) 355-6947 *(For a Touchpoints professional in your area)*
www.touchpoints.org

Zero to Three: National Center for Infants, Toddlers and Families

734 15th St., NW; Suite 1000
Washington, DC 20005
(202) 638-1144
Fax: (202) 638-0851
www.zerotothree.org

Child Health (General Resources)

Health Oasis

The Mayo Clinic
www.mayohealth.org
General health information site

International Food Information Council

1100 Connecticut Ave., NW
Suite 430
Washington, DC 20036
(202) 296-6540
Fax: (202) 296-6547
www.ificinfo.health.org
Information on food allergies, nutrition, and food safety

National Health Information Center

Office of Disease Prevention and Health Promotion (ODPHP)
Department of Health and Human Services
PO Box 1133
Washington, DC 20013-1133
(800) 336-4797 or (301) 565-4167
Fax: (301) 984-4256
http://nhic-nt.health.org
Health information referral service

National Maternal and Child Health Clearinghouse

2070 Chain Bridge Rd., Suite 450
Vienna, VA 22182-2536
(703) 356-1964 or (888) 434-4624
Fax: (703) 821-2098
www.nmchc.org

NetWellness

www.netwellness.org
"Ask an expert" section addressing questions on health, caring for a newborn, and breast-feeding

*Pan American Health
    Organization*
Regional Office of the World
    Health Organization
Office of Information and Public
    Affairs
525 23rd St., NW
Washington, DC 20037
(202) 974-3000
Fax: (202) 974-3663
www.paho.org
*International public health agency;
health care outreach*

Pediatric Projects
PO Box 571555
Tarzana, CA 91357
(800) 947-0947
Phone/fax: (818) 705-3660
www.pediatricmentalhealth.org
*Free "Pediatric Mental Health"
newsletter sample copy and information on medical toys and books
that help explain health care to
children*

Dental Health

*American Academy of Pediatric
    Dentistry (AAPD)*
211 E. Chicago Ave., Suite 700
Chicago, IL 60611-2616
(312) 337-2169
Fax: (312) 337-6329
www.aapd.org
Information on tooth-grinding

American Dental Association
211 E. Chicago Ave., Suite 1200
Chicago, IL 60611
(312) 440-2617
Fax: (312) 440-2800
www.ada.org

*American Dental Hygienists'
    Association*
444 N. Michigan Ave., Suite 3400
Chicago, IL 60611
(800) 847-6718 or (312) 440-8900
Fax: (312) 440-6780
www.adha.org

*National Institute of Dental
    Research*
Public Inquiries and Reports
    Branch
Bldg. 31, Room 51349
31 Center Dr., MSC-2190
Bethesda, MD 20892-2190
(301) 496-4261
www.nidr.nih.gov

*National Oral Health Information
    Clearinghouse (NOHIC)*
1 NOHIC Way
Bethesda, MD 20892-3500
(301) 402-7364
TTY: (301) 656-7581
Fax: (301) 907-8830
www.aerie.com/nohicweb

Disabilities/
Special Needs

Ability Online Support Network
503-1120 Finch Ave. West
Toronto, ON M3J 3H7, Canada
(416) 650-6207
Fax: (416) 650-5073
www.ablelink.org

*American Psychological
    Association*
750 First St., NE
Washington, DC 20002
(800) 374-2721 or (202) 336-5500
www.apa.org
*Learning disabilities, dyslexia,
mental health*

American Self-Help Clearinghouse
100 Hanover Ave., Suite 202
Cedar Knolls, NJ 07927
(800) 367-6274 (in NJ only) or
(973) 326-8853
www.selfhelpgroups.org
*Provides information on organiza-
tions for single parents or parents of
children with disabilities, rare illnesses, etc., and helps people find
support groups*

*American Speech-Language-
    Hearing Association (ASLHA)*
10801 Rockville Pike
Rockville, MD 20852
(800) 498-2071
Phone/TTY: (301) 571-0457
Fax: (877) 541-5035
www.asha.org

Arc of the United States, The
1010 Wayne Ave., Suite 658
Silver Spring, MD 20910
(301) 565-3842
Fax: (301) 565-5342
http://thearc.org
Mental retardation

Autism Society of America
7910 Woodmont Ave., Suite 300
Bethesda, MD 20814-3015
(800) 3AUTISM, x150
(301) 657-0881
Fax: (301) 657-0869
www.autism-society.org

*Birth Defect Research for Children,
    Inc.*
930 Woodcock Rd., Suite 225
Orlando, FL 32803
(407) 895-0802
www.birthdefects.org

*Center on Human Development
   Disability (CHDD)*
University of Washington
Box 357920
Seattle, WA 98195-7920
(206) 685-1242
Fax: (206) 543-5771
www.depts.washington.edu/chdd
*Referrals and information on devel-
opment disabilities*

*Children and Adults with
   Attention Deficit
   Disorders (CHADD)*
8181 Professional Place, Suite 201
Landover, MD 20785
(800) 233-4050 or (301) 306-7070
Fax: (301) 306-7090
www.chadd.org

*Council for
   Exceptional Children*
Education Resources Information
   Center (ERIC)
Clearinghouse on Disabilities and
   Gifted Education
1920 Association Dr.
Reston, VA 20191-1589
(800) 328-0272 or (703) 620-3660
www.cec.sped.org

*Davis Dyslexia Association
   International (DDAI)*
1601 Old Bayshore Highway
Suite 245
Burlingame, CA 94010
(888) 999-3324 or (650) 692-7141
Fax: (650) 692-7075
www.dyslexia.com

Exceptional Parent Magazine
555 Kinderkamack Rd.
Oradell, NJ 07649-1517
(201) 634-6550
Fax: (201) 634-6599
www.eparent.com
*Web site provides links to over 100
special needs-related associations
and organizations*

*Federation for Children
   with Special Needs*
1135 Tremont St., Suite 420
Boston, MA 02120
(617) 236-7210
www.fcsn.org
*Operates CAPP/National Parent
Resource Center*

*Interdisciplinary Council on
   Developmental and Learning
   Disorders*
4938 Hampden Lane, Suite 800
Bethesda, MD 20814
(301) 656-2667
www.icdl.com

International Dyslexia Association
Chester Bldg., Suite 382
8600 La Salle Rd.
Baltimore, MD 21286-2044
(800) ABCD-123 or
(410) 296-0232
Fax: (410) 321-5069
www.interdys.org
*Provides information on dyslexia,
answers questions, and provides
referrals to local resources*

*Internet Resources for Special
   Children*
www.irsc.org

*Learning Disabilities Association
   of America (LDA)*
4156 Library Rd.
Pittsburgh, PA 15234-1349
(412) 341-1515 or (888) 300-6710
Fax: (412) 344-0224
www.ldanatl.org

March of Dimes
Birth Defects Foundation
1275 Mamaroneck Ave.
White Plains, NY 10605
(888) 663-4637, (914) 428-7100,
or (914) 997-4763
www.modimes.org

*National Attention Deficit
   Disorders Association*
1788 Second St., Suite 200
Highland Park, IL 60035
(847) 432-ADDA
Fax: (847) 432-5874
www.add.org

National Birth Defects Center
40 Second Ave., Suite 520
Waltham, MA 02451
(781) 466-9555
(800) 322-5014 *(Pregnancy
environmental hot line)*
www.thegenesisfund.org

*National Center for
   Learning Disabilities*
381 Park Ave. S.; Suite 1401
New York, NY 10016
(888) 575-7373 or (212) 545-7510
Fax: (212) 545-9665
www.ncld.org
*Referrals and resources for special
education programs*

*National Down
   Syndrome Congress*
7000 Peachtree-Dunwoody Rd. NE
Lake Ridge 400 Office Park Bldg. 5,
Suite 100
Atlanta, GA 30328
(800) 232-6372
www.ndsccenter.org

*National Information Center
   for Children and Youth
   with Disabilities*
PO Box 1492
Washington, DC 20013
(800) 695-0285 or (202) 884-8200
Fax: (202) 884-8441
www.nichcy.org
*Information on special education
legislation and other services*

National Resource Library
National Center for Youth with
  Disabilities (NCYD)
www.peds.umn.edu/centers/ihd/nc
  yd.html

Parents Helping Parents
3041 Olcott St.
Santa Clara, CA 95054-3222
(408) 727-5775
Fax: (408) 727-0181
www.php.com
*Assists parents of children with
special needs*

*Spina Bifida Association
  of America*
4590 MacArthur Blvd. NW,
Suite 250
Washington, D.C. 20007-4226
(800) 621-3141 or (202) 944-3285
www.sbaa.org

United Cerebral Palsy Association
1660 L St., NW; Suite 700
Washington, DC 20036
(800) 872-5827 or (202) 776-0406
Fax: (800) 776-0414 or
(202) 776-0414
www.ucpa.org

Hearing Problems

Auditory-Verbal International
2121 Eisenhower Ave., Suite 402
Alexandria, VA 22314
(703) 739-1049
TDD: (703) 739-0874
Fax: (703) 739-0395
www.auditory-verbal.org
Deaf or hard-of-hearing

*Alexander Graham Bell
  Association for the Deaf
  and Hard-of-Hearing*
3417 Volta Pl., NW
Washington, DC 20007-2778
Phone/TTY: (202) 337-5220
Fax: (202) 337-8314
www.agbell.org

*American Academy
  of Audiology*
8300 Greensboro Dr., Suite 750
McLean, VA 22102
(800) AAA-2336 or (703) 790-8466
Fax: (703) 790-8631
www.audiology.org

*American Society
  for Deaf Children*
PO Box 3355
Gettysburg, PA 17325
(800) 942-ASDC (*Parent hot line*)
Phone/TTY: (717) 334-7922
Fax: (717) 334-8808
www.deafchildren.org

*American Speech-Language-
  Hearing Association (ASLHA)*
10801 Rockville Pike
Rockville, MD 20852
(800) 498-2071
Phone/TTY: (301) 571-0457
Fax: (877) 541-5035
www.asha.org

American Tinnitus Association
PO Box 5
Portland, OR 97207-0005
(800) 634-8978
Fax: (503) 248-0024
www.ata.org
Ringing in the ears

*Boys Town Research Registry for
  Hereditary Hearing Loss*
555 N. 30th St.
Omaha, NE 68131
(402) 498-6388

Phone/TDD: (800) 320-1171
Fax: (402) 498-6331
www.boystown.org/deafgene.reg

Deaf Education Web Site
Council on Education of the Deaf
www.educ.kent.edu/deafed

Deafness Research Foundation
12575 Fifth Ave., 11th fl.
New York, NY 10017
(800) 535-3323
Phone/TDD: (212) 599-0027
Fax: (212) 599-0039

Dial-a-Hearing Screening Test
(800) 222-EARS
*Over-the-phone screening and local
referrals*

HiP Magazine
www.hipmag.org
*On-line magazine for deaf and
hard-of-hearing children*

House Ear Institute
2100 W. 3rd St.
Los Angeles, CA 90057
(213) 483-4431
Phone/TDD: (800) 287-4763 or
(800) 352-8888 (*The Lead Line*)
www.hei.org
*Information about hearing and
related disorders*

Listen Up!
www.listen-up.org
*Information and resources for deaf
and hard-of-hearing children*

*National Association
  of the Deaf*
814 Thayer Ave.
Silver Spring, MD 20910-4500
(301) 587-1788
TTY: (301) 587-1789
Fax: (301) 587-1791
www.nad.org

*Self Help for Hard
of Hearing People, Inc.*
7910 Woodmont Ave., Suite 1200
Bethesda, MD 20814
(301) 657-2248
TTY: (301) 657-2249
Fax: (301) 913-9413
www.shhh.org

Sign Media, Inc.
4020 Blackburn La.
Burtonsville, MD 20866-1167
Phone/TTY: (800) 475-4756
Fax: (301) 421-0270
www.signmedia.com
*Information about American deaf
culture; sign language instruction*

Where Do We Go from Hear?
www.gohear.org
Deafness, hearing disorders

Medical Conditions

*AIDS Treatment
Information Service*
PO Box 6303
Rockville, MD 20849-6003
(800) HIV-0440
Fax: (301) 519-6616
www.hivatis.org
In Spanish or English

*American Academy of
Dermatology*
PO Box 4014
Schaumburg, IL 60168-4014
(Include a self-addressed stamped
envelope indicating topics of
interest)
(888) 462-DERM or
(847) 330-0230
www.aad.org
*Educational pamphlets on hair,
skin, and nail conditions; connects
people with dermatologists*

*American Academy of
Otolaryngology-Head
and Neck Surgery*
One Prince St.
Alexandria, VA 22314-3357
(703) 836-4444
Fax: (703) 683-5100
www.entnet.org
*List of ear, nose, and throat doctors
in your area*

*American Academy of Sleep
Medicine*
6301 Bandel Rd. NW, Suite 101
Rochester, MN 55901
(507) 287-6006
Fax: (507) 287-6008
www.asda.org

*American Association for Pediatric
Ophthalmology and Strabismus*
PO Box 193832
San Francisco, CA 94119-3832
http://med-aapos.bu.edu
Lazy eye, strabismus, crossed eyes

American Cancer Society
National Home Office
1599 Clifton Rd., NE
Atlanta, GA 30329
(800) ACS-2345
www.cancer.org

*American Chronic Pain
Association*
PO Box 850
Rocklin, CA 95677
(916) 632-0922
Fax: (916) 632-3208
www.theacpa.org

*American Cleft Palate-Craniofacial
Association (ACPA)/Cleft Palate
Foundation (CPF)*
104 S. Estes Dr. #204
Chapel Hill, NC 27514
(800) 24-CLEFT or (919) 933-9044
Fax: (919) 933-9604
www.cleft.com

American Diabetes Association
National Office
1701 N. Beauregard St.
Alexandria, VA 22311
(800) 342-2383
www.diabetes.org

American Epilepsy Society
342 North Main St.
West Hartford, CT 06117-2507
(860) 586-7505
Fax: (860) 586-7550
www.aesnet.org

*American Foundation
for Urologic Disease*
1128 N. Charles St.
Baltimore, MD 21201
(800) 242-2383 or (410) 468-1800
Fax: (410) 468-1808
www.afud.org

American Heart Association
National Center
7272 Greenville Ave.
Dallas, TX 75231
(800) AHA-USA1 or
(214) 373-6300
www.americanheart.org

*American Juvenile Arthritis
Organization*
Arthritis Foundation
1330 W. Peachtree St.
Atlanta, GA 30309
(800) 283-7800
www.arthritis.org
*Publications and answers to ques-
tions on joint pain and arthritis*

American Liver Foundation
75 Maiden Lane, Suite 603
New York, NY 10038
(800) 223-0179 (*Hepatitis/liver
disease hot line*)
(800) 465-4837
www.liverfoundation.org
Jaundice, hepatitis

American Lung Association
1740 Broadway
New York, NY 10019
(800) LUNG-USA or
(212) 315-8700
Fax: (212) 315-8870
www.lungusa.org

**American Lyme Disease
Foundation, Inc. (ALDF)**
Mill Pond Offices
293 Route 100, Suite 204
Somers, NY 10589
(800) 876-LYME or
(914) 277-6970
Fax: (914) 277-6974
www.aldf.com
*Physician referrals; information on
tick-borne illnesses*

**American Podiatric Medical
Association**
9312 Old Georgetown Rd.
Bethesda, MD 20814-1698
(800) FOOT-CARE *(Foot care
information center)*
(301) 571-9200
Fax: (301) 530-2752
www.apma.org
*Sprains and strains, toeing-in, flat
feet, athlete's foot, ringworm, nail
problems, footwear*

**American Pseudo-Obstruction and
Hirschsprung's Disease Society**
158 Pleasant St.
North Andover, MA 01845-2797
(978) 685-4477
Fax: (978) 685-4488
www.tiac.net/users/aphs
*Pediatric gastrointestinal motility
disorders, including gastroesophageal reflux and other pediatric bowel
disorders*

American Skin Association
150 E. 58th St., 33rd Floor
New York, NY 10155-0002
(800) 499-SKIN or (212) 753-8260
Fax: (212) 688-6547
www.skinassn.org
*General information on all skin dis-
orders, including rashes*

Children's Heart Foundation
200 W. Jackson Blvd.
Suite 1550
Chicago, IL 60606
(312) 957-0445
www.childrensheart.com

**Candlelighters Childhood Cancer
Foundation**
3910 Warner St.
Kensington, MD 20895
(800) 366-2223 or (301) 962-3520
Fax: (301) 962-3521
www.candlelighters.org
Cancer support for children

Children's Hospice International
2202 Mount Vernon Ave., Suite 3C
Alexandria, VA 22301
(800) 242-4453 or (703) 684-0330
Fax: (703) 684-0226
www.chionline.org
Home care for dying children

Cooley's Anemia Foundation
129-09 26th Ave., No. 203
Flushing, NY 11354
(800) 522-7222 or (718) 321-2873
Fax: (718) 321-3340
www.thalassemia.org

Cystic Fibrosis Foundation
6931 Arlington Rd.
Bethesda, MD 20814
Phone: 800-344-4823
www.cff.org

Division of Parasitic Diseases
Centers for Disease Control and
Prevention
4770 Buford Highway, NE
Atlanta, GA 30341-3724
(770) 488-7760
Fax: (770) 488-7761
www.cdc.gov/ncidod/dpd
Chronic diarrhea, pinworm, scabies

**Elizabeth Glaser Pediatric
AIDS Foundation**
2950 31st St., Suite 125
Santa Monica, CA 90405
(888) 499-HOPE or
(310) 314-1459
Fax: (310) 314-1469
www.pedaids.org

**Fanconi Anemia Research
Fund, Inc.**
1801 Willamette St., Suite 200
Eugene, OR 97401
(800) 828-4891 *(Family support)*
(541) 687-4658
www.fanconi.org

Human Growth Foundation
997 Glen Cove Ave.
Glen Head, NY 11545
(800) 451-6434
Fax: (516) 671-4055
www.hgfound.org
Growth disorders

Joslin Diabetes Center
One Joslin Pl.
Boston, MA 02215
(800) JOSLIN-1 or (617) 732-2400
Fax: (617) 732-2500
www.joslin.harvard.edu

Juvenile Diabetes Foundation
120 Wall St.
New York, NY 10005
(212) 785-9500
Fax: (212) 785-9595
www.jdfcure.org

Kids AIDS Site, The
720 Olive Way, Suite 1800
Seattle, WA 98101
www.thekidsaidssite.com

Leukemia & Lymphoma Society
1311 Mamaroneck Ave.
White Plains, NY 10605
(800) 955-4572 *(Hot line)*
(914) 949-5213
Fax: (914) 949-6691
www.leukemia.org

Little People's Research Fund
80 Sister Pierre Dr.
Towson, MD 21204
(800) 232-5773 or (410) 494-0055
Fax: (410) 494-0062
www.lprf.org
Growth disorders

Lyme Disease Foundation
1 Financial Plaza, 18th Floor
Hartford, CT 06103-2601
(860) 525-2000
(800) 886-LYME *(Lyme disease
information hot line)*
Fax: (860) 525-TICK
www.lyme.org

*Lymphoma Research Foundation
of America*
8800 Venice Blvd., No. 207
Los Angeles, CA 90034
(800) 500-9976 or (310) 204-7040
Fax: (310) 204-7043
www.lymphoma.org

*National Arthritis and
Musculoskeletal and Skin
Diseases Information
Clearinghouse (NAMSIC)*
1 AMS Circle
Bethesda, MD 20892-3675
(301) 495-4484
TDD: (301) 565-2966
Fax: (301) 718-6366

Fax back system: (301) 881-2731
(24-hour service)
www.nih.gov/niams
*Arthritis, dermatology, acne/
pimples, impetigo*

National Cancer Institute
Bldg 31, Rm. 10A03
31 Center Dr., MSC 2580
Bethesda, MD 20892-2580
(800) 4-CANCER *(Cancer information service)*
www.nci.nih.gov

*National Childhood Cancer
Foundation*
440 E. Huntington Dr., Suite 300
Arcadia, CA 91066-6012
(800) 458-6223
www.nccf.org

*National Chronic Pain Outreach
Association*
7979 Old Georgetown Rd.
Suite 100
Bethesda, MD 20814-2429
http://neurosurgery.mgh.harvard.
edu/ncpainoa.htm

*National Digestive Disease
Information Clearinghouse
(NDDIC)*
National Institute of Diabetes and
Digestive and Kidney Diseases
2 Information Way
Bethesda, MD 20892-3570
(301) 654-3810
Fax: (301) 907-8906
www.niddk.nih.gov

*National Eczema Association for
Science & Education*
1220 SW Morrison, Suite 433
Portland, OR 97205
(800) 818-7546 or (503) 228-4430
Fax: (503) 224-3363
www.eczema-assn.org

*National Foundation for Infectious
Diseases*
4733 Bethesda Ave., Suite 750
Bethesda, MD 20814
(301) 656-0003
Fax: (301) 907-0878
www.nfid.org

*National Headache
Foundation (NHF)*
428 W. Saint James Pl., 2nd Floor
Chicago, IL 60614-2750
(888) NHF-5552
Fax: (773) 525-7357
www.headaches.org

*National Heart, Lung, and Blood
Institute Information Center*
PO Box 30105
Bethesda, MD 20824-0105
(301) 251-1222
www.nhlbi.nih.gov/health/public/
lung

National Hypertension Association
324 E. 30th St.
New York, NY 10016
(212) 889-3557
Fax: (212) 447-7032
www.nathypertension.org
*Distributes information about high
blood pressure for the public*

*National Immunization
Information Hotline*
CDC
(800) 232-2522 *(English)*
(800) 232-0233 *(Spanish)*

*National Institute of Neurological
Disorders and Stroke*
NIH Neurological Institute
PO Box 5801
Bethesda, MD 20824
(800) 352-9424
www.ninds.nih.gov

National Jewish Medical and Research Center

1400 Jackson St.
Denver, CO 80206
(800) 222-LUNG *(Lung Line)*
(303) 388-4461
Fax: (303) 270-2162
www.njc.org
Information on respiratory, allergic, and immune system diseases

National Kidney Foundation

30 E. 33rd St., Suite 1100
New York, NY 10016
(800) 622-9010 or (212) 889-2210
Fax: (212) 689-9261
www.kidney.org

National Organization for Rare Disorders, Inc. (NORD)

PO Box 8923
New Fairfield, CT 06812-8923
(800) 999-6673 or (203) 746-6518
TDD: (203) 746-6927
Fax: (203) 746-6481
www.rarediseases.org

National Pediculosis Association

PO Box 610189
Newton, MA 02461
(781) 449-6487
Fax: (781) 449-8129
www.headlice.org
Lice, scabies

National Prevention Information Network (AIDS Prevention)

Centers for Disease Control and Prevention
PO Box 6003
Rockville, MD 20849-6003
(800) 458-5231
Fax: (888) 282-7681
www.cdcnpin.org

National Scoliosis Foundation

5 Cabot Pl.
Stoughton, MA 02072
(800) 673-6922 or (781) 341-6333
Fax: (781) 341-8333
www.scoliosis.org

Parents of Kids with Infectious Diseases

PO Box 5666
Vancouver, WA 98668
(877) 557-5437
(360) 695-0293
Fax: (360) 695-6941
www.pkids.org
Resources for parents of children with chronic viral infectious diseases

Pulmonary Hypertension Association (PHA)

850 Sligo Ave., Suite 800
Silver Spring, MD 20907-8277
(800) 748-7274
(301) 565-3004
Fax: (301) 565-3994
www.phassociation.org

Scoliosis Association, Inc.

PO Box 811705
Boca Raton, FL 33481-1705
(800) 800-0669 or (561) 994-0669
Fax: (561) 994-2455
www.spine-surgery.com

Sickle Cell Disease Association of America

200 Corporate Pointe, Suite 495
Culver City, CA 90230-7633
(800) 421-8453
Fax: (310) 215-3722
www.sicklecelldisease.org

Sturge-Weber Foundation

PO Box 418
Mount Freedom, NJ 07970
(800) 627-5482 or (973) 895-4445
Fax: (973) 895-4846
www.sturge-weber.com
Information on, and support for, Sturge-Weber syndrome, capillary vascular malformations, and Klippel Trenaunay

Vestibular Disorders Association

PO Box 4467
Portland, OR 97208-4467
(800) 837-8428
(503) 229-7705
Fax: (503) 229-8064
www.vestibular.org
Information on and support for dizziness and balance disorders

The VZV Research Foundation

40 E. 72nd St.
New York, NY 10021
(800) 472-VIRUS or (212) 472-3181
Fax: (212) 861-7033
Chicken pox, shingles

Weight Control Information Network

1 WIN Way
Bethesda, MD 20892
(202) 828-1025
(877) 946-4627
Fax: (202) 828-1028
www.niddk.nih.gov/health/nutrit/win.htm

Medical/Financial Assistance

Administration for Children and Families

370 L'Enfant Promenade SW
Washington, DC 20447
(877) 696-6775
www.acf.dhhs.gov

American Accreditation Healthcare Commission/ Utilization Review Accreditation Commission (URAC)

1275 K St., NW; Suite 1100
Washington, DC 20005
(202) 216-9010
Fax: (202) 216-9006
www.urac.org

Families USA Foundation
1334 G St., NW
Washington, DC 20005
(800) 593-5041 or (202) 628-3030
Fax: (202) 347-2417
www.familiesusa.org
*Health care and Medicaid
information*

*Health Care Financing
Administration (HCFA)*
7500 Security Blvd.
Baltimore, MD 21244
(410) 786-3000
www.hcfa.gov
*Operates regional Medicare and
Medicaid offices throughout the
country*

*Health Insurance Association
of America*
555 13th St., NW; Suite 600 E
Washington, DC 20004
(800) 879-4422 or (202) 824-1600
Fax: (202) 824-1722
www.hiaa.org

Hospital Free Care Programs
*Contact the hospital in your area to
inquire about these services; for children with hospital bills not covered
by other programs*

*Joint Commission on Accreditation
of Health Care Organizations
(JCAHO)*
1 Renaissance Blvd.
Oakbrook Terrace, IL 60181
(630) 792-5541
Fax: (630) 792-5005
www.jcaho.org
*Evaluates health care programs,
hospitals*

*National Association of Children's
Hospitals and Related
Institutions (NACHRI)*
401 Wythe St.
Alexandria, VA 22314
(703) 684-1355
Fax: (703) 684-1589
www.childrenshospitals.net
Parent's guide to health care

*National Committee for Quality
Assurance (NCQA)*
2000 L Street, NW; Suite 500
Washington, DC 20036
(202) 955-3500
Fax: (202) 955-3599
www.ncqa.org

*Supplemental Security
Income (SSI)*
Social Security
(800) 772-1213
www.ssa.gov/notices/supplemen
tal-security-income
*Cash benefits and health insurance
for children with disabilities*

*Women, Infants and
Children Program*
Supplemental Food Programs
Division
3101 Park Center Dr.
Alexandria, VA 22303
(703) 305-2746
Fax: (703) 305-2196
www.fns1.usda.gov/uic
*Supplemental food for women,
infants, and children who qualify*

Mental Health

*American Academy of
Child and Adolescent
Psychiatry (AACAP)*
3615 Wisconsin Ave., NW
Washington, DC 20016-3007
(202) 966-7300
Fax: (202) 966-2891
www.aacap.org
Eating disorders

*Anxiety Disorders
Association of America*
11900 Parklawn Dr., Suite 100
Rockville, MD 20852-2624
(301) 231-9350
Fax: (301) 231-7392
www.adaa.org

*Center for Effective Collaboration
and Practice*
The American Institutes for
Research
1000 Thomas Jefferson St. NW
Suite 400
Washington, DC 20007
(888) 457-1551 or (202) 944-5400
Fax: (202) 944-5454
www.air.org/cecp

*Eating Disorders Awareness and
Prevention, Inc.*
603 Stewart St.; Suite 803
Seattle, WA 98101
(800) 931-2237 *(Information and
referral hot line)*
(206) 382-3587
Fax: (206) 829-8501
www.edap.org

*Federation of Families for
Children's Mental Health*
1101 King St.; Suite 120
Alexandria, VA 22314-2971
(703) 684-7710
Fax: (703) 836-1040
www.ffcmh.org

Knowledge Exchange Network
National Mental Health Services
PO Box 42490
Washington, DC 20015
(800) 789-2647
(800) 790-2647 *(Electronic bulletin board)*
Fax: (301) 984-8796
TDD: (301) 443 9006
www.mentalhealth.org

National Association of Anorexia Nervosa and Associated Disorders (ANAD)
Box 7
Highland Park, IL 60035
(847) 831-3438 *(Hot line)*
Fax: (847) 433-4632
www.anad.org

Research and Training Center on Family Support and Children's Mental Health
Portland State University
PO Box 751
Portland, OR 97207-0751
(503) 725-4040
Fax: (503) 725-4180
www.rtc.pdx.edu

Parenting

Baby Bag Online
www.babybag.com

Childhelp USA
15757 N. 78th St.
Scottsdale, AZ 85260
(800) 4-ACHILD or
TDD (800) 2-ACHILD *(24-hour crisis hot line)*
(480) 922-8212
Fax: (480) 922-7061
www.childhelpusa.org
Intervention, information, and referrals for children, troubled parents, and adult survivors of abuse

Families and Work Institute
330 7th Ave.
New York, NY 10001
(212) 465-2044
Fax: (212) 465-8637
www.familiesandwork.org
Support for balancing family and work

Family Education Network
Learning Network Parent Channel
575 Market Street, 17th Floor
San Francisco, CA 94105
800-323-4776
www.familyeducation.com

Fatherhood Project
c/o Families and Work Institute
330 7th Ave.
New York, NY 10001
(212) 465-2044
Fax: (212) 465-8637
www.familiesandwork.org

FEMALE (Formerly Employed Mothers at the Leading Edge)
PO Box 31
Elmhurst, IL 60126
(Send a self-addressed stamped envelope)
(630) 941-3553
Fax: (630) 941-3551
www.femalehome.org

Federal Communications Commission V-Chip Task Force
www.fcc.gov/vchip
(877) 2-VCHIP-TV *(For informational brochures)*

iVillage
www.parentsoup.com

KidsCom Company, The
131 W. Seeboth St., 2nd fl.
Milwaukee, WI 53204
(414) 271-KIDS
Fax: (414) 272-2728
www.kidscom.com
Educational web site for kids ages 4–15 to explore

Kids First!
The Coalition for Quality Children's Media (CQCM)
112 W. San Francisco St.
Suite 305A
Santa Fe, NM 87501
(505) 989-8076
Fax: (505) 986-8477
www.cqcm.org
Information on child-appropriate videos, CD-ROMs, and television shows

National Association of Mothers' Centers
64 Division Ave.
Levittown, NY 11756
(800) 645-3828 or (516) 520-2929
Fax: (516) 520 1639
Information on parenting groups

National Center for Fathering
PO Box 413888
Kansas City, MO 64141
(800) 593-DADS
FAX: (913) 384-4665
www.fathers.com

National Organization of Mothers of Twins Clubs, Inc.
PO Box 438
Thompson Station, TN 37179
(615) 595-0936
(877) 540-2200
www.nomotc.org

National Parenting Center, The
22801 Ventura Blvd., No. 110
Woodland Hills, CA 91367
(800) 753-6667
www.tnpc.com/
Parenting information from prenatal through adolescence

New Parents Network
PO Box 64237
Tucson, AZ 85728-4237
(520) 327-1451
Fax: (520) 881-7104
www.npn.org

National Child Abuse Hotline
(800) 422-4453

Parental Stress Line
Parents' and Children's Services
The United Way
(800) 632-8188

Parents Anonymous
675 W. Foothill Blvd., Suite 220
Claremont, CA 91711
(909) 621-6184
Fax: (909) 625-6304
www.parentsanonymous-natl.org
Provides a toll-free hot line number for each state

Recovery, Inc.
802 N. Dearborn St.
Chicago, IL 60610
(312) 337-5661
Fax: (312) 337-5756
www.recovery-inc.com
Recognizing/preventing child abuse; self-help training for controlling anger, anxiety, and depression

Single Mothers by Choice
PO Box 1642
Gracie Square Station
New York, NY 10028
(212) 988-0993
www.autocyt.com/chinaseas/
     single.html
Support for 30- to 45-year-old single mothers

Single Parent Resource Center
31 E. 28th St., 2nd Floor
New York, NY 10016
(212) 951-7030
Fax: (212) 951-7037

Stepfamily Association of America
650 J St., Suite 205
Lincoln, NE 68508
(800) 735-0329
Fax: (402) 477-8317
www.stepfam.org

Triplet Connection, The
PO Box 99571
Stockton, CA 95209
(209) 474-0885
Fax: (209) 474-9243
www.tripletconnection.org
Support for parents of multiples

U.S. Information Agency
301 Fourth St., SW
Washington, DC 20547
(202) 401-9810
Fax on demand service:
     (202) 205-8237, #203
www.usia.gov

Poison Control

American Association of Poison Control Centers
www. aapcc.org
Information for parents and a directory of poison control centers

Pregnancy/Childbirth

American Dietetic Association
216 W. Jackson Blvd., Suite 800
Chicago, IL 60606-6995
(800) 366-1655 or (312) 899-0040
www.eatright.org
Local registered dietitian referrals and recorded nutrition message

Doulas of North America
13513 North Grove Drive
Alpine, UT 84004
(801) 756-7331
Fax: (801) 763-1847
www.dona.com

International Association of Parents and Professionals for Safe Alternatives in Childbirth (NAPSAC)
Route 4, Box 646
Marble Hill, MO 63764
Phone/fax: (573) 238-2010
Information on childbirth options, breast-feeding, and parenting issues

International Cesarean Awareness Network, Inc. (ICAN, Inc.)
1304 Kingsdale Ave.
Redondo Beach, CA 90278
(310) 542-6400
Fax: (310) 542-5368
www.childbirth.org

International Childbirth Education Association, Inc.
PO Box 20048
Minneapolis, MN 55420
(800) 624-4934 *(Mail-order bookstore)*
(952) 854-8660
Fax: (952) 854-8772
www.icea.org
Information on childbirth classes

Lamaze International
2025 M Street, Suite 800
Washington, DC 20036-3309
(800) 368-4404 or
(202) 367-1128
Fax: (202) 367-2128
www.lamaze-childbirth.com

ParentsPlace.com
subsidiary of iVillage, Inc.
www.parentsplace.com

Pregnancy RiskLine
PO Box 142106
Salt Lake City, UT 84114-2106
(801) 328-2229
Fax: (801) 538-9448
*Referrals to local information about
exposures that may affect pregnancy;
information on breast-feeding*

*Sidelines National Support
    Network*
PO Box 1808
Laguna Beach, CA 92652
(949) 497-2265
Fax: (949) 497-5598
www.sidelines.org
*Support network for women experi-
encing complicated pregnancies*

Safety

Alisa Ann Ruch Burn Foundation
3600 Ocean View Blvd., No. 1
Glendale, CA 91208
(800) 242-BURN
(818) 249-2230
Fax: (818) 249-2488
www.aarbf.org

American Red Cross
431 18th Street, NW
Washington, DC 20006
(202) 639-3520
www.redcross.org
*Emergency training, child safety,
child care options, and birth classes*

American Trauma Society
8903 Presidential Pkwy., Suite 512
Upper Marlboro, MD 20772
(800) 556-7890 or (301) 420-4189
Fax: (301) 420-0617
www.amtrauma.org
*Injury prevention information and
programs*

Auto Safety Hot Line
U.S. Department of Transportation
Office of the Administrator
400 Seventh St., SW
Washington, DC 20590
(888) 327-4238
www.nhtsa.dot.gov

Brain Injury Association, Inc.
105 N. Alfred St.
Alexandria, VA 22314
(800) 444-NHIF *(Family help line)*
(703) 236-6000
Fax: (703) 236-6001
www.biausa.org

*Children's Health Environmental
    Coalition Network*
PO Box 1540
Princeton, NJ 08542
(609) 252-1915
Fax: (609) 252-1536
www.checnet.org

Clinical Pharmacology Online
www.cp.gsm.com
Information on medications

Food Safety and Inspection Service
U.S. Department of Agriculture
Meat and Poultry Hotline, Room
    2925S
1400 Independence Ave., SW
Washington, DC 20250-9860
(800) 535-4555 or (202) 720-5604
(Meat and poultry hot line)
Fax: (202) 690-2859
www.usda.gov
Answers questions on food poisoning

*Foundation for Aquatic Injury
    Prevention*
1310 Ford Bldg.
Detroit, MI 48226
(800) 342-0330
Fax: (313) 963-1330
www.aquaticisf.org

*Foundation for Spinal Cord Injury
    Prevention, Care, and Cure*
1310 Ford Building
Detroit, MI 48226-3901
(800) 342-0330
Fax: (313) 963-1330
www.fscip.org

*Mothers and Others for a
    Liveable Planet*
40 West 20th St.
New York, NY 10011
www.mothers.org

National Burn Victim Foundation
246A Madisonville Rd.
PO Box 409
Basking Ridge, NJ 07920
(800) 803-5879 or (908) 953-9091
Fax: (908) 953-9099
www.nbvf.org

*National Center for Education in
    Maternal and Child Health*
2000 15th St. North; Suite 701
Arlington, VA 22201-2617
(703) 524-7802
Fax: (703) 524-9335
www.ncemch.org

*National Center for Injury
    Prevention and Control*
4770 Buford Highway NE
Mail Stop K63
Atlanta, GA 30341-3724
(770) 488-1506
Fax: (770) 488-1667
www.cdc.gov/ncipc

National Center for Lead-Safe Housing, The
10227 Wincopin Circle, Suite 205
Columbia, MD 21044
(410) 992-0712
Fax: (410) 715-2310
www.leadsafehousing.org

National Clearinghouse for Alcohol and Drug Information
PO Box 2345
Rockville, MD 20847-2345
(800) 729-6686
Fax: (301) 468-6433
www.health.org

National Fire Protection Association
Fire Education Department
One Batterymarch Park
PO Box 9101
Quincy, MA 02269
(617) 770-3000
Fax: (617) 770-0200
www.nfpa.org
Fire safety for children

National Highway Traffic Safety Administration
400 7th St., NW, Room 2318
Washington, DC 20590
Auto Safety Hotline:
888-DASH-2-DOT
www.nhtsa.dot.gov/people/injury/
    childps

National Lead Information Center and Clearinghouse
(800) 424-LEAD or
(800) LEAD-FYI
www.epa.gov/opptintr/lead

National Program for Playground Safety
University of Northern Iowa
School for HPELS
Cedar Falls, IA 50614-0618

(800) 554-PLAY
(319) 273-2416
Fax: (319) 273-7308
www.uni.edu/playground

National Safe Kids Campaign
1301 Pennsylvania Ave., NW
Suite 1000
Washington, DC 20004-1707
(800) 441-1888 or (202) 662-0600
Fax: (202) 393-2072
www.safekids.org

National Safety Council
1121 Spring Lake Dr.
Itasca, IL 60143-3201
(800) 621-7615 or (630) 285-1121
Fax: (630) 285-1315
www.nsc.org

National SIDS Resource Center
2070 Chain Bridge Rd., Suite 450
Vienna, VA 22182
(703) 821-8955
(800) 505-CRIB
(Back-to-Sleep Information Line)

National Spinal Cord Injury Association
8701 Georgia Avenue, Suite 500
Silver Spring, MD 20851
(301) 588-6959
Fax: (301) 588-9414
www.spinalcord.org

National Youth Sports Safety Foundation
333 Longwood Avenue, Suite 202
Boston, MA 02115
(617) 277-1171
Fax: (617) 277-2278
www.nyssf.org
Sports safety, coaching

Ozone Protection Hotline
U.S. Environmental Protection
    Agency
EPA, Mail Stop 6205J
401 M St., SW
Washington, DC 20460
(800) 296-1996
Fax: (301) 614-3396
www.epa.gov/docs/ozone
Sun protection tips and information regarding UV levels

Pew Environmental Health Commission at the Johns Hopkins School of Public Health
111 Market Ave., Suite 850
Baltimore, MD 21202
(410) 659-2690
Fax: (410) 659-2699
www.pewenvirohealth.jhsph.edu

Safe Drinking Water Hotline
U.S. Environmental Protection
    Agency
EPA, Mail Stop 4604
401 M St., SW
Washington, DC 20460
(800) 426-4791 or (703) 285-1101
www.epa.gov/OGWDW

SmartParent.com
www.smartparent.com
Resources for protecting children from Internet dangers

Sudden Infant Death Syndrome Alliance
1314 Bedford Ave., Suite 210
Baltimore, MD 21208
(800) 221-SIDS *(24 hours a day)*
(410) 653-8226
Fax: (410) 653-8709
www.sidsalliance.org

*Sudden Infant Death
    Syndrome Network*
PO Box 520
Ledyard, CT 06339
(860) 339-7042, ext. 551
Fax: (860) 887-7309
www.sids-network.org

Toy Safety Hotline
Toy Manufacturers of America
1115 Broadway, Suite 400
New York, NY 10010
(800) 851-9955
Fax: (212) 633-1429
www.toy-tma.com

Travelers' Health Hotline
National Center for Infectious
    Diseases: Travelers' Health
(877) FYI-TRIP
Fax: (888) 232-3299
www.cdc.gov/travel

*U.S. Consumer Product Safety
    Commission*
Washington, DC 20207-0001
(800) 638-2772 *(Hot line)*
TTY: (800) 638-8270
Fax: (301) 504-0124
www.cpsc.gov
*Product recall information, product
safety information*

*U.S. Food and Drug
    Administration*
200 C St., SW
Washington, DC 20204
(888) 723-3366 *(Food information)*
www.fda.gov
Answers to food safety questions

United States Olympic Committee
One Olympic Plaza
Colorado Springs, CO 80909
(719) 632-5551
www.olympic-usa.org
*Referrals to sports organizations for
safety tips*

Vision Problems

*American Association for Pediatric
    Ophthalmology and Strabismus*
PO Box 193832
San Francisco, CA 94119-3832
http://med-aapos.bu.edu

*National Association for Parents
    of the Visually Impaired*
PO Box 317
Watertown, MA 02272-0317
(800) 562-6265
(617) 972-7441
Fax: (617) 972-7444
www.spedex.com/napvi

National Center for the Blind
National Federation of the Blind
1800 Johnson St.
Baltimore, MD 21230
(410) 659-9314
Fax: (410) 685-5653
www.nfb.org

National Eye Institute
Bldg. 31, Room 6A32
31 Center Dr.
Bethesda, MD 20892
(301) 496-5248
Fax: (301) 402-1065
www.nei.nih.gov

*Recording for the Blind
    and Dyslexic*
20 Roszel Rd.
Princeton, NJ 08540
(800) 803-7201, (800) 221-4792, or
(609) 452-0606
Fax: (609) 987-8116
www.rfbd.org

You and Your Child's Doctor

American Academy of Pediatrics
141 NW Point Blvd.
Elk Grove Village, IL 60007-1098
(847) 434-4000
Fax: (847) 434-8000
www.aap.org

*American Board of
    Family Practice*
2228 Young Dr.
Lexington, KY 40505
(888) 995-5700
(859) 269-5626
Fax: (859) 335-7501
www.abfp.org
*To verify the certification status of
physicians; service is free through
the Web site, but there is a charge for
written requests*

American Board of Pediatrics
111 Silver Cedar Ct.
Chapel Hill, NC 27514
(919) 929-0461
Fax: (919) 929-9255
www.abp.org
*To verify if a doctor is board
certified*

*American College of
    Sports Medicine*
401 W. Michigan St.
PO Box 1440
Indianapolis, IN 46202-3233
(317) 637-9200
Fax: (317) 634-7817
www.acsm.org

Family Voices
PO Box 769
Algodones, NM 87001
(888) 835-5669 or (505) 867-2368
Fax: (505) 867-6517
www.familyvoices.org

Glossary of Common Medical Terms

Consult the index for terms that do not appear on this list.

Acquired Any disease or disorder that was not present at birth.

Acute Any disorder or symptom (often severe) that begins suddenly.

Amino acids Chemical compounds essential to the chemical reactions within cells. Some amino acids can be created by the body, others must be obtained in the diet. Amino acids are the building blocks of proteins.

Androgen The male hormone produced naturally by the body, or synthetically as a drug, necessary for normal male sexual development and reproductive function.

Anesthesia A procedure using medication (injected, inhaled, or oral) that causes loss of sensation or loss of consciousness. Used to prevent discomfort and pain, especially during surgery.

Antibiotic Medication used to treat bacterial infections. Some antibiotics are effective only against certain types of bacteria.

Antibodies Proteins made by white blood cells to destroy foreign proteins (created by bacteria, viruses, and other microorganisms) in the body. Part of the immune system.

Anticoagulant Medication that decreases the blood's clotting ability. Used to prevent harmful clots by halting the production of certain enzymes.

Anti-inflammatory Medication that reduces pain, redness, swelling, and heat in body tissues.

Apnea Any period during which breathing stops, particularly during sleep.

Bacteria A group of living, single-celled organisms too small to be seen without a microscope. Some can cause disease by producing poisons that harm cells. Bacteria can enter the body through skin injuries or the lungs, mouth, genitals, or nose.

Benign A mild or noncancerous form of a disease.

Biopsy A procedure in which skin, muscle, organ, or tumor tissue or cells are removed to be examined under a microscope.

CAT or CT (computed tomography) scan A test in which X rays are sent through the body at different angles to produce computer-generated pictures, showing a cross-section of an organ or anatomical area.

Catheterization, cardiac A procedure in which a thin tube, called a catheter, is inserted through a blood vessel into the heart to assess its condition.

Chronic A disorder or set of symptoms that has persisted for a long time.

Cognition Mental or intellectual activity, such as thinking, learning, remembering, or speaking.

Compression A technique in which a pad is applied to the skin with pressure and held in place by a bandage to alleviate bleeding, pain, or swelling.

Congenital A condition that is present at birth. Congenital conditions may be inherited or occur in the womb or during delivery.

Convulsion Another word for a seizure. A person in a convulsion may lose consciousness or have twitching and shaking for several seconds or minutes.

Coronary Of or pertaining to the arteries encircling the heart. Coronary arteries supply the heart with blood.

Culture Cells, microorganisms, or bacteria grown in the laboratory to diagnose infections.

Development The natural process of physical and intellectual growth.

Dietary supplement Additional calories, vitamins, minerals, proteins, or other nutrients. Usually taken in the form of pills, powders, or drinks.

Disease An abnormal condition or illness that impairs body functions, systems, or organs.

Disorder A disturbance of structure, function, or both. Disorders can be either acquired or congenital.

Echocardiogram A painless diagnostic procedure in which a device is placed on the chest. Ultrasound (sound with a higher frequency than what the human ear can detect) is bounced off the heart to obtain a picture of the heart and its valves and vessels.

Electrocardiogram (ECG or EKG) A painless test in which electrodes (metal disks) are connected to the chest, wrists, and ankles and to a recording machine that displays electrical impulses of the heart. ECGs can be taken at home, in a doctor's office, or in the hospital using special equipment. They may provide information about how the heart is functioning.

Electroencephalogram (EEG) A painless procedure in which a patient lies on a table with electrodes (metal disks) connected to various parts of his or her scalp and to a machine that records the brain's electrical activity.

Endocrine Pertaining to the endocrine system, a collection of glands that secrete hormones into the bloodstream to regulate metabolism, growth, temperature control, stress response, and sexual development rate and functioning. Essential for normal body functioning.

Endoscopy A procedure to investigate disorders in which a body cavity, such as the larynx, bladder, or abdomen, is examined by inserting a lighted tubelike instrument (endoscope). In some cases, general anesthesia is given. A camera or video recorder may record the exam.

Enzymes Proteins that regulate chemical reaction rates.

Estrogen The female hormone produced naturally by the body, or synthetically as a drug, necessary for normal female sexual development and reproductive function.

Family health history A record of the health conditions or disorders of family members, including all blood-related parents, grandparents, aunts, uncles, siblings, and cousins. Doctors use family histories to consider genetic factors in diagnosis.

Fever A body temperature above 100°F measured in the ear or rectum, or 99°F measured in the mouth or under the arm.

Fiber Indigestible plant parts. Fiber helps normal bowel functioning by passing through the digestive system almost unchanged. It does not provide energy or nutrients.

Fungus Fungi are simple, ubiquitous organisms that are usually harmless and occasionally beneficial. In the natural world, they are usually beneficial decomposers, breaking down and hence recycling dead organic material. Some fungi are parasitic, however, feeding off of living tissue, and can cause disease and death among humans. Molds, mildews, yeasts (e.g., *Candida*), and mushrooms are all different types of fungi.

Gastrointestinal Of or pertaining to the digestive system, which includes the esophagus (a tube connecting the throat and stomach), stomach, intestines, and rectum.

General Affecting most or all parts of the body (e.g., general anesthesia).

Genetic A condition or characteristic passed from parent to child. Refers to genes (the building blocks of inheritance), which influence personal characteristics and cell functioning in all body organs and systems.

Gestation The period from conception through birth.

Hemorrhage A medical term for bleeding.

Hormones Body chemicals released into the bloodstream to have a specific effect on the body. Hormones can influence growth, sexual development, metabolism, and the body's response to stress or illness. They are essential for normal body functioning.

Immune system The proteins and cells constituting the body's natural defense system, which protects against infection and abnormal cells by destroying invading microorganisms or tumor cells.

Immunization A disease prevention method that prepares the immune system by causing the creation of antibodies directed toward certain microorganisms. Immunizations can be either short- or long-term.

Immunosuppression Reduced immune system activity.

Incidence A measure of how common a disease is in a certain group of people; the number of new cases of disease that occurs during a particular period.

Incubation period The time between the first introduction of a bacterium, a virus, or another microorganism into the body until symptoms appear, during which time a person can sometimes infect others unknowingly. Varies for different organisms.

Infection A population of microorganisms, such as viruses, bacteria, or fungi, that causes disease by damaging cells or releasing toxins in the body.

Infertility, fertility Infertility refers to the inability to reproduce. Women are generally fertile (and able to conceive) from puberty to menopause. Men are generally fertile (and able to impregnate) from puberty into old age.

Intelligence quotient (IQ) A measurement of the ability to learn, understand, problem solve, and think out concepts. IQ is measured by intelligence tests, although new theories of intelligence recommend less reliance on numbers alone for this measurement.

Intramuscular Describes an injection given deeply into the muscle, where medication can be absorbed into the bloodstream.

Intravenous (IV) A thin, plastic tube inserted into a vein, which drips medication, blood or plasma, nutrients, or fluids into the bloodstream.

Intussusception A telescoping of the bowel wall into another segment of the bowel, cutting off part of the blood supply and leading to injury or even destruction of part of the bowel.

Local Affecting only part of the body. For instance, local anesthesia is the induced loss of pain only in the area being treated.

Lymph glands (lymph nodes) Small, immune-system filtering organs that trap microorganisms and pus cells, limiting the spread of infection. They are most visible in the neck, groin, and armpit.

Magnetic resonance imaging (MRI) A procedure in which a patient lies inside a hollow magnetic cylinder while bursts of a magnetic field create high-quality images of body organs and structures without exposing the patient to radiation.

Malignant Becoming more severe over time, often resulting in death.

Malocclusion A condition in which the upper and lower teeth do not meet properly.

Medical health history A record of a patient's past health disorders, vaccinations, treatments, tests, and examination results, usually kept as part of the medical records.

Metabolism All of the body's chemical processes, including the breakdown or buildup of complex substances, the production of energy, and the elimination of waste products.

Milestones Skills or abilities that a child acquires at predetermined age ranges, indicating that the child is learning and has progressed to a new development stage.

Motor skills (fine, gross) Skills involving muscle and nerve movement. Fine motor skills are slight movements requiring precision, such as the ability to pick up a raisin. Gross motor skills involve a larger portion of the body, such as an infant's ability to keep her head steady when held in a sitting position.

Mucus A thick, slimy fluid that lubricates and protects parts of the body (including the digestive tract and the airways) from acid and enzymes, dry air, pollutants, and abrasion.

Nausea The queasy feeling of needing to vomit.

Nebulized Medication made into a mist. Usually given through a face mask or an inhaler.

Neonate A newborn infant of up to 4 weeks old.

Neurological A term referring to the nervous system (which gathers, interprets, transmits, and stores information), including the brain, nerves, spinal cord, and parts of the sensory organs.

Nutrition The study of nutrients that are not made in the body but are essential for body functioning. Nutrients include fat, fiber, carbohydrates, minerals, vitamins, protein, and water.

Occlusion The blocking of a vessel, a canal, an opening, or a passage. Occlusions can be caused by disease or created for medical purposes.

Oral Relating to the mouth, usually applied to swallowing medication or holding a thermometer under the tongue.

Otoscope A lighted instrument with a funnel-shaped tip, which health professionals use to magnify and observe the ear canal and eardrum.

Parenteral A method of giving medication that doesn't involve the stomach or intestines. Parenteral medication is usually given by needle.

Pediatrics The branch of medicine relating to the care, development, diagnosis, and treatment of newborns, infants, toddlers, children, and adolescents.

Preterm (premature) A term referring to any birth that occurs before 37 weeks of pregnancy.

Prevalence The number of cases of an illness or a condition in a group of people.

Progesterone A female sex hormone produced naturally by the body, or synthetically as a drug. Progesterone is necessary for the proper functioning of the female reproductive system.

Protein One of many complex essential molecules. Consists of linked amino acids. Used to build cells and to carry out cellular metabolism.

Pulmonary Associated with the lungs.

Reflux An abnormal backflow of fluid in a body passage. For example, when acidic fluid from the stomach goes up the feeding tube (the esophagus) into the back of the throat and sometimes the lungs, the condition is known as esophageal reflux.

Relapse The recurrence of a disease or symptoms after a period of better health or apparent recovery.

Renal Relating to the kidneys.

Rupture The tearing of tissue, sometimes causing an organ or a tissue to protrude through the tissue containing it (e.g., a hernia).

Saline Containing salt.

Seizure Sudden, temporary changes (convulsions) in physical movement or behavior caused by abnormal electrical brain activity. In one type of seizure, a person loses consciousness, twitching and shaking for several seconds or minutes.

Septic A bacterial condition in which tissues are infected and pus forms or bacteria spread throughout the body.

Sign An indication of a disease or disorder seen by the doctor during a physical examination.

Sonogram An image created by sound with a higher frequency than that which the human ear can detect (ultrasound). Sonograms are often used to evaluate the condition of a fetus or to diagnose other conditions, such as stones in the gallbladder.

Sphygmomanometers An instrument used to measure blood pressure. A rubber ball inflates a cuff with an inflatable bladder, and a pressure gauge is attached to the bladder.

Sputum (phlegm) Saliva and respiratory discharges coughed up from airway glands.

Steroids A group of molecules that include hormones produced in the adrenal glands. Steroids control the body's electrolyte balance, energy, metabolism, kidney function, growth, and sexual function. Three classes of steroidal hormones have different functions in the body. They are corticosteroids, anabolic steroids, and mineralocorticoids. Synthetic steroids are used to treat a variety of different diseases, from asthma to autoimmune disorders.

Stethoscope An instrument with a cup-shaped piece that amplifies body sounds, including the heartbeat and breathing, and conveys them to the ears through tubing and ear pieces.

Subacute Lasting for an intermediate length of time between acute and chronic, usually from several days to up to a few weeks.

Suppositories A solid medication placed in a body passage or cavity, such as the anus or vagina. Suppositories dissolve at body temperature, releasing the active ingredient.

Surgery The use of physical means (often involving skin-cutting instruments) to remove a tumor or to alleviate or diagnose a disease, an injury, or a disorder.

Suture A surgical stitch made with specialized fiber or thread to sew incision or wound edges together. Sutures are meant to promote healing.

Symptom Evidence of a disease or condition that is noticed by the patient.

Systemic Affecting the entire body.

Therapist A professional trained in the treatment of a disease or another condition.

Topical A term referring to medication applied to the surface of a body part. Topical drugs can be placed on the skin, in the ear canal, in the vagina, in the rectum, or on the surface of the eye.

Transfusion The transferring of blood or blood components into a vein or an artery, usually because of blood loss or anemia.

Trauma A severe physical, cognitive, or emotional shock or injury.

Tumor An abnormal cell mass. Tumors are produced when cells in one area reproduce too fast; they can be either cancerous or noncancerous.

Urinalysis Analysis of urine by various tests to detect a condition or disease of the kidneys or bladder.

Urinary Pertaining to the body organs that form and discharge fluid waste, excess water, or chemical substances (kidney, bladder, and associated structures).

Vaccination One type of immunization in which microorganisms rendered harmless are introduced into the body, usually by injection, to produce long-term immunity to those microorganisms.

Virus One of the smallest types of infectious agents capable of causing disease.

Vitamin One of a group of complex chemicals essential for normal body functioning. Most vitamins cannot be produced by the body.

Wheezing Breathing with difficulty, often with a high-pitched whistling sound from the chest. Caused by a narrowing of the small airways in the lungs. Wheezing is typically associated with allergic conditions.

X ray A procedure using certain wavelengths of electromagnetic radiation to form pictures of bones, organs, and tissues inside the body. Usually used for diagnosis.

Index

Note: Page numbers in **boldface** refer to key topics in the sections on Emergencies and Common Childhood Illnesses.

Abdomen
  swelling of
    arthritis and, 616
    mumps and, 646
  tenderness in, mononucleosis and, 643, 644
  trauma to, 392, 423
Abdominal pain, **422–24**
  advice for parents, 424
  anxiety disorders and, 442
  appendicitis and, 446, 447
  assessment of, 423–24
  causes of, 422–23, 485
  colic, 82–83, 84, 423, **510–12**
  constipation and, 512
  depression and, 527
  fever with, 422, 446
  food poisoning and, 570
  gastroesophageal reflux and, 576
  lead poisoning and, 621
  mononucleosis and, 643
  pneumonia and, 662
  during pregnancy, 5
  prevention of, 424
  relieving, 511–12
  requiring medical attention, 344, 422
  stomach flu and, 447
  worms and, 727
Abdominal thrusts, for choking intervention, 403, 404
Abnormal heart rhythm. See Dysrhythmia
Abrasions. See Scrape(s)
Abscesses, 476
Absence seizure, 682
Abuse. See Child abuse
Academic performance, 255
Accreditation, NAECP, 321
ACE (angiotensin converting enzyme) inhibitors, 601
Acetaminophen, 350–51
  for abdominal pain, 424
  for burns, 396
  for fever reduction, 568
  in first aid kit, 376
  for headaches, 585
  liquid, 23, 351
  and liver inflammation, 595
  for mouth ulcers, 488, 489

use during immunization, 115
use during pregnancy, 7
Acid(s), and eye injury, 408
Acid-fast bacilli, 713
Acidic foods, avoiding during mumps, 647
Acne, **429–31**, 670
  advice for parents, 430–31
  anabolic steroids and, 276
  causes of, 429
  prevention of, 431
  treatment of, 429–30
  types of, 429
Aconite, risks associated with, 304
Acquired immunodeficiency syndrome. See HIV/AIDS infection
Activated charcoal, for poisoning intervention, 417
Active sleep, in newborn, 38
Activities
  for 2-year-olds, 185, 187
  for 4-year-olds, 227
  for 5-year-olds, 251
Acupressure, 304
Acupuncture, 304
Acute lymphoblastic leukemia (ALL), 484
Acute mastoiditis, 549
Acute myelogenous leukemia (AML), 484
Acyclovir, for cold sores, 506
ADD. See Attention-deficit disorder
Addiction. See Substance abuse
Additives, avoiding in baby foods, 132
Adenoids. See Tonsils
ADH. See Antidiuretic hormone
ADHD. See Attention-deficit disorder
Adoption
  health concerns, 305–7
  information sources, 742
Adrenal glands, tumors of, 485
Affective disorder. See Depression
Afrin (oxymetazoline), for nosebleed, 650
Afterbirth, expelling, 30
Age of child. See also specific age groups
  and heart rate, 426, 427
  and length/height percentiles, 734–35
  and permanent tooth eruption, 632
  and sexual attraction, 280
  and sleep requirements, 108–9, 266
  and weight percentiles, 732–33
Aggressiveness

anabolic steroids and, 276
depression and, 527
physical, 467
play as outlet for, 232
of preschoolers, 220
of toddlers, discouraging, 204
verbal, 467
AIDS. See HIV/AIDS infection
Air travel
  with preschooler, 247
  with toddler, 210
Airway(s)
  during asthma episode, 450
  obstruction of
    and choking, 397
    clearing, 398–405
    loss of consciousness and, 379
    signs of, 398, 402
    and wheezing, 451
  opening of, 379, 380, 384, 400
Alarm, bed-wetting, 463
Albuterol, 7, 452
Alcohol use
  during breast-feeding, risks associated with, 66
  discussing with child, 281–82
  during pregnancy, risks associated with, 7–8, 10, 456, 459, 640
Alert inactivity, in newborn, 38
Alkalis, and eye injury, 408
ALL. See Acute lymphoblastic leukemia
Allergic dermatitis, 531
Allergic shock (anaphylaxis), **389–91**, 432
  prevention of, 391
  signs and symptoms of, 390
  treatment of, 390–91
Allergies, **431–36**
  advice for parents, 434–35
  and asthma, 432, 450
  blisters caused by, 475
  breast-feeding and decreased risk of, 48
  causes of, 432
  eczema and, 531
  food. See Food allergies
  and hives, 606
  information sources, 743
  and laryngitis, 619
  and pinkeye, 660
  prevention of, 435–36
  signs and symptoms of, 130, 431
  smoke exposure and increased risk of, 86
  testing for, 433

signs of, 5
tobacco use and, 8
Mite bites, 611, 612
Mites (scabies), 671, **676–77**
sources of information on, 751
Mitral valve prolapse, and dental visit
precautions, 209
MMR. *See* Measles, mumps, rubella
vaccine
Mobiles, safety considerations, 88, 117
Molds
allergies to, preventing, 435
and asthma, 450
Moles, 471
Molluscum contagiosum, **642**
Money management skills, developing,
268–69
Mongolian spots, 471
Monkey bars, avoiding, 210
Mononucleosis, **642–44**, 692
advice for parents, 644
causes of, 643
diagnosis of, 643
and hives, 606
signs and symptoms of, 643
and swollen glands, 703
Monosodium glutamate (MSG), and
headaches, 584
Montelukast, 452
Mood swings, anabolic steroids and,
276
Moraxella catarrhalis, and pinkeye, 660
Mosquito bites, 611, 612
Mother(s)
breast-feeding and advantages for, 48
of newborn, needs of, 89–90
newborn's ability to recognize, 56, 60
resources for, 753
rooming in with newborn, 47
and sick-child care, 345–46
Motion sickness, 546, **644–45**, 724
Motor development. *See* Fine motor
development; Gross motor
development; Movement
Mouth
cleft roof of, **502–4**
dry, as symptom of dehydration,
524, 525
exploring with, infant and, 122
of newborn, examination of, 41
pain in
mumps and, 646
thrush and, 708
pale spots in, measles and, 636
poison in, treating, 416
ulcers of, 488
canker sores, **487–89**
cold sores, **506–7**
hand-foot-and-mouth disease,
579–80

Mouth-to-mouth rescue breathing,
379, 381, 384–85
after choking, 400, 402
after drowning, 407
Movement
at 1 month, 58
at 1 to 3 months, 99
at 4 to 7 months, 120–23
at 8 to 12 months, 152–55
at 1 year, 173–75
at 2 years, 181–82
at 3 years, 216–17
at 4 years, 223–25
at 5 years, 251
encouraging, 122
impaired control of. *See* Cerebral
palsy
top-down development of, 99
MSG. *See* Monosodium glutamate
MSUD. *See* Maple syrup urine disease
Mucins, in breast milk, 69
Mucus
asthma and, 450
clearing from infant's nose, 481
colds/flu and, 509
cystic fibrosis and, 523
Mumps, 113, **646–47**
avoiding during pregnancy, 11
cause of, 646
complications of, 110
diagnosis of, 646
and meningitis, 638, 646
signs and symptoms of, 646
treatment of, 646–47
vaccination, 110, 113
side effects of, 114
Muscle aches
colds/flu and, 507, 508
fifth disease and, 569
hepatitis and, 594
Lyme disease and, 633
Muscle strains, **697–98**
and back pain, 460
Muscle tone
of newborn, evaluation of, 31
poor, cerebral palsy and, 494
Muscle tumors, 485
Mycobacterium tuberculosis, 713
Mycoplasma pneumonia, 663
Myocarditis, 498
colds/flu and, 508
Myoclonic seizure, 683
Myopia (nearsightedness), 721, 722
diagnosis of, 269
Myringotomy, 550

Nagging, ineffectiveness of, 266–67
Nails. *See* Fingernails; Toenails
Nakedness, toddlers and, 189, 195

Nanny, 314, 315
defining expectations for, 316–17
determining salary and benefits for,
317
interviewing, 317–19
supervision of, 319
Naps/napping
enforced, and sleep problems,
197–98
infants and, 135
preschoolers and, 240
vs. quiet time, 198
toddlers and, 196
National Academy of Early Childhood
Programs (NAECP), 321
National Association for the Education
of Young Children (NAEYC),
321
Natural childbirth, 4
Nausea
abdominal pain and, 422
appendicitis and, 446
dizziness and, 545, 546
dysrhythmia and, 425
food poisoning and, 570
headache and, 583
jaundice and, 613
medications for, avoiding, 725
treatment of, during pregnancy, 7
Navel
cleaning of, 74
examination of, 41
hernia of, **598–99**
infection of, 74, **714**
Nearsightedness (myopia), 721, 722
diagnosis of, 269
Nebulizer, for asthma medication,
453–54
Neck
boils on, 477
of newborn, examination of, 41
stiff, meningitis and, 637
swollen glands in, 485, 507, 643, 675
Neck injury, first aid response to, 387
Neck pain, **647–49**
causes of, 648
diagnosis of, 648
Lyme disease and, 633
treatment of, 649
Nedocromil, 452
Neglect, and mental retardation, 640
Neonatal acne, 429
Neonatal intensive care unit (NICU),
666, 668
multidisciplinary team in, 667
Nephritis, 715
Nervousness. *See* Anxiety
Neural tube defects, 693
factors contributing to, 695
prevention of, 3, 13, 696

Children's Hospital Boston

Children's Hospital Boston, the primary pediatric teaching hospital for Harvard Medical School, is the nation's premier pediatric medical center and the world's leading pediatric research center. Consistently rated as the best children's hospital in the country, it enjoys an extraordinary reputation among physicians, parents, and children. Over 80 distinguished physicians and pediatric specialists, on the staff of the hospital and among the Harvard Medical School faculty, contributed to the research and advice in this book.

Medical Editors

Alan D. Woolf, M.D., M.P.H., is Associate Professor of Pediatrics at Harvard Medical School and an attending physician at Children's Hospital Boston. A board-certified toxicologist, he directs the hospital's clinical and fellowship training programs in medical toxicology, and codirects the pediatric environmental health center. He is also Director of the Massachusetts/Rhode Island poison control center, and President of the American Association of Poison Control Centers. Dr. Woolf has lectured widely both nationally and internationally on childhood poisoning and pediatric environmental toxic exposures. His research interests include poisoning and childhood injury prevention, and he has authored or co-authored more than 150 published research reports, reviews, and other articles.

Margaret A. Kenna, M.D., is Associate Professor of Otology and Laryngology at Harvard Medical School and a full-time pediatric otolaryngologist at Children's Hospital Boston. She is Director of the Pediatric Cochlear Implant Program at Children's Hospital and also Director of the Hearing Impaired program in the department of Otolaryn-gology and Communication Disorders. Dr. Kenna is an editor of one of the major textbooks in pediatric otolaryngology and has published over 100 journal articles, book chapters, and other types of publications in the field of pediatric otolaryngology. Her areas of research include otitis media and sensorineural hearing loss in children.

Howard C. Shane, Ph.D., is Associate Professor of Otolaryngology at Harvard Medical School and Director of Speech Pathology services at Children's Hospital Boston. He directs the Communication Enhancement Center, the oldest and largest clinical program in the country having as its exclusive purpose the evaluation for and prescription of alternative and augmentative communication. Dr. Shane is a Fellow of the American Speech and Hearing Association and the recipient of the Goldenson Award for Innovations in Technology from the United Cerebral Palsy Association. Author of numerous papers and chapters on severe speech impairment, he has lectured internationally, and has produced many computer innovations enjoyed by persons with communication disorders.